EIGHTH EDITION

MANUAL OF
ANTIBIOTICS
AND
INFECTIOUS
DISEASES

D1227215

EIGHTH EDITION

MANUAL OF ANTIBIOTICS AND INFECTIOUS DISEASES

John E. Conte, Jr., M.D.

Clinical Professor of Epidemiology and Biostatistics,
Medicine, and Microbiology and Immunology

Director, Hospital Epidemiology and Infection Control
University of California, San Francisco
San Francisco, California

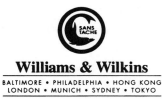

Williams & Wilkins

BALTIMORE • PHILADELPHIA • HONG KONG
LONDON • MUNICH • SYDNEY • TOKYO

A WAVERLY COMPANY

Editor: Jonathan W. Pine, Jr.
Managing Editor: Molly L. Mullen
Copy Editors: Klementyna Bryte; Margaret D. Hanson, RN; Stephen Siegforth
Designer: Norman W. Och
Illustration Planner: Wayne Hubbel
Production Coordinator: Kim Nawrozki

Copyright © 1995
Williams & Wilkins
428 East Preston Street
Baltimore, Maryland 21202, USA

Printed in the United States of America

Library of Congress Cataloging-in-Publication Data

Conte, John E.
    Manual of Antibiotics and Infectious diseases / John E. Conte, Jr.—8th ed.
        p.   cm.
    Includes bibliographical references and index.
    ISBN 0-683-02068-4
        1. Antibiotics—Handbooks, manuals, etc.   2. Communicable diseases—Hand-
        books, manuals, etc.   I. Title
    [DNLM: 1. Antibiotics—therapeutic use—handbooks.   2. Antibiotics—admin-
    istration & dosage—handbooks.   3. Communicable Diseases—drug therapy—hand-
    books.   QV 39C761m 1995]
    RM267.C63   1995
    615'.329—dc20
    DNLM/DLC
    for Library of Congress   94-23078
                                                                                         CIP

                                                                          94 95 96 97 98
                                                                          1 2 3 4 5 6 7 8 9 10

PREFACE

This manual is designed for students, house staff, practicing physicians, and other health professionals involved in the day-to-day care of patients with infectious diseases. An attempt has been made to incorporate into one book a variety of important source materials that ordinarily can be found in many different locations.

The manual is divided into eleven sections.

Section 1. Antibiotics

Clinically important information is presented for each antibiotic. This section includes the availability and trade names of each drug, its clinical use, adult and pediatric dosage, adverse reactions, and drug interactions. A table detailing the pharmacology of the various drugs including dosage in renal insufficiency is also provided.

Section 2. Empiric Antibiotic Therapy

Recommendations are made for drugs of choice, alternative therapy, and appropriate dosages for various clinical situations in which infection is suspected but the organism and its susceptibilities have not yet been determined.

Section 3. Therapy of Established Infection

Empiric antibiotic therapy is continued until Gram stains and cultures from the laboratory reveal one or more specific agents. At this point, specific therapy is begun; this section summarizes antibiotic choices, dosages, route of administration, and duration of therapy for patients for whom the etiology of the infection has been determined.

Section 4. Prophylactic Antibiotics

This section provides guidelines for the use of antibiotic prophylaxis during various surgical procedures and in medical situations.

Section 5. AIDS and HIV Infection

This is a new section that summarizes the use of drugs in patients with HIV infection or AIDS. It includes protocols for the management of patients with early HIV infection.

Section 6. Antibiotic Susceptibilities

This is a tabular summary of organisms commonly encountered in human infectious diseases and their susceptibility to antimicrobial agents.

Section 7. Bacterial Resistance

This is a new section that has been added in response to the increasing problem of bacterial resistance. Graphical and tabular summaries of the epidemiology and resistance patterns of organisms such as methicillin-resistant *Staphylococcus aureus,* antibiotic-resistant enterococci penicillin-resistant pneumococci, and resistant Gram-negative rods are presented.

Section 8. Clinical Use of Immunobiologic Agents

These agents are available by request from Immunobiologics, Biologic Products Division, Bureau of Laboratories of the Centers for Disease Control and Prevention. Guidelines are given for the use of immune serum globulin and hepatitis B immune globulin, influenza vaccine, pneumococcal vaccine, polio vaccine, rabies immune globulin, tetanus prophylaxis, immunobiologic agents, and drugs distributed by the CDC.

Section 9. Drugs for Parasitic Infections

This section summarizes the agents of choice and dosage and toxicity of drugs used for the treatment of parasitic infection.

Section 10. Tuberculosis

This section provides information regarding the epidemiology, diagnosis, treatment, and infection control aspects of tuberculosis.

Section 11. Sexually Transmitted Diseases

United States Public Health Service recommendations for the treatment of sexually transmitted diseases are provided.

ACKNOWLEDGMENTS

This book is dedicated to my wife, Michelle; my daughter, Sarah; and my son, Jack. They provide great strength for everything I do.

Special recognition is given to Nancy Polkinghorne for her well-organized and dedicated work on this edition. I would like to thank Jennifer Kaae and Eve Benton for their assistance.

Although Steve Barriere is no longer a co-editor, many of his important contributions to earlier editions remain in this one and they continue to add value to the manual. However, I am responsible for all shortcomings or errors presented in the eighth edition.

John E. Conte, Jr., M.D.
1994

CONTENTS

ABBREVIATIONS

ADA	Americans with Disabilities Act
AFB	acid-fast bacilli
AIDS	acquired immunodeficiency syndrome
APF	assigned protection factor
ARC	AIDS-related complex
AUG	area under the curve
bid	twice a day
BUN	blood urea nitrogen
BV	bacterial vaginosis
C	cramps
CAPD	chronic ambulatory peritoneal dialysis
cc	cubic centimeter
CDC	Centers for Disease Control and Prevention
CMV	cytomegalovirus
CNS	central nervous system
CL_{CR}	creatinine clearance
Cp	plasma concentration
Cr_s	serum creatinine
CSF	cerebrospinal fluid
D	diarrhea
DFM	dust-fume-mist
DGI	disseminated gonococcal infection
dl	deciliter(s)
DM	dust-mist
EIA	enzyme immunoassay
eIPV	enhanced inactivated polio vaccine
F	fever
°F	fahrenheit
FDA	Food and Drug Administration
FTA-ABS	fluorescent treponemal antibody absorption (test)
gm	gram(s)
GABHS	group A β-hemolytic streptococcus
GI	gastrointestinal
GNR	Gram-negative rods
G-6-PD	glucose-6-phosphate dehydrogenase (deficiency)
HCW	health-care worker
HD	hemodialysis
HEPA	high-efficiency particulate air
HIV	human immunodeficiency virus
HPF	high-powered field

HPV	human *Papillomavirus* infection
hr	hour(s)
HSV	herpes simplex virus
i.d.	intradermal
i.m.	intramuscular
i.t.	intrathecal
IU	international unit(s)
i.v.	intravenous
kg	kilogram(s)
KOH	potassium hydroxide
L	liter
lb	pound
LD	loading dose
LET	leukocyte esterase test
LGV	lymphogranuloma venereum
LP	lumbar puncture
M	molar
MAC	*Mycobacterium avium* complex
MBC	minimum bactericidal concentration
μg	microgram(s)
MD	maintenance dose
mEq	milliequivalent
mg	milligram(s)
MIC	minimum inhibitory concentration
min	minute(s)
MLC	minimum lethal concentration
ml	milliliter(s)
MPC	mucopurulent cervicitis
mo	month
mos	months
MU	million units
N	nausea
NGU	nongonococcal urethritis
NIH	National Institutes of Health
NIOSH	National Institute for Occupational Safety and Health
OSHA	Occupational Safety and Health Administration
OTC	over-the-counter
OPV	oral polio vaccine
PAPR	powered air-purifying respirators
PCP	*Pneumocystis carinii* pneumonia
PID	pelvic inflammatory disease
p.o.	by mouth
PPD	purified protein derivative (of tuberculin)
qd	daily, once a day
qid	4 times a day
qod	every other day
q2h	every 2 hours
q4h	every 4 hours

q6h	every 6 hours
q8h	every 8 hours
q12h	every 12 hours
RBC	red blood cell
RPR	rapid protein reagin
RVVC	recurrent vulvovaginal candidiasis
s.c.	subcutaneous
SIADH	syndrome of inappropriate antidiuretic hormone
STD	sexually transmitted disease(s)
$t_{1/2}$	half-life
TB	tuberculosis
TCA	trichloroacetic acid
Td	tetanus, diphtheria
TGC	third-generation cephalosporin
tid	3 times a day
TMP/SMX	trimethoprim-sulfamethoxazole
U	unit(s)
μg/ml	micrograms/milliliter
μM	micromolar
UTI	urinary tract infection
UVGI	ultraviolet germicidal irradiation
V_D	volume of distribution
VDRL	Venereal Disease Research Laboratories
VVC	vulvovaginal candidiasis
VZV	varicella-zoster virus

SECTION 1
Antibiotics

The summaries that follow are designed to provide the clinician with important dosage and pharmacological data, as well as information regarding adverse reactions and drug interactions. In general, orally administered antimicrobials are subject to the vagaries of absorption from the GI tract, and interactions with other medications or substances may significantly reduce the amount of drug carried into the bloodstream (e.g., tetracyclines or quinolones with multivalent cations, ketoconazole with antacids, or H_2-receptor blockers). Additionally, seriously ill patients may have reduced blood flow to the GI tract, which will also compromise absorption of oral medications. Under these circumstances, intravenous formulations, if available, are recommended.

An attempt is made to provide information on all currently useful antibiotics (Tables 1.1–1.6). Older drugs that have fallen into relative disuse are not included. For example, semisynthetic penicillins such as methicillin, aminoglycosides such as neomycin or kanamycin, or agents such as triacetyloleandomycin and colistin play little to no role in current clinical medicine and are either less effective or more toxic than new agents. Several tetracycline and sulfonamide derivatives

Table 1.1. Aminoglycoside Dosing Chart[a]

Aminoglycoside	Usual Loading Doses (mg/kg)	Expected Peak Serum Levels (μg/ml)
Tobramycin		
Gentamicin	1.5–2.0	4–10
Amikacin	7.5	20–30
Netilmicin	2–3.0	8–12

1. Select loading dose in mg/kg (ideal weight) to provide peak serum levels in range listed in the table for desired aminoglycoside.
2. Select maintenance dose (as percentage of chosen loading dose) to continue peak serum levels indicated in the table, according to desired dosing interval and the patient's corrected creatinine clearance.*
*Calculate corrected creatinine clearance ($Cl(c)_{CR}$) as:
$Cl(c)_{CR}$ male = 140 − age/serum creatinine
$Cl(c)_{CR}$ female = 0.85 × $Cl(c)_{CR}$ male

Adapted from Hull JH, Sarubbi FA. Amikacin serum concentrations: prediction of levels and dosage guidelines. Ann Intern Med 1978; 89:612.
[a] Assumptions made using this nomogram:
 1. Use in adult patients only (not pediatrics).
 2. Patient has volume of distribution = 0.25 L/kg.

Table 1.2. Percentage of Loading Dose Required for Dosage Interval Selected

CL(c)$_{CR}$ (ml/min)	Half-life* (hr)	8 hr (%)	12 hr (%)	24 hr (%)
90	3.1	84		
80	3.4	80	91	
70	3.9	76	88	
60	4.5	71	84	
50	5.3	65	79	
40	6.5	57	72	92
30	8.4	48	63	86
25	9.9	43	57	81
20	11.9	37	50	75
17	13.6	33	46	70
15	15.1	31	42	67
12	17.9	27	37	61
10	20.4	24	34	56
7	25.9	19	28	47
5	31.5	16	23	41
2	46.8	11	16	30
0	69.3	8	11	21

*From Hull JH, Sarubbi FA: Amikacin serum concentrations: prediction of levels and dosage guidelines. Ann Intern Med 1978; 89:612.
ªAlternatively, half the chosen loading dose may be given at an interval approximately equal to the estimated half-life.

are deliberately excluded, because these analogs offer no advantage over tetracycline or sulfisoxazole in the treatment of infectious diseases. Data are also supplied on agents that are investigational at the time of this writing but may soon be available.

Definitions

SERUM CONCENTRATIONS

The values provided are the expected maximal concentrations achieved after administration of the listed dose.

HALF-LIFE ($t_{1/2}$)

When absorption and distribution are complete, the plasma concentrations for most antibiotics decline exponentially; thus, drug elimination follows first-order kinetics. The slope of the curve obtained during this phase is equal to the elimination rate constant (k). Half-life is related to the slope k by the equation:

$$t_{1/2} = \frac{\text{Ln } 2}{k} = \frac{0.693}{k}$$

The slope of the curve and half-life can be estimated by a plot of drug concentration (log scale) versus time (linear scale) (Fig. 1.1).

Table 1.3. Antimicrobial Agents: Use in Adult Patients

Generic Name	Trade Names	Route	Adult Dosage	Dose Change in Renal Impairment (See Tables 1.1, 1.2, 1.5)
Antituberculous Agents				
Capreomycin	Capastat	i.m.	15 mg/kg/d	Yes
Cycloserine	Seromycin	Oral	250–500 mg/d	Yes
Ethambutol	Myambutol	Oral	15–25 mg/kg/d	Yes
Ethionamide	Tecator-SC	Oral	250–500 mg/d	No
Isoniazid	INH, Nydrazid	Oral, i.m.	300 mg/d	Yes
Para-aminosalicylic acid		Oral	4–6 g/d	Not recommended
Pyrazinamide		Oral	1–2 g/d	Yes
Rifampin	Rifadin, Rimactane	Oral, i.v.	600 mg/d	Yes
Streptomycin		i.m.	15 mg/kg/d	Yes
Antifungal Agents				
Amphotericin B	Fungizone	i.v.	0.3–1 mg/kg/d	No
Miconazole	Monistat	i.v.	0.2–1.2 g q8h	No
Ketoconazole	Nizoral	Oral	0.2–4 g q24h	No
Fluconazole	Diflucan	i.v.	0.1–0.4 g q24h	Yes
		Oral	0.1–0.4 g q24h	Yes
Itraconazole	Sporanox	Oral	0.1–0.2 g q12h	No
Flucytosine	Ancobon	i.v.	0.75–2.5 g q6h	Yes
		Oral	0.75–2.5 g q6h	Yes
Antiviral Agents				
Acyclovir	Zovirax	i.v.	5–10 mg/kg q8h	Yes
		Oral	0.2–0.8 g q4h × 5/d	Yes
Ganciclovir	Cytovene	i.v.	5 mg/kg q12h	Yes
Amantadine	Symmetrel	Oral	0.2 g q24h	Yes
Rimantidine	Flumadine	Oral	0.2 g q24h	Yes
Antiparasitic agents (see Section 9)				

Table 1.3—continued

Generic Name	Trade Names	Route	Adult Dosage	Dose Change in Renal Impairment (See Tables 1.1, 1.2, 1.5)
Antibiotics Aminoglycosides				
Amikacin	Amikin	i.m., i.v.	5 mg/kg q8h or 7.5 mg/kg q12h	Yes
Gentamicin	Garamycin	i.m., i.v.	1–1.7 mg/kg q8h	Yes
Tobramycin	Nebcin	i.m., i.v.	1–1.7 mg/kg q8h	Yes
Netilmicin	Netromycin	i.m., i.v.	1.3–2.2 mg/kg q8h or 2–3.25 mg/kg q/12h	Yes
Cephalosporins				
1st Generation				
Cefadroxil	Duricef	Oral	0.5–1 gm q12h	Yes
Cefazolin	Ancef, Kefzol	i.m., i.v.	0.5–1.5 gm q8h	Yes
Cephalexin	Keflex	Oral	250–500 mg q6h	No
2nd Generation				
Cefaclor	Ceclor	Oral	250–500 mg q8h	Yes
Cefamandole	Mandol	i.m., i.v.	1–2 gm q4–6h	Yes
Cefmetazole	Zefasone	i.v.	2 gm q6–8h	Yes
Cefonicid	Monocid	i.m., i.v.	1–2 gm q24h	Yes
Cefotetan	Cefotan	i.m., i.v.	1–2 gm q12h	Yes
Cefoxitin	Mefoxin	i.m., i.v.	1–2 gm q4–6h	Yes
Cefprozil	Cefzil	Oral	0.25–0.5 gm q12h	No
Loracarbef	Lorabid	Oral	0.2–0.4 gm q12h	No
Cefuroxime	Zinacef	i.m., i.v.	0.75–1.5 gm q8h	Yes
	Ceftin	Oral	0.25–0.5 gm q12h	No
3rd Generation				
Cefepime	Axepim	i.v.	1 gm q12h	Yes
Cefixime	Suprax	Oral	0.4 gm q24h	No
Cefoperazone	Cefobid	i.m., i.v.	1–2 gm q8–12h	No
Cefotaxime	Claforan	i.m., i.v.	1–2 gm q6–12h	Yes

Drug	Trade name	Route	Dosage	Oral
Cefpodoxime	Vantin	Oral	0.1–0.4 gm q12	Yes
Ceftazidime	Fortaz, Tazidime, Tazicef	i.m., i.v.	1–2 gm q8h	Yes
Ceftizoxime	Cefizox	i.v.	1–2 gm q8–12h	Yes
Ceftriaxone	Rocephin	i.m., i.v.	1–2 gm q12–24h	No
Penicillins				
Penicillin G potassium	Pfizerpen	i.m., i.v.	2–3 MU q4h	Yes
Penicillin G tablets		Oral	0.5–1 gm q6h	No
Penicillin V	Pen-Vee K	Oral	0.25–0.5 gm q6h	No
Ampicillin	Omnipen	i.m., i.v.	0.5–1.5 gm q4–6h	Yes
		Oral	0.5–1 gm q6h	Yes
Ampicillin/sulbactam	Unasyn	i.v.	1.5–3 gm q6h	Yes
Amoxicillin	Amoxil	Oral	0.25–0.5 gm q8h	Yes
Amoxicillin/clavulanate	Augmentin	Oral	0.25–0.5 gm q8h	Yes
Oxacillin	Bactocil	i.m., i.v.	1–2 gm q4h	No
Nafcillin	Unipen	i.m., i.v.	1–2 gm q4h	No
Cloxacillin	Tegopen	Oral	0.25 gm q4–6h	No
Dicloxacillin	Pathocil	Oral	0.25–0.5 gm q6h; 0.25–0.75 gm q6h	No
Ticarcillin	Ticar	i.m., i.v.	3 gm q4–6h	Yes
Ticarcillin/clavulanate	Timentin	i.v.	3.1 gm q4–6h	Yes
Mezlocillin	Mezlin	i.m., i.v.	3–4 gm q4–6h	Yes
Piperacillin	Pipracil	i.m., i.v.	3–4 gm q4–6h	Yes
Piperacillin/tazobactam	Zosyn	i.v.	3 gm/375 mg q6h	Yes
Other betalactams				
Aztreonam	Azactam	i.m., i.v.	1 gm q8–12h	Yes
Imipenem-cilastatin	Primaxin	i.v.	1 gm q6–8h	Yes
Tetracyclines				
Tetracycline HCl	Achromycin	i.v., oral	0.25–0.5 gm q6–8h	Yes
Doxycycline	Vibramycin	i.v., oral	0.1 gm q12–24h	No
Trimethoprim-sulfonamides				
Sulfisoxazole	Gantrisin	i.v., oral	1 gm q6h	Yes

Table 1.3—continued

Generic Name	Trade Names	Route	Adult Dosage	Dose Change in Renal Impairment (See Tables 1.1, 1.2, 1.5)
Trimethoprim-Sulfamethoxazole	Septra, Bactrim	i.v.	10–20 mg/kg/d	Yes
		Oral	1–2 DS tablets q12h	Yes
Trimethoprim	Proloprim	Oral	100 mg q12h	Yes
Macrolides				
Erythromycin	many	i.v.	0.25–1 gm q6h	No
		Oral	0.25–0.5 gm q6h	No
Clarithromycin	Biaxin	Oral	0.25–0.5 gm q12h	?
Azithromycin	Zithromax	Oral	0.5 g, then 0.25 gm/day	?
Quinolones				
Norfloxacin	Noroxin	Oral	0.4 gm q12h	Yes
Ciprofloxacin	Cipro	Oral	0.25–0.75 gm q12h	Yes
		i.v.	0.2–0.4 gm q12h	Yes
Ofloxacin	Floxin	Oral	0.2–0.4 gm q12h	Yes
		i.v.	0.2–0.4 gm q12h	Yes
Enoxacin	Penetrex	Oral	0.2–0.4 gm q12h	Yes
Lomefloxacin	Maxaquin	Oral	0.4 gm q24h	Yes
Others				
Clindamycin	Cleocin	Oral	0.15–0.45 gm q6h	No
		i.v.	0.6–0.9 gm q6–8h	No
Chloramphenicol	Chloromycetin	i.v., oral	0.25–0.75 gm q6h	Yes
Vancomycin	Vancocin, Vancoled	i.v.	1 gm q12h	Yes

Table 1.4. Daily Dosage Schedules for Antimicrobial Agents in Pediatric Patients Beyond the Newborn Period

Agent, Generic (Trade Name)	Route	Dosage/kg/24 hr	
		Mild-to-Moderate Infection	Severe Infection
Penicillins			
Penicillin G, crystalline (numerous)	i.v., i.m.	25,000–50,000 units in 4 doses	100,000–300,000 units in 4–6 doses
Penicillin G, procaine (numerous)	i.m.	25,000–50,000 units in 1–2 doses	Inappropriate
Penicillin G, benzathine (Bicillin, Permapen)	i.m.	<30 lb = 600,000 units; 30–60 lb = 1,200,000 units; >60 lb = 2,400,000 units	Inappropriate
Penicillin G, potassium (numerous)	Oral	25,000–50,000 units in 4 doses	Inappropriate
Phenoxymethyl penicillin (numerous)	Oral	25,000–50,000 units in 4 doses	Inappropriate
Penicillinase-resistant penicillins			
Methicillin (Staphcillin, Celbenin)	i.v., i.m.	100–200 mg in 4 doses	200–300 mg in 4–6 doses
Oxacillin (Prostaphlin, Bactocill)	i.v., i.m.	50–100 mg in 4 doses	100–200 mg in 4–6 doses
	Oral	50–100 mg in 4 doses	Inappropriate
Nafcillin (Unipen)	i.v., i.m.	50–100 mg in 4 doses	100–200 mg in 4–6 doses
	Oral	50–100 mg in 4 doses	Inappropriate
Cloxacillin (Tegopen)	Oral	25–50 mg in 4 doses	Inappropriate
Dicloxacillin (Dynapen, Pathocil, Veracillin)	Oral	12.5–25 mg in 4 doses	Inappropriate
Broad-spectrum penicillins			
Ampicillin (numerous)	i.v., i.m.	50–100 mg in 4 doses	200–400 mg in 4 doses
	Oral	50–100 mg in 4 doses	Inappropriate
Amoxicillin (Amoxil, Larotid, Polymox)	Oral	20–40 mg in 3 doses	Inappropriate
Amoxicillin and potassium clavulanate (Augmentin)	Oral	20–40 mg in 3 doses	Inappropriate
Bacampicillin (Spectrobid)	Oral	25–50 mg in 2 doses	Inappropriate

Table 1.4—continued

Agent, Generic (Trade Name)	Route	Dosage/kg/24 hr	
		Mild-to-Moderate Infection	Severe Infection
Cyclacillin (Cyclapen-W)	Oral	50–100 mg in 3 doses	Inappropriate
Carbenicillin (Geopen, Pyopen)	i.v., i.m.	100–200 mg in 4 doses	400–600 mg in 4–6 doses
Ticarcillin (Ticar)	i.v., i.m.	50–100 mg in 4 doses	200–300 mg in 4–6 doses
Mezlocillin (Mezlin)	i.v.	Inappropriate	200–300 mg in 4–6 doses
Azlocillin (Azlin)	i.v.	Inappropriate	200–450 mg in 4–6 doses
Cephalosporins			
Cephalothin (Keflin)	i.v., i.m.	40–80 mg in 4 doses	100–150 mg in 4–6 doses
Cefazolin (Kefzol, Ancef)	i.v., i.m.	50 mg in 4 doses	50–100 mg in 4 doses
Cephalexin (Keflex)	Oral	25–50 mg in 4 doses	Inappropriate
Cefoxitin (Mefoxin)	i.v., i.m.	Inappropriate	80–160 mg in 4–6 doses
Cefaclor (Ceclor)	Oral	40 mg in 3 doses	Inappropriate
Cefuroxime (Zinacef)	i.v., i.m.	Inappropriate	75–200 mg in 3 doses
Moxalactam (Moxam)	i.v.	Inappropriate	150–200 mg in 3–4 doses
Cefotaxime (Claforan)	i.v., i.m.	Inappropriate	100–200 mg in 4 doses
Ceftriaxone (Rocephin)	i.v., i.m.	Inappropriate	100 mg in 2 doses
Ceftazidime (Fortaz, Tazidime, Tazicef)	i.v., i.m.	Inappropriate	90–150 mg in 3 doses
Erythromycin			
Erythromycin glucoheptonate (Ilotycin, IV)	i.v.	Inappropriate	15–20 mg in 3–4 doses
Erythromycin lactobionate (Erythrocin, IV)		Inappropriate	Inappropriate
Erythromycin base (Ilotycin, E-mycin)	Oral	20–50 mg in 3–4 doses	Inappropriate
Erythromycin ethyl succinate (Pediamycin, Erythrocin)		Inappropriate	Inappropriate
Erythromycin stearate (Erythrocin)		Inappropriate	Inappropriate
Erythromycin estolate (Ilosone)		Inappropriate	Inappropriate

	Route		
Lincosamines			
Lincomycin (Lincocin)	i.v., i.m.	10 mg in 2 doses	20 mg in 2 doses
Clindamycin (Cleocin)	i.v., i.m.	10–25 mg in 4 doses	25–40 mg in 4 doses
	Oral	8–16 mg in 4 doses	Inappropriate
Aminoglycosides			
Streptomycin (numerous)	i.m.	Inappropriate	20–40 mg in 3 doses
Kanamycin (Kantrex)	i.v., i.m.	15 mg in 2–3 doses	15 mg in 2–3 doses
Gentamicin (Garamycin)	i.v.,[a] i.m.	Inappropriate	3–7 mg in 3 doses
Tobramycin (Nebcin)	i.v.,[a] i.m.	Inappropriate	3–7 mg in 3 doses
Amikacin (Amikin)	i.v.,[a] i.m.	Inappropriate	15 mg in 2 doses
Netilmicin	i.v., i.m.	Inappropriate	3–7.5 mg in 3 doses
Polymyxins			
Polymyxin B (Aerosporin)	i.m.	Inappropriate	25,000–40,000 units in 4 doses
Colistin sodium colistimethate (Coly-Mycin M)	i.m.	Inappropriate	2.5–5 mg in 4 doses
Others			
Tetracyclines (numerous)	i.v.	Inappropriate	10–20 mg in 2–3 doses
	Oral	20–40 mg in 4 doses	Inappropriate
Chloramphenicol (Chloromycetin)	i.v.	Inappropriate	50–100 mg in 3–4 doses
	Oral	Inappropriate	50–100 mg in 3–4 doses
Sulfadiazine	i.v., s.c.	120 mg in 4 doses	120 mg in 4 doses
Sulfisoxazole (Gantrisin)	i.v., s.c.	120 mg in 4 doses	120 mg in 4 doses
	Oral	120 mg in 4 doses	Inappropriate
Triple sulfonamides	iv., s.c.	120 mg in 4 doses	120 mg in 4 doses
Trimethoprim-sulfamethoxazole (Bactrim, Septra)	Oral	8 mg trimethoprim, 40 mg sulfamethoxazole in 2 doses	15–20 mg trimethoprim and 75–100 mg sulfamethoxazole in 3 doses[b] or 8–10 mg or trimethoprim and 40–50 mg sulfamethoxazole in 3 doses[c]
	i.v.	Inappropriate	
Vancomycin (Vancocin)	i.v.	Inappropriate	15–50 mg in 4 doses

Reprinted and modified with permission from Feigin R.D., Cherry J.D. *Textbook of Pediatric Infectious Diseases*, 2nd ed.
[a]Intravenous administration over 30–60 minutes.
[b]For *Pneumocystis carinii* pneumonitis.
[c]For other severe urinary, respiratory, and gastrointestinal tract infections.

Table 1.5. Daily Dosage Schedules for Antibiotics of Value in Treating Infections in Newborn Infants

Agent, Generic (Trade Name)	Route	Dosage/kg/24 hr	
		< 7 Days of Age	7–28 Days of Age
Penicillin G, crystalline (numerous)	i.v., i.m. 2 doses	50,000–100,000 units in 3 doses	100,000–200,000 units
Penicillinase-resistant penicillins			
Methicillin (Staphcillin, Celbenin)	i.v., i.m.	50–100 mg in 2 doses	100–200 mg in 3 doses
Oxacillin (Prostaphlin, Bactocill)	i.v., i.m.	50–100 mg in 2 doses	100–200 mg in 3 doses
Nafcillin (Unipen)	i.m.[a]	50–100 mg in 2 doses	100–200 mg in 3 doses
Broad-spectrum penicillins			
Ampicillin (numerous)	i.v., i.m.	100 mg in 2 doses	200 mg in 3 doses
Carbenicillin (Geopen, Pyopen)	i.v., i.m.	200–300 mg in 4 doses	400 mg in 4 doses
Ticarcillin (Ticar)	i.v., i.m.	150–225 mg in 2–3 doses	225–300 mg in 3 doses
Cephalosporins			
Moxalactam (Moxam)	i.v.	100 mg in 2 doses	150 mg in 3 doses
Cefotaxime (Claforan)	i.v., i.m.	100 mg in 2 doses	150 mg in 3 doses
Aminoglycosides			
Kanamycin (Kantrex)	i.v.,[b] i.m.	15 mg in 2 doses	15 mg in 2 doses
Gentamicin (Garamycin)	i.v.,[b] i.m.	6 mg in 2 doses	7.5 mg in 3 doses
Tobramycin (Nebcin)	i.v.,[b] i.m.	4 mg in 2 doses	5 mg in 3 doses
Amikacin (Amikin)	i.v.,[b] i.m.	15 mg in 2 doses	15 mg in 2 doses
Chloramphenicol (Chloromycetin)	i.v.	Premature—25 mg in 2 doses Term—25 mg in 2 doses	Premature—25 mg in 2 doses Term—50 mg in 2 doses
Vancomycin (Vancocin)	i.v.	30 mg in 2 doses	30–45 mg in 3 doses

Reprinted and modified with permission from Feigin RD, Cherry, JD (eds). Textbook of Pediatric Infectious Diseases. 2nd ed.
[a] No clinical experience available for use intravenously in newborn infants.
[b] Intravenous administration over 30–60 minutes.

Table 1.6. Pharmacological Characteristics of Selected Antimicrobials

Drug	C_{max} (mg/L)	$t_{1/2}$ (hr) (Normal)	$t_{1/2}$ (hr) (Anuria)	PB (%)	Fe (%)	CSF (%)	Dosage in Renal Failure[a]	Comments
Acyclovir 5 mg kg i.v. 200 mg p.o.	34–50 2.5	3	20	15	95	50	CL_{cr} >50 = full dose 25–50 every 12 hr 10–24 = every 24 hr <10 = 50% dose every 24 hr	Oral doses need not be reduced for renal failure; 50% removed by HD
Amantadine	NA	12	>100	Low	>90	High	CL_{cr} >80 = full dose 60–80 = 200/100 mg daily on alternate days 40–59 = 100 mg daily 20–39 = 100 mg 3 × wk <20 = 200/100 mg alternate wk	Serum concentrations have not been correlated with therapeutic effect; HD has little effect
Amoxicillin 500 mg p.o.	8	1	16	Low	40–70	Low	See ampicillin	Oral doses generally need not be reduced for renal failure, unless severe; 50% removed by HD
Amphotericin B 0.5 mg/kg i.v.	1	24–48 (15 d)	Same	>90	<5	Low	No dosage reduction	If sodium loading does not ameliorate renal dysfunction, alternate day dosing may be useful; no effect by HD

Table 1.6—continued

Drug	C_{max} (mg/L)	$t_{1/2}$ (hr) (Normal)	$t_{1/2}$ (hr) (Anuria)	PB (%)	Fe (%)	CSF (%)	Dosage in Renal Failure[a]	Comments
Ampicillin 1 g i.v. 500 mg p.o.	40 4	0.75	12	20	>90	25	CL_{cr} >50 = full dose; 25–50 = 75% of dose; 10–24 = 50% of dose; <10 = 25% of dose	Pharmacokinetics not affected by sulbactam (Unasyn)
Aztreonam 1 g i.v.	100	1.7	6	56	65	25	CL_{cr} >30 = full dose; <30 = 50% of dose	50% removed by HD
Capreomycin 1 g i.m.	30	2.5	50–100	?	70?	Very low	CL_{cr} >50 = full dose; 25–50 = 50% of dose Q 24h; 10–24 = 50% of dose Q 48h; <10 = 50% of dose 2 x week	No data on HD
Carbenicillin 5 g i.v. 764 mg p.o.	300 8	0.75	16	50	>90	20	CL_{cr} >30 = full dose; 20–30 = 50–75% of dose; 10–19 = 25–50% of dose; <10 = 15% of dose	Reduce dose to 7.5% for hepatic failure + severe renal failure; 50% removed by hemodialysis
Cefaclor 500 mg p.o.	14	0.75	3	Low	70	NA	Reduce dose by 50% in severe renal failure (CL_{cr} <10)	
Cefadroxil 500 mg p.o.	16	1.25	15–20	Low	90	NA	Reduce dose by 50% in severe renal failure (CL_{cr} <10)	

Drug							Dosing adjustment	Hemodialysis
Cefamandole 1 g i.v.	70	1	16–18	70	<90	Low	CL_{cr} >80 = full dose 50–80 = 50–75% of dose 25–49 = 25–50% of dose 10–24 = 15–25% of dose <10 = 10% of dose	50% removed by HD
Cefazolin 1 g i.v.	120	1.5	36–60	85	95	Low	CL_{cr} >50 = full dose 25–50 = 50% of dose 15–24 = 25% of dose 5–14 = 12.5% of dose <5 = 6.25% of dose	Supplemental dose after HD
Cefepime	70	2	32	20	80	?	CL_{cr} >80 = full dose 40–80 = 50–75% of dose 20–39 = 25–50% of dose 10–20 = 12.5–25% of dose <10 = 5–10% of dose	Supplemental dose after HD
Cefixime 400 mg p.o.	4	3.5	12	70	20	NA	Administer 50% of dose in patients with CL_{cr} <20 ml/min	No effect by HD
Cefmetazole 1 g i.v.	180	1.3	15–33	85	65–75	NA	CL_{cr} >50 = full dose 30–49 = 75% of dose 10–29 = 50% of dose <10 = 25% of dose	
Cefonicid 1 g i.v.	200	4.5	70	98	>90	Low	CL_{cr} >80 = full dose 40–80 = 50–75% of dose 20–39 = 25–50% of dose 10–20 = 12.5–25% of dose <10 = 5–10% of dose	No effect by HD

Table 1.6—continued

Drug	C_{max} (mg/L)	$t_{1/2}$ (hr) (Normal)	$t_{1/2}$ (hr) (Anuria)	PB (%)	Fe (%)	CSF (%)	Dosage in Renal Failure[a]	Comments
Cefoperazone 1 g i.v.	150	2	2	90	25	Low	No dosage reduction	No effect by HD
Cefotaxime 1 g i.v. (desacetyl-)	60 / 10	1 / 2	2.5 / 20–30	40 / Low	50 / >90	30–40 / ?	Reduce dose by 50% in severe renal failure (CL_{cr} <20)	40% removed by HD
Cefotetan 1 g i.v.	100	3.5	24–48	85	90	Low	CL_{cr} >30 = full dose; 10–30 = 50% of dose; <10 = 25% of dose	25–50% removed by HD
Cefoxitin 1 g i.v.	70	1	20	70	80	Low	CL_{cr} >80 = full dose; 50–80 = 50–75% of dose; 25–49 = 25–50% of dose; 10–24 = 15–25% of dose; <10 = 10% of dose	50% removed by HD
Ceftazidime 1 g i.v.	80	1.9	30	Low	80	30–40	CL_{cr} >50 = full dose; 30–50 = 65% of dose; 15–29 = 33% of dose; 5–14 = 17% of dose; <5 = 8% of dose	50% removed by HD
Ceftizoxime 1 g i.v.	80	1.3	36	Low	95	20–30	CL_{cr} >80 = full dose; 40–80 = 67% of dose; 10–39 = 33% of dose; <10 = 10% of dose	50% removed by HD

Drug							Dosage adjustment in renal failure	HD
Ceftriaxone 1 g i.v.	150	8	10	96	40	10	No dosage reduction	Minimal effect by HD
Cefuroxime 0.75 g i.v.	80	1.3	15	Low	90	30	CL_{cr} >80 = full dose 50–80 = 50–75% of dose 25–49 = 25–50% of dose 10–24 = 15–25% of dose <10 = 10% of dose	50% removed by HD
Cephalexin 500 mg p.o.	15	0.75	24	Low	<90	NA	CL_{cr} <50 = full dose 20–50 = 50% of dose <20 = 25% of dose	50% removed by HD; same data apply to cephradine
Cephalothin 1 g i.v.	50	0.5	3	65	65	Low	Reduce dose by 50% in severe renal failure (CL_{cr} <20)	Minimal effect by HD; same data apply to cephapirin
Chloramphenicol 500 mg i.v. 250 mg p.o.	10 8	3	3	50	<10	75	No dosage reduction	>50% reduction by HD
Clavulanic acid 100 mg i.v. 125 mg p.o.	8 4	1.2	3	15	35	?	See amoxicillin and ticarcillin	See amoxicillin and ticarcillin
Clindamycin 600 mg i.v. 300 mg p.o.	25 4	3	3	90	10	40	No dosage reduction	Minimal effect by HD
Clofazimine 200 mg p.o.	0.5–1	200	Same?	?	Low	Low?	No dosage reduction	Food enhances absorption by as much as 60%
Cloxacillin 500 mg p.o.	8	0.5	0.8	90–95	75	NA	No dosage reduction	No effect by HD

Table 1.6—continued

Drug	C_{max} (mg/L)	$t_{1/2}$ (hr) (Normal)	$t_{1/2}$ (hr) (Anuria)	PB (%)	Fe (%)	CSF (%)	Dosage in Renal Failure[a]	Comments
Cycloserine 500 mg p.o.	20	10	?	?	60	100	Reduce dosage by 50% in severe renal failure	Best to avoid in renal failure
Doxycycline 100 mg p.o. 100 mg i.v.	1.5 2	16	20	90	20	20	No dosage reduction	
Erythromycin 500 mg p.o. 1 g i.v.	1.5 10	1.5	1.5	80	15	10	No dosage reduction	No effect by HD
Ethambutol 1 g p.o.	4	4	18	20–30	60–80	25–50	CL_{cr} >30 = full dose 10–30 = 50% of dose <10 = 35% of dose	35% removed by HD
Fluconazole 100 mg p.o. 200 mg i.v.	6 9	22	98	10	65	60–90	CL_{cr} >50 = full dose 20–50 = 50% of dose 10–19 = 25% of dose <10 = 12.5% of dose	
Flucytosine 30 mg/kg p.o.	40	4	>80	10	>90	>50	CL_{cr} >40 = full dose 20–40 = 50% of dose 10–19 = 25% of dose <10 = 15% of dose	50–75% reduction by HD
Ganciclovir 5 mg/kg i.v.	45 μmol/L	2.5	28	Low	>90	25–65	CL_{cr} >50 = full dose 20–50 = 50% of dose 10–19 = 25% of dose <10 = 12.5% of dose	50% removed by HD

Drug						Dosage adjustment	Hemodialysis
Griseofulvin 1 g p.o.	1.5	16	16	?	<1	NA	No dosage reduction	No effect by HD
Imipenem 500 mg i.v.	30	1	4	20	70	?	CL_{cr} >70 = full dose 30–70 = 50–75% of dose 10–29 = 25–50% of dose <10 = 15–25% of dose	50% removed by HD
Isoniazid 300 mg p.o.	2.5	1 (rapid) 3 (slow)	4	Low	<25	50–100	Dosage reduction to 200 mg in slow acetylators only	No effect by HD
Ketoconazole 200 mg p.o.	3	6	6	99	<10	Low	No dosage reduction	No effect by HD
Metronidazole 250 mg p.o. 500 mg i.v.	6 14	8	10	20	30–40	>100	No dosage reduction	Parent compound and active metabolite are >50% removed by HD
Mezlocillin 60 mg/kg	260	1	3	25–50	40–70	?	CL_{cr} >30 = full dose 20–30 = 50–75% of dose <20 = 35% of dose	Minimal effect by HD
Miconazole 600 mg i.v.	10	24	24	85	<10	Low	No dosage reduction	No effect by HD
Minocycline 100 mg p.o.	1.5	18	30	75	10	50	Minimal effect by HD	Minimal effect by HD
Nafcillin 1 g i.v.	40	0.75	1.5	92	40	20	No dosage reduction	Minimal effect by HD
Oxacillin 1 g i.v.	40	0.5	1	94	50	?	No dosage reduction	No effect by HD

Table 1.6—continued

Drug	C_{max} (mg/L)	$t_{1/2}$ (hr) (Normal)	$t_{1/2}$ (hr) (Anuria)	PB (%)	Fe (%)	CSF (%)	Dosage in Renal Failure[a]	Comments
Penicillin G 1 mU i.v. 500 mg p.o. procaine 1.2 mU i.m. benzathine 1.2 mU i.m.	0.5 2 3 0.1	10	65	>90	30–40		Cl_{cr} <10 = 1/2 usual dose	50% removed by HD
Penicillin V 500 mg p.o.	5	0.5	10	80	>90	NA	Reduce dosage by 50% in severe renal failure	
Pentamidine 4 mg kg i.v.	0.5–3	120	?	?	<10	?	No dosage reduction	No effect by HD
Piperacillin 60 mg/kg	240	1	3	20	50–90	?	CL_{cr} >30 = full dose 20–30 = 65% of dose <20 = 35–50% of dose	50% removed by HD pharmacokinetics not affected be tazobactam (Zosyn)
Polymyxin B 50 mg i.v.	5	4	36	High	60	Low	CL_{cr} >40 = full dose 20–40 = 75% of dose 5–20 = 50% of dose <5 = 25% of dose	No effect by HD
Pyrazinamide 20 mg/kg p.o.	60	6	?	?	20	100	No data	No data on HD
Quinolones Ciprofloxacin 500 mg p.o. 200 mg i.v.	2 3	4	10	Low	60	Low	Reduce dosage by 50% in severe renal failure	Minimal reduction by HD

Drug/Dose	C_{max}	$t_{1/2}$		PB	Fe	CSF	Renal failure dosing	Hemodialysis / comments
Norfloxacin 400 mg p.o.	1.5	4	9	Low	30	NA	No dosage reduction	No effect by HD
Ofloxacin 400 mg p.o.	5	7	30	Low	90	?	Reduce dose by 50% in severe renal failure	
Rifampin 600 mg p.o.	8	3	3	75	<20	50	No effect by HD	
Sulfisoxazole 1 g p.o.	75	6	12	85	50	30	Removed by HD	
Tetracycline 500 mg p.o. / 250 mg i.v.	2.5 / 3.5	8	>48	60	50	10	Avoid	Do not use in renal failure
Ticarcillin 3 g i.v.	320	1	20	50	80	30–50	CL_{cr} >60 = full dose; 30–60 = 35–65% of dose; 10–29 = 25–35% of dose; 10 = 25% of dose	Removed by HD; pharmacokinetics not affected by clavulanic acid (Timentin)
Trimethoprim 160 mg p.o. / 5 mg/kg i.v.	2 / 6	10	36	55	75	>50	CL_{cr} >50 = full dose; 20–40 = 60–75% of dose; 10–20 = 50–60% of dose; <10 = 25–50% of dose	Dosage reduction is only necessary for doses of 10/50 mg/kg per day or greater; 30–40% reduction by HD
Sulfamethoxazole 800 mg p.o. / 25 mg/kg i.v.	40 / 120	9	20	60	30	>50	As above	
Vancomycin 1 g i.v.	20	6	>100	low	>95	20–30	Monitor serum levels	No effect by HD

a Loading dose should always be administered. C_{max}, Average peak serum concentration; $t_{1/2}$, elimination half-life; PB, serum protein-binding; Fe, fraction of dose excreted unchanged in urine; HD, hemodialysis; CSF-CSF, penetration.

Protein Binding

The values listed are the average reported for percentage of drug bound to plasma proteins. These data are potentially important, because highly protein-bound drugs are generally not cleared by hemodialysis. Additionally, the protein-bound drug is not microbiologically active, and the bound fraction is not diffusible.

Percentage of Drug Excreted Unchanged

The fraction of a dose of an antibiotic that is eliminated in the unchanged (nonmetabolized) form by the kidneys is reflected in the percentage of drug excreted unchanged. This value is important for two reasons: Drugs that are minimally removed by urinary excretion may not be effective in the treatment of urinary tract infection, particularly in patients with reduced renal function, and drugs that are predominantly eliminated unchanged generally require dosage adjustment in renal failure. The extent of this adjustment depends on several factors, including the extent of renal elimination (the half-life of a drug that is 50% excreted unchanged will double in anuria, whereas the half-life of aminoglycosides [95% excreted unchanged] will increase 20-fold) and the toxicity of the compound. For example, although ampicillin accumulates to a significant extent in renal failure, it is relatively nontoxic, and dosage adjustment need not be as rigorous as for aminoglycosides.

Estimating Renal Function

Creatinine clearance is the most frequently used measure of renal function. The clearances of most antibiotics have been correlated to creatinine clearance. Thus, it is important to be able to estimate an individual patient's endogenous renal function. This estimation is the first step in the approach to modifying a dosage regimen in renal failure. The most reliable method for estimating creatinine clearance (CL_{CR}) in adults is the following equation developed by Cockcroft and Gault:

$$CL_{CR} = \frac{(140 - \text{Age}) (\text{Wgt in kg}) [\text{x } 0.85 \text{ for women}]}{(72) (Cr_S)}$$

where Wgt and Cr_S are weight and serum creatinine, respectively. Various methods are available for this estimation in infants and young children, but the most useful equation is:

$$CL_{CR} = \frac{(0.48) \times \text{Hgt(cm)}}{Cr_S}$$

where Hgt is the height of the infant.

The equation for adults should be used with lean (ideal) body weight in kilograms. The estimate may be erroneous in patients who are malnourished or cachectic, in those with changing renal function, or in the elderly. Height is expressed in centimeters for the pediatric equation. The loading and maintenance dose recommendations for the use of aminoglycosides in patients with impaired renal function are summarized in Tables 1.1 and 1.2.

Testing for Synergy

Various methods are used for in vitro testing of synergy. The most commonly used technique involves testing a combination of antibiotics at one-fourth the minimum inhibitory concentration (MIC) for each drug alone. If the organism is inhibited with the combination at these concentrations, the combination is deemed synergistic. This simple test does not provide information regarding bactericidal synergy. This would be provided by testing the drugs at one-fourth the minimum bactericidal concentration (MBC) and measuring lethality rather than inhibition. An alternative method, which many clinicians feel is more clinically applicable, measures the rate of bactericidal action by serially sampling bacterial colony counts during incubation with a combination of drugs and comparing the rate of kill with each drug alone. Clinical situations in which it would be desirable to use a synergistically bactericidal combination include bacterial infection in the profoundly neutropenic patient and systemic infection with *Pseudomonas aeruginosa*.

Antibiotic Blood Levels

The "blood level" is the plasma or serum concentration of an antibiotic. This determination may provide useful clinical information as (1) a guide to dosage in patients with uncertain or changing renal function; (2) an aid in evaluating antibiotic toxicity; and (3) a guide to adjusting the oral dosage of an antibiotic.

Determination of the blood levels of the following antibiotics is frequently helpful:

gentamicin	chloramphenicol
tobramycin	flucytosine
netilmicin	vancomycin
amikacin	

In general, at least one blood level determination is necessary to be useful for (2) or (3). Two or more determinations are necessary for (1). Peak and trough levels are the minimum number of points needed to ascertain the half-life of an antibiotic (see Fig. 1.1). For the approximate times to obtain blood levels, a rule of thumb is to obtain a "peak" concentration 1 hour after the start of an IV infusion, therefore, 30 minutes after a 30-minute infusion or immediately after a 60-minute infusion. The presence of a second or third antibiotic in serum may prevent assay by biological methods, owing to cross-sensitivity of test organisms.

Serum Antimicrobial Activity

A few studies have indicated that measurement of the antibiotic activity of serial dilutions of a patient's serum during therapy may predict recovery from certain infectious diseases, such as endocarditis or perhaps osteomyelitis. The test is performed by taking the patient's serum at a peak or a trough level. The serum is serially diluted and inoculated with the organism that is infecting the patient. The dilutions are then tested for bactericidal activity (Fig. 1.2). Presumed favorable prognostic value is associated with bactericidal dilutions of 1:8 or greater. Additionally, the test should be performed when oral antibiotics are substituted for parenteral therapy in the treatment of serious infections, such as osteomyelitis or endocarditis. This procedure will help to ensure the adequacy of the therapy.

There is much controversy regarding the timing of blood samples for this test. Collection of blood at peak concentrations results in a determination of the maximum bactericidal activity of the patient's serum. However, trough measurements reveal the duration of bactericidal activity. Unfortunately, if the half-life of the antibiotic being used is short and the dosing interval is greater than 4–6 half-lives, the bactericidal activity at the trough level may be zero; peak concentrations, however, may be adequate, and the patient will respond to therapy.

Acyclovir

ADVERSE REACTIONS

Nephrotoxicity

Precipitation of acyclovir crystals in renal tubules occurs if solubility of drug is exceeded (2.5 mg/ml at 37°C), or if drug is given by bolus injection. Patients should be appropriately hydrated so that adequate urine flow is achieved, especially in the first 2 hours after dose.

CNS Toxicity

Tremors, confusion, hallucination, lethargy, and agitation have been reported rarely. May be increased in patients with prior neurological complications of cytotoxic therapy.

DRUG INTERACTIONS

Probenecid

Renal excretion is decreased, resulting in prolonged half-life and higher serum concentrations.

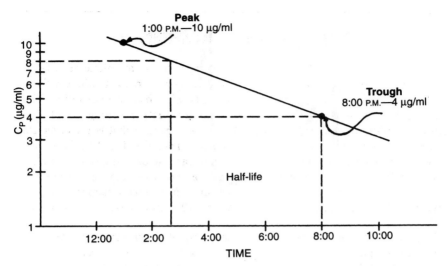

Figure 1.1. In order to estimate the half-life of a drug, one should (1) draw a straight line connecting the two measured plasma levels at the appropriate time, and then (2) choose two points along the line, the first of which is half the concentration of the second. The time it takes for the C_p to decline by half (from 8 to 4 ml) is 5½ hours.

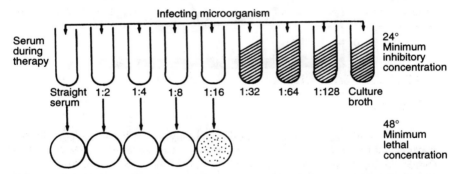

Figure 1.2. The test for serum antimicrobial activity determines the maximum dilution of serum that will show bacteriostatic or bactericidal (lethal) activity against an infecting organism. Interpretation of results: Bacteriostatic at 1 : 16 dilution, bactericidal at 1 : 8 dilution. (Adapted from Youmans, G.P., Paterson, P.Y., and Sommers, H.: The biologic and clinical basis of infectious diseases. Philadelphia: W.B. Saunders, 1975.)

Amantadine

ADVERSE REACTIONS

CNS Toxicity

Nervousness, dizziness, agitation or ataxia, drowsiness, and insomnia may result.

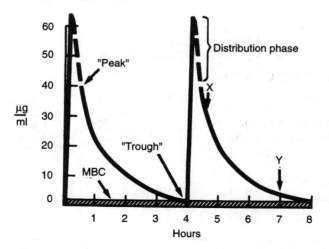

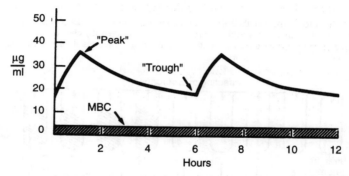

Figure 1.3. Typical antibiotic serum concentration curves for a 70-kg adult with normal renal function. (MBC = minimum bactericidal concentration.) *A*, Nafcillin (1 g i.v. q4h) is infused rapidly (10–15 minutes), and true peak levels occur after a distribution phase. Serum bactericidal level taken at point X should be 1 : 16, whereas at point Y it may be 1 : 2 or less. *B*, Vancomycin (500 mg i.v. q6h—steady state) is infused over 60 minutes. A peak level may be taken shortly after the end of the infusion. Because of longer $t_{1/2}$, serum bactericidal levels taken at trough should be 1 : 4 or more.

Anticholinergic Reactions

Blurred vision, dry mouth, and tachycardia may occur.

Gastrointestinal Disturbance

Anorexia and nausea are mild.

Teratogenic Reactions

None are reported.

DRUG INTERACTIONS
CNS Toxicity

It may be increased in patients receiving other CNS stimulants such as amphetamines.

Amikacin

ADVERSE REACTIONS

Ototoxicity

High-frequency hearing loss and tinnitus occur after prolonged (>10–14 days) therapy. Hearing loss in the conversational range and vestibular damage are rare but may be irreversible.

Nephrotoxicity

Acute tubular necrosis occurs in 5–10% of patients and is manifested by increases in serum creatinine and BUN.

Neuromuscular Blockade

This has only been reported with aminoglycosides administered by intraperitoneal lavage and in patients with myasthenia gravis.

DRUG INTERACTIONS

Diuretics (Furosemide, Ethacrynic Acid)

These are felt to potentiate oto- or nephrotoxicity, presumably due to volume contraction, although some clinical data suggest that furosemide does not produce these effects.

Penicillins

Inactivation of the aminoglycosides is caused in vitro and in vivo. Caution should be exercised in patients with renal insufficiency, in whom excessive concentrations of penicillins may result in decreased aminoglycoside concentrations. Amikacin is inactivated to a lesser extent than the other agents. The clinical significance of this interaction may lead to excessive dosage escalation, particularly if reaction occurs in vitro.

Miscellaneous

Aminoglycosides may enhance the nephrotoxicity of platinum compounds, amphotericin B, and cyclosporine.

Amoxicillin

ADVERSE REACTIONS

Hypersensitivity Reactions

As with all penicillins, rash, urticaria, anaphylaxis, and serum sickness are possible but are uncommon.

Gastrointestinal Disturbances

In children, amoxicillin may produce less diarrhea than ampicillin when given in oral suspensions.

DRUG INTERACTIONS

See penicillin G.

Amphotericin B

ADVERSE REACTIONS

Acute

Fever, chills, nausea/vomiting/anorexia, and headache may occur. These symptoms may be caused by deoxycholate, used to form colloidal solution, or by colloidal suspension itself; recent data suggest amphotericin B-induced release of TNF may be responsible. Analgesics, antiemetics, ibuprofen, meperidine, antipyretics, heparin, or hydrocortisone may be useful treatments, but none has been systematically studied.

Chronic

Anemia—Suppression of erythropoietin? Hypokalemia, hypomagnesemia, renal tubular acidosis: disruption of renal tubular cell membrane

Renal Failure

Renal artery spasm leading to ischemia Sodium loading (500 ml 0.9% saline) prior to Ampho B shown to decrease renal toxicity.

Hypokalemia and hypomagnesemia require replacement with appropriate salts (KCl or $KHCO_3$ and $MgSO_4$). Anemia does not respond to replacement therapy with iron or folates. RBC transfusions or erythropoietin may be needed if hematocrit falls excessively.

DRUG INTERACTIONS

Digitalis

Caution must be taken to monitor hypokalemia carefully.

Penicillins

Carbenicillin or ticarcillin given concomitantly may exacerbate hypokalemia.

Ampicillin

ADVERSE REACTIONS

See also penicillin G.

Drug Eruptions

A characteristic nonurticarial maculopapular rash that is nonallergic may appear 3–4 days after the onset of therapy. This reaction is more frequent in patients with viral infections, especially mononucleosis, or when ampicillin is taken together with allopurinol. The mechanism for this increased incidence is unknown. The reaction fades with continued therapy.

Antibiotic-associated Diarrhea Colitis

Surveys have demonstrated that ampicillin is the most frequently implicated drug in producing this adverse effect.

DRUG INTERACTIONS

See penicillin G.

Mezlocillin/Piperacillin

ADVERSE REACTIONS

See carbenicillin/ticarcillin.

DRUG INTERACTIONS

See penicillin.

Aminoglycosides

These drugs can inactivate aminoglycosides in vitro. In vivo, clinically significant inactivation of aminoglycosides by extend-spectrum penicillin has occurred in patients with renal failure.

Aztreonam

ADVERSE REACTIONS

No significant adverse effects have been reported to date. Transient elevation of liver enzymes has been reported without clinical evidence of liver injury.

DRUG INTERACTIONS

Phlebitis following intravenous administration (1.9%). Monitor renal function carefully if administered with aminoglycosides. Activity may be reduced by betalactamase-inducing antibiotics.

Capreomycin

ADVERSE REACTIONS

Nephrotoxicity

Acute tubular necrosis occurs frequently, if daily administration is prolonged beyond the recommended duration. Renal tubular dysfunction that results in electrolyte disturbances may occur.

Ototoxicity

Deafness or vertigo occur frequently, if therapy is prolonged.

DRUG INTERACTIONS

See amikacin.

Carbenicillin

ADVERSE REACTIONS

See also penicillin G.

Hepatotoxicity

Hepatitis has been described, usually as mild elevation of transaminase.

Hypokalemia

This reaction is caused by tubular excretion of potassium with carbenicillin as a nonreabsorbable anion.

Decreased Platelet Aggregation

This drug inhibits platelet aggregation at high concentration, possibly predisposing to bleeding diatheses.

Drug Interactions

See penicillin G.

Cefaclor, Cefadroxil, Cefpodoxime, Cefprozil

ADVERSE REACTIONS

See cephalexin.

DRUG INTERACTIONS

See cephalexin.

Cefamandole

ADVERSE REACTIONS

See cephalothin and cefotetan.

DRUG INTERACTIONS

Alcohol

The *N*-methylthiotetrazol side chain can produce a disulfiram-like reaction in patients who ingest ethanol or ethanol-containing medication while receiving any drug that contains this moiety.

Cefixime

ADVERSE REACTIONS

Diarrhea occurs in 16% of patients. Nausea and vomiting are uncommon. See also cephalothin and cephalexin.

DRUG INTERACTIONS

See cephalothin. False-positive tests for ketonuria, glycosuria, and positive Coombs'.

Cefmetazole

ADVERSE REACTIONS

Hypoprothrombinemia

Like cefotetan, cefamandole, and cefoperazone, this drug contains the N-methylthiotetrazol (NMTT) side chain that may lead to hypoprothrombinemia. Pharmacokinetic studies have shown that less NMTT is produced from cefmetazole than the other cephalosporins; however, prophylactic vitamin K should be given to patients at high risk of bleeding, regardless of the types of antibiotics administered. See also cephalothin.

DRUG INTERACTIONS

See cephalothin.

Cefonicid

ADVERSE REACTIONS

See cephalothin.

DRUG INTERACTIONS

Probenecid

Decreases the clearance of cefonicid.

Cefoperazone

ADVERSE REACTIONS

See cefazolin and cefotaxime.

DRUG INTERACTIONS

See cefamandole.

Cefotaxime, Cefazolin, Cefoxitin, Ceftazidime, Ceftizoxime, Cefuroxime/Cefuroxime Axetil

ADVERSE REACTIONS

See cephalothin.

DRUG INTERACTIONS

See cephalothin.

Cefotetan

ADVERSE REACTIONS

See cephalothin.

Hypoprothrombinemia

Like other cephalosporins with the N-methylthiotetrazole moiety in their structures, hypoprothrombinemia has been reported, which is prevented by prophylactic vitamin K. This has been seen predominantly in patients receiving 4 to 6 g/day of cefotetan, but would be expected to occur with lower doses in patients with renal insufficiency. Patients at high risk for bleeding should receive prophylactic vitamin K, regardless of the type of antibiotic administered.

DRUG INTERACTIONS

See cefamandole.

Ceftriaxone

ADVERSE REACTIONS

See cephalothin. Biliary pseudolithiasis has been reported in adults and children receiving high doses, presumably due to deposition of a calcium salt of ceftriaxone.

DRUG INTERACTIONS

See cephalothin.

Cephalexin

ADVERSE REACTIONS

Gastrointestinal Disturbance

Nausea, vomiting, and diarrhea may occur. See also cephalothin.

DRUG INTERACTIONS

See cephalothin.

Cephalothin/Cephapirin

ADVERSE REACTIONS

Hypersensitivity Reactions

As with penicillins, rash, hives, anaphylaxis, and serum sickness reactions have been described. (Less than 1% cross-sensitivity with penicillins?)

Nephrotoxicity

Interstitial nephritis (probably allergic) has been described with cephalothin.

Neurotoxicity

Confusion and convulsions may occur. This reaction is similar to that with penicillin G with high doses in the presence of renal failure.

Hematologic Reaction

Hemolytic anemia (Coombs' test positive) is rarely reported.

Thrombophlebitis

Frequent changes of IV site may be necessary. The usefulness of intravenous filters in the prevention of thrombophlebitis is controversial.

DRUG INTERACTIONS

Uricosurics (Probenecid, Sulfinpyrazone)

These drugs block renal tubular secretion and decrease clearance of most cephalosporins.

Chloramphenicol

ADVERSE REACTIONS

Aplastic Anemia

The incidence of this reaction is approximately 1 in 40,000, but mortality from the reaction is >50%. Bone marrow transplantation is the recommended management.

Dose-related Bone Marrow Suppression

Doses in excess of 50 mg/kg/day or serum levels above 20–25 µg/ml have been associated with reduced iron utilization by bone marrow and with vacuolization of erythroblasts, megakaryocytes, and leukocyte precursors, with resultant anemia, thrombocytopenia, and leukopenia. This type of marrow toxicity is reversible and responds to reduction in dosage and to discontinuance of the drug.

Gray Baby Syndrome

Circulatory collapse occurs in premature infants and neonates who are given excessive doses of chloramphenicol (>25–50 mg/kg/day).

DRUG INTERACTIONS

Inhibition of the metabolism of phenytoin, oral hypoglycemic agents, and oral anticoagulants may result in phenytoin toxicity, hypoglycemia, and hemorrhage.

Clavulanic Acid/Sulbactam

ADVERSE REACTIONS

See amoxicillin, ampicillin, and ticarcillin.

Gastrointestinal Disturbance

The combination of amoxicillin and clavulanic acid produces a higher incidence of diarrhea than amoxicillin alone. Nausea and vomiting have been reported in 5–40% of patients.

DRUG INTERACTION

See penicillin G.

Clindamycin

ADVERSE REACTIONS

Gastrointestinal Disturbance

Diarrhea, which may occur in 20–30% of patients, is reversible and subsides promptly with discontinuance of therapy. Pseudomembranous colitis (antibiotic-associated colitis) is a complication caused by overgrowth of toxin-producing *Clostridium difficile* in stool. This reaction may occur with oral or parenteral therapy. Penicillins, cephalosporins, sulfonamides, and other antibiotics have also produced this reaction.

Hepatotoxicity

Elevated SGOT may be due to intramuscular administration. Clinical hepatitis has not been reported.

DRUG INTERACTIONS

No significant interactions are reported.

Clofazimine

ADVERSE REACTIONS

Skin

Pink-to-brown-black discoloration occurs in nearly all patients within a few weeks. This reaction is slowly reversible. Ichthyosis, rash, and dryness occur in 5–25% of patients.

Gastrointestinal Disturbance

Abdominal pain, nausea, vomiting, and diarrhea occur in approximately 50% of patients; bowel obstruction and GI bleeding are rare.

Ocular

Irritation, dryness, and conjunctival pigmentation may occur.

Miscellaneous

Discoloration of body secretions is common; splenic infarction and thrombo-embolism are rare.

DRUG INTERACTIONS

None described.

Cloxacillin/Dicloxacillin

ADVERSE REACTIONS

See also penicillin G.

Gastrointestinal Disturbance

Nausea, vomiting, or diarrhea may occasionally occur.

DRUG INTERACTIONS

See also penicillin G.

Cycloserine

ADVERSE REACTIONS

Neurotoxicity

Psychoses, delirium, confusion, headache, convulsions, and tremor have all been reported. Neurotoxicity appears to be more frequent and severe at the higher dosages. Pyridoxine may help to prevent these effects.

DRUG INTERACTIONS

Concurrent administration with other antituberculous agents may result in folate or vitamin B_{12} deficiency.

Doxycycline

ADVERSE REACTIONS

See tetracycline.

DRUG INTERACTIONS

See tetracycline.

Erythromycin

ADVERSE REACTIONS

Gastrointestinal Disturbance

Nausea, vomiting, and diarrhea may occur.

Hepatotoxicity

This has been documented with the estolate and ethyl succinate salts of the drug. Allergic symptoms such as fever, rash, and eosinophilia may occur. Cholestatic jaundice and hepatocellular necrosis may resolve on withdrawal of the drug. Hepatotoxicity apparently occurs only after prolonged therapy (10–14 days).

Thrombophlebitis

This condition is associated with intravenous administration.

DRUG INTERACTIONS

The clearance of several drugs may be reduced owing to the inhibitory effects of erythromycin on hepatic metabolism. These include theophylline, warfarin, carbamazepine, and cyclosporine.

Ethambutol

ADVERSE REACTIONS

Ocular Toxicity

Reversible retrobulbar neuropathy, which causes defects in red-green vision, may occur. The incidence of this reaction is approximately 5% at doses of 25–50 mg/kg/day. It is rare at 15 mg/kg/day.

Hyperuricemia

There are only two reports of increased uric acid as a result of ethambutol therapy.

DRUG INTERACTIONS

None are reported.

Ethionamide

ADVERSE REACTIONS

Gastrointestinal Disturbance

Nausea, vomiting, cramps, and diarrhea are common.

Hepatotoxicity

Hepatocellular necrosis may occur but is uncommon.

Neurotoxicity

Psychoses, depression, and anxiety may occur and may be reversible with nicotinamide therapy.

DRUG INTERACTIONS

None are reported.

Fluconazole

ADVERSE REACTIONS

Gastrointestinal Disturbance

Two to four percent of patients experience nausea, vomiting, or diarrhea. Hepatitis is rare, but liver function abnormalities occur commonly. Stevens-Johnson syndrome has been reported in one patient.

DRUG INTERACTIONS

As with ketoconazole, fluconazole can inhibit the metabolism of certain drugs but to a lesser extent. The most significant interactions have been reported with phenytoin and sulfonylureas. Cyclosporin clearance may be reduced in patients receiving larger doses of fluconazole, so that serum levels should be monitored more carefully.

Flucytosine (5-Fluorocytosine)

ADVERSE REACTIONS

Gastrointestinal Disturbance

Nausea and vomiting are frequent, owing to the size of the dose. Administering the capsules individually at 5- to 10-minute intervals may help to alleviate this problem.

Hematologic Toxicity

This is felt to be dose-related. Conversion of flucytosine to 5-fluorouracil has been demonstrated in vivo. Excessive serum levels of flucytosine may lead to concentrations of antimetabolite that produce bone marrow toxicity. Agranulocytosis and aplastic anemia have been reported.

Hepatotoxicity

Hepatic necrosis has been reported but is rare. This reaction also is probably dose-related.

DRUG INTERACTIONS

Antifungal activity may be reduced by cytosine arabinoside. Half-life is prolonged by drugs that decrease glomerular filtration rate.

Ganciclovir

ADVERSE REACTIONS

Hematopoietic

Reversible granulocytopenia and thrombocytopenia are common and appear to be dose-related. G-CSF has been used successfully to ameliorate the leukopenia. Anemia may also occur.

Miscellaneous

Fever, rash, and abnormal liver function tests occur occasionally.

DRUG INTERACTIONS

Cytotoxic or marrow-suppressive drugs exacerbate the leukopenia. Probenecid reduces the clearance of ganciclovir. A high incidence of seizures has been reported with concomitant imipenem use.

Gentamicin

ADVERSE REACTIONS

See amikacin.

DRUG INTERACTIONS

See amikacin.

Griseofulvin

ADVERSE REACTIONS

Gastrointestinal Disturbance

Nausea, vomiting, and diarrhea are uncommon when the drug is taken after eating.

Neurotoxicity

Headaches are relatively common but often subside spontaneously. Fatigue, irritability, and confusion have been reported but are rare. Peripheral neuropathy is rare.

Porphyria

The drug may potentially aggravate acute intermittent porphyria, although the clinical significance of this reaction is unclear.

DRUG INTERACTIONS

Barbiturates

The administration of barbiturates, particularly phenobarbital, may increase the metabolism of griseofulvin.

Oral Contraceptives and Warfarin

Griseofulvin may induce microsomal liver enzymes and may increase the metabolism of warfarin and oral contraceptives, thus negating the hypoprothrombinemic effect of warfarin and contraceptive effects.

Imipenem-Cilastatin

ADVERSE REACTIONS

CNS Toxicity

Seizures have been reported in small numbers of patients, primarily those with predisposing CNS disease or in whom dosage was not carefully adjusted for renal insufficiency.

Nausea/Vomiting

Larger doses and more rapid infusions lead to frequent GI distress. Slowing the rate of infusion appears to alleviate this problem.

DRUG INTERACTIONS

See penicillin G.

Isoniazid

ADVERSE REACTIONS

Gastrointestinal Upset

Nausea, vomiting, and diarrhea are relatively uncommon with recommended doses.

Neurotoxicity

Psychosis, confusion, convulsions, and coma may occur with overdosage. Peripheral neuropathy rarely occurs at doses of 5 mg/kg/day but may occur frequently with larger doses and in patients who are malnourished (pyridoxine deficiency) or who are predisposed to neuritis (alcoholics, diabetics, uremics). The administration of 10 mg of pyridoxine for every 100 mg of isoniazid prevents this toxicity. If neuritis occurs, it may be slowly reversible with the administration of pyridoxine.

Hepatotoxicity

An age-related occurrence, this condition results in hepatitis with hepatocellular necrosis and jaundice, if the drug is not discontinued early. The incidence of clinical hepatitis increases with age and is at least 2.3% in patients >50 years old.

Alcoholics do not appear to be more prone to liver injury. The role of acetylation in the predisposition to hepatic toxicity is unclear. Some reports suggest greater toxicity with rifampin/INH combinations in slow acetylators. At least 15–20% of patients manifest an early transient rise in SGOT that does not necessitate discontinuance of isoniazid. Patients should be encouraged to report the early signs and symptoms of toxicity (see Section V).

Hyperglycemia

The impairment of glucose tolerance is significant in diabetics only.

DRUG INTERACTIONS

Anticonvulsants

Isoniazid may inhibit the metabolism of phenytoin, thereby causing excessive serum levels.

Antacids

Aluminum or other antacids may interfere with the absorption of isoniazid.

Itraconazole

ADVERSE REACTIONS

Gastrointestinal

Nausea (10.6%), vomiting (5.1%), diarrhea (3.3%).

Skin

Rash (8.6%), pruritus (2.5%).

CNS

Headache (3.8%), dizziness (1.7%).

Liver

Impaired function (2.7%).

DRUG INTERACTIONS

Should not be administered with terfenadine or aztemizole. Serious or fatal cardiac arrhythmias may occur.

Ketoconazole

ADVERSE REACTIONS

Gastrointestinal Disturbances

Nausea and vomiting are common. The drug can be given with food, but absorption is reduced.

Hepatotoxicity

Reversible hepatitis has been observed and does not appear to be dose-related; some fatalities.

Adrenal Suppression/Gynecomastia/Oligospermia

These reactions have been reported and are probably due to inhibition of steroid synthesis.

DRUG INTERACTIONS

Antacids/Cimetidine

Elevation of gastric pH results in retarded dissolution of the drug and impaired absorption. Drug administration should be at least 2 hours before antacid administration or in an acidic fluid such as fruit juice or dilute HCl.

Cyclosporin/Rifampin/Corticosteroids

Ketoconazole inhibits oxidative drug metabolism in the liver, leading to an increased pharmacological effect (or toxicity) of these compounds.

Coadministration with terfenadine or astemizole may lead to serious or fatal cardiac arrhythmias.

Methenamine

ADVERSE REACTIONS

Gastrointestinal Disturbance

Nausea and vomiting are frequent, since formaldehyde may be liberated in the stomach. The mandelate salt is enteric-coated to attempt to prevent this, but suspensions and hippurate tablets are not. To ameliorate this problem, doses should be given with food.

DRUG INTERACTIONS

Alkalinizing Agents

Any disease state or drug, such as acetazolamide, that produces an alkaline urine negates the effects of methenamine.

Metronidazole

ADVERSE REACTIONS

Gastrointestinal Disturbance

Nausea and vomiting occur infrequently. A metallic taste is a common finding.

Neurotoxicity

Ataxia and vertigo are uncommon; headache is more frequent. Slow reversible peripheral neuropathy may occur with prolonged administration of high doses. Seizures occur rarely.

Urine

Dark urine, caused by photosensitive metabolites, may be reported by the patient.

Carcinogenicity

The drug has been implicated in producing tumors in animals and may also be mutagenic. Therefore, it should not be given to pregnant women.

DRUG INTERACTIONS

"Antabuse" Reaction

When alcohol is taken after metronidazole, a disulfiram-like reaction may occur.

Miconazole

ADVERSE REACTIONS

Thrombophlebitis

This reaction is probably a result of vehicle.

Anemia

Normochromic or normocytic anemia may occur.

Thrombocytosis

The mechanism for this is unknown, but platelet counts may reach 1 million/mm^3.

Hyponatremia

This abnormality is observed in patients with CNS infection and may be due to syndrome of inappropriate antidiuretic hormone secretion (SIADH).

Hyperactivity

This finding is probably a result of a polyethoxylated castor oil vehicle.

Cardiorespiratory Toxicity

Severe reactions (anaphylactoid) have been reported after first doses.

DRUG INTERACTION

Warfarin

Prolongation of prothrombin time may occur.

Minocycline

ADVERSE REACTIONS

See also tetracycline.

Neurotoxicity

This agent is unique among the tetracyclines, in that it causes nausea, dizziness, weakness, ataxia, and vertigo in many patients receiving the drug. These reactions occur within the first day or so of therapy.

DRUG INTERACTIONS

See tetracycline.

Nafcillin

ADVERSE REACTIONS

See also penicillin G.

Hematological Reaction

Neutropenia, which is immediately reversible on discontinuance of the drug, is seen in 10–20% of patients receiving 150–200 mg/kg/day for 10–14 days or longer.

Phlebitis

This drug appears to be relatively irritating, so intravenous sites should be inspected and rotated frequently.

DRUG INTERACTIONS

See penicillin G.

Netilmicin

ADVERSE REACTIONS

See also amikacin.

Hepatic Toxicity

Elevations of transaminase and alkaline phosphatase have been frequently seen with netilmicin, unlike other aminoglycosides.

Ototoxicity

Netilmicin appears to be less toxic to the cochlear portions of the inner ear than other aminoglycosides.

DRUG INTERACTIONS

See amikacin.

Nitrofurantoin

ADVERSE REACTIONS

Gastrointestinal Disturbance

Frequent and dose-related nausea and vomiting can be severe. The drug should be taken with food. Use of the macrocrystalline form may reduce this effect, but it is more expensive.

Hypersensitivity Reactions

Eosinophilia, rash, and drug fever have been reported in about 4% of patients.

Peripheral Neuritis

This condition usually occurs only in patients with renal failure who have been given the drug. Slow in onset and recovery, it causes ascending motor and sensory polyneuropathy. Patients who are to receive long-term therapy should be warned to report symptoms such as paresthesias.

Pulmonary Toxicity

A pneumonitis that may progress to interstitial fibrosis has been reported primarily in elderly patients. Acute and chronic reactions have been described. The acute reaction has been associated with allergic symptoms and signs such as eosinophilia. The more chronic reaction may also produce hepatic damage.

However, the causal relationship of nitrofurantoin in the chronic reaction is unclear.

Hepatic Toxicity

Several cases of cholestasis or hepatocellular damage have been described, but this reaction appears to be rare, and the causal relationship is unclear.

Hematological Toxicity

Patients with severe glucose-6-phosphate dehydrogenase (G-6-PD) deficiency may develop hemolytic anemia when given the drug.

DRUG INTERACTIONS

Probenecid

Uricosuric agents appear to decrease the renal clearance of nitrofurantoin; this decrease results in lower urinary concentrations and in potentially toxic serum levels.

Oxacillin

ADVERSE REACTIONS

See also penicillin G.

Hepatotoxicity

Elevated SGOT and other clinical findings of hepatitis have been associated with oxacillin. Hepatic necrosis has also been described.

DRUG INTERACTIONS

See penicillin G.

Penicillin G

ADVERSE REACTIONS

Hypersensitivity Reactions

Rash, urticaria, serum sickness, anaphylaxis, nephritis, and drug fever may occur. Minor antigenic determinants (metabolites and penicillin itself) are the mediators of immediate and accelerated hypersensitivity reactions. Major determinants (penicilloyl and others) are responsible for delayed reactions.

The incidence of anaphylaxis appears to be 0.004–0.04%. However, mortality may be as high as 10%.

Skin testing with the major determinant mixture cannot detect immediate or accelerated reactions. The procedure for adding penicillin G to the skin test (minor determinants) is not standardized, may be unreliable, and may itself produce anaphylaxis. Similarly, desensitization procedures are dangerous. If a patient gives a strong history of immediate or accelerated penicillin reaction, a nonpenicillin, noncephalosporin antibiotic should be administered, unless penicillin absolutely *must* be given (e.g., CNS syphilis).

Neurotoxicity

Convulsions and other forms of encephalopathy have occurred when doses of penicillin G in excess of 20,000,000 U/day are administered in the presence of moderate-to-severe renal insufficiency, or when doses of 60,000,000–100,000,000 U/day are given.

Nephrotoxicity

Although interstitial nephritis appears to occur most frequently with methicillin, it has been reported during the course of therapy with a number of penicillins, including penicillin G.

Hematologic Toxicity

Coombs' test positive hemolytic anemia may occur with doses in excess of 10,000,000 U/day.

DRUG INTERACTIONS

Aminoglycosides

High concentrations of penicillin, carbenicillin, and ticarcillin bind and inactivate aminoglycosides in vitro and in vivo. Caution should be taken in interpreting aminoglycoside levels in the circumstance of renal failure and the concomitant administration of these drugs.

Bacteriostatic Agents

In two reports, the combination of penicillin G and a bacteriostatic agent (tetracycline or chloramphenicol) produced a poorer response in the treatment of meningitis than did penicillin alone. This presumed antagonism between penicillins and bacteriostatic agents is reproducible in vitro but requires prior exposure of the bacteria to the bacteriostatic agent and other manipulations.

Uricosuric Agents

Probenecid, indomethacin, sulfinpyrazone, and high-dose aspirin (>3–4 g/day) can block the tubular secretion of many penicillins and may lead to prolonged high serum levels. This secretory blockade also occurs in the CNS. Removal of pencillins from the CSF is slowed, potentially leading to neurotoxicity.

Penicillin V (Phenoxymethyl Penicillin)

ADVERSE REACTIONS

See penicillin G.

DRUG INTERACTIONS

See penicillin G.

Pentamidine

ADVERSE REACTIONS

Acute Systemic Reactions

Most of the following occur after intravenous administration: hypotension, syncope, dizziness, salivation, nausea, vomiting, flushing, incontinence, edema, tachycardia, dyspnea, epileptiform movements, headache, lethargy, hypoglycemia.

Subacute Toxicity

Nephrotoxicity

Acute tubular necrosis.

Hepatotoxicity

Slight elevations of SGOT.

Hypocalcemia

Pancreatitis

Thrombocytopenia and Anemia

Hyperglycemia and Diabetes Mellitus

DRUG INTERACTIONS

None are reported.

Polymyxin B

ADVERSE REACTIONS

Neurotoxicity

Paresthesias and peripheral neuropathies may occur transiently. Severe reactions, such as ataxia or convulsions, may occur with large doses in the presence of renal insufficiency. Neuromuscular blockade, which also appears to be dose-related, is a noncompetitive type that is not reversible by cholinesterase inhibitors. Artificial ventilation and calcium administration may be beneficial. Administration of the antibiotic should be discontinued.

Nephrotoxicity

Acute tubular necrosis with renal failure is encountered with high dosages of these agents. The toxicity is nearly uniform at doses greater than those recommended.

DRUG INTERACTIONS

Neuromuscular blocking agents or general anesthetics may be potentiated by the neurotoxic effects of these drugs, when given perioperatively.

Pyrazinamide

ADVERSE REACTIONS

Hepatotoxicity

Hepatic toxicity appears to occur in at least 5% of patients receiving doses > 30 mg/kg/day. The incidence is much less with the use of recommended dosages.

Gastrointestinal Disturbance

Frequent nausea and vomiting may prevent administration of appropriate dosages.

Hyperuricemia

A few episodes of acute gout have been reported.

DRUG INTERACTIONS

None are reported.

Pyrimethamine

ADVERSE REACTIONS

Gastrointestinal Disturbance

Frequent nausea and vomiting occur with daily dosage.

Hematological Toxicity

Because the drug may interfere with human folate metabolism, megaloblastic anemia, leukopenia, and thrombocytopenia may occur. Folinic acid (leucovorin) may be used in doses of 6–10 mg/day to reverse this toxicity.

DRUG INTERACTIONS

None are reported.

Quinolones

ADVERSE REACTIONS

Extensive experience with oral administration of these drugs has revealed that GI disturbance occurs in approximately 5% of patients and CNS toxicity (dizziness, headache) only rarely. Seizures have been reported in patients taking other agents associated with seizures, such as imipenem and theophylline, and in patients receiving high doses, especially intravenously.

DRUG INTERACTIONS

Theophylline

Ciprofloxacin may inhibit the metabolism of theophylline, leading to toxic serum concentrations. This reaction occurs to a limited extent with norfloxacin but not with the others.

Multivalent Cations

Like tetracyclines, cations may chelate the quinolones and interfere with absorption. Doses of antacids, iron, or sucralfate should be given at least 2 hours and, preferably, 4 hours apart from the quinolone administration.

Ribavirin

ADVERSE REACTIONS

Pulmonary

Worsening of respiratory status is common, especially in patients being mechanically ventilated. This reaction may be caused by precipitation of the drug within the ventilatory apparatus. Accumulation of fluid in the tubing has also been noted.

Cardiovascular

Hypotension and cardiac arrest have been noted.

Carcinogenesis/Mutagenesis

Ribavirin induces cell transformation in mammalian systems and is listed as a Category X teratogen.

Miscellaneous

Caregivers have reported rashes and conjunctivitis from exposure to the aerosol.

DRUG INTERACTIONS

None described.

Rifampin

ADVERSE REACTIONS

Hypersensitivity Reactions

These include dermatitis and a "flu-like" syndrome with occasional thrombocytopenia, hemolytic anemia, and acute renal failure. Clinical evidence suggests that this syndrome may be antibody-mediated. High-antibody titers may be responsible for the "flu-like" syndrome during intermittent or interrupted therapy.

Hepatotoxicity

This reaction has been reported to be predominantly cholestatic; it may occur more frequently in older patients, and there may be enhanced toxicity when administered with isoniazid. However, there is no consistent evidence of the significance of this interaction.

Discoloration

Bodily secretions such as saliva, sweat, tears, and urine may be tinged reddish-orange during therapy.

DRUG INTERACTIONS

Rifampin enhances the metabolism of cyclosporine, oral anticoagulants, oral contraceptives, corticosteroids, sulfonylureas, and methadone, resulting in a decreased pharmacological effect of these drugs. It may also enhance the metabolism of thyroxine and digoxin.

Streptomycin

ADVERSE REACTIONS

Ototoxicity

Primarily vestibular; toxicity may be more severe in the elderly.

Nephrotoxicity

This reaction does not appear to be a problem with usual dosages.

DRUG INTERACTIONS

See amikacin.

Sulfadoxine

ADVERSE REACTIONS

See sulfisoxazole. Additionally, sulfadoxine is an ultra-long-acting sulfonamide. Stevens-Johnson syndrome has been observed occasionally.

DRUG INTERACTIONS

See sulfisoxazole.

Sulfisoxazole

ADVERSE REACTIONS

Hypersensitivity Reactions

Rash, exfoliative dermatitis and, rarely, Stevens-Johnson syndrome. The last reaction has been associated primarily with the use of long-acting sulfonamides but also has been reported with sulfisoxazole.

Hematological Toxicity

The most common manifestation, although rare itself, is agranulocytosis, which is reversible on discontinuance of the drug. Extremely rare reactions such as aplastic anemia have also been noted. Hemolytic anemia may develop in patients with severe G-6-PD deficiency.

Kernicterus

Sulfonamides may displace bilirubin from protein-binding sites. Infants born to mothers being treated with sulfonamides or who are given sulfas in the postnatal period may develop jaundice or, rarely, kernicterus.

Renal Damage

This condition was common when less-soluble sulfonamides were used, and patients developed crystalluria, which led to obstruction. This complication occurs seldom, if at all, with the more-soluble congeners.

DRUG INTERACTIONS

Oral Hypoglycemics

There may be transient hypoglycemia by displacement from protein. The clinical significance is questionable.

Oral Anticoagulants

Transient hypoprothrombinemia due to displacement from protein or inhibition of metabolism may occur. The clinical significance of this interaction is questionable.

Phenytoin

Sulfonamides may inhibit the metabolism of phenytoin; this leads to excessive serum levels.

Tetracycline

ADVERSE REACTIONS

Hypersensitivity Reactions

Uncommon.

Gastrointestinal Disturbance

Nausea and vomiting occur frequently. Diarrhea is common, and pseudomembranous colitis has been reported.

Yeast Overgrowth

Although this complication occurs with many antibiotics, it appears to occur more frequently with tetracyclines. Thrush and vaginitis are particular problems. Preparations of antifungal agents in combination with tetracycline are ineffective and should not be used.

Staphylococcal Enterocolitis

Tetracycline-resistant staphylococci often appear in the feces of patients treated with tetracyclines; however, enterocolitis with severe diarrhea, dehydration, and circulatory collapse is rare.

Photosensitivity

Although this reaction appears to be peculiar to demeclocycline and doxycycline, all tetracyclines are felt to have this potential.

Tooth and Bone Deposition

These drugs are deposited in calcifying areas of tooth and bone, and they may discolor either deciduous or permanent teeth. Bone deposition has been shown to result in temporary cessation of bone growth. This effect is reversible on discontinuance of therapy. For these reasons, tetracyclines should not be given to pregnant or nursing women, or to children under the age of 8 years.

Hepatotoxicity

Fatty infiltration of the liver is associated primarily with intravenous tetracycline and appears to be particularly significant in pregnant women who are given large doses (>2 g/day).

Nephrotoxicity

In patients with renal failure, the antianabolic effects of tetracyclines may result in further increases in BUN and in creatinine. A ''Fanconi-like syndrome,'' consisting of acidosis, nephrosis, and aminoaciduria, has been associated with the ingestion of outdated tetracyclines. This reaction has not been reported since the reformulation of tetracycline products.

Increased Intracranial Pressure

Observed in both infants and adults, this appears to be reversible on discontinuance of therapy.

DRUG INTERACTIONS

Diuretics

The administration of potent diuretics to patients receiving tetracyclines may aggravate the increases in BUN by volume depletion.

Antacids

Tetracyclines bind to divalent cations, and absorption from the GI tract is diminished (e.g., Ca_{2+}, Al_{2+}, Mg_{2+}, Fe_{2+}).

Penicillins

See penicillin G.

Ticarcillin

ADVERSE REACTIONS

See penicillin G and carbenicillin.

DRUG INTERACTIONS

See penicillin G.

Tobramycin

ADVERSE REACTIONS

See section on clinical use; see also amikacin.

DRUG INTERACTIONS

See amikacin.

Trimethoprim and Sulfamethoxazole

ADVERSE REACTIONS

Gastrointestinal Disturbance

The oral formulation may produce nausea and vomiting.

Hematological Toxicity

Both agents have been associated with various blood dyscrasias, including agranulocytosis, thrombocytopenia, and hemolytic anemia (especially in G-6-PD deficiency). Inhibition of folate synthesis that leads to anemia is a problem only in patients who are already folate-deficient and are receiving large doses of the drugs. The anemia is reversible with administration of folates, preferably folinic acid (calcium leucovorin). The administration of exogenous folates has no effect on the treatment of the infection. Leukopenia seen in patients with AIDS is not associated with folate deficiency and is not prevented or treated with exogenous folates.

Renal Disease

Crystalluria leading to obstruction is not a problem with the more-soluble sulfonamides such as sulfamethoxazole. Serum creatinine elevations during therapy may reflect an inhibition of creatinine secretion by trimethoprim. Acute tubular necrosis has been reported but only in patients with preexisting renal damage.

Hypersensitivity Reactions

These may vary from mild dermatitis to Stevens-Johnson syndrome. The latter complication is very rare with the more-soluble sulfonamides.

Kernicterus

Sulfonamides, which displace bilirubin from protein-binding sites, may cause jaundice and perhaps kernicterus.

DRUG INTERACTIONS

See sulfonamides.

Vancomycin

ADVERSE REACTIONS

Ototoxicity

Hearing loss has been associated with high (>60–80 μg/ ml), prolonged serum concentrations.

Nephrotoxicity

This appears to be infrequent to rare at recommended doses. Early reports may have been due to an impurity in the formulation.

Hypotension/Flushing/Pruritus

This is caused by too rapid an infusion of the drug (redman syndrome). A 1-hour infusion time is recommended.

DRUG INTERACTIONS

Concurrent administration with aminoglycoside may result in increased oto- or nephrotoxicity.

Vidarabine

ADVERSE REACTIONS

Gastrointestinal Disturbance

Nausea, vomiting, and anorexia are relatively common.

DRUG INTERACTIONS

None reported.

SELECTED READINGS

Andriole VT. The future of the quinolones. Drugs 1993;45 (Suppl. 3):1–7.

Buckley MM, Brogden RN, Barradell LB, Goa KL. Imipenem/cilastatin. A reappraisal of its antibacterial activity, pharmacokinetic properties and therapeutic efficacy. Drugs 1992;44(6):1012.

Centers for Disease Control. Control of influenza A outbreaks in nursing homes: amantadine as adjunct to vaccine—1989–1990. JAMA 1992;267(3):344–46.

Cleary JD, Taylor JW, Chapman SW. Imidazoles and triazoles in antifungal therapy. DICP 1990;24(2):148–52.

Fass RJ. Erythromycin, clarithromycin, and azithromycin: Use of frequency distribution curves, scattergrams, and regression analyses to compare in vitro activities and describe cross-resistance. Antimicrob Agents Chemother 1993;37(10):2080–6.

Leehy DJ, Braun BI, Tholl DA, Chung LS, Gross CA, Roback JA, Lentino JR. Can pharmacokinetic dosing decrease nephrotoxicity associated with aminoglycoside therapy? J Am Soc Nephrol 1993;4(1):81–90.

Medical Letter Drugs Therapy. Piperacillin/tazobactam. 1994;36(914):7–9.

Medical Letter Drugs Therapy. Rimantadine for prevention and treatment of influenza. Med Lett Drug Ther 1993;35(910):109–10.

Sanders CC. Cefepime the next generation. Clin Infect Dis 1993;17(3):369–79.

Schmitt HJ. New methods of delivery of amphotericin B. Clin Infect Dis 1993;17 (Suppl. 2):S501–6.

SECTION 2
Empiric Antibiotic Therapy

Empiric antibiotic therapy should not be confused with antibiotic prophylaxis. The former consists of the early institution of antibiotic therapy, pending the results of cultures and clinical response. Empiric treatment is begun in patients who have an illness and in whom there is an expectation of an infectious cause. Such treatment, which may be lifesaving, should be directed against the organisms most likely to cause the illness. Examination of the gram-stained smear is important and frequently allows one to choose antibiotic therapy more specific for the infection. Definitive therapy (Section 4) is then instituted when the results of culture and sensitivity tests become available.

Antibiotic prophylaxis is the administration of an antibiotic prior to the onset of symptoms in order to prevent clinical infection. Examples of rational medical prophylaxis include the prevention of rheumatic fever, isoniazid prophylaxis for tuberculin-positive individuals, and meningococcal prophylaxis. Examples of rational surgical prophylaxis include the prevention of infection associated with vaginal hysterectomy, abdominal surgery, and prosthetic implant surgery.

Tables 2.1 through 2.7 attempt to guide clinicians in the choice of empiric antibiotics for specific clinical situations. The tables are arranged by organ system and by organisms most likely to cause the infection. When cultures are available and a definitive diagnosis is made, therapy should be instituted as outlined in Section 3 (Therapy of Established Infection).

Table 2.1. Cardiovascular Infection

Disorder	Possible Organisms	Antibiotic of Choice	Alternative Regimen
Acute bacterial endocarditis Native valve	S. aureus, enterococci, S. pyogenes, aerobic GNR[a] (drug use)	Penicillin and nafcillin and gentamicin	Vancomycin and gentamicin
Prosthetic valve or vascular graft infection	S. aureus, S. epidermidis, aerobic GNR	Vancomycin and gentamicin	Nafcillin[b] and gentamicin
Subacute bacterial endocarditis or "culture-negative" endocarditis	S. viridans, enterococci, HACEK organisms (Haemophilus, Actinobacillus, Cardiobacterium, Eikenella, Kingella)	Penicillin G and gentamicin	Vancomycin and gentamicin
Pyogenic pericarditis	S. pneumoniae, N. meningitidis, group A streptococci, S. aureus, and aerobic GNR	Nafcillin and gentamicin	Vancomycin and TGC[c]
Septic thrombophlebitis associated with i.v. catheter or intravascular shunts	S. aureus, S. epidermidis, and aerobic GNR	Vancomycin and gentamicin	Vancomycin and TGC
Septic thrombophlebitis associated with pelvic surgery or abortion	Bacteroides sp., aerobic GNR, and streptococci	Clindamycin and gentamicin	Metronidazole and TGC

Note: Oxacillin can be substituted for nafcillin in this and the subsequent tables in this chapter.
[a] GNR, Gram-negative rods.
[b] Nafcillin or cephalosporin will not be effective for S. epidermis, two-thirds of which are resistant to these drugs.
[c] TGC, third-generation cephalosporin.

Table 2.2. Musculoskeletal Infection

Disorder	Possible Organisms	Antibiotic of Choice	Alternative Regimen
Osteomyelitis (age < 6 months)	Group A or B streptococci *S. aureus,* aerobic GNR[a]	Nafcillin and gentamicin	Nafcillin and TGC[b]
Osteomyelitis (age > 6 months and adults)	*S. aureus, H. influenzae,* streptococci	Cefuroxime or TGC	Vancomycin or clindamycin
Septic arthritis (age <2 months)	*S. aureus,* streptococci, aerobic GNR	Nafcillin and gentamicin	Nafcillin and TGC
(2 months–5 yr)	*H. influenzae, S. aureus,* streptococci, aerobic GNR	Cefuroxime or TGC	TGC and vancomycin
> 5 yr and adults	*S. aureus* or *N. gonorrhoeae* (older children and adults)	Nafcillin or penicillin G (gonorrhea)	Clindamycin or tetracycline
Septic arthritis, postoperative or traumatic	*S. aureus, S. epidermidis,* and aerobic GNR, streptococci	Vancomycin and gentamicin	Imipenem

[a] GNR, Gram-negative rods.
[b] TGC, third-generation cephalosporin.

Table 2.3. CNS Infection

Disorder	Possible Organisms	Antibiotic of Choice	Alternative Regimen
Meningitis (age < 2 months)	E. coli, group B streptococci, S. faecalis, N. meningitidis, S. pneumoniae listeria	Ampicillin and TGC[a]	Ampicillin and gentamicin
age > 2 months < 10 yrs	H. influenzae, S. pneumoniae, N. meningitidis	TGC	Ampicillin, and chloramphenicol
adults	S. pneumoniae, N. meningitidis	TGC	Chloramphenicol (not effective for aerobic GNR[b])
Meningitis associated with open head trauma, or hospital-acquired infection	S. aureus, S. pneumoniae, GNR	Vancomycin and TGC	Vancomycin and gentamicin
Meningitis associated with closed head trauma	S. pneumoniae	Penicillin G	Chloramphenicol
Brain abscess	S. pneumoniae, streptococci, mixed anaerobes	Nafcillin, TGC, and metronidazole	Chloramphenicol
Brain abscess associated with trauma or postoperative infection	S. pneumoniae, streptococci, S. aureus, GNR, and mixed anaerobes	Vancomycin, TGC, and metronidazole	Vancomycin, TGC, and rifampin

[a] TGC, third-generation cephalosporin.
[b] GNR, Gram-negative rods.

Table 2.4. Gastrointestinal Infection

Disorder	Possible Organisms	Antibiotic of Choice	Alternative Regimen
Gastroenteritis	Shigella, Salmonella, Campylobacter, toxigenic or invasive E. coli	Quinolone	TMP/SMX[a] and erythromycin
Typhoid fever	Salmonella	TMP-SMX, TGC,[b] or chloramphenicol	Ampicillin, amoxicillin, quinolone
Necrotizing enterocolitis	S. aureus, S. epidermidis, aerobic GNR,[c] C. perfringens	Vancomycin and TGC and metronidazole	Vancomycin and TGC and clindamycin
Cholecystitis	E. coli, other GNR S. faecalis, anaerobes	Gentamicin and ampicillin	TGC and metronidazole
Peritonitis; ruptured viscus; perirectal abscess	B. fragilis, other anaerobes, E. coli, other GNR, S. faecalis	Ampicillin, clindamycin, gentamicin	TGC and gentamicin, ± metronidazole
Perirectal abscess (leukemic or neutropenic)	B. fragilis, other anaerobes, E. coli, Pseudomonas, other GNR, S. faecalis	Piperacillin and tobramycin ± metronidazole	Ceftazidime and tobramycin ± metronidazole

[a] TMP/SMX, trimethoprim-sulfamethoxazole; not effective for Campylobacter.
[b] TGC, third-generation cephalosporin.
[c] GNR, Gram-negative rods.

Table 2.5. Urinary Tract Infection

Disorder	Possible Organisms	Antibiotic of Choice	Alternative Regimen
Cystitis, outpatient-acquired	E. coli, other GNR[a] enterococcus, chlamydia	TMP/SMX[b]	Cephalexin, quinolone, or nitrofurantoin
Cystitis, nosocomial, not "septic"	Antibiotic-resistant GNR, enterococcus	Gentamicin or TGC[c] or quinolone	Ampicillin and gentamicin
Pyelonephritis, first episode, not "septic"	E. coli, other aerobic GNR, enterococcus	TMP/SMX[d]	Tetracycline or quinolone or nitrofurantoin
Pyelonephritis, recurrent or with "sepsis"	E. coli, proteus, Klebsiella, other aerobic GNR	TGC[d] and gentamicin	Imipenem

[a] GNR, Gram-negative rods.
[b] Use tetracycline or doxycycline if risk factors for chlamydia are present. TMP/SMX, trimethoprim-sulfamethoxazole.
[c] TGC, third-generation cephalosporin.
[d] Use ampicillin and gentamicin if enterococci are suspected.

Table 2.6. Respiratory Infection

Disorder	Possible Organisms	Antibiotic of Choice	Alternative Regimen
Pharyngitis	Group A and C streptococci, C. diphtheriae	Penicillin G	Erythromycin
Epiglottitis	H. influenzae	TGC[a]	Chloramphenicol
Otitis (<4 yrs)	H. influenzae, S. pneumoniae, group A streptococci	Erythromycin and sulfisoxazole, or amoxicillin	TMP/SMX[b]
Otitis (>4 yrs)	S. pneumoniae, group A streptococci	Amoxicillin	TMP/SMX
Sinusitis	S. pneumoniae, group A streptococci, S. aureus	Amoxicillin	TMP/SMX, cefuroxime, amoxicillin/clavulanate
Bronchitis	S. pneumoniae, streptococci, H. influenzae	TMP/SMX or TGC	Azithromycin, clarithromycin or quinolone
Aspiration pneumonia or lung abscess (outpatient)	Mixed oropharyngeal flora, anaerobes	Clindamycin	Penicillin G
Adult pneumonia Outpatient-acquired, no lung disease, alcoholism or influenza	S. pneumoniae, M. pneumoniae	Erythromycin (penicillin G for S. pneumoniae identified)	Clarithromycin or azithromycin
pneumonia alcoholism	S. pneumoniae, klebsiella, S. aureus	Cefuroxime	Gentamicin and vancomycin
influenza	S. pneumoniae, S. aureus	Nafcillin	Vancomycin
chronic lung disease	S. pneumoniae, H. influenzae, S. aureus	Cefuroxime	TMP/SMX alone or with vancomycin

Pediatric pneumonia			
neonates <2 mos	S. pneumoniae, H. influenzae, GNR[c]	Ampicillin and gentamicin	TGC
2–14 wk (afebrile patient; nonbacterial pneumonia)	C. trachomatis	Erythromycin	Sulfisoxazole
2 months–6 yrs	H. influenzae, S. pneumoniae	Amoxicillin or cefuroxime	TGC
>6 yrs	S. pneumoniae, M. pneumoniae	Penicillin G or erythromycin	Azithromycin or clarithromycin
Cystic fibrosis	P. aeruginosa, S. aureus	Nafcillin, piperacillin, and tobramycin	TGC and tobramycin

[a] TGC, third-generation cephalosporin.
[b] TMP/SMX, trimethoprim-sulfamethoxazole.
[c] GNR, Gram-negative rods.

Table 2.7. Skin Infection

Disorder	Possible Organisms	Antibiotic of Choice	Alternative Regimen
Erysipelas, impetigo, or cellulitis unassociated with trauma or i.v. catheter	Group A streptococci, S. aureus	Phenoxymethyl penicillin or penicillin G (inpatients)	Erythromycin or cephalexin
Ascending lymphangitis	Group A streptococci	Phenoxymethyl penicillin or penicillin G (inpatients)	Erythromycin or cephalexin
Cellulitis secondary to infected i.v. catheter or postoperative wound infection	S. aureus, group A streptococci, aerobic GNR[a]	Nafcillin and gentamicin	TGC[b] and gentamicin
Cellulitis associated with GI or pelvic surgery	S. aureus, group A streptococci, aerobic GNR, anaerobes	Nafcillin, gentamicin, and clindamycin	TGC, gentamicin, and clindamycin
Cellulitis associated with trauma, myonecrosis, with sepsis	Group A streptococci, S. aureus, aerobic GNR, anaerobes	Imipenem	TGC, gentamicin, and clindamycin
Furuncle without surrounding cellulitis	S. aureus	None	Clindamycin
Furuncle with surrounding cellulitis	S. aureus	Dicloxacillin	Clindamycin or gentamicin
Decubitus ulcer	Streptococci, S. aureus, GNR, anaerobes	Ampicillin/sulbactam, ticarcillin/clavulanic acid, or imipenem	Clindamycin or gentamicin
Infected burns	S. aureus, GNR	Nafcillin and gentamicin	Vancomycin and gentamicin

[a] GNR, Gram-negative rods.
[b] TGC, third-generation cephalosporin.

SECTION 3
Therapy of Established Infection

There are many divergent opinions among authoritative sources regarding the treatment of infectious diseases. Nevertheless, at some point the clinician must choose an antibiotic in a given dose and route of administration to treat a specific infection. The purpose of Tables 3.1 through 3.7 is to provide a guideline for the choice of antibiotic therapy when the infecting organism has been identified. The current organism-specific recommendations of the Medical Letter are presented in Table 3.8. This definitive phase of therapy follows the institution of empiric antibiotic therapy outlined in Section 2.

Table 3.1. Infective Endocarditis

Site	Organism	Suggested Regimen	Alternative Regimen	Comments
Native valve	S. viridans or S. bovis	Penicillin G[a] for 4 wk; penicillin G plus gentamicin for 2 wk; penicillin G for 4 wk plus gentamicin for 2 wk	Vancomycin[b] or ceftriaxone[b] for 4 wk	Optimal therapy is parenteral penicillin G for 4 wk. The duration of therapy can be shortened by adding gentamicin to the regimen. Penicillin-gentamicin combination recommended for minimum inhibitory concentration (MIC) > 0.1 to < 0.5µg/ml. Avoid gentamicin for ages > 65, renal failure, or previous 8th nerve damages.
	E. faecalis, streptococci with MIC >0.5 µg/ml	Penicillin G[e] and gentamicin[f] for 6 wk	Vancomycin[d] and gentamicin[f] for 6 wk	Optimal therapy is parenteral penicillin G and gentamicin for 6 wk. Some authors recommend penicillin G for 6 wk and gentamicin for 4 wk.
	S. aureus	Nafcillin[c] or nafcillin plus gentamicin	Vancomycin[d]	Some authors suggest adding gentamicin to the regimen for 5 days.
	S. pneumoniae, S. pyogenes, N. meningitidis, N. gonorrhoeae	Penicillin G[e] for 6 wk	Vancomycin[d] for all Gram-positives	The treatment of meningococcal and gonococcal endocarditis in patients with serious penicillin allergy has not been studied. Penicillin, penicillin congeners, and cephalosporins should not be used in patients with major penicillin allergy.
	S. faecalis	Penicillin G[e] and gentamicin[f]	Vancomycin[d] and gentamicin[f]	A reduced or "synergistic" dose of gentamicin should be used to minimize toxicity. Gentamicin (1 mg/kg q8h, normal renal function).

Pseudomonas and *Serratia*; other aerobic Gram-negative rods (GNR)	Mezlocillin[g] or piperacillin plus tobramycin/gentamicin	Tobramycin or trimethoprim/sulfamethoxazole[i] (*Serratia*)	Gram-negative endocarditis should be treated with synergistic antibiotic combinations whenever possible. Blood levels of aminoglycosides must be monitored and the dose adjusted for renal function. *Serratia* infections may be treated with trimethoprim/sulfamethoxazole alone or in combination with other antibiotics such as polymyxin B.
Prosthetic valve infection			
S. aureus	Nafcillin	Vancomycin[d]	Any of the organisms involved in acute or subacute endocarditis can cause prosthetic valve infection. There is a possibility of cure of prosthetic valve endocarditis with medical therapy alone; however, if bacteremia continues or relapse occurs, valve replacement should be performed and therapy continued for an additional 6 wk.
S. epidermidis or nafcillin-resistant *S. aureus* (NRSA)	Vancomycin	Vancomycin,[d] gentamicin[k] and rifampin[j]	Some authors recommend adding gentamicin[k] and rifampin[j].
Fungal endocarditis			
Candida, Aspergillus	Amphotericin B[l]		Most, if not all, patients with fungal endocarditis require surgical resection of the lesion and valve replacement. Medical therapy rarely, if ever, is curative.

Table 3.1—continued

[a] Penicillin G, 2–3 mU i.v. q4h for 4 weeks.

[b] Vancomycin, 15 mg/kg i.v. q12h for 4 weeks; ceftriaxone 2 gm i.v. q24h for 4 weeks.

[c] Nafcillin, 1.5 g i.v. q4h for 6 weeks alone or add gentamicin, 1.5 mg/kg q8h, for first 5 days. Right-sided endocarditis in intravenous drug users (IVDU) responds to 2 weeks of nafcillin plus tobramycin.

[d] Vancomycin, 15 mg/kg i.v. q12h for 6 weeks.

[e] Penicillin G, 3 mU i.v. q4h for 6 weeks.

[f] Gentamicin, 1.0 mg/kg q8h for 6 weeks in patients with normal renal function. Check blood levels and serum creatinine at least once a week.

[g] Mezlocillin or piperacillin, 5 g i.v. q8h for 6 weeks.

[h] Tobramycin/gentamicin, 1.75 mg/kg i.v. q8h for 6 weeks.

[i] Trimethoprim/sulfamethoxazole, 10 mg/kg/day i.v. in two divided doses for 6 weeks.

[j] Rifampin, 600 mg/day.

[k] Gentamicin, 1 mg/kg i.v. q8h for 2 weeks.

[l] Amphotericin B, 0.75 mg/kg/day i.v. for 8–10 weeks. When fungemia is cleared, therapy can be changed to the same dose on an every other day basis.

Table 3.2. Musculoskeletal Infection

	Organism	Suggested Regimen	Alternative Regimen	Comment
Osteomyelitis/septic arthritis (infant <3 months old)	S. aureus, aerobic GNR,[a] group A, B streptococci	Nafcillin and TGC		Adjust therapy for specific organism: S. aureus, nafcillin; group A, B streptococci, penicillin G; aerobic GNR, TGC, depending on sensitivity. Duration: 4–6 weeks.
Osteomyelitis/septic arthritis (age <6 years)	S. aureus, streptococci, H. influenzae	Nafcillin and TGC	Clindamycin or vancomycin; ±TGC	Adjust therapy for specific organism. (See above.) Blood culture, aspiration/biopsy for culture. Duration: 4–6 weeks.
Osteomyelitis/septic arthritis (older children and adults)	S. aureus, aerobic GNR, and H. influenzae uncommon	Nafcillin; ±TGC	Clindamycin or vancomycin; ±TGC	Adjust therapy for specific organism. Clindamycin has been used successfully in the treatment of osteomyelitis in children and is preferred by many pediatricians. In adults, clindamycin can also be used, but vancomycin is preferred, especially in the acute phases of the illness. Ciprofloxacin should not be used in pregnant women or children. Duration: 4–6 weeks. Joint drainage is necessary, either by repeated needle aspiration or, if unsuccessful, by open surgical drainage.
Septic arthritis (older children and adults)	N. gonorrhoeae	Ceftriaxone, cefotaxime, or ceftizoxime	Spectinomycin	Primary therapy with cephalosporins or spectinomycin (β-lactam allergy) followed by oral cefixime or ciprofloxacin.

Table 3.2—continued

	Organism	Suggested Regimen	Alternative Regimen	Comment
Septic arthritis (postoperative, traumatic, association with drug use)	S. aureus	Nafcillin	Clindamycin or vancomycin	Therapy for septic arthritis should be based on specific organism sensitivities. Duration: 3–4 weeks with needle or open drainage. Treatment, especially due to *Pseudomonas* or *Serratia*, should be with synergistic antibiotic combinations whenever possible.
	S. epidermidis	Vancomycin	Nafcillin (if sensitive)	
	Aerobic GNR (not *Pseudomonas* or *Acinetobacter*)	TGC		
	Pseudomonas	Ticarcillin, mezlocillin or piperacillin, and tobramycin	Ceftazidime or imipenem, and tobramycin	
	Acinetobacter	Imipenem and gentamicin	TMP/SMX and gentamicin	*Acinetobacter* is also susceptible to piperacillin (MIC$_{90}$ = 16 mg/ml) which should be used with gentamicin.

*Aerobic GNR, Gram-negative rods; TGC, third-generation cephalosporin; MIC, minimum inhibitory concentration; TMP/SMX, trimethoprim-sulfamethoxazole.

Table 3.3. Pediatric Meningitis

Organism	Antibiotic of Choice[a]	Alternative Regimen	Comment
N. meningitidis	Penicillin G	TGC[b] or chloramphenicol	Pediatric patients with meningitis should be treated until afebrile for 3–5 days and for a total of at least 7–10 days. Close contacts should receive rifampin prophylaxis. (See Section 4.)
S. pneumoniae	Penicillin G	TGC or chloramphenicol	S. pneumonia in CNS should be tested for penicillin susceptibility. Treat resistant strains with chloramphenicol or TGC.
H. influenzae	TGC	Ampicillin (if sensitive) or chloramphenicol	Isolates should be tested for β-lactamase production. Give rifampin prophylaxis at completion of therapy. Duration of therapy is as described for N. meningitidis.
E. coli	TGC		Meningitis in neonates should be treated for 2 weeks and often longer, depending on the clinical response.
Group B streptococcus	Penicillin G ± gentamicin	TGC and gentamicin	
E. faecalis	Ampicillin and gentamicin	Vancomycin and gentamicin	CNS strains should be tested for ampicillin and vancomycin susceptibility and high level of gentamicin resistance.[a]
Listeria	Ampicillin and gentamicin	TMP/SMX	As with most meningitis in neonates, therapy should usually be continued for 2 or more weeks.

[a] See Section 1, Tables 4a and 4b for dosages.
[b] TGC, third-generation cephalosporin; TMP/SMX, trimethoprim-sulfamethoxazole.

Table 3.4. Adult Meningitis

Organism	Antibiotic of Choice	Penicillin-Allergic Patients	Comment
S. pneumoniae	Penicillin G	TGC[a] or chloramphenicol	Antibiotic therapy should be continued for at least 10 days. CNS isolates should be tested for penicillin susceptibility.
N. meningitidis	Penicillin G	TGC or chloramphenicol	Close contacts should receive rifampin prophylaxis. (See Section 4.)
H. influenzae	TGC	Ampicillin (if susceptible)	Isolates should be tested for β-lactamase production.
S. aureus, NRSA, *S. epidermidis*	Vancomycin	Nafcillin	Most cases of *S. aureus* meningitis are secondary to trauma or are postsurgical. Treatment may be necessary for 2 weeks or longer. If response is slow and/or cultures remain positive, vancomycin may be given intrathecally in a dose of 20 mg/day. Use nafcillin only if *S. aureus* is susceptible.
Aerobic GNR (not *Pseudomonas*)	TGC		Gram-negative meningitis is usually the result of trauma or is postsurgical. Chloramphenicol is not recommended for the treatment of meningitis due to *Enterobacteriaceae*.
Pseudomonas	Ceftazidime and tobramycin	Piperacillin and tobramycin	Aminoglycoside must be given i.v. and intrathecally (4 mg q12–18hr).

[a]TGC, third-generation cephalosporin; NRSA, nafcillin-resistant *S. aureus*; aerobic GNR, Gram-negative rods.

Table 3.5. Acute Gastroenteritis

Organism	Source	Vehicle	Mechanism	Incubation Period	Severity and Duration	N^a V C D F	Laboratory	Treatment
Staphylococcus aureus	Human skin; animals	Food (ice cream, cream fillings, etc.), frozen foods, cheese, meats	Ingestion of performed toxin; no effect on mucosa, direct effect on CNS	1–8 hr	Moderate to severe; 2–24 hr	$4+^b$ 4+ 1+ 1+ 0	Special studies required	No antibiotic, self-limited
Bacillus cereus	Soil, raw vegetables	Same	1. Emetic toxin (fried rice) 2. Intestinal toxin	1–6 hr 10–12 hr	<24 hr 12–24 hr	4+ 4+ 4+ 1+ 0 2+ 1+ 4+ 4+ 0	Special studies; food culture	No antibiotic, self-limited
Clostridium perifringens	Normal bowel flora	Food (meats, gravies, especially stews)	Ingestion of performed toxin	8–24 hr	Mild to moderate, 1–2 days	1+ 1+ 3+ 3+ 0	Special studies required	No antibiotic, self-limited
Escherichia coli	Normal bowel flora	Food; water; person to person	1. Toxin 2. Mucosal invasion	6–72 hr	Mild; 1–3 days	1+ 1+ 2+ 3+ 1+	Special studies required	Quinolone and loperamide
Salmonella (nontyphi)	Animal bowel flora	Poultry, eggs, or their products	Infection	8–48 hr	Moderate to very severe, 1–5 days	3+ 3+ 4+ 4+ 4+	Routinely isolated	No antibiotics in uncomplicated cases: treat bacteremia, metastatic foci or immune compromised host; no opiates
Shigella	Human bowel flora	Person to person; occasionally food	1. Infection 2. Toxin	12–72 hr	Moderate to very severe; 2–7 days	1+ 1+ 4+ 4+ 4+	Routinely isolated	Ciprofloxacin, norfloxacin, ofloxacin, or TMP/SMX

Table 3.5—continued

Organism	Source	Vehicle	Mechanism	Incubation Period	Severity and Duration	Nᵃ V C D F	Laboratory	Treatment
Vibrio parahaemolyticus	Ocean water	Undercooked seafood, raw fish	Uncertain	4–96 hr	Moderate to severe; 1–5 days	3+ 2+ 3+ 4+ 1+	Special studies	Role of antibiotics unclear, may use quinolone, doxycycline, or TMP/SMX
Vibrio el tor (cholera); not in United States, except Louisiana	Human bowel; carriers and victims	Water or direct contamination	Toxin	6–48 hr	Mild to severe; 2–7 days	0 1+ 0 4+ 0	Special studies; not routinely available	Tetracyclineᶜ or doxycycline; TMP/SMX; quinolone
Campylobacter jejuni	Human bowel; ? poultry and other animals	Water or direct contamination	Infection	2–10 days	Mild to severe; 1–4 days	3+ 2+ 4+ 4+ 2+	Routinely isolated	Erythromycin or quinolone; tetracyclineᶜ

ᵃ N, nausea; V, vomiting; C, cramps; D, diarrhea; F, fever.
ᵇ 4+, always present; 3+, usually present; 2+, irregularly present; 1+, infrequently present; 0, always absent.
ᶜ Tetracycline contraindicated in pregnant women or children ≤8 years old.

Table 3.6. Gastrointestinal Infection

	Organism(s)	Antibiotic of Choice	Alternative Regimen	Comment
Typhoid fever	S. typhosa, S. paratyphi	Ceftriaxone or ciprofloxacin or ofloxacin	Ampicillin, TMP/SMX, or chloramphenicol	Treatment should be continued for 14 days. Salicylates should be avoided. Relapses occur in 10–20% of patients, despite adequate therapy. Treatment should be based on susceptibilities. Ampicillin, chloramphenicol, and TMP/SMX resistance reported.
Cholecystitis, cholangitis	E. coli, other aerobic GNR,[a] E. faecalis, anaerobes	Ampicillin and gentamicin and metronidazole	Imipenem	Alternative regimens include ampicillin/sulbactam, ticarcillin/clavulanate, or piperacillin/tazobactam. Therapy should be continued 7–10 days. Most patients should undergo cholecystectomy when stable.
Peritonitis, primary SBP	S. pneumoniae, aerobic GNR, S. aureus	TGC and gentamicin	Ampicillin/sulbactam, ticarcillin/ clavulanate, or piperacillin/ tazobactam, and gentamicin	Treatment should be based upon the identification and susceptibilities of the isolated pathogens.
Peritonitis, ruptured viscus, perirectal abscess	B. fragilis, other anaerobes, E. coli, other aerobic GNR, E. faecalis	Ampicillin and gentamicin and metronidazole	Imipenem or TGC and metronidazole	Combined therapy should be continued 10–14 days, depending on the clinical response. In neutropenic or immunosuppressed patients, mezlocillin or piperacillin should be substituted for ampicillin, and tobramycin for gentamicin.
CAPD	Candida, S. epidermidis, aerobic GNR, S. aureus	Amphotericin B or vancomycin		Use intraperitoneal vancomycin, 1 gm/L, and gentamicin, 100 mg/L, initial dose, then vancomycin, 25 mg/L, and gentamicin, 8 mg/L, until organism identified. Add i.v. antibiotics for severely ill patient. Use amphotericin B, 4 mg/L, for Candida.

Table 3.6—continued

	Organism(s)	Antibiotic of Choice	Alternative Regimen	Comment
Liver abscess	E. coli, other aerobic GNR, E. faecalis, mixed anaerobes, rarely aerobic positive cocci	Ampicillin and gentamicin and metronidazole	Imipenem or TGC and metronidazole	Surgical drainage is the most important aspect of treatment. Therapy should be adjusted according to the results of aerobic and anaerobic cultures. Optimum duration of antibiotic therapy for liver abscess after successful drainage is unknown; 1 week is suggested. With multiple liver abscesses, therapy may have to be continued for months.
Alcohol-related or idiopathic pancreatitis	None			Pancreatitis is not known to be a bacterial disease; antibiotic therapy is not recommended.
Infected pancreatic pseudocyst or abscess	Aerobic GNR, anaerobes, S. aureus, Enterococcus	Ampicillin/sulbactam, ticarcillin/clavulanate, or piperacillin/ tazobactam and gentamicin	Imipenem ± gentamicin	Surgical drainage necessary.

ᵃ Aerobic GNR, Gram-negative rods; TGC, third-generation cephalosporin; SBP, spontaneous bacterial peritonitis; CAPD, chronic ambulatory peritoneal dialysis.

Table 3.7. Urinary Tract Infection

Organism	Antibiotic of Choice	Alternative Regimen	Comment
Cystitis, outpatient-acquired (dysuria) *E. coli*, other aerobic GNR, *C. trachomatis*, *S. saprophyticus*	TMP/SMX[a] or tetracycline (for *C. trachomatis*); see Comment	TMP, quinolone, nitrofurantoin, oral cephalosporin	Less than 8 WBC/HPF in unspun urine (or negative esterase test): no treatment indicated; >8 WBC/HPF (positive esterase test) and no bacteria seen on Gram stain (spun urine): treat for *C. trachomatis* with 1 week of tetracycline. If bacteria present, treat for 3 days. Single-dose treatment acceptable but higher rate of failure.
Cystitis, hospital-acquired, patient not "septic" Antibiotic-resistant aerobic GNR, *Enterococcus*	TGC (use ampicillin and gentamicin if *Enterococcus* suspected)	Ampicillin and gentamicin	Parenteral therapy should be continued until results of cultures and sensitivities are available. If organism isolated is sensitive to a less toxic antibiotic, therapy should be changed accordingly and continued for 10 days. Urinary catheter should be removed as soon as possible.
Pyelonephritis, first episode, patient not "septic" *E. coli*, other aerobic GNR, *Enterococcus*	TMP/SMX, TGC (use ampicillin and gentamicin if *Enterococcus* suspected)	Ampicillin and gentamicin, or quinolone, or oral cephalosporin	Patients who have no previous episodes of urinary tract infection and who are mildly ill can be managed as outpatients. Therapy should be continued for 10–14 days.

Table 3.7—continued

	Organism	Antibiotic of Choice	Alternative Regimen	Comment
Pyelonephritis, recurrent, or patient is "septic"	E. coli, other aerobic GNR, Enterococcus	TGC and gentamicin	Imipenem or ampicillin and gentamicin	Patients in this category must be hospitalized and treated parenterally until cultures and sensitivities are available. Blood cultures should be obtained. If urine Gram stain reveals Gram-positive cocci in chains, therapy with ampicillin and gentamicin should be initiated and continued for 10–14 days. Urological investigation is recommended.

[a]TMP/SMX, trimethoprim-sulfamethoxazole; aerobic GNR, Gram-negative rods; TGC, third-generation cephalosporin.

Table 3.8. Respiratory Infection

	Organism	Antibiotic of Choice	Alternative Regimen	Comment
Pharyngitis	Group A streptococcus (C. haemolyticum, Mycoplasma, viruses, group C, G streptococci	Benzathine, penicillin G or penicillin V	Erythromycin, azithromycin, clarithromycin, oral cephalosporin	Treat symptomatic patient with positive rapid test for GABHS or when follow-up is unlikely or impossible, an antibiotic has been administered prior to culture, or the patient has a history of rheumatic fever or has rheumatic heart disease. Otherwise, treat for positive culture.
	C. diphtheriae	Erythromycin	Penicillin G	Antibiotic treatment should be continued 10–12 days. Diphtheria antitoxin should be administered as soon as possible. Antibiotic therapy is not known to alter the complications or the clinical course of diphtheria.
	N. gonorrhoeae	Ceftriaxone (125 mg i.m.)	Ciprofloxacin (500 mg p.o.)	Quinolone contraindicated for nursing or pregnant women and patients <17 years old. Quinolones not effective for syphilis.
Epiglottitis	H. influenzae, group A streptococci, S. pneumoniae	TGC	Ampicillin and chloramphenicol	Intubation should be available immediately. For H. influenzae close contacts <4 years old should receive rifampin prophylaxis.
Otitis, sinusitis	See Table 2.7			Refer to Table 2.7 for the treatment of otitis and sinusitis. Unless special procedures are performed, specific organisms and sensitivities are not usually available to guide therapy.
Aspiration pneumonia	Mixed oropharyngeal flora, anaerobes	Clindamycin	Cefoxitin or ampicillin/ sulbactam	Continue therapy 10–14 days, depending on patient's response.
Lung abscess	Mixed oropharyngeal flora, anaerobes	Clindamycin	Cefoxitin or ampicillin/ sulbactam	After acute phase of illness, therapy may be given orally and should be continued for 2–3 months, depending on the patient's response.

Table 3.8—continued

	Organism	Antibiotic of Choice	Alternative Regimen	Comment
Pneumonia	S. pneumoniae	Penicillin G	Erythromycin or cefuroxime	Treat for 7–10 days. Most patients with pneumococcal pneumonia should be hospitalized and treated parenterally during the acute phase of illness.
	S. aureus	Nafcillin	Vancomycin or cefazolin	S. aureus pneumonia is a life-threatening infection. Because of the tendency for abscess development and relapse, treatment should be continued for a minimum of 2 weeks and preferably for 3 weeks.
	H. influenzae	TGC	TMP/SMX, ampicillin/sulbactam	H. influenzae pneumonia usually occurs in children and in elderly adults, or in those with chronic lung disease or alcoholism. If the organism's sensitivity is known, ampicillin should be used. When it is unknown and in areas of high ampicillin resistance, a β-lactamase stable cephalosporin is recommended. Therapy should be continued 10–14 days.
	Serratia, pseudomonas, other aerobic GNR	Mezlocillin or piperacillin and tobramycin; (Pseudomonas) or gentamicin (Serratia)	Ceftazidime and tobramycin or gentamicin	Most consultants recommend combined antibiotic therapy for Gram-negative pneumonia. Treatment should be continued 2–3 weeks, depending on the patient's response.
	Mycoplasma	Erythromycin, azithromycin, or clarithromycin	Tetracycline	Tetracycline is also effective, but should not be used in children; 10 days of treatment is recommended.
	Chlamydia trachomatis	Erythromycin		Occurs in infants from 2 to 15 weeks of age. Patients are frequently afebrile and appear to have nonbacterial pneumonia. Treatment should be continued for 10 days.

[a] GABHS, group A β-hemolytic streptococcus; TGC, third-generation cephalosporin.

Table 3.9. Miscellaneous Infections

Organism	Therapy	Comment
Actinomyces (actinomycosis)	Antibiotic of choice: penicillin G Alternate therapy: tetracycline	Most patients, particularly those with extensive disease, require 6–8 months of therapy with or without surgical debridement. Initial treatment should be in hospital, with penicillin G i.v. 4–6 weeks, followed by outpatient therapy with oral penicillin.
Anthrax	Antibiotic of choice: penicillin G Alternate therapy: erythromycin	Uncomplicated cutaneous anthrax may be treated orally or with low parental doses of penicillin. In severe disseminated infection, with pulmonary and/or CNS involvement, high-dose therapy (20 MU/day) is recommended. Treatment should be continued for 7–10 days.
Bordetella (whooping cough)	Antibiotic of choice: erythromycin Alternate therapy: TMP/SMX[a] or ampicillin	Treatment has no effect on the clinical course of whooping cough. However, the organism is eliminated from secretions, and the patient is thereby rendered noninfectious. Asymptomatic carriers with cultures positive for *Bordetella* should be treated for 2 weeks.
Brucella (brucellosis)	Antibiotics of choice: tetracycline and gentamicin Alternate therapy: TMP/SMX	In patients who are severely ill, streptomycin should be given in addition to tetracycline. Duration of therapy should be at least 3 weeks. Relapse occurs in approximately 10–20% of patients and necessitates retreatment. In children under 8 years old, chloramphenicol or trimethoprim/sulfamethoxazole may be substituted for tetracycline.

Table 3.9—continued

Organism	Therapy	Comment
Erysipelothrix (erysipeloid)	Antibiotic of choice: penicillin G Alternate therapy: erythromycin	Predominant form is an acute localized cellulitis. Bacteremia and endocarditis are rare complications. The cellulitic form of the infection may be treated with oral therapy for 10–14 days. Systemic infection and endocarditis should be treated with penicillin G i.v. in higher doses (12 MU/day) for 4–6 weeks.
Francisella tularensis (tularemia)	Antibiotic of choice: streptomycin or gentamicin Alternate therapy: tetracycline or chloramphenicol	Treatment should be continued for 10 days. Tetracycline or chloramphenicol may be used in patients who cannot tolerate aminoglycosides, but these drugs may not be as effective. Relapses do occur, requiring treatment. Resistant organisms do not emerge.
Legionella pneumophila (Legionnaires' disease)	Antibiotics of choice: erythromycin Alternate therapy: add rifampin	Legionnaires' disease is known to occur in outpatients sporadically and in epidemics, as well as in hospitalized and immunosuppressed hosts. It should be considered in any patient with apparent nonbacterial pneumonia. Treatment should be continued for 10–14 days, depending on patient response. Rifampin should be added in patients who are slow to respond.
Leptospira (leptospirosis)	Antibiotic of choice: penicillin G Alternate therapy: tetracycline	Therapy early in the course of illness may favorably affect the signs and symptoms of leptospirosis. Penicillin G or tetracycline, parenterally or orally, is recommended for 1 week.

Organism	Therapy	Comments
Listeria (listeriosis)	Antibiotics of choice: ampicillin ± gentamicin Alternate therapy: TMP/SMX	Controversy exists as to whether ampicillin is superior to penicillin; 2 weeks of therapy appears adequate in most patients, but treatment may have to be prolonged in immunosuppressed patients. It may be necessary to vary dosage and duration, depending on site involved, severity of infection, and clinical response.
Nocardia asteroids	Antibiotics of choice: sulfisoxazole or TMP/SMX Alternate therapy: imipenem and amikacin	Parenteral administration of sulfonamide or TMP/SMX is the treatment of choice for acutely ill patients. After 2–3 weeks of i.v. therapy, and with a good clinical response, oral treatment may be given, usually for 3–6 months, depending on the extent and severity of the infection.
Pseudomonas pseudomallei (melioidosis)	Antibiotics of choice: ceftazidime Alternate therapy: imipenem	Treatment may have to be continued for many months because of the tendency to relapse.
Spirillum minus (rat-bite fever)	Antibiotic of choice: penicillin G Alternate therapy: tetracycline	Seven to ten days of treatment is recommended. Response is usually rapid.
Streptobacillus moniliformis (rat-bite fever)	Antibiotic of choice: penicillin G Alternate therapy: tetracycline	Seven to ten days of treatment is recommended. Patients with S. moniliformis endocarditis should be treated for 4–6 weeks, with dosage guided by serum bactericidal assays.
Yersinia pestis (plague)	Antibiotics of choice: streptomycin or tetracycline Alternate therapy: chloramphenicol	Household contacts of patients with plague should be treated with tetracycline or sulfisoxazole for 1 week. Patients with plague should be treated with 10 days of streptomycin or tetracycline. In the presence of meningitis, chloramphenicol should be added to the regimen.

ªTMP/SMX, trimethoprim-sulfamethoxazole.

Table 3.10. Antibacterial Drugs of Choice

Infecting Organism	Drug of First Choice	Alternative Drugs
GRAM-POSITIVE COCCI		
Enterococcus		
Endocarditis or other severe infection	Penicillin G or ampicillin + gentamicin or streptomycin	Vancomycin + gentamicin or streptomycin; ampicillin/sulbactam + gentamicin or streptomycin; teicoplanin[2]
Uncomplicated urinary tract infection	Ampicillin or amoxicillin	Nitrofurantoin; a fluoroquinolone[3]
Staphylococcus aureus or epidermidis		
Non-penicillinase-producing	Penicillin G or V[4]	A cephalosporin[5,6]; vancomycin; imipenem; clindamycin; a fluoroquinolone[3]
Penicillinase-producing	A penicillinase-resistant penicillin[7]	A cephalosporin[5,6]; vancomycin; amoxicillin/clavulanic acid; ticarcillin/clavulanic acid; piperacillin/tazobactam; ampicillin/sulbactam; imipenem; clindamycin; a fluoroquinolone[3]
Methicillin-resistant[8]	Vancomycin ± gentamicin ± rifampin	Trimethoprim-sulfamethoxazole; minocycline[9]; a fluoroquinolone[3]
Streptococcus pyogenes (Group A) and Groups C and G	Penicillin G or V[4]	An erythromycin[10], a cephalosporin[5,6]; vancomycin; clarithromycin; azithromycin; clindamycin[10]
Streptococcus, Group B	Penicillin G or ampicillin	A cephalosporin[5,6]; vancomycin; an erythromycin
Streptococcus, viridans group[1]	Penicillin G ± gentamicin	A cephalosporin[5,6]; vancomycin
Streptococcus bovis[1]	Penicillin G	A cephalosporin[5,6]; vancomycin
Streptococcus, anaerobic or *Peptostreptococcus*	Penicillin G	Clindamycin; a cephalosporin[5,6]; vancomycin
Streptococcus pneumoniae[11] (pneumococcus)	Penicillin G or V[4]	An erythromycin; a cephalosporin[5,6]; vancomycin ± rifampin; trimethoprim-sulfamethoxazole; azithromycin; clarithromycin; clindamycin; chloramphenicol[12]

Reprinted with permission from *Medical Letter* 1994;36(925).

* Resistance may be a problem; susceptibility tests should be performed.

[1] Disk sensitivity testing may not provide adequate information; β-lactamase assays and dilution tests for susceptibility should be used in serious infections and in endocarditis should assess bactericidal as well as inhibitory end-points.

[2] Investigational drug in United States available through Marion Merrell Dow; Telephone (800) 362-7466.

[3] For most infections, ofloxacin or ciprofloxacin. For urinary tract infections, norfloxacin, lomefloxacin, or enoxacin can be used. Ciprofloxacin and ofloxacin are available for intravenous use. None of these agents is recommended for children.

[4] Penicillin V is preferred for oral treatment of infections caused by nonpenicillinase-producing staphylococci and other Gram-positive cocci. For initial therapy of severe infections, penicillin G, administered parenterally, is first choice. For somewhat longer action in less severe infections due to Group A streptococci, pneumococci, or *Treponema pallidum*, procaine penicillin G, an intramuscular formulation, is given once or twice daily. Benzathine penicillin G, a slowly absorbed preparation, is usually given in a single monthly injection for prophylaxis of rheumatic fever, once for treatment of Group A streptococcal pharyngitis and once or more for treatment of syphilis.

[5] The cephalosporins have been used as alternatives to penicillins in patients allergic to penicillins, but such patients may also have allergic reactions to cephalosporins.

[6] For parenteral treatment of staphylococcal or nonenterococcal streptococcal infections, a "first-generation" cephalosporin such as cephalothin or cefazolin can be used; for staphylococcal endocarditis, some *Medical Letter* consultants prefer cephalothin. For oral therapy, cephalexin or cephradine can be used. The "second-generation" cephalosporins cefamandole, cefprozil, cefuroxime, cefuroxime axetil, cefonicid, cefotetan, cefmetazole, cefoxitin, and loracarbef are more active than the first-generation drugs against Gram-negative bacteria. Cefuroxime and cefamandole are active against ampicillin-resistant strains of *H. influenzae*, but cefamandole has been associated with prothrombin deficiency and occasional bleeding. Cefoxitin, cefotetan, and cefmetazole are active against *B. fragilis*. The "third-generation" cephalosporins cefotaxime, cefoperazone, ceftizoxime, ceftriaxone, and ceftazidime have greater activity than the second-generation drugs against enteric Gram-negative bacilli. Cefixime and cefpodoxime (Med Lett 1989;31:73 and 1992;34:107) are oral cephalosporins with more activity than second-generation cephalosporins against facultative Gram-negative bacilli. They have no useful activity against anaerobes or *Pseudomonas aeruginosa*, and cefixime has no useful activity against staphylococci. With the exception of cefoperazone (which, like cefamandole, can cause bleeding) and ceftazidime, the activity of all currently available cephalosporins against *Pseudomonas aeruginosa* is poor or inconsistent.

[7] For oral use against penicillinase-producing staphylococci, cloxacillin or dicloxacillin is preferred; for severe infections, a parenteral formulation of methicillin, nafcillin, or oxacillin should be used. Neither ampicillin, amoxicillin, bacampicillin, carbenicillin, ticarcillin, mezlocillin, nor piperacillin is effective against penicillinase-producing staphylococci. The combinations of clavulanic acid with amoxicillin or ticarcillin, sulbactam with ampicillin, and tazobactam with piperacillin are active against these organisms.

[8] Many strains of coagulase-positive staphylococci and coagulase-negative staphylococci are resistant to penicillinase-resistant penicillins; these strains are also resistant to cephalosporins and imipenem.

[9] Tetracyclines are generally not recommended for pregnant women or children less than 8 years old.

[10] Group A streptococcus may be resistant to erythromycins and clindamycin (Seppälä, H., et al. N Engl J Med 1992;326:292.

[11] Some strains may show intermediate resistance or high-level resistance to penicillin. Infections caused by strains with intermediate sensitivity to penicillin may respond to cefotaxime or ceftriaxone. Highly resistant strains should be treated with vancomycin with or without rifampin. In patients allergic to penicillin, erythromycin, azithromycin, or clarithromycin are often useful for respiratory infections, but vancomycin with or without rifampin is recommended for meningitis. Some strains of *S. pneumoniae* are resistant to erythromycin, trimethoprim-sulfamethoxazole, clarithromycin, azithromycin, and chloramphenicol.

[12] Because of the possibility of serious adverse effects, this drug should be used only for severe infections when less hazardous drugs are ineffective.

Table 3.10—continued

Infecting Organism	Drug of First Choice	Alternative Drugs
GRAM-NEGATIVE COCCI		
Moraxella (Branhamella) catarrhalis	Trimethoprim-sulfamethoxazole	Amoxicillin/clavulanic acid; an erythromycin; clarithromycin; azithromycin; a tetracycline[9]; cefuroxime[5]; cefotaxime[5]; ceftizoxime[5]; ceftriaxone[5]; cefuroxime axetil[5]; cefixime[5]
*Neisseria gonorrhoeae (gonococcus)	Ceftriaxone[5]	Cefixime[5]; cefotaxime[5]; a fluoroquinolone[3]; spectinomycin; penicillin G; chloramphenicol[12]
Neisseria meningitidis[13] (meningococcus)	Penicillin G	Cefotaxime[5]; ceftizoxime[5]; ceftriaxone[5]; chloramphenicol[12]; a sulfonamide[14]
GRAM-POSITIVE BACILLI		
Bacillus anthracis (anthrax)	Penicillin G	An erythromycin; a tetracycline[9]
Bacillus cereus, subtilis	Vancomycin	Imipenem
Clostridium perfringens[15]	Penicillin G	Metronidazole; clindamycin; imipenem; a tetracycline[9]; chloramphenicol[12]
Clostridium tetani[16]	Penicillin G	A tetracycline[9]
Clostridium difficile[17]	Metronidazole	Vancomycin; bacitracin
Corynebacterium diphtheriae[18]	An erythromycin	Penicillin G
Corynebacterium, JK group	Vancomycin	Penicillin G + gentamicin; erythromycin
Listeria monocytogenes	Ampicillin ± gentamicin	Trimethoprim-sulfamethoxazole
ENTERIC GRAM-NEGATIVE BACILLI		
*Bacteroides		
Oropharyngeal strains	Penicillin G[19]	Clindamycin; cefoxitin[5]; metronidazole; chloramphenicol[12]; cefotetan[5]
Gastrointestinal strains[20]	Metronidazole	Clindamycin; imipenem; ticarcillin/clavulanic acid; piperacillin/tazobactam; cefoxitin[5]; cefotetan[5]; ampicillin/sulbactam; piperacillin; chloramphenicol[12]; ceftizoxime[5]; cefmetazole[5]
*Campylobacter fetus	Imipenem	Gentamicin
*Campylobacter jejuni	A fluoroquinolone[3] or an erythromycin	A tetracycline[9]; gentamicin

ENTERIC GRAM-NEGATIVE BACILLI—continued

Enterobacter	Imipenem[21]	Cefotaxime,[5,21] ceftizoxime,[5,21] ceftriaxone,[5,21] or ceftazidime[5,21]; gentamicin, tobramycin, or amikacin; trimethoprim-sulfamethoxazole; carbenicillin,[22] ticarcillin,[22] mezlocillin,[22] or piperacillin[22]; aztreonam[21]; a fluoroquinolone[3]
Escherichia coli[23]	Cefotaxime, ceftizoxime, ceftriaxone, or ceftazidime[5,21]	Ampicillin ± gentamicin, tobramycin, or amikacin; carbenicillin,[22] ticarcillin,[22] mezlocillin,[22] or piperacillin[22]; gentamicin, tobramycin, or amikacin; amoxicillin/clavulanic acid[22]; ticarcillin/clavulanic acid[22]; piperacillin/tazobactam[22]; ampicillin/sulbactam[22]; trimethoprim-sulfamethoxazole; imipenem[21]; aztreonam[21]; a fluoroquinolone[3]; another cephalosporin[5,6]
Helicobacter pylori[24]	Tetracycline HCl[9] + metronidazole + bismuth subsalicylate	Amoxicillin + metronidazole + bismuth subsalicylate; tetracycline HCl + clarithromycin + bismuth subsalicylate

[13] Rare strains of N. meningitidis are resistant or relatively resistant to penicillin (Riley G et al. N Engl J Med 1991;324:997.) Rifampin is recommended for prophylaxis in close contacts of patients infected by sulfonamide-resistant organisms.

[14] Sulfonamide-resistant strains are frequent in the United States, and sulfonamides should be used only when susceptibility is established by susceptibility tests.

[15] Debridement is primary. Large doses of penicillin G are required. Hyperbaric oxygen therapy may be a useful adjunct to surgical debridement in management of the spreading necrotic type.

[16] For prophylaxis, a tetanus toxoid booster and, for some patients, tetanus immune globulin (human) are required.

[17] In order to decrease the selection of vancomycin-resistant enterococci in hospitals, many *Medical Letter* consultants now recommend use of metronidazole first in treatment of most patients with C. *difficile* colitis with oral vancomycin used only for seriously ill patients or those who do not respond to metronidazole. Also see Med Lett 1989;31:94.

[18] Antitoxin is primary; antimicrobials are used only to halt further toxin production and to prevent the carrier state.

[19] *Bacteroides* species from the oropharynx may be resistant to penicillin; for patients seriously ill with infections that may be due to these organisms, or when response to penicillin is delayed, clindamycin is preferred.

[20] When infection is in the central nervous system, either intravenous metronidazole or chloramphenicol is recommended.

[21] In severely ill patients, some *Medical Letter* consultants would add gentamicin, tobramycin, or amikacin.

[22] In severely ill patients, some *Medical Letter* consultants would add gentamicin, tobramycin, or amikacin (but see Footnote 32).

[23] For an acute, uncomplicated urinary tract infection, before the infecting organism is known, the drug of first choice is trimethoprim-sulfamethoxazole.

[24] Graham DY et al. Ann Intern Med 1992;116:705. Hentschel E et al. N Engl J Med 1993;328:308.

Table 3.10—continued

Infecting Organism	Drug of First Choice	Alternative Drugs
ENTERIC GRAM-NEGATIVE BACILLI—continued		
*Klebsiella pneumoniae[23]	Cefotaxime, ceftizoxime, ceftriaxone, or ceftazidime[5,21]	Imipenem[21]; gentamicin, tobramycin, or amikacin; amoxicillin/clavulanic acid[21]; ticarcillin/clavulanic acid[22]; piperacillin/tazobactam[22]; ampicillin/sulbactam[21]; trimethoprim-sulfamethoxazole; aztreonam[21]; a fluoroquinolone[3]; mezlocillin[22] or piperacillin[22]; another cephalosporin[5,6]
*Proteus mirabilis[23]	Ampicillin[25]	A cephalosporin[5,6,21]; ticarcillin,[22] mezlocillin,[22] or piperacillin[22]; gentamicin, tobramycin, or amikacin; trimethoprim-sulfamethoxazole; imipenem[21]; aztreonam[21]; a fluoroquinolone[3]; chloramphenicol[12]
*Proteus, indole-positive (including Providencia rettgeri, Morganella morganii, and Proteus vulgaris)	Cefotaxime, ceftizoxime, ceftriaxone, or ceftazidime[5,21]	Imipenem[21]; gentamicin, tobramycin, or amikacin; carbenicillin,[22] ticarcillin,[22] mezlocillin,[22] or piperacillin[22]; amoxicillin/clavulanic acid[21]; ticarcillin/clavulanic acid[22]; piperacillin/tazobactam[22]; ampicillin/sulbactam[21]; aztreonam[21]; trimethoprim-sulfamethoxazole; a fluoroquinolone[3]
*Providencia stuartii	Cefotaxime, ceftizoxime, ceftriaxone, or ceftazidime[5,21]	Imipenem[21]; ticarcillin/clavulanic acid[22]; piperacillin/tazobactam[22]; gentamicin, tobramycin, or amikacin; carbenicillin[22], ticarcillin,[22] mezlocillin,[22] or piperacillin[22]; aztreonam[21]; trimethoprim-sulfamethoxazole; a fluoroquinolone[3]
*Salmonella typhi[26]	Ceftriaxone[5] or a fluoroquinolone[3]	Chloramphenicol[12]; trimethoprim-sulfamethoxazole; ampicillin; amoxicillin
*Other Salmonella[27]	Cefotaxime[5] or ceftriaxone[5] or a fluoroquinolone[3]	Ampicillin or amoxicillin; trimethoprim-sulfamethoxazole; chloramphenicol[12]

ENTERIC GRAM-NEGATIVE BACILLI—*continued*

Serratia	Cefotaxime, ceftizoxime, ceftriaxone, or ceftazidime[5,28]	Gentamicin or amikacin; imipenem[28]; aztreonam[28]; trimethoprim-sulfamethoxazole; carbenicillin,[29] ticarcillin,[29] mezlocillin,[29] or piperacillin[29]; a fluoroquinolone[3]
Shigella	A fluoroquinolone[3]	Trimethoprim-sulfamethoxazole; ampicillin; ceftriaxone[5]; cefixime[5]
Yersinia enterocolitica	Trimethoprim-sulfamethoxazole	A fluoroquinolone[3]; gentamicin, tobramycin, or amikacin; cefotaxime or ceftizoxime[5]

OTHER GRAM-NEGATIVE BACILLI

Acinetobacter	Imipenem[21]	Tobramycin, gentamicin, or amikacin; ticarcillin,[22] mezlocillin,[22] or piperacillin[22]; ceftazidime[21]; trimethoprim-sulfamethoxazole; a fluoroquinolone[3]; minocycline[9]; doxycycline[9]
Aeromonas	Trimethoprim-sulfamethoxazole	Gentamicin or tobramycin; imipenem; a fluoroquinolone[3]
Bordetella pertussis (whooping cough)	An erythromycin	Trimethoprim-sulfamethoxazole; ampicillin
Brucella	A tetracycline[9] + streptomycin or gentamicin	A tetracycline[9] + rifampin; chloramphenicol[12] ± streptomycin; trimethoprim-sulfamethoxazole ± gentamicin; rifampin + a tetracycline[9]
Calymmatobacterium granulomatis (granuloma inguinale)	A tetracycline[9]	Streptomycin or gentamicin; trimethoprim-sulfamethoxazole; an erythromycin
Eikenella corrodens	Ampicillin	An erythromycin; a tetracycline[9]; amoxicillin/clavulanic acid; ampicillin/sulbactam; ceftriaxone

[25] Large doses (6 gm or more daily) are usually necessary for systemic infections. In severely ill patients, some *Medical Letter* consultants would add gentamicin, tobramycin, or amikacin.

[26] Ampicillin or amoxicillin may be effective in milder cases. Ciprofloxacin or ampicillin is the drug of choice for *S. typhi* carriers.

[27] Most cases of *Salmonella* gastroenteritis subside spontaneously without antimicrobial therapy.

[28] In severely ill patients, some consultants would add gentamicin or amikacin.

[29] In severely ill patients, some *Medical Letter* consultants would add gentamicin or amikacin (but see Footnote 32).

Table 3.10—continued

Infecting Organism	Drug of First Choice	Alternative Drugs
OTHER GRAM-NEGATIVE BACILLI—continued		
*Francisella tularensis (tularemia)	Streptomycin or gentamicin	A tetracycline[9]; chloramphenicol[12]
*Fusobacterium	Penicillin G	Metronidazole; clindamycin; cefoxitin[5]; chloramphenicol[12]
Gardnerella vaginalis (bacterial vaginosis)	Oral metronidazole[30]	Topical clindamycin or metronidazole; oral clindamycin
*Haemophilus ducreyi (chancroid)	Erythromycin or ceftriaxone or azithromycin	A fluoroquinolone[3]
*Haemophilus influenzae		
Meningitis, epiglottitis, arthritis, and other serious infections	Cefotaxime or ceftriaxone[5]	Cefuroxime[5] (but not for meningitis); chloramphenicol[12]
Upper respiratory infections and bronchitis	Trimethoprim-sulfamethoxazole	Ampicillin or amoxicillin; cefuroxime[5]; amoxicillin/clavulanic acid; cefuroxime axetil[5]; cefaclor[5]; cefotaxime[5]; ceftizoxime[5]; ceftriaxone[5]; cefixime[5]; a tetracycline[9]; clarithromycin; azithromycin
Legionella species	An erythromycin + rifampin	Trimethoprim-sulfamethoxazole; clarithromycin; azithromycin; ciprofloxacin[31]
Leptotrichia buccalis	Penicillin G	A tetracycline[9]; clindamycin; an erythromycin
Pasteurella multocida	Penicillin G	A tetracycline[9]; a cephalosporin[5,6]; amoxicillin/clavulanic acid; ampicillin/sulbactam
*Pseudomonas aeruginosa		
Urinary tract infection	A fluoroquinolone[3]	Carbenicillin, ticarcillin, piperacillin, or mezlocillin; ceftazidime[5]; imipenem; aztreonam; tobramycin; gentamicin; amikacin
Other infections	Ticarcillin, mezlocillin, or piperacillin + tobramycin, gentamicin, or amikacin[32]	Ceftazidime,[5] imipenem, or aztreonam + tobramycin, gentamicin, or amikacin; a fluoroquinolone[3]
Pseudomonas mallei (glanders)	Streptomycin + a tetracycline[9]	Streptomycin + chloramphenicol[12]

OTHER GRAM-NEGATIVE BACILLI—continued

Organism	First Choice	Alternatives
*Pseudomonas pseudomallei (melioidosis)	Ceftazidime[5]	Chloramphenicol[12] + doxycycline[9] + trimethoprim-sulfamethoxazole; amoxicillin/clavulanic acid; imipenem
*Pseudomonas cepacia	Trimethoprim-sulfamethoxazole	Ceftazidime[5]; chloramphenicol[12]
Spirillum minus (rat-bite fever)	Penicillin G	A tetracycline[9]; streptomycin
Streptobacillus moniliformis (rat-bite fever; Haverhill fever)	Penicillin G	A tetracycline[9]; streptomycin
Vibrio cholerae (cholera)[33]	A tetracycline[9]	Trimethoprim-sulfamethoxazole; a fluoroquinolone[3]
Vibrio vulnificus	A tetracycline[9]	Cefotaxime[5]
*Xanthomonas maltophilia (Pseudomonas maltophilia)	Trimethoprim-sulfamethoxazole	Minocycline[9]; ceftazidime[5]; a fluoroquinolone[3]
Yersinia pestis (plague)	Streptomycin	A tetracycline[9]; chloramphenicol[12]; gentamicin

ACID FAST BACILLI

Organism	First Choice	Alternatives
*Mycobacterium tuberculosis[34]	Isoniazid + rifampin + pyrazinamide ± ethambutol or streptomycin[12]	Ciprofloxacin or ofloxacin[31]; cycloserine[12]; capreomycin[12] or kanamycin[12] or amikacin[12]; ethionamide[12]; clofazimine[12]; para-aminosalicylic acid[12]
*Mycobacterium kansasii	Isoniazid + rifampin ± ethambutol or streptomycin[12]	Ethionamide[12]; cycloserine[12]
*Mycobacterium avium complex	Clarithromycin or azithromycin + one or more of the following: ethambutol; clofazimine[12]; ciprofloxacin[31]; amikacin[12]	Rifabutin; rifampin; ethionamide[12]; cycloserine[12]; imipenem
Prophylaxis	Rifabutin	
*Mycobacterium fortuitum complex	Amikacin + doxycycline[9]	Cefoxitin[5]; rifampin; a sulfonamide

[30] Metronidazole is effective for bacterial vaginosis, even though it is not usually active against Gardnerella in vitro.
[31] Usually not recommended for use in children.
[32] Neither gentamicin, tobramycin, netilmicin, nor amikacin should be mixed in the same bottle with carbenicillin, ticarcillin, mezlocillin, or piperacillin for intravenous administration. When used in high doses or in patients with renal impairment, these penicillins may inactivate the aminoglycosides.
[33] Antibiotic therapy is an adjunct to and not a substitute for prompt fluid and electrolyte replacement.
[34] For more details, see Medical Letter 1993;35:99.

Table 3.10—continued

Infecting Organism	Drug of First Choice	Alternative Drugs
ACID FAST BACILLI—continued		
Mycobacterium marinum (balnei)[35]	Minocycline[9]	Trimethoprim-sulfamethoxazole; rifampin; clarithromycin
Mycobacterium leprae (leprosy)	Dapsone + rifampin ± clofazimine	Minocycline[9]; protionamide[12,36], ofloxacin[31,37]; clarithromycin[38]
ACTINOMYCETES		
Actinomyces israelii (actinomycosis)	Penicillin G	A tetracycline[9]; erythromycin; clindamycin
Nocardia	Trimethoprim-sulfamethoxazole	Sulfisoxazole; amikacin[12]; minocycline[9]; imipenem; cycloserine[12]
CHLAMYDIAE		
Chlamydia psittaci (psittacosis; ornithosis)	A tetracycline[9]	Chloramphenicol[12]
Chlamydia trachomatis (Trachoma)	Azithromycin	A tetracycline[9] (topical plus oral); a sulfonamide (topical plus oral)
(Inclusion conjunctivitis)	An erythromycin (oral or i.v.)	A sulfonamide
(Pneumonia)	An erythromycin	A sulfonamide
(Urethritis, cervicitis)	Doxycycline[9] or azithromycin	Erythromycin; ofloxacin[31]; sulfisoxazole; amoxicillin
(Lymphogranuloma venereum)	A tetracycline[9]	Erythromycin
Chlamydia pneumoniae (TWAR strain)	A tetracycline[9]	An erythromycin; clarithromycin
MYCOPLASMA		
Mycoplasma pneumoniae	An erythromycin or a tetracycline[9]	Clarithromycin; azithromycin
Ureaplasma urealyticum	An erythromycin	A tetracycline[9]; clarithromycin

Organism	Drug of first choice	Alternative drugs
RICKETTSIA—Rocky Mountain spotted fever, endemic typhus (murine), epidemic typhus (louse-borne), scrub typhus, trench fever, Q fever, human ehrlichiosis[39]	A tetracycline[9]	Chloramphenicol[12,40]; a fluoroquinolone[3]
ROCHALIMAEA		
Agent of bacillary angiomatosis (*Rochalimaea henselae or quintana*)[41]	An erythromycin	Doxycycline[9]
Cat-scratch bacillus (*Rochalimaea henselae*)[41,42]	Ciprofloxacin[43]	Trimethoprim-sulfamethoxazole; gentamicin; rifampin
SPIROCHETES		
Borrelia burgdorferi (Lyme disease)[44]	Doxycycline[9] or amoxicillin	Cefuroxime axetil[5]; ceftriaxone[5]; cefotaxime[5]; penicillin G; azithromycin; clarithromycin
Borrelia recurrentis (relapsing fever)	A tetracycline[9]	Penicillin G
Leptospira	Penicillin G	A tetracycline[9]
Treponema pallidum	Penicillin G[4]	A tetracycline[9]; ceftriaxone[5]
Treponema pertenue (yaws)	Penicillin G	A tetracycline[9]

[35] Most infections are self-limited without drug treatment.
[36] An investigational drug in the United States.
[37] Ji B et al. Antimicrob Agents Chemother April 1994;38:662.
[38] Chan GP et al. Antimicrob Agents Chemother March 1994;38:515.
[39] Raoult D, Drancourt M. Antimicrob Agents Chemother 1991;35:2457.
[40] Not recommended for human ehrlichiosis.
[41] Adal KA et al. N Engl J Med May 26, 1994;330:1509.
[42] Role of antibiotics is not clear (Margileth AM. Pediatr Infect Dis J, 1992;11:474).
[43] Ciprofloxacin is not recommended for use in children.
[44] For treatment of early infection in nonpregnant adults, tetracycline is preferred; for fully developed infection with arthritis or meningitis, ceftriaxone is preferred.

SECTION 4
Prophylactic Antibiotics

Surgical Prophylaxis[a]

Antimicrobial prophylaxis can decrease the incidence of infection, particularly wound infection, after certain operations, but this benefit must be weighed against the risks of toxic and allergic reactions, emergence of resistant bacteria, and superinfection (1). *Medical Letter* consultants generally recommend antimicrobial prophylaxis only for procedures with high infection rates and those involving implantation of prosthetic material.

TIMING

With many antimicrobials, a single dose given just before the procedure provides adequate tissue concentrations throughout the operation. When surgery is prolonged or massive blood loss occurs, or when an antimicrobial with a short half-life is used, such as cefoxitin (Mefoxin), giving a second dose during the procedure may be advisable. Postoperative doses of prophylactic drugs are generally unnecessary.

CARDIAC

Prophylactic antibiotics can decrease the incidence of infection after open-heart surgery, including valvular procedures and coronary artery bypass grafts (2). Single doses appear to be as effective as multiple doses, provided that high concentrations are maintained in the blood throughout the operation. Prophylaxis may not be necessary for pacemaker implantation in centers with a low incidence of infection.

NONCARDIAC THORACIC

Controlled trials of antimicrobial prophylaxis have produced conflicting results in pulmonary resection; some have shown a decrease in wound infection, but not in pneumonia or empyema (3, 4). Prophylactic antimicrobials may prevent empyema after closed-tube thoracostomy for chest trauma, but the evidence is limited (5).

---

[a] Modified and reprinted with permission from The Medical Letter, Inc. Oct. 1, 1993;35(906):91–94.

VASCULAR

Preoperative administration of a cephalosporin decreases the incidence of postoperative wound infection after arterial reconstructive surgery on the abdominal aorta; vascular operations on the leg, which include a groin incision; and amputation of the lower extremity for ischemia (6). Many clinicians also recommend prophylaxis for implantation of any vascular prosthetic material, including grafts for vascular access in hemodialysis.

ORTHOPAEDIC

Prophylactic antistaphylococcal drugs can decrease the incidence of both early and late infection in prosthetic joints following total hip replacement (7, 8). They also decrease the rate of infection when hip and other fractures are treated with internal fixation by nails, plates, screws, or wires. *Medical Letter* consultants disagree on whether patients with indwelling prosthetic joints should receive antimicrobial prophylaxis routinely when undergoing dental, gastrointestinal, or genitourinary procedures; for long procedures, surgery in an infected area, or other procedures with a high risk of bacteremia, administration of an antistaphylococcal agent may be advisable.

NEUROSURGERY

Studies of antimicrobial prophylaxis for implantation of cerebrospinal fluid shunts have produced conflicting results (9). In spinal surgery, the postoperative infection rate after conventional lumbar discectomy is so low that antibiotics have not been shown to be effective; infection rates are higher after spinal procedures involving fusion or prolonged spinal surgery; and use of prophylactic antibiotics is common, but controlled trials of such use are lacking. An antistaphylococcal antibiotic may decrease the incidence of infection after craniotomy (9–11).

OPHTHALMIC

Data are limited on the effectiveness of antimicrobial prophylaxis for ophthalmic surgery, but postoperative endophthalmitis can be devastating. Most ophthalmologists use antimicrobial eyedrops for prophylaxis, and many also give a subconjunctival injection at the end of the procedure.

HEAD AND NECK

Prophylaxis with antimicrobials has decreased the high incidence of wound infection after head and neck operations that involve an incision through the oral or pharyngeal mucosa (12). Gentamicin eardrops may decrease the incidence of purulent otorrhea after placement of a tympanostomy tube (13).

GASTRODUODENAL

The risk of infection after gastroduodenal surgery is high when gastric acidity and gastrointestinal motility are diminished by obstruction, hemorrhage, gastric ulcer, or malignancy, or by therapy with histamine H_2-receptor agonists, such as cimetidine (Tagamet), ranitidine (Zantac), nizatidine (Axid), or famotidine (Pepcid). Preoperative use of a cephalosporin can decrease the incidence of postoperative infection in these circumstances and also after gastric bypass surgery for obesity or percutaneous endoscopic gastrostomy (14).

BILIARY TRACT

Antimicrobials are recommended before biliary tract surgery only for patients with an increased risk of infection—those more than 70 years old and those with acute cholecystitis, obstructive jaundice, or common duct stones.

COLORECTAL

Preoperative antibiotics can decrease the incidence of infection after colorectal surgery; for elective operations, an oral regimen appears to be as effective as parenteral drugs (15). Whether a combination of oral and parenteral agents would be more effective than either alone is unclear. The prophylactic regimen should include antimicrobials effective against both facultative Gram-negative bacilli and anaerobes such as *Bacteroides fragilis*.

APPENDECTOMY

Preoperative antimicrobials can decrease the incidence of infection after appendectomy. Regimens with activity against both facultative Gram-negative bacilli and anaerobes are more effective than those active against either alone (16).

GYNECOLOGY AND OBSTETRICS

Antimicrobial prophylaxis decreases the incidence of infection after vaginal hysterectomy and possibly after abdominal hysterectomy (17). Perioperative or preoperative antimicrobials can prevent infection after emergency cesarean section in high-risk situations such as active labor or premature rupture of membranes, after first-trimester abortion in high-risk women, and also after midtrimester abortions (18).

UROLOGY

Infectious disease experts do not recommend antimicrobials before urological operations in patients with sterile urine. When the urine culture is positive or unavailable, patients should be treated to sterilize the urine before surgery or receive a single preoperative dose of an appropriate agent (19).

OTHER PROCEDURES

Prophylaxis with antimicrobial drugs is not routinely recommended for cardiac catheterization, gastrointestinal endoscopy, arterial puncture, thoracentesis, paracentesis, repair of simple lacerations, or outpatient treatment of burns.

Table 4.1. Antibiotic Prophylaxis for Surgical Procedures

Procedure	Likely Pathogens	Recommended Regimen	Adult Dosage before Surgery[a]
Clean			
Cardiac			
Prosthetic valve, coronary artery bypass, other open-heart surgery, pacemaker implant	Staphylococcus epidermidis, S. aureus, Corynebacterium, enteric Gram-negative bacilli	Cefazolin or cefuroxime OR vancomycin[c]	1–2 gm i.v.[b] 1 gm i.v.
Vascular			
Arterial surgery involving the abdominal aorta, a prosthesis, or a groin incision	S. aureus, S. epidermidis, enteric Gram-negative bacilli	Cefazolin OR vancomycin[c]	1–2 gm i.v. 1 gm i.v.
Lower extremity amputation for ischemia	S. aureus, S. epidermidis, enteric Gram-negative bacilli, clostridia	Cefazolin OR vancomycin[c]	1 gm i.v. 1 gm i.v.
Neurosurgery			
Craniotomy	S. aureus, S. epidermidis	Cefazolin OR vancomycin[c]	1 gm i.v. 1 gm i.v.
Orthopaedic			
Total joint replacement, internal fixation of fractures	S. aureus, S. epidermidis	Cefazolin OR vancomycin[c]	1–2 gm i.v. 1 gm i.v.
Ophthalmic	S. aureus, S. epidermidis, streptococci, enteric Gram-negative bacilli, Pseudomonas	Gentamicin OR tobramycin OR neomycin-gramicidin-polymyxin B Cefazolin	Multiple drops topically over 2–24 hr 100 mg subconjunctivally at end of procedure

Table 4.1—continued

Procedure	Likely Pathogens	Recommended Regimen	Adult Dosage before Surgery[a]
Clean-contaminated			
Head and neck			
Entering oral cavity or pharynx	S. aureus, streptococci, oral anaerobes	Cefazolin OR clindamycin	1–2 gm i.v. 600–900 mg i.v.
Abdominal			
Gastroduodenal	Enteric Gram-negative bacilli, Gram-positive cocci	High risk, gastric bypass, or percutaneous endoscopic gastrostomy only: cefazolin	1 gm i.v.
Biliary tract	Enteric Gram-negative bacilli, enterococci, clostridia	High risk only: cefazolin	1 gm i.v.
Colorectal	Enteric Gram-negative bacilli, anaerobes	Oral: neomycin + erythromycin base[d]	
Appendectomy	Enteric Gram-negative bacilli, anaerobes	Parenteral: cefoxitin OR cefotetan Cefoxitin OR cefotetan	1 gm i.v. 1 gm i.v.
Gynecologic			
Vaginal or abdominal hysterectomy	Enteric Gram-negatives, anaerobes, group B streptococci enterococci	Cefazolin	1 gm i.v.
Cesarean section	Same as for hysterectomy	High risk only: cefazolin	1 gm i.v. after cord clamping
Abortion	Same as for hysterectomy	First trimester high risk:[e] aqueous penicillin G OR doxycycline Second trimester: cefazolin	1 million units i.v. 300 mg po[f] 1 gm i.v.

Dirty Surgery

Ruptured viscus[g]	Enteric Gram-negative bacilli, anaerobes, enterococci	Cefoxitin	2 gm i.v. q6h
		OR cefotetan	1–2 gm i.v. q12h
		either + gentamicin	1.5 mg/kg i.v. q8h
		OR clindamycin	600 mg i.v. q6h
		+ gentamicin	1.5 mg/kg i.v. q8h
Traumatic wound[g,h]	S. aureus, group A streptococci, clostridia	Cefazolin	1–2 gm i.v. q8h

[a] Parenteral prophylactic antimicrobials can be given as a single intravenous dose just before the operation. Cefazolin can also be given intramuscularly. For prolonged operations, additional intraoperative doses should be given q4–8h for the duration of the procedure.

[b] Some consultants recommend an additional dose when patients are removed from bypass during open-heart surgery.

[c] For hospitals in which methicillin-resistant S. aureus and S. epidermidis frequently cause wound infection or for patients allergic to penicillins or cephalosporins. Rapid intravenous administration may cause hypotension, which could be especially dangerous during induction of anesthesia. Even if the drug is given over 60 minutes, hypotension may occur. Treatment with diphenhydramine (Benadryl and others) and further slowing of the infusion rate may be helpful. (Maki DG et al. J Thorac Cardiovasc Surg 1992;104:1423.) For procedures in which enteric Gram-negative bacilli are likely pathogens, such as vascular surgery involving a groin incision, cefazolin should be included in the prophylaxis regimen.

[d] After appropriate diet and catharsis, 1 gm of each at 1 PM, 2 PM, and 11 PM the day before a morning operation.

[e] Patients with previous pelvic inflammatory disease, previous gonorrhea, or multiple sex partners.

[f] Divided into 100 mg 1 hour before the abortion and 200 mg ½ hour after.

[g] For dirty surgery, therapy should usually be continued for 5 to 10 days.

[h] For bite wounds, in which likely pathogens may also include oral anaerobes,ᵃ Eikenella corrodens (human), and Pasteurella multocida (dog and cat), some Medical Letter consultants recommend use of amoxicillin-clavulanic acid (Augmentin) or ampicillin-sulbactam (Unasyn).

"DIRTY" SURGERY

"Dirty" surgery, such as that for a perforated abdominal viscus, a compound fracture, or a laceration due to an animal or human bite, is often followed by infection; use of antimicrobial drugs for these operations is considered treatment rather than prophylaxis and should be continued postoperatively for several days.

CHOICE OF A PROPHYLACTIC AGENT

An effective prophylactic regimen should be directed against the most likely infecting organisms; it need not eradicate every potential pathogen; rather, the goal is to decrease their numbers below critical levels necessary to cause infection. For most procedures, cefazolin (Ancef and others), which has a moderately long serum half-life, has been effective. In institutions where methicillin-resistant *Staphylococcus aureus* or methicillin-resistant coagulase-negative staphylococci have become important pathogens, vancomycin (Vancocin and others) should be used. For colorectal surgery and appendectomy, *Medical Letter* consultants prefer cefoxitin (Mefoxin) or cefotetan (Cefotan), because they are more active than cefazolin against bowel anaerobes, including *B. fragilis*. For other abdominal and pelvic procedures, including obstetrical and gynecological operations, cefazolin has been equally effective and is less expensive. Third-generation cephalosporins, such as cefotaxime (Claforan), ceftriaxone (Rocephin), cefoperazone (Cefobid), ceftazidime (Fortaz; Tazicef; Tazidime), or ceftizoxime (Cefizox), should not be used for surgical prophylaxis. They are expensive; their activity against staphylococci is often less than that of cefazolin; their spectrum of activity against facultative Gram-negative bacilli includes organisms rarely encountered in elective surgery; and their widespread use for prophylaxis promotes emergence of resistance to these potentially valuable drugs. See Table 4.1.

REFERENCES

1. Kaiser AB. Postoperative infections and antimicrobial prophylaxis. In: Mandell GL, Douglas RG, Bennett JE, eds. Principles and practice of infectious diseases. 3rd ed. New York: Churchill Livingstone, 1990:2245.
2. Ariano RE, Zhanel GG. Antimicrobial prophylaxis in coronary bypass surgery: a critical appraisal (published erratum appears in DICP 1991). DICP Ann Pharmacother 1991;25(7–8):876.
3. Aznar R, Mateu M, Miro JM, Gatell JM, et al. Antibiotic prophylaxis in non-cardiac thoracic surgery: cefazolin versus placebo. Eur J Cardiothorac Surg 1991;5:515.
4. Hopkins CC. Antibiotic prophylaxis in clean surgery: peripheral vascular surgery, noncardiovascular thoracic surgery, herniorrhaphy, and mastectomy. Rev Infect Dis 1991;13(suppl 10):S869–873.
5. Fallon WF Jr, Wears RL. Prophylactic antibiotics for the prevention of infectious complications including empyema following tube thoracostomy for trauma: results of meta-analysis. J Trauma 1992;33(1):110–116.
6. Strachan CJ. Antibiotic prophylaxis in peripheral vascular and orthopaedic prosthetic surgery. J Antimicrob Chemother 1993;31(suppl B):65–78.
7. Fitzgerald RH Jr. Infections of hip prostheses and artificial joints. Infect Dis Clin North Am 1989;3(2):329–338.
8. Heath AF. Antimicrobial prophylaxis for arthroplasty and total joint replacement: discussion and review of published clinical trials. Pharmacotherapy 1991;11:157–163.
9. Brown EM. Antimicrobial prophylaxis in neurosurgery. J Antimicrob Chemother 1993;31(suppl B):49–63.

10. van Ek B, Dijkmans BA, van Dulken H, et al. Effect of cloxacillin prophylaxis on the bacterial flora of craniotomy wounds. Scand J Infect Dis 1990;22(3):345–352.
11. Djindjian M, Ayache P, Brugieres P, Malapert D, Baudrimont M, Poirier J. Giant gangliocytic paraganglioma of the filum terminale. J Neurosurg 1990;73(3):459–461.
12. Weber RS, Callender DL. Antibiotic prophylaxis in clean-contaminated head and neck oncologic surgery. Ann Otol Rhinol Laryngol 1992;101:16–20.
13. Baker RS, Chole RA. A randomized clinical trial of topical gentamicin after tympanostomy tube placement. Arch Otolaryngol 1988;114:755–757.
14. Jain NK, Larson DE, Schroeder KW, et al. Antibiotic prophylaxis for percutaneous endoscopic gastrostomy. A prospective, randomized, double-blind clinical trial. Ann Intern Med 1987;107(6):824–828.
15. Gorbach SL, Condon RE, Conte JE Jr, et al. Evaluation of new anti-infective drugs for surgical prophylaxis. Clin Infect Dis 1992;15(suppl 1):S313–338.
16. Browder W, Smith JW, Vivoda LM, Nichols RL. Nonperforative appendicitis: a continuing surgical dilemma. J Infect Dis 1989;159(6):1088–1094.
17. Hemsell DL. Prophylactic antibiotics in gynecologic and obstetric surgery. Rev Infect Dis 1991;13(suppl 10):S821–S841.
18. Houang ET. Antibiotic prophylaxis in hysterectomy and induced abortion. A review of the evidence. Drugs 1991;41(1):19–37.
19. Kunin CM. Detection, prevention and management of urinary tract infections. 4th ed. Philadelphia: Lea & Febiger, 1987:361.

Prevention of Bacterial Endocarditis[b]

Surgical and dental procedures and instrumentations involving mucosal surfaces or contaminated tissue commonly cause transient bacteremia that rarely persists for more than 15 minutes. Blood-borne bacteria may lodge on damaged or abnormal heart valves or on the endocardium or the endothelium near congenital anatomical defects, resulting in bacterial endocarditis or endarteritis. Although bacteremia is common following many invasive procedures, only a limited number of bacterial species commonly cause endocarditis. It is impossible to predict which patient will develop this infection or which particular procedure will be responsible.

Certain cardiac conditions are more often associated with endocarditis than others (Table 4.2). Furthermore, certain dental and surgical procedures are much more likely to initiate the bacteremia that results in endocarditis than are other procedures (Table 4.3). Prophylactic antibiotics are recommended for patients at risk for developing endocarditis who are undergoing those procedures most likely to produce bacteremia with organisms that commonly cause endocarditis.

Prophylaxis is most effective when given perioperatively in doses that are sufficient to ensure adequate antibiotic concentrations in the serum during and after the procedure. To reduce the likelihood of microbial resistance, it is important that prophylactic antibiotics be used only during the perioperative period. They should be initiated shortly before a procedure (1 to 2 hours) and should not be continued for an extended period (no more than 6 to 8 hours). In the case of delayed healing, or of a procedure that involves infected tissue, it may be necessary to provide additional doses of antibiotics.

[b] Reprinted from Committee on Rheumatic Fever, Endocarditis and Kawasaki Disease of the Council on Cardiovascular Disease in the Young, American Heart Association. JAMA 1990;204:2919.

Table 4.2.   Cardiac Conditions[a]

Endocarditis prophylaxis recommended

Prosthetic cardiac valves, including bioprosthetic and homograft valves
Previous bacterial endocarditis, even in the absence of heart disease
Most congenital cardiac malformations
Rheumatic and other acquired valvular dysfunction, even after valvular surgery
Hypertrophic cardiomyopathy
Mitral valve prolapse with valvular regurgitation

Endocarditis prophylaxis not recommended

Isolated secundum atrial septal defect
Surgical repair without residua beyond 6 months of secundum atrial septal defect, ventricular septal defect, or patent ductus arteriosus
Previous coronary artery bypass graft surgery
Mitral valve prolapse without valvular regurgitation
Physiological, functional, or innocent heart murmurs
Previous Kawasaki disease without valvular dysfunction
Previous rheumatic fever without valvular dysfunction
Cardiac pacemakers and implanted defibrillators

[a] This table lists selected conditions but is not meant to be all-inclusive.

In addition to using a prophylactic regimen for genitourinary procedures, antibiotic therapy should be directed against the most likely bacterial pathogen.

In patients who have prosthetic heart valves, a previous history of endocarditis, or surgically constructed systemic-pulmonary shunts or conduits, physicians may choose to administer prophylactic antibiotics, even for low-risk procedures that involve the lower respiratory, genitourinary, or gastrointestinal tracts.

This statement represents recommended guidelines to supplement practitioners in the exercise of their clinical judgment and is not intended as a standard of care for all cases. It is impossible to make recommendations for all clinical situations in which endocarditis may develop. Practitioners must exercise their own clinical judgment in determining the choice of antibiotics and number of doses that are to be administered in individual cases or special circumstances. Furthermore, because endocarditis may occur despite appropriate antibiotic prophylaxis, physicians and dentists should maintain a high index of suspicion regarding any unusual clinical events (such as unexplained fever, weakness, lethargy, or malaise) following dental or other surgical procedures in patients who are at risk for developing bacterial endocarditis.

Because no adequate, controlled clinical trials of antibiotic regimens for the prevention of bacterial endocarditis in humans have been done, recommendations are based on in vitro studies, clinical experience, data from experimental animal models, and assessment of both the bacteria most likely to produce bacteremia from a given site and those most likely to result in endocarditis. The substantial morbidity and mortality in patients who have endocarditis and the paucity of controlled clinical studies emphasize the need for continuing research into the epidemiology, pathogenesis, prevention, and therapy of endocarditis.

Table 4.3.   Dental or Surgical Procedures[a]

Endocarditis prophylaxis recommended

    Dental procedures known to induce gingival or mucosal bleeding, including professional cleaning
    Tonsillectomy and/or adenoidectomy
    Surgical operations that involve intestinal or respiratory mucosa
    Bronchoscopy with a rigid bronchoscope
    Sclerotherapy for esophageal varices
    Esophageal dilation
    Gallbladder surgery
    Cystoscopy
    Urethral dilatation
    Urethral catheterization if urinary tract infection is present
    Urinary tract surgery if urinary tract infection is present
    Prostatic surgery
    Incision and drainage of infected tissue
    Vaginal hysterectomy
    Vaginal delivery in the presence of infection

Endocarditis prophylaxis not recommended

    Dental procedures not likely to induce gingival bleeding, such as simple adjustment of orthodontic appliances or fillings above the gum line
    Injection of local intraoral anesthetic (except intraligamentary injections)
    Shedding of primary teeth
    Tympanotomy tube insertion
    Endotracheal intubation
    Bronchoscopy with a flexible bronchoscope, with or without biopsy
    Cardiac catheterization
    Endoscopy with or without gastrointestinal biopsy
    Cesarean section
    In the absence of infection for urethral catheterization, dilatation and curettage, uncomplicated vaginal delivery, therapeutic abortion, sterilization procedures, or insertion or removal of intrauterine devices

[a] This table lists selected procedures but is not meant to be all-inclusive.

The current recommendations are an update of those made by the Committee in 1984. They incorporate new data and include opinions of national and international experts.

Standard Prophylactic Regimen for Dental, Oral, and Upper Respiratory Tract Procedures

Poor dental hygiene and periodontal or periapical infections may produce bacteremia, even in the absence of dental procedures. Individuals who are at risk for developing bacterial endocarditis should establish and maintain the best possible oral health to reduce potential sources of bacterial seeding. Dentists should make every attempt to reduce gingival inflammation in patients who are at risk by means of brushing, flossing, fluoride rinse, chlorhexidine gluconate mouth rinse, and professional cleaning before proceeding with routine dental procedures. Chlorhexidine that is painted on isolated and dried gingiva 3 to 5 minutes prior to tooth extraction has been shown to reduce postextraction bacteremia. Other agents such as povidone-iodine or iodine and glycerin may also be appropriate. Furthermore, irrigation of the gingival sulcus with chlorhexidine prior to tooth extraction has been shown to reduce postextraction bacteremia in adults. Application of chlorhexidine may be used as an adjunct to antibiotic prophylaxis, particularly in patients who are at high risk and/or have poor dental hygiene.

Antibiotic prophylaxis is recommended with all dental procedures likely to cause gingival bleeding, including routine professional cleaning. If a series of dental procedures is required, it may be prudent to observe an interval of 7 days between procedures to reduce the potential for the emergence of resistant strains of organisms. If possible, a combination of procedures should be planned in the same period of prophylaxis. Edentulous patients may develop bacteremia from ulcers caused by ill-fitting dentures; therefore, denture wearers should be encouraged to have periodic examinations or to return to the practitioner if soreness develops. When new dentures are inserted, it is advisable to have the patient return to the practitioner to correct any overextension that could cause mucosal ulceration. Because the spontaneous shedding of primary teeth or simple adjustment of orthodontic appliances does not present a significant risk of endocarditis, antibiotic prophylaxis is not necessary in these situations. Similarly, endotracheal intubation is not an indication for antibiotic prophylaxis unless it is associated with another procedure for which prophylaxis is recommended.

α-Hemolytic (viridans) streptococci are the most common cause of endocarditis following dental procedures, and prophylaxis should be specifically directed against these organisms. Certain upper respiratory tract procedures, such as tonsillectomy and/or adenoidectomy, bronchoscopy with a rigid bronchoscope, and surgical procedures that involve the respiratory mucosa, may also cause bacteremia with organisms that commonly cause endocarditis and have antibiotic susceptibilities similar to those producing bacteremia following dental procedures. Therefore, the same regimen is recommended for these procedures as is recommended for dental procedures. Endocarditis has not been reported in association with insertion of tympanotomy tubes.

The recommended standard prophylactic regimen for all dental, oral, and upper respiratory tract procedures is amoxicillin (Table 4.4). The antibiotics amoxicillin, ampicillin, and penicillin V are equally effective in vitro against α-hemolytic streptococci; however, amoxicillin is now recommended because it is better absorbed from the gastrointestinal tract and provides higher and more sustained serum levels. The choice of penicillin V rather than amoxicillin as prophylaxis against α-hemolytic streptococcal bacteremia following dental, oral, and upper respiratory tract procedures is rational and acceptable.

Individuals who are allergic to penicillins (such as amoxicillin, ampicillin, or penicillin) should be treated with the provided alternative oral regimens. Erythromycin ethylsuccinate and erythromycin stearate are recommended because of more rapid and reliable absorption than other erythromycin formulations, resulting in higher and more sustained serum levels. For individuals who cannot

Table 4.4. Recommended Standard Prophylactic Regimen for Dental, Oral, or Upper Respiratory Tract Procedures in Patients Who Are at Risk[a]

Drug	Dosing Regimen
Standard regimen	
Amoxicillin	3.0 gm orally 1 hr before procedure; then 1.5 q6h after initial dose
Regimen for amoxicillin/penicillin-allergic patients	
Erythromycin	Erythromycin ethylsuccinate, 800 mg, or erythromycin stearate, 1.0 gm, orally 2 hr before procedure, then half the dose 6 hr after initial dose
or	
Clindamycin	300 mg orally 1 hr before procedure and 150 mg 6 hr after initial dose

[a] Includes those with prosthetic heart valves and other high-risk patients.

tolerate either penicillins or erythromycin, clindamycin hydrochloride is the recommended alternative. Tetracyclines and sulfonamides are not recommended for endocarditis prophylaxis.

Alternate Prophylactic Regimens for Dental, Oral, and Upper Respiratory Tract Procedures

Table 4.5 lists alternate prophylactic regimens for individuals who may not be candidates to receive the standard prophylactic regimen. For individuals who are unable to take oral medications, a parenteral agent may be necessary. Ampicillin sodium is recommended because parenteral amoxicillin is not available in the United States. When parenteral administration is needed in an individual who is allergic to penicillin, clindamycin phosphate is recommended.

Individuals who have prosthetic heart valves, a previous history of endocarditis, or surgically constructed systemic-pulmonary shunts or conduits are at high risk for developing endocarditis, and endocardial infection in such individuals is associated with substantial morbidity and mortality. For this reason, previous recommendations of this committee emphasized the use of stringent prophylactic regimens, with a strong preference for the parenteral route of administration. In practice, there are substantial logistic and financial barriers to the use of parenteral regimens. Moreover, oral regimens have now been used in individuals in other countries who have prosthetic heart valves, and failures in prophylaxis have not been a problem. Consequently, the Committee recommends the use of the standard prophylactic regimen (Table 4.4) in patients who have prosthetic heart valves and in the other high-risk groups. It is recognized that some practitioners may prefer to use parenteral prophylaxis in these high-risk groups of patients. Accordingly, an alternate regimen is also provided in Table 4.5.

Table 4.5. Alternate Prophylactic Regimens for Dental, Oral, or Upper Respiratory Tract Procedures in Patients Who Are at Risk

Drug	Dosing Regimen[a]
Patients unable to take oral medications	
Ampicillin	Intravenous or intramuscular administration of ampicillin, 2.0 gm, 30 min before procedure; then intravenous or intramuscular administration of ampicillin, 1.0 gm, or oral administration of amoxicillin, 1.5 gm, 6 hr after initial dose
Ampicillin/amoxicillin/penicillin-allergic patients unable to take oral medications	
Clindamycin	Intravenous administration of 300 mg 30 min before procedure and an intravenous or oral administration of 150 mg 6 hr after initial dose
Patients considered high risk and not candidates for standard regimen	
Ampicillin, gentamicin, and amoxicillin	Intravenous or intramuscular administration of ampicillin, 2.0 gm, plus gentamicin, 1.5 mg/kg (not to exceed 80 mg), 30 min before procedure; followed by amoxicillin, 1.5 gm, orally 6 hr after initial dose; alternatively, the parenteral regimen may be repeated 8 hr after initial dose
Ampicillin/amoxicillin/penicillin-allergic patients considered high risk	
Vancomycin	Intravenous administration of 1.0 gm over 1 hr, starting 1 hr before procedure; no repeated dose necessary

[a] Initial pediatric doses are as follows: ampicillin, 50 mg/kg; clindamycin, 10 mg/kg, gentamicin, 2.0 mg/kg; and vancomycin, 20 mg/kg. Follow-up doses should be one half the initial dose. *Total pediatric dose should not exceed total adult dose.* No initial dose is recommended in this table for amoxicillin (25 mg/kg is the follow-up dose).

Regimens for Genitourinary and Gastrointestinal Procedures

Surgery, instrumentation, or diagnostic procedures that involve the genitourinary or gastrointestinal tracts may cause bacteremia. The rate of bacteremia that is found following urinary tract procedures is high if urinary tract infection is present. Although the risk that any particular patient will develop endocarditis is low, the genitourinary tract is second only to the oral cavity as a portal of entry for organisms that cause endocarditis. The instrumented gastrointestinal tract seems to be less important as a portal of entry for organisms that cause bacterial endocarditis than the oral cavity or genitourinary tract.

Bacterial endocarditis that occurs following genitourinary and gastrointestinal tract surgery or instrumentation is most often caused by *Enterococcus faecalis* (enterococci). Although Gram-negative bacillary bacteremia may follow these procedures, Gram-negative bacilli are only rarely responsible for endocarditis. Thus, antibiotic prophylaxis to prevent endocarditis that occurs following genitourinary or gastrointestinal procedures should be directed primarily against entero-cocci.

Table 4.6 outlines the recommended regimens for prophylaxis for genitouri-nary or gastrointestinal tract procedures. The Committee continues to recommend parenteral antibiotics, particularly in high-risk patients (e.g., those with prosthetic heart valves or a previous history of endocarditis). In low-risk patients, an alterna-tive oral regimen is provided.

Specific Situations and Circumstances

RHEUMATIC FEVER

Antibiotic regimens used to prevent the recurrence of acute rheumatic fever are inadequate to the prevention of bacterial endocarditis. Individuals who take an oral penicillin for secondary prevention of rheumatic fever or for other purposes may have viridans streptococci in their oral cavities that are relatively resistant to penicillin, amoxicillin, or ampicillin. In such cases, the physician or dentist should select erythromycin or another of the alternative regimens (listed in Tables 4.4 and 4.5), instead of amoxicillin (or another penicillin) for endocarditis prophy-laxis.

Table 4.6.   Regimens for Genitourinary/Gastrointestinal Procedures

Drug	Dosing Regimen[a]
Standard regimen	
Ampicillin, gentamicin, and amoxicillin	Intravenous or intramuscular administration of ampicillin, 2.0 gm, plus gentamicin, 1.5 mg/kg (not to exceed 80 mg), 30 min before procedure; followed by amoxicillin, 1.5 gm, orally 6 hr after initial dose; alternatively, the parenteral regimen may be repeated once 8 hr after initial dose
Ampicillin/amoxicillin/penicillin-allergic patient regimen	
Vancomycin and gentamicin	Intravenous administration of vancomycin, 1.0 gm over 1 hr plus intravenous or intramuscular administration of gentamicin, 1.5 mg/kg (not to exceed 80 mg), 1 hr before procedure; may be repeated once 8 hr after initial dose
Alternate low-risk patient/regimen	
Amoxicillin	3.0 gm orally 1 hr before procedure; then 1.5 gm 6 hr after initial dose

[a] Initial pediatric doses are as follows: ampicillin, 50 mg/kg; amoxicillin, 50 mg/kg; gentamicin, 2.0 mg/kg; and vancomycin, 20 mg/kg. Follow-up doses should be half the initial dose. *Total pediatric dose should not exceed total adult dose.*

PATIENTS WHO RECEIVE ANTICOAGULANTS

Intramuscular injections for endocarditis prophylaxis should be avoided in patients who receive heparin. The use of warfarin sodium is a relative contraindication to intramuscular injections. Intravenous or oral regimens should be used whenever possible.

PATIENTS WHO HAVE RENAL DYSFUNCTION

In patients who have a markedly compromised renal function, it may be necessary to modify or omit the second dose of gentamicin sulfate or vancomycin hydrochloride.

PATIENTS WHO UNDERGO CARDIAC SURGERY

Patients who have cardiac conditions (Table 4.2) that predispose them to endocarditis are at risk for developing bacterial endocarditis when undergoing open heart surgery. Similarly, patients who undergo surgery for placement of prosthetic heart valves or prosthetic intravascular or intracardiac materials are also at risk for the development of bacterial endocarditis. Because the morbidity and mortality of endocarditis in such patients are high, perioperative prophylactic antibiotics are recommended.

Endocarditis associated with open-heart surgery is most often caused by *S. aureus*, coagulase-negative staphylococci, or diphtheroids; streptococci, Gram-negative bacteria, and fungi are less common. No single antibiotic regimen is effective against all these organisms. Furthermore, prolonged use of broad-spectrum antibiotics may predispose to superinfection with unusual or resistant microorganisms.

Prophylaxis at the time of cardiac surgery should be directed primarily against staphylococci and should be of short duration. First-generation cephalosporins are most often used, but the choice of an antibiotic should be influenced by the antibiotic's susceptibility patterns at each hospital. For example, high prevalence of infection by methicillin-resistant *S. aureus* in a particular institution should prompt consideration of vancomycin for perioperative prophylaxis. Prophylaxis with the chosen antibiotic should be started immediately before the operative procedure, repeated during prolonged procedures to maintain levels intraoperatively, and continued for no more than 24 hours postoperatively to minimize emergence of resistant microorganisms. The effects of cardiopulmonary bypass and compromised postoperative renal function on antibiotic levels in the serum should be considered, and doses should be timed appropriately before and during the procedure.

A careful preoperative dental evaluation is recommended so that required dental treatment can be completed before cardiac surgery whenever possible. Such measures may decrease the incidence of late postoperative endocarditis.

STATUS FOLLOWING CARDIAC SURGERY

The same precautions that have been outlined for the patient who has not undergone a surgical procedure but is undergoing dental, gastrointestinal, genitourinary, or other procedures should be observed in the years following most heart or valvular surgery. The risk of developing endocarditis appears to continue indefinitely and is particularly significant for patients who have prosthetic heart valves. Furthermore, the morbidity and mortality that result from prosthetic valve endocarditis are high. Patients who have an isolated secundum atrial septal defect that has been surgically repaired, a ventricular septal defect, or patent ductus arteriosus do not seem to be at risk of developing endocarditis following a 6-month healing period after surgery. Data are insufficient to allow recommendations for prophylactic therapy after closure of these lesions by nonsurgical devices. There is no evidence that coronary artery bypass graft surgery introduces a risk for a patient's developing endocarditis. Therefore, antibiotic prophylaxis is not needed for this condition.

CARDIAC TRANSPLANTATION

There are insufficient data to support specific recommendations for patients who have had heart transplants. Some physicians place these patients in the category of people who will need prophylaxis, however.

SELECTED READINGS

Bisno AL, Dismukes WE, Durack DT, et al. Antimicrobial treatment of infective endocarditis due to viridans streptococci, enterococci, and staphylococci. JAMA 1989;261:1471–1477.

Dajani AS, Bisno AL, Chung KJ, et al. Prevention of rheumatic fever. Circulation. 1988;78:1082–1086.

Durack DT. Infective and noninfective endocarditis. In: Hurst JW, Schlant RC, Rackley CE, Sonnenblick EH, Wenger NK, eds. The heart. 7th ed. New York: McGraw-Hill Information Services Co., 1990:1230–1255.

Durack DT. Prophylaxis for infective endocarditis. In: Mandell GL, Douglas RG Jr, Bennett JE, eds. Principles and practice of infectious diseases. 3rd ed. New York: Churchill Livingstone, 1990:716–721.

Endocarditis Working Party of the British Society for Antimicrobial Chemotherapy. Antibiotic prophylaxis of infective endocarditis. Lancet 1990;335:88–89.

Horstkotte D, Friedrichs W, Pippert H, Bircks W, Loogen F. Benefit of prophylaxis for infectious endocarditis in patients with prosthetic heart valves [in German with English abstract]. Z Kardiol 1986;75:8–11.

Imperiale TF, Horwitz RI. Does prophylaxis prevent postdental infective endocarditis. Am J Med 1990;88:131–136.

Kaplan EL, Shulman ST. Endocarditis. In: Adams FH, Emmanouilides GC, Riemenschneider TA, eds. Moss' heart disease in infants, children, and adolescents. 4th ed. Baltimore: Williams & Wilkins, 1989:718–730.

Prevention of Rheumatic Fever[c]

Prevention of both initial and recurrent attacks of acute rheumatic fever depends on control of group A β-hemolytic streptococcal upper respiratory tract infections. These include tonsillopharyngitis (strep throat) and associated conditions such as otitis, sinusitis, and mastoiditis. Prevention of first attacks (primary

[c]Reprinted with permission from the report of the American Heart Association's Committee. A Statement for Health Professionals Prepared by the Committee on Rheumatic Fever and Infective Endocarditis of the Council of Cardiovascular Disease in the Young—1988. Circulation 71-1008 (CP).

prevention) is accomplished by proper identification and adequate antibiotic treatment of these streptococcal infections. The individual who has suffered an attack of rheumatic fever is inordinately susceptible to recurrences following subsequent group A streptococcal upper respiratory tract infections and needs continuous protection to prevent recurrences (secondary prevention).

The current recommendations reflect the fact that the incidence of rheumatic fever remains quite low in most areas of the country. These recommendations may not apply to certain areas of the United States where sharp increases in incidence of rheumatic fever have been noted recently or regions of the world that continue to have a high incidence of the disease. Reappearance of acute rheumatic fever in a specific geographic region should draw attention to therapeutic, preventive, and epidemiological measures as well as stimulate use of these recommendations.

PREVENTION OF INITIAL ATTACKS (PRIMARY PREVENTION)

Group A streptococcal infections of the upper respiratory tract are the precipitating cause of rheumatic fever. During epidemics, as many as 3% of untreated acute streptococcal sore throats may be followed by rheumatic fever; in endemic infections, attacks of rheumatic fever may be fewer. Appropriate antibiotic treatment of streptococcal upper respiratory tract infection prevents acute rheumatic fever in most cases. Unfortunately, it is not uncommon for episodes of acute rheumatic fever to result from inapparent streptococcal infections for which patients do not seek medical care. These episodes, therefore, are not preventable.

Diagnosis of Streptococcal Infections

Prevention of initial episodes of acute rheumatic fever requires accurate recognition and proper antibiotic treatment of group A streptococcal upper respiratory tract infections. Streptococcal skin infections (impetigo or pyoderma) do not lead to acute rheumatic fever and are not discussed here.

Symptoms common in individuals with streptococcal pharyngitis or tonsillitis include sore throat (generally of sudden onset), headache, and fever of varying degree (usually from 101 to 104°F). Abdominal pain, nausea, and vomiting may occur, especially in children. Clinical signs suggesting streptococcal infection include anterior cervical lymphadenitis (tender lymph nodes), inflamed throat, tonsillopharyngeal exudate, excoriated nares (especially in infants), and a scarlatiniform rash. However, most of these manifestations are nonspecific and may be associated with respiratory tract infections from other causes. Signs and symptoms usually not associated with streptococcal infection are simple coryza, hoarseness, cough, conjunctivitis, anterior stomatitis, and diarrhea.

Throat Culture.   Acute pharyngitis is more often caused by a virus rather than by group A streptococci. It is often difficult to differentiate on clinical grounds alone among infections caused by these etiologic agents. Group A streptococci are not a common cause of pharyngitis in children less than 3 years of age, and rheumatic fever is rare in this age group in the United States. First attacks of rheumatic fever are also rare in older adults.

Throat cultures are valuable in establishing diagnosis of streptococcal infection and management of the patient with pharyngitis. Group A streptococci are virtually always found on a throat culture obtained during an active infection in an untreated patient. Unfortunately, the culture does not reliably distinguish between acute streptococcal infections and streptococcal carriers with concomitant viral infections. Nevertheless, the culture allows the physician to withhold antibiotic therapy safely in the majority of patients with sore throat, that is, those with negative cultures for group A streptococci.

Rapid antigen detection tests for diagnosis of group A streptococcal pharyngitis are now available commercially and can provide results in minutes compared with the 24 to 48 hours required to obtain results of a throat culture. Most of these tests have a high degree of specificity; therefore, treatment is indicated for the patient with acute pharyngitis who has a positive test result. Physicians should be aware that most of these tests have less than the desired degree of sensitivity, particularly in instances where simultaneously obtained throat cultures show a sparse growth of group A streptococci. Therefore, negative test results must be confirmed with a throat culture. Sparse growth of group A streptococci does not necessarily reflect the carrier state and may indicate acute infection.

Streptococcal Antibody Tests. Streptococcal antibody tests are of no immediate value in diagnosis or management of acute streptococcal respiratory tract infections. However, antistreptolysin O (ASO), antideoxyribonuclease B (anti-DNase B), and other streptococcal antibody tests are useful in confirming a recent group A streptococcal infection. The tests are, therefore, helpful in patients who have possible nonsuppurative complications of streptococcal infections (acute rheumatic fever or acute glomerulonephritis). A commercially available agglutination test (such as the Streptozyme test), which is based on antibody agglutination of erythrocytes coated with a mixture of streptococcal antigens, is simpler to perform than traditional streptococcal antibody tests. However, the test suffers from significant variation in the potency of various lots, apparent lack of standardization, and poorly characterized antigenic composition and is not recommended.

Recommended Treatment Schedules

Prevention of rheumatic fever requires eradication of group A streptococci from the throat. Treatment should begin as soon as a definite diagnosis of group A streptococcal infection is made (Table 4.7). Penicillin, even when started several days after onset of acute illness, effectively prevents primary attacks of rheumatic fever; however, early diagnosis and therapy may reduce the period of infectivity as well as that of morbidity, allowing the patient to return to normal activity sooner. Virtually all patients are noncontagious 24 hours after initiation of therapy and may return to normal activities at that time, assuming that they complete the course of therapy.

Table 4.7. Primary Prevention of Rheumatic Fever (Treatment of Streptococcal Tonsillopharyngitis)

Agent[a]	Dose	Mode	Duration
Benzathine penicillin G	600,000 units for patients <60 lb 1,200,000 units for patients >60 lb	Intramuscular	Once
	or		
Penicillin V (phenoxymethyl penicillin)	250 mg 3 times daily	Oral	10 days
For individuals allergic to penicillin:			
Erythromycin estolate	20–40 mg/kg/day 2–4 times daily (maximum 1 gm/day)	Oral	10 days
	or		
Ethylsuccinate	40 mg/kg/day 2–4 times daily (maximum 1 gm/day)	Oral	10 days

[a] The following agents are acceptable but usually not recommended: amoxicillin, dicloxacillin, oral cephalosporins, and clindamycin. The following are not acceptable: sulfonamides, trimethoprim, tetracyclines, and chloramphenicol.

Penicillin is the drug of choice, except in patients with allergic reactions.[d] Broad-spectrum penicillins such as ampicillin and amoxicillin offer no advantages over penicillin in treatment of streptococcal pharyngitis. Penicillin may be administered intramuscularly or orally. Intramuscular administration of a single dose of benzathine penicillin G ensures adequate duration of treatment. If oral therapy is used, a full 10 days of treatment is necessary. Oral therapy requires patient compliance but may be associated with fewer allergic reactions. The choice between intramuscular and oral penicillin depends on the physician's assessment of the patient's likely compliance with an oral regimen and the risks of rheumatic fever in a particular population.

Intramuscular Benzathine Penicillin G.   This formulation is preferred for patients who are unlikely to complete a 10-day course of oral therapy, patients with a personal or family history of rheumatic fever, and patients whose geographic or socioeconomic environment is at substantial risk for development of rheumatic fever. Injections that contain procaine penicillin in addition to benzathine penicillin G are less painful. If such mixtures are used, they should contain benzathine penicillin G in the following doses:

The recommended dosage of benzathine penicillin G is 600,000 units intramuscularly for patients weighing 60 lb (27 kg) or less, and 1,200,000 units for patients weighing more than 60 lb. The combination of 900,000 units of benzathine penicillin G and 300,000 units of procaine penicillin G may be satisfactory in many smaller patients, but this dosage is based on limited data. The efficacy of

[d] Published reports conflict as to whether penicillin. especially ampicillin, interferes with effectiveness of oral contraceptives. The physician should advise the patient of childbearing age of possible drug interaction. The patient may choose to use a supplementary method of contraception while taking these antibiotics.

this combination for heavier patients such as teenagers or adults requires further study.

Oral Penicillin.   The oral antibiotic of choice is penicillin V. Dosage for both children and adults is 250 mg three times daily for 10 days. It is important to emphasize that patients should continue to take penicillin regularly for the entire 10-day period, even though they will likely be asymptomatic after the first few days.

Other Antimicrobial Agents.   Antibiotics other than penicillin should be prescribed only for patients who are allergic to penicillin. Erythromycin is indicated for such patients and should be prescribed for 10 days. Erythromycin estolate (20 to 40 mg/kg/day) in two to four divided doses, or erythromycin ethyl succinate (40 mg/kg/day in two to four divided doses) is effective in treating streptococcal pharyngitis; however, efficacy of a twice daily regimen in adults requires further study. The maximum dose of erythromycin is 1 gm/day. Although strains of group A streptococci resistant to erythromycin are prevalent in some areas of the world, they are rare in the United States.

Oral cephalosporins, also given for 10 days, are acceptable alternatives for the patient allergic to penicillin. However, they should not be used in patients with immediate hypersensitivity to penicillin and are more expensive.

Certain antimicrobials are not recommended for treatment of streptococcal upper respiratory tract infections. Tetracyclines should not be used because of the high prevalence of strains resistant to this antibiotic. Sulfonamide drugs will not eradicate the streptococcus and should not be used to treat streptococcal infection, although they are effective as continuous prophylaxis for recurrent attacks of rheumatic fever (see below). Similarly, trimethoprim-sulfamethoxazole should not be used to treat streptococcal pharyngitis.

PREVENTION OF RECURRENT ATTACKS OF RHEUMATIC FEVER (SECONDARY PREVENTION)

General Considerations

A rheumatic patient who develops a streptococcal upper respiratory tract infection is at high risk of developing a recurrent attack of acute rheumatic fever. An infection need not be symptomatic to trigger a recurrence, which can strike even in optimally treated symptomatic infections. For these reasons, prevention of recurrent rheumatic fever depends on continuous antimicrobial medication rather than solely on recognition and treatment of acute episodes of streptococcal pharyngitis. In general, continuous antimicrobial prophylaxis is recommended for patients with a well-documented history of rheumatic fever (including cases manifested solely by Sydenham's chorea) and those with definite evidence of rheumatic heart disease. Such prophylaxis should be initiated as soon as acute rheumatic fever or rheumatic heart disease is diagnosed. A full therapeutic course of penicillin (as outlined under Recommended Treatment Schedules) should first be given to patients with acute rheumatic fever to eradicate group A streptococci that may or may not be recovered on throat culture. Streptococcal infections

Table 4.8.   Secondary Prevention of Rheumatic Fever (Prevention of Recurrent Attacks)

Agent	Dose	Mode
Benzathine penicillin G	1,200,000 units	Intramuscular every 4 weeks[a]
	or	
Penicillin V	250 mg twice daily	Oral
	or	
Sulfadiazine	0.5 gm once daily for patients <60 lb 1.0 gm once daily for patients >60 lb	Oral
For individuals allergic to penicillin and sulfadiazine:		
Erythromycin	250 mg twice daily	Oral

[a] In high-risk situations, administration every 3 weeks is advised.

occurring in family members of rheumatic patients should be treated appropriately (Table 4.8).

Duration of Prophylaxis

Continuous antimicrobial prophylaxis provides the most effective protection from rheumatic fever recurrences. Risk of recurrence depends on several factors. For example, risk decreases as the interval since the most recent attack lengthens, while risk increases with multiple previous attacks. In addition, the patient's risk of acquiring a streptococcal upper respiratory tract infection must be considered. Adults with a high risk of exposure to streptococcal infections include parents of young children, teachers, physicians, nurses and allied health personnel, military recruits, and others living in crowded situations. Data also indicate a higher risk of recurrences in economically disadvantaged populations. Physicians must consider each patient's situation when determining appropriate duration of prophylaxis.

Patients who have had rheumatic carditis are at a relatively high risk for recurrences of carditis and are likely to sustain serious cardiac involvement with each recurrence. Therefore, patients who have had rheumatic carditis should receive long-term antibiotic prophylaxis well into adulthood and perhaps for life. Prophylaxis should continue even after valve surgery, including prosthetic valve replacement, because these patients remain at risk of recurrence of rheumatic fever.

In contrast, patients who have not had rheumatic carditis are at considerably less risk of cardiac involvement with a recurrence. Therefore, a physician may wish to discontinue prophylaxis in these patients after several years. In general, prophylaxis should continue until the patient is in his or her early 20s and five years have elapsed since the last rheumatic attack. The decision to continue prophylaxis should be made after discussion with the patient of potential risks and benefits and careful consideration of the epidemiological risk factors enumerated above.

Choice of Program for Prevention of Recurrent Rheumatic Fever

Intramuscular Benzathine Penicillin G.   An injection of 1,200,000 units of this long-acting penicillin preparation every 4 weeks is the recommended method of secondary prevention. In countries where incidence of acute rheumatic fever is particularly high, or in certain high-risk patients, use of benzathine penicillin G every 3 weeks may be warranted. Long-acting penicillin is of particular value in patients with a high risk of rheumatic fever recurrence, especially those with rheumatic heart disease in whom recurrence is more dangerous. In each patient, the advantages of benzathine penicillin G must be weighed against inconvenience to the patient and pain of injection, which may cause some patients to discontinue prophylaxis.

Oral Agents.   Successful oral prophylaxis depends primarily on patient compliance. Patients need careful and repeated instructions about the importance of continuing prophylaxis. Most failures of prophylaxis occur in noncompliant patients. Even with optimal compliance, risk of recurrence is still higher in those on regular oral prophylaxis compared to those receiving intramuscular benzathine penicillin G. Oral agents are more appropriate for patients at lower risk for rheumatic recurrence. Accordingly, some physicians elect to switch patients to oral prophylaxis when they have reached late adolescence or young adulthood and have remained free of rheumatic attacks for at least 5 years. In the doses recommended below, sulfadiazine and oral penicillin are about equally effective.

Sulfadiazine.   The dosage is 1.0 gm once daily for patients over 60 lb (27 kg) and 0.5 gm once daily for patients under 60 lb. Reactions are infrequent and usually minor. Blood counts may be advisable 2 weeks after starting prophylaxis, as leukopenia has been reported. Prophylaxis with sulfonamides is contraindicated in late pregnancy because of transplacental passage and competition with bilirubin for neonatal albumin-binding sites. Data comparing sulfadiazine and other sulfonamides are not available.

Penicillin V.   The dosage is 250 mg twice daily. Penicillin V is the preferred form of oral penicillin because it is relatively resistant to gastric acid. Allergic reactions are similar to those with intramuscular penicillin. Anaphylaxis is rare in patients receiving oral penicillin. NOTE: Allergic reactions to penicillin are more common in adults than they are in children. They occur in only a small percentage of patients, are more frequent after injection, and include urticaria and angioneurotic edema. A serum sickness-like reaction characterized by fever and joint pains may be mistaken for acute rheumatic fever. As with all penicillins, anaphylaxis, although rare, may occur. A careful history for allergic reactions to penicillin should be obtained.

Other Drugs.   For the exceptional patient who may be allergic to both penicillin and sulfonamides, erythromycin may be used. An appropriate dose has not been established, but 250 mg twice daily is suggested.

Bacterial Endocarditis Prophylaxis

Patients with evidence of rheumatic valvular heart disease also require additional short-term antibiotic prophylaxis before some surgical and dental procedures to prevent possible development of bacterial endocarditis. Antibiotic regimens used to prevent recurrences of acute rheumatic fever are inadequate for prevention of bacterial endocarditis. These patients should be protected by administration of appropriate antibiotics in recommended doses. Patients with prosthetic valves are at particularly high risk. The current recommendations of the American Heart Association concerning prevention of bacterial endocarditis should be followed. Patients who have had rheumatic fever but do not have evidence of rheumatic heart disease do not need endocarditis prophylaxis.

Special Problems

There is uncertainty about the most appropriate management of treatment failures, chronic carriers, and contacts.

Treatment Failures

Failure to eradicate group A streptococci from the throat usually occurs more frequently after oral antibiotic treatment than after administration of intramuscular benzathine penicillin G.

Because risk of acute rheumatic fever is low in most U.S. populations and most patients who fail treatment are streptococcal carriers, posttreatment throat cultures are now indicated only in patients who are at unusually high risk for rheumatic fever, who remain symptomatic, or who develop recurring symptoms. Repeated courses of antibiotic therapy are not indicated in asymptomatic patients who continue to harbor group A streptococci after appropriate therapy, except in rheumatic individuals, members of their families, or other epidemiological circumstances.

Carriers

Chronic carriers usually do not need antibiotic treatment. However, a difficult diagnostic problem arises when carriers develop symptomatic upper respiratory tract viral infections. It is frequently not possible to determine whether group A streptococci isolated from a carrier indicates current streptococcal infection or identifies that individual as a chronic carrier. Thus, it is often reasonable to administer a single course of therapy.

Streptococcal carriers appear to pose little threat to themselves in developing sequelae of streptococcal infection or in disseminating the organism to those who live and work around them. Therefore, streptococcal carriers usually do not need to be identified or treated.

Asymptomatic Contacts

In most circumstances, identification and treatment of asymptomatic household contacts are not indicated. However, in households with a rheumatic individual, or special epidemiological circumstances, it is advisable to obtain cultures and treat those with positive cultures.

SELECTED READINGS

Books

Breese BB, Hall C. Beta hemolytic streptococcal diseases. Boston: Houghton Mifflin, 1980.
Markowitz M, Gordis L. Rheumatic fever. 2nd ed. Philadelphia: WB Saunders, 1972.
Shulman ST, ed. Pharyngitis: management in an era of declining rheumatic fever. Philadelphia: Praeger, 1984.
Stollerman GH. Rheumatic fever and streptococcal infection. New York: Grune & Stratton, 1975.

Book Chapters and Articles

Bisno AL. Rheumatic fever. In: Wyngaarden JB, Smith LH, eds. Cecil's textbook of medicine. 18th ed. Philadelphia: WB Saunders, 1988:1580–1586.
Krause RM. Streptococcal diseases. In: Wyngaarden JB, Smith LH, eds. Cecil's textbook of medicine. 18th ed. Philadelphia: WB Saunders, 1988:1572–1580.
Markowitz M. Rheumatic fever. In: Behrman RE, Vaughn VC III, eds. Nelson textbook of pediatrics. 13th ed. Philadelphia: WB Saunders, 1987:539–543.
Veasy GL, Wiedmeier SE, Orsmond GS, Ruttenburg HD, Boucek MM, Roth SJ, Tait VF, Thompson JA, Daly JA, Kaplan EL, Hill HR. Resurgence of acute rheumatic fever in the intermountain area of the United States. N Engl J Med 1987;316:421–427.
Wannamaker LW, Kaplan EL. Acute rheumatic fever. In: Adams FH, Emmanouilides GC, eds. Moss' heart disease in infants, children, and adolescents. 3rd ed. Baltimore: Williams & Wilkins, 1983:534–552.

American Heart Association Publications

Ad hoc committee to revise the Jones Criteria (modified) of the Council on Rheumatic Fever and Congenital Heart Disease of the American Heart Association: Jones criteria (revised) for guidance in the diagnosis of rheumatic fever. Circulation 1984;69:203A–208A.
Prevention of bacterial endocarditis. A statement for health professionals by the Committee on Rheumatic Fever and Infective Endocarditis of the Council on Cardiovascular Disease in the Young. Shulman ST, Amren DPS, Bisno AL, Dajani AS, Durack DT, Gerber MA, Kaplan EL, Millard HD, Sanders WE, Schwartz RH, Watanakunakorn C. Special report. Circulation 1984;70:1123A–1127A.
Wannamaker LW. A method for culturing beta hemolytic streptococci from the throat. Circulation 1965;32:1054–1058.

Guidelines for Meningococcal Prophylaxis[e](1–3)

Antimicrobial chemoprophylaxis of intimate contacts remains the chief preventive measure in sporadic cases of *N. meningitidis* disease in the United States. Intimate contacts include (1) household members, (2) day-care center contacts, and (3) anyone directly exposed to the patient's oral secretions, such as through mouth-to-mouth resuscitation or kissing. The attack rate for household contacts is 0.3 to 1%, 300 to 1000 times the rate in the general population.

Unless the causative organism is known to be sensitive to sulfadiazine, the drug of choice is rifampin, given twice daily for 2 days (600 mg every 12 hours to adults; 10 mg/kg every 12 hours to children 1 month of age or older; 5 mg/kg every 12 hours to children under 1 month of age). Rifampin has been shown

---

[e] Modified from Immunization Practices Advisory Committee. MMWR 1985;34:259–260.

to be 90% effective in eradicating nasopharyngeal carriage. No serious adverse effects have been noted. However, rifampin prophylaxis is not recommended for pregnant women, as the drug is teratogenic in laboratory animals. As well as turning urine orange, rifampin is excreted in tears, resulting in staining of contact lenses; thus, they should not be used during the course of therapy.

Because systemic antimicrobial therapy of meningococcal disease does not reliably eradicate nasopharyngeal carriage of *N. meningitidis*, it is also important to give chemoprophylaxis to the index patient before discharge from the hospital (4).

Nasopharyngeal cultures are not helpful in determining who warrants chemoprophylaxis and unnecessarily delay institution of this preventive measure.

REFERENCES

1. Band JD, Chamberland ME, Platt T, Weaver RE, Thornsberry C, Fraser DW. Trends in meningococcal disease in the United States, 1975–1980. J Infect Dis 1983;148:754–758.
2. Ross SC, Densen P. Complement deficiency states and infection: epidemiology, pathogenesis and consequences of neisserial and other infections in an immune deficiency. Medicine 1984;63:243–73.
3. Francke EL, Neu HC. Postsplenectomy infection. Surg Clin North Am 1981;61:135–55.
4. Abramson JS, Spika JS. Persistence of *Neisseria meningitidis* in the upper respiratory tract after intravenous antibiotic therapy for systemic meningococcal disease. J Infect Dis 1985;151:370–1.

SELECTED READINGS

Dworzack DL, Sanders CC, Horowitz EA, Allais JM, Sookpranee M, Sanders WE Jr, Ferraro FM. Evaluation of single-dose ciprofloxacin in the eradication of *Neisseria meningitidis* from nasopharyngeal carriers. Antimicrob Agents Chemother 1988;32(11):1740–1741.
Schwartz B. Chemoprophylaxis for bacterial infections: principles of and application to meningococcal infections. Rev Infect Dis 1991;13(suppl 12):S170–S173.

Prevention of Recurrent Bacterial Urinary Tract Infections (Reinfections) in Women[f]

Young to middle-aged nonpregnant women with three or more recurrent episodes of new infection (reinfection) per year are candidates for long-term antimicrobial chemoprophylaxis. There should be no history of prior urological surgery, renal calculi, or genitourinary tract abnormality (1–9).

Prophylactic Regimen(s)

Preferred Regimen

Trimethoprim (40 mg)/**sulfamethoxazole** (200 mg), i.e., one-half of a regular strength tablet orally at bedtime three times per week on Sunday, Wednesday, and Friday. (A daily regimen also is effective.)

Alternative Regimens

---

[f]Modified and reprinted with permission from Drug Evaluations Annual 1994, American Medical Association.

Nitrofurantoin 50 mg (or nitrofurantoin macrocrystals, 100 mg) orally once daily at bedtime
or
Trimethoprim 50 to 100 mg orally once daily at bedtime.

Remarks

1. Duration of prophylaxis generally is 6 months. If recurrence of infection then occurs within 3 months, prophylaxis frequently is reinstituted for 2 years.
2. Trimethoprim-sulfamethoxazole penetrates vaginal secretions very well and effectively eradicates *Enterobacteriaceae* from the fecal reservoir and prevents perineal colonization. Emergence of resistant bacterial strains has not been a problem. Serious adverse reactions have been rare.
3. In one study, serious adverse reactions (e.g., pulmonary toxicity) were reported with long-term nitrofurantoin administration (10).
4. Whether the use of trimethoprim alone will lead to more rapid emergence of trimethoprim-resistant bacterial strains than the combination is still unresolved. Many experts prefer to reserve trimethoprim alone for patients who are allergic to sulfonamides.
5. Long-term, low-dose norfloxacin (200 mg once daily at bedtime) also has been effective for the prevention of recurrent urinary tract infections (11). Some urological consultants like this agent because it has not been associated with plasmid-mediated, transferable resistance.
6. Prior to beginning chemoprophylaxis, any acute urinary tract infection should be treated with appropriate antimicrobial agents, and a sterile urine culture should be obtained (usually 2 weeks after treatment).
7. A screening intravenous pyelogram (IVP) is no longer considered necessary for the majority of women who are candidates for long-term chemoprophylaxis. An exception is relapsing urinary tract infections due to urease-producing bacteria (e.g., *Proteus*), where infected urinary calculi must be considered.
8. Recurrences of urinary tract infection in some women appear to correlate temporally with sexual intercourse. For such patients, a single prophylactic dose of an appropriate antimicrobial agent taken immediately after intercourse appears to prevent active infections. In a randomized, double-blind, placebo-controlled trial, postcoital antimicrobial prophylaxis with trimethoprim (40 mg)/sulfamethoxazole (200 mg) was shown to be effective in patients with both low (<2/week) or high (>3/week) intercourse frequencies; side effects were few, and compliance was excellent (12). Thus, this approach may be an acceptable alternative to long-term chemoprophylaxis for selected women.
9. Another strategy for managing recurrent urinary tract infections is to prescribe antimicrobial drugs for susceptible women to keep at home and self-administer when symptoms arise. Intermittent self-therapy with single-dose trimethoprim (320 mg)/sulfamethoxazole (1600 mg) was shown to be efficacious and economical in selected women (e.g., those in whom the symptomatic episode was most likely acute cystitis rather than urethritis or vaginitis, those with ability to accurately self-diagnose acute cystitis) (13).

REFERENCES

1. Stamm WE et al. Antimicrobial prophylaxis of recurrent urinary tract infections: double-blind, placebo-controlled trial. Ann Intern Med 1980;92:770–775.
2. Stamm WE et al. Is antimicrobial prophylaxis of urinary tract infections cost effective? Ann Intern Med 1981;94:251–255.
3. Stamm WE et al. Urinary prophylaxis with trimethoprim and trimethoprim/sulfamethoxazole: efficacy, influence on natural history of recurrent bacteriuria, and cost control. Rev Infect Dis 1982;4:450–455.
4. Treatment of urinary tract infections. Med Lett Drugs Ther 1981;23:69–70.
5. Ronald AR, Harding GKM. Urinary infection prophylaxis in women. Ann Intern Med 1981;94:268–270.
6. Fang LST et al. Clinical management of urinary tract infection. Pharmacotherapy 1982;2:91–99.
7. Farrar WE Jr. Infections of urinary tract. Med Clin North Am 1983;67:187–201.
8. Fowler JE. Urinary tract infections in women. Urol Clin North Am 1986;13:673–683.
9. Valenti WM, Reese RE. Genitourinary tract infections. In: Reese RE, Douglas RG Jr, eds. A practical approach to infectious diseases. ed 2. Boston: Little, Brown & Co, 1986;327–358.
10. Holmberg L et al. Adverse reactions to nitrofurantoin: analysis of 921 reports. Am J Med 1980;69:733–738.
11. Nicolle LE et al. Prospective, randomized, placebo-controlled trial of norfloxacin for prophylaxis of recurrent urinary tract infection in women. Antimicrob Agents Chemother 1989;33:1032–1035.
12. Stapleton A et al. Postcoital antimicrobial prophylaxis for recurrent urinary tract infection: a randomized, double-blind, placebo-controlled trial. JAMA 1990;264:703–706.
13. Wong ES et al. Management of recurrent urinary tract infections with patient-administered single-dose therapy. Ann Intern Med 1985;102:302–307.

Prevention of Pneumococcal Infection in Asplenic Patients[g]

Anatomical or functionally asplenic patients (e.g., those with sickle cell disease), particularly children, are susceptible to overwhelming infection with encapsulated bacteria, including *Streptococcus pneumoniae*, *Haemophilus influenzae* type b, and *Neisseria meningitidis*. *S. pneumoniae* is the most frequent and important cause of septicemia in the asplenic child, and continuous antimicrobial chemoprophylaxis directed against this organism traditionally has been recommended for children and adolescents after splenectomy or diagnosis of chronic splenic dysfunction. Whether to use similar chemoprophylaxis in adult patients is less clear (1–4).

Prophylactic Regimen(s)

Preferred Regimen

Penicillin V (oral: children less than 5 years, 125 mg twice daily; adults and children 5 years and older, 250 mg twice daily).

Remarks

1. The efficacy of this regimen in preventing pneumococcal septicemia in infants and young children with sickle cell anemia has been demonstrated in a randomized, double-blind, placebo controlled trial (5).

ᵍ Modified and reprinted with permission from Drug Evaluations Annual 1994, American Medical Association.

2. Some experts recommend use of ampicillin (25 to 50 mg/kg/day), amoxicillin (20 mg/kg/day), or trimethoprim-sulfamethoxazole (4 mg/20 mg/kg/day) for children less than 5 years of age to include coverage against *H. influenzae*.

3. Penicillin G benzathine (intramuscularly, 1.2 million units every 4 weeks) also has been suggested for this indication (6). Monthly injections of this long-acting penicillin appeared to be effective in preventing pneumococcal infections in young Jamaican children with sickle cell anemia (7). Pain at the site of intramuscular injection is a disadvantage of this regimen. Also, there is some concern that adequate serum concentrations of penicillin G are not maintained during the latter part of the dosing interval (7).

4. The optimum duration of prophylaxis is unknown, but in children it traditionally has ranged from 2 to 4 years. An unacceptably high incidence of pneumococcal infections in children with sickle cell anemia after they had terminated penicillin prophylaxis at 3 years of age suggests that prophylaxis should continue beyond the age of 3 years and perhaps indefinitely (7). There also is concern that penicillin prophylaxis may prevent the development of naturally acquired immunity against pneumococcal infections in young children and, therefore, increase their susceptibility to infection if the prophylactic regimen is terminated (5, 7, 8).

5. Suboptimal compliance has been associated with failure of prophylaxis (8). Therefore, the necessity for strict compliance to the prophylactic regimen should be emphasized to the patient and/or parents. It also should be stressed that continuous prophylaxis has limitations. Some bacteria that can cause fulminant bacteremia are not susceptible to the antimicrobial agent selected for prophylaxis. Patients and/or parents should be aware that any febrile illness is potentially serious and that immediate medical attention should be sought. When septicemia is a possibility, the physician should hospitalize the patient, obtain blood and other appropriate body fluid (e.g., cerebrospinal fluid) specimens for culture, and initiate antimicrobial therapy (e.g., intravenous cefotaxime in children less than 5 years.)

6. Anatomically or functionally asplenic, including sickle cell disease, patients 2 years of age or older also should receive pneumococcal 23-valent polysaccharide vaccine (9) and quadrivalent (A, C, Y, W-135) meningococcal vaccine (10). Anatomically or functionally asplenic, including sickle cell disease, patients also should receive *Haemophilus* b polysaccharide conjugate vaccine (11).

REFERENCES

1. Prevention of serious infections after splenectomy. Med Lett Drugs Ther 1977;19:2–4.
2. Reese RE, Betts RF. Antibiotic use. In: Reese RE, Douglas RG Jr, eds: A practical approach to infectious diseases. ed 2. Boston: Little, Brown & Co, 1986;559–679.
3. Powars D, Overturf G. Penicillin in sickle cell anemia: panacea for lost spleen? [Editorial]. Am J Dis Child 1987;141:250–252.
4. Report of the Committee on Infectious Diseases. American Academy of Pediatrics Redbook, ed 21. Elk Grove Village, IL: American Academy of Pediatrics, 1988;46–48.
5. Gaston MA et al. Prophylaxis with oral penicillin in children with sickle cell anemia: randomized trial. N Engl J Med 1986;314:1593–1599.

6. Sanford JP. Guide to antimicrobial therapy, 1989. West Bethesda, MD: Antimicrobial Therapy Inc, 1989;93–97.
7. John AB et al. Prevention of pneumococcal infection in children with homozygous sickle cell disease. Br Med J 1984;288:1567–1570.
8. Buchanan GR, Smith SJ. Pneumococcal septicemia despite pneumococcal vaccine and prescription of penicillin prophylaxis in children with sickle cell anemia. Am J Dis Child 1986;140:428–432.
9. Recommendations of the Immunization Practices Advisory Committee (ACIP). Pneumococcal polysaccharide vaccine. MMWR 1989;38:64–76.
10. Meningococcal vaccines. MMWR 1985;34:255–259.
11. Recommendations of the Immunization Practices Advisory Committee (ACIP). *Haemophilus* b conjugate vaccine for prevention of *Haemophilus influenzae* type b disease among infants and children 2 months of age and older. MMWR 1991;40(RR-1):1–7.

Prevention of Pertussis in Exposed Persons[h]

Exposure to pertussis can result in clinical disease in both immunized and unimmunized contacts. Infants (less than 1 year of age) and unimmunized children less than 7 years of age are at greatest risk, and some experts recommend antimicrobial chemoprophylaxis only for these high-risk children (1). However, the Committee on Infectious Diseases of the American Academy of Pediatrics currently recommends chemoprophylaxis for all household and other close contacts less than 7 years of age, regardless of immunization status, and encourages chemoprophylaxis for household and other close contacts 7 years old or older because older children and adults can transmit infection (2). The index case also should receive antimicrobials to prevent spread (2–4).

Prophylactic Regimen(s)

Preferred Regimen

Erythromycin orally 40 to 50 mg/kg/day (maximum, 2 gm/day), divided into four doses for 14 days after contact is broken.

Remarks

1. Erythromycin has been shown to eliminate carriage of *Bordetella pertussis*, but efficacy in preventing disease is not fully established. (Note: A retrospective analysis of the literature suggests that erythromycin estolate has been more effective than erythromycin ethylsuccinate or erythromycin stearate in eliminating *B. pertussis* carriage, presumably due to better penetration of the estolate into respiratory secretions (4)).
2. Trimethoprim-sulfamethoxazole (orally 8 mg/40 mg/kg/day) is recommended as an alternative by some experts, but its value is less well-established.
3. In addition to chemoprophylaxis, the Committee on Infectious Diseases of the American Academy of Pediatrics also recommends the following: (*a*) Exposed children, especially those incompletely immunized, should be observed carefully for respiratory symptoms for 14 days after contact is broken.

[h]Modified and reprinted with permission from Drug Evaluations Annual 1994, American Medical Association.

(*b*) Household and other close contacts (such as those in day care or classrooms) less than 7 years of age who have had at least four doses of pertussis vaccine should receive a booster dose of vaccine, preferably as DTP (diphtheria, tetanus, pertussis), unless they have received a dose within the previous 3 years. (*c*) Household and other close contacts less than 7 years of age who are unimmunized or who have received less than four doses of DTP should have DTP immunization initiated or continued according to the recommended schedule. Children who have received their third dose 6 months or more before exposure should be given their fourth dose at this time (2).

REFERENCES

1. Recommendations of the Immunization Practices Advisory Committee (ACIP). Diphtheria, tetanus, and pertussis: guidelines for vaccine prophylaxis and other preventive measures. MMWR 1985;34:405–426.
2. Report of the Committee on Infectious Diseases: American Academy of Pediatrics Redbook, ed 21. Elk Grove Village, IL: American Academy of Pediatrics, 1988;315–325.
3. Feder HM Jr. Chemoprophylaxis in ambulatory pediatrics. Pediatr Infect Dis 1983;2:251–257.
4. Bass JW. Pertussis: current status of prevention and treatment. Pediatr Infect Dis 1985;4:614–619.

Prevention of Recurrent Acute Otitis Media[i]

Antimicrobial chemoprophylaxis has decreased the number of recurrent episodes of acute otitis media in children in various studies, but conclusive evidence that the advantages outweigh the disadvantages for this management option are lacking. Furthermore, the indications for prophylaxis, the most effective drugs, and the optimum duration of prophylaxis have not been clearly established. Although more definitive clinical studies are necessary, many infectious disease experts currently recommend antimicrobial chemoprophylaxis (as outlined below) as a reasonable approach in children with at least three episodes of acute otitis media in the previous 6 months or four episodes in 1 year (1–6).

Prophylactic Regimen(s)

Preferred Regimens

Amoxicillin orally 20 mg/kg once daily at bedtime
or
Sulfisoxazole orally 50 mg/kg once daily at bedtime.

Remarks

1. Duration of prophylaxis is about 6 months or during the winter and spring when the incidence of respiratory tract infections is high.
2. Amoxicillin or sulfisoxazole generally is preferred because of proven effectiveness, safety, and low cost. Although some experts have suggested trimethoprim (4 mg/kg)/sulfamethoxazole (20 mg/kg) orally once daily at bedtime as a

[i]Modified and reprinted with permission from Drug Evaluations Annual 1994, American Medical Association.

possible alternative, others do not recommend this combination regimen (4, 6, 7).

3. If episodes of acute otitis media occur during prophylaxis, an alternative regimen should be used for treatment.

4. If episodes of acute otitis media recur after conclusion of prophylaxis, reinstitution of chemoprophylaxis and myringotomy with insertion of tympanotomy tubes are alternative management options.

5. Hazards of antimicrobial chemoprophylaxis include potential for adverse drug reactions and emergence of resistant bacterial strains.

6. Because chemoprophylaxis could alleviate symptoms of acute otitis media without eliminating middle ear effusion, monthly evaluation of patients for middle ear effusion is recommended.

REFERENCES

1. Paradise JL. Antimicrobial prophylaxis for recurrent acute otitis media. Ann Otol Rhinol Laryngol 1981;(suppl 84):53–57.
2. Paradise JL. Chemoprophylaxis of recurrent otitis media in early infancy (Q and A). Pediatr Infect Dis J 1988;7:78–79.
3. Klein JO, Bluestone CD. Acute otitis media. Pediatr Infect Dis J 1982;1:66–73.
4. Chemoprophylaxis for recurrent acute otitis media. Med Lett Drugs Ther 1983;25:102–103.
5. Klein JO. Antimicrobial prophylaxis for recurrent acute otitis media. Pediatr Ann 1984;13:398–403.
6. Bluestone CD. Otitis media and sinusitis: management and when to refer to otolaryngologist. Pediatr Infect Dis J 1987;6:100–106.
7. Sanford JP. Guide to antimicrobial therapy, 1990. West Bethesda, MD: Antimicrobial Therapy, Inc, 1990;90–94.

Prevention of Travelers' Diarrhea[j]

ADVICE FOR TRAVELERS

Patients planning to travel to other countries often ask physicians for advice about immunizations and prevention of diarrhea and malaria. Legal requirements for entry and epidemiological conditions in different countries vary from time to time, often unpredictably, but some reasonable recommendations can be made. More detailed information is available in *Health Information for International Travel*, published annually by the Centers for Disease Control and Prevention (CDC), which can be obtained from the Superintendent of Documents, U.S. Government Printing Office, Washington, DC 20402. Up-to-date automated information is available from the CDC by telephone (404-332-4559) or by fax (404-332-4565).

TRAVELERS' DIARRHEA

The most common cause of travelers' diarrhea, usually a self-limited illness lasting several days, is infection with enterotoxigenic *Escherichia coli, Campylobacter, Shigella, Salmonella*; viruses and parasites are less common causes of

[j]Modified and reprinted with permission from The Medical Letter, Inc., May 13, 1994;36:922.

this disorder. Travelers to areas where hygiene is poor should be advised to avoid foods that are not steaming hot, raw vegetables, fruit they have not peeled themselves, and tap water, including ice.

Prophylaxis

Medical Letter consultants generally do not prescribe drugs prophylactically, but rather instruct the patient to begin treatment promptly when symptoms occur. When prophylaxis is indicated, ciprofloxacin (Cipro), 500 mg once daily, ofloxacin (Floxin), 300 mg once daily, or norfloxacin (Noroxin), 400 mg once daily, is recommended (1). Pepto-Bismol, an over-the-counter formulation of bismuth subsalicylate, can also prevent diarrhea in travelers who take two tablets four times daily with meals and at bedtime. Pepto-Bismol turns the tongue and stool black and sometimes can cause mild tinnitus. Patients who are allergic to salicylates or are taking therapeutic doses of salicylates or anticoagulants should not take Pepto-Bismol, and no one should take it for more than 3 weeks. Bismuth subsalicylate may decrease the bioavailability of doxycycline (Vibramycin and others), which is sometimes used for malaria prophylaxis.

Treatment

Oral rehydration solutions, available in pharmacies and grocery stores in many countries, can help maintain fluid balance (2). Loperamide hydrochloride (Imodium), a synthetic opioid (4-mg loading dose, then 2 mg orally after each loose stool, to a maximum of 16 mg/day) can relieve symptoms. If diarrhea is moderate or severe, ciprofloxacin (500 mg twice a day), norfloxacin (400 mg twice a day), or ofloxacin (300 mg twice a day) is recommended until symptoms resolve, for up to 3 days (3). Trimethoprim-sulfamethoxazole (Bactrim, Septra, and others), 160/800 mg twice a day, is an alternative, but resistance to this drug has become common in many areas (4).

IMMUNIZATION

Cholera

The risk of cholera to tourists is very low; the currently licensed parenteral vaccine, which is prepared from killed bacteria, has limited effectiveness, often causes reactions, and is generally not recommended for travelers (5).

Hepatitis A

To prevent hepatitis A, immune globulin may be advisable for susceptible travelers going to areas where hygiene is poor, particularly those going outside the usual tourist routes. It should be given close to the time of departure in a dose for adults of 2 ml intramuscularly for a stay of less than 3 months, and 5 ml for a longer stay, repeated every 5 months. The dose for children is 0.02 ml/kg for a stay of less than 3 months, and 0.06 ml/kg for a longer period. Immune globulin made in the United States will not transmit HIV (6). An inactivated whole virus vaccine against hepatitis A (SKB HAVrix) may soon be available here (7). A controlled trial of a similar vaccine demonstrated a high degree of effectiveness (8).

Hepatitis B

Vaccination against hepatitis B is not ordinarily recommended for foreign travel, except for medical personnel whose work could require handling of body fluids or for people who expect to have sexual contacts, receive medical or dental care, or stay for more than 6 months in areas such as Southeast Asia or sub-Saharan Africa, where hepatitis B is highly endemic. Hepatitis B vaccine is less effective when injected into the gluteal area, where it may not reach muscle; it should be injected into the deltoid in a series of three doses over 2 to (preferably) 6 months.

Japanese Encephalitis

Vaccination against Japanese encephalitis, a frequently fatal mosquito-borne disease that occurs in rural Asia, should be considered for travelers who anticipate spending a month or longer in rural rice-growing areas where they will be heavily exposed to mosquitoes. Countries where the disease may be a problem include Bangladesh, Cambodia, China, India, Indonesia, Korea, Laos, Malaysia, Myanmar (Burma), Nepal, Pakistan, the Philippines, Singapore, Sri Lanka, Taiwan, Thailand, Vietnam, and eastern areas of Russia. The disease now occurs only rarely on the main islands of Japan or in Hong Kong. The attack rate in travelers is very low; in the past 10 years, fewer than 10 cases, most of them in military personnel, have been documented in U.S. citizens. A formalin-inactivated, purified mouse-brain-derived vaccine that has been shown to protect against the disease is now available in the United States (JE-Vax, Connaught). Allergic reactions, including urticaria and angioedema, have been reported (9). When indicated, a primary series of three doses, given over 2 to (preferably) 4 weeks, is recommended.

Measles

People born after 1956 who have not received two doses of measles vaccine (after their first birthday) and do not have a physician-documented history of infection or laboratory evidence of immunity should receive a single dose of measles (or measles-mumps-rubella) vaccine before traveling anywhere, but at least 2 weeks before or 3 months after immune globulin.

Meningococcal Disease

Meningococcal vaccine is recommended only for tourists traveling to areas where epidemics are occurring. Epidemics occur frequently in sub-Saharan Africa from December to June, and also in northern India and Nepal. Saudi Arabia requires a certificate of immunization for pilgrims to Mecca. A single-dose vial of quadrivalent meningococcal polysaccharide vaccine against *N. meningitidis* serogroups A, C, Y, and W135 is available from Connaught Laboratories (10).

Polio

Adult travelers to tropical or developing countries who have not previously been immunized against polio should receive a primary series of enhanced inactivated polio vaccine (eIPV). If protection is needed within 4 weeks, a single dose of eIPV or trivalent (live) oral polio vaccine (OPV) is recommended, but OPV rarely can cause vaccine-induced polio (one case per million first doses distributed), particularly in previously unimmunized adults. Previously unimmunized children should receive a primary series of OPV. Travelers who have previously completed a primary series should receive a booster dose of OPV or eIPV.

Rabies

Pre-exposure immunization against rabies is recommended for travelers with an occupational risk of exposure or those traveling for extended periods in endemic areas. People at high risk of being exposed should receive three injections of rabies vaccine over 3 or 4 weeks (11).

Tetanus and Diphtheria

Whether traveling or not, everyone should receive a tetanus-diphtheria toxoid (Td) booster injection every 10 years. For travelers, the Td booster is especially important for those going to developing countries and to Russia and the Ukraine, where a large outbreak of diphtheria has been occurring in recent years (12).

Typhoid

In the past, parenteral typhoid vaccine prepared from killed bacteria was recommended for travel to rural areas of tropical countries, where typhoid tends to be endemic, or to any area where an outbreak was occurring. The parenteral vaccine is not fully protective, however, and often causes 1 to 2 days of pain at the site of injection, sometimes accompanied by fever, malaise, and headache. A live oral vaccine (Vivotif Berna-Swiss Serum and Vaccine Institute), reported to be equally effective, protective longer, and better tolerated, is now available in the United States from Berna Products (800-533-5899). The traveler takes one enteric-coated capsule every other day for a total of four capsules, beginning at least 2 weeks before departure. A new purified capsular polysaccharide vaccine (Typhim Vi, Connaught Pasteur Merieux) is also effective and requires only a single parenteral dose (13).

Yellow Fever

Yellow fever vaccine, an attenuated live virus vaccine prepared in eggs, is recommended for travel to rural areas in the yellow fever endemic zones, which include most of tropical South America and most of Africa between 15°N and 15°S. An outbreak of the disease was recently reported in Kenya (14). The vaccine is available in the United States only in centers designated by state health departments. Boosters are given every 10 years. Some countries in Africa require a certificate of yellow fever vaccination from all entering travelers; other countries in Africa, South America, and Asia require evidence of vaccination from travelers coming from infected or endemic areas.

Other Recommendations

More than one vaccine can be given at the same time. Antibiotics should be avoided, if possible, for 1 week before and 3 weeks after oral typhoid vaccine. Immunocompromised or pregnant patients generally should not receive live virus vaccines, but measles vaccine is recommended for HIV-infected patients (15).

Malaria

Countries with a risk of malaria are listed in Table 4.9; additional information is available from the CDC at 404-332-4555. Some countries with both urban and rural malaria may not have any malaria in major cities most frequently visited by tourists. Kenya, for example, has no malaria in Nairobi, and Brazil has none in Rio de Janeiro. Bombay, on the other hand, has recently had some epidemics.

Recommendations for prevention of malaria were published in the *Medical Letter* (Drugs for parasitic infections. 1993;35:111). Mefloquine (Lariam), 250 mg once a week, is the drug of choice for travel to areas with chloroquine-resistant malaria, except the Thai-Cambodian and Thai-Burmese border areas, where mefloquine resistance is common, and doxycycline, 100 mg daily, is preferred. Chloroquine resistance has been reported in all areas where malaria occurs, except for Central America west of the Panama Canal Zone, Mexico, Haiti, the Dominican Republic, and parts of the Mideast (including Egypt, Syria, and Iraq). In chloroquine-sensitive areas, chloroquine (Aralen and others), 300 mg base once a week, is the drug of choice. In all malarious areas, use of room sprays, mosquito nets, window screens, clothing with long sleeves and long pants, and insect repellents containing up to 35% diethyltoluamide (DEET) is recommended, especially during evening and night hours. DEET can, however, cause severe reactions, particularly in higher concentrations or with prolonged or excessive use in children. Spraying clothing with permethrin (Permanone) and using permethrin-impregnated mosquito nets are also helpful. Since none of these measures is 100% effective, travelers to malarious areas should be advised to seek prompt medical attention for febrile illness while traveling or for up to a year afterwards.

Table 4.9. Countries with a Risk of Malaria

Africa	Americas	Asia	Oceania
Angola	Argentina[a]	Afghanistan	Papua New
Benin	Belize[a]	Azerbaijan	Guinea
Botswana	Bolivia[a]	Bangladesh	Solomon Islands
Burkina Faso	Brazil	Bhutan[a]	Vanuatu
Burundi	Colombia[a]	Cambodia	
Cameroon	Costa Rica[a]	China, People's	
Central African	Dominican	Republic[a]	
Republic	Republic[a]	India	
Chad	Ecuador	Indonesia	
Comoros	El Salvador[a]	Iran[a]	
Congo	French Guiana	Iraq	
Cote d'Ivoire	Guatemala[a]	Laos	
Djibouti	Guyana[a]	Malaysia	
Egypt[a]	Haiti	Myanmar[a]	
Equatorial Guinea	Honduras[a]	Nepal[a]	
Ethiopia	Mexico[a]	Oman	
Gabon	Nicaragua	Pakistan	
Gambia	Panama[a]	Philippines[a]	
Ghana	Paraguay[a]	Saudi Arabia	
Guinea	Peru[a]	Sri Lanka	
Guinea-Bissau	Suriname[a]	Syrian Arab	
Kenya	Venezuela[a]	Republic[a]	
Liberia		Tajikistan	
Madagascar		Thailand[a]	
Malawi		Turkey	
Mali		United Arab	
Mauritania		Emirates	
Mauritius[a]		Vietnam[a]	
Mayotte (French		Yemen	
territorial			
collectivity)			
Mozambique			
Namibia			
Niger			
Nigeria			
Rwanda			
Sao Tome and			
Principe			
Senegal			
Sierra Leone			
Somalia			
South Africa[a]			
Sudan			
Swaziland			
Tanzania			
Togo			
Uganda			
Zaire			
Zambia			
Zimbabwe			

Adapted from Health Information for International Travel, 1993. Includes only countries for which prophylaxis is recommended. Modified and reprinted with permission from The Medical Letter, Inc., May 13, 1994;36:922.
[a] No malaria in urban areas.

REFERENCES

1. DuPont HL, Ericsson CD. Prevention and treatment of traveler's diarrhea. N Engl J Med 1993;328:1821.
2. Ericsson CD, DuPont HL. Travelers' diarrhea: approaches to prevention and treatment. Clin Infect Dis 1993;16:616.
3. Murphy GS et al. Ann Intern Med 1993;118:582.
4. DuPont HL. Travellers' diarrhoea. Which antimicrobial? Drugs 1993;45:910.
5. Med Lett 1991;33:107.
6. MMWR 1990;39(no. RR-2):1.
7. Andre FE, Dhondt E, et al. Clinical assessment of the safety and efficacy of an inactivated hepatitis A vaccine: rationale and summary of findings. Vaccine 1992;10 (suppl 1992):S160.
8. Werzberger A, Mensch B, Kuter B, Brown L, et al. A controlled trial of a formalin-inactivated hepatitis A vaccine in healthy children. N Engl J Med 1992;327:453.
9. MMWR 1993;42(no. RR-1):12.
10. Wolfe MS. Eosinophilia in the returning traveler. Infect Dis Clin North Am 1992;6(2);489.
11. Med Lett 1990;32:117.
12. MMWR 1993;42:840.
13. Arnold WS et al. Experience with Vi typhoid capsular polysaccharide vaccine in the U.K. J Infect 1992;25:63.
14. U.S. Public Health Service Advisory Memorandum No. 104, March 24, 1993.
15. MMWR 1994;43(no. RR-1):21.

SECTION 5
AIDS and HIV Infection[a]

Drugs for AIDS and Associated Infections

Results of recently completed clinical trials have led to some changes in recommendations for treatment of human immunodeficiency virus (HIV) and other infections associated with AIDS.

HIV INFECTION

None of the drugs currently available to treat HIV-infected patients can eradicate the infection; all should be considered palliative.

Zidovudine

Zidovudine (Retrovir, also called AZT), a nucleoside analog that inhibits HIV reverse transcriptase, has transiently decreased circulating p24 antigen titers, increased circulating CD4 T-cells, and decreased the frequency of opportunistic infections in patients with advanced HIV disease. The drug has been associated with an increase in median survival from less than 9 months to more than 2 years after diagnosis of AIDS (1). Use of zidovudine in symptomatic HIV-infected patients has slowed progression to AIDS and prolonged survival (2, 3). Early use in asymptomatic HIV-infected patients remains controversial; the drug has slowed progression to symptomatic disease in some studies, but a beneficial effect on survival has not been demonstrated (4, 5).

Adverse effects of zidovudine include anemia, neutropenia, nausea, vomiting, headache, fatigue, confusion, malaise, myopathy, and hepatitis. Recently, findings similar to those with Reye's syndrome have been reported in a few HIV-infected patients who had taken zidovudine (6, 7). Erythropoietin (Epogen, Procrit) may be helpful for anemia but only in patients with low (<500 IU/L) erythropoietin levels (8, 9). GM-CSF (Leukine, Prokine) or G-CSF (Neupogen) may increase the number of neutrophils in patients with zidovudine-induced neutropenia (10). One study of 43 women who took zidovudine during pregnancy found that the drug was well-tolerated and apparently not associated with malformations or other untoward effects on the fetus (11).

---

[a]Modified and reprinted with permission from The Medical Letter, Inc. September 3, 1993;35:904.

With continued use of zidovudine, in vitro resistance to the drug often develops and has been associated with clinical deterioration (12). Strains of HIV resistant in vitro to zidovudine may be susceptible to DDI or DDC (13).

DDI

Didanosine (dideoxyinosine, DDI, Videx), another reverse-transcriptase inhibitor, has been approved by the U.S. Food and Drug Administration (FDA) for use in patients unresponsive to or intolerant of zidovudine. Use of DDI can transiently decrease serum p24 antigen levels, increase CD4 T-cell counts, and lead to weight gain in patients with AIDS or AIDS-related complex (ARC) (14–16). Sequential use of zidovudine and DDI, rather than continuous use of zidovudine, appears to delay clinical deterioration (17).

Major treatment-limiting toxicities have been painful peripheral neuropathy, acute pancreatitis, and gastrointestinal disturbances; hepatic failure has also occurred (18). DDI decreases gastrointestinal absorption of itraconazole, ketoconazole, and possibly dapsone (19).

In vitro resistance to DDI may occur. Some DDI-resistant isolates of HIV are also resistant in vitro to DDC.

DDC

Zalcitabine (dideoxycytidine, DDC, Hivid), a third inhibitor of HIV reverse transcriptase, has been approved by the U.S. Food and Drug Administration for concurrent use with zidovudine in patients with advanced HIV infection. One study in patients with advanced disease found concurrent use of zidovudine and DDC more effective than use of zidovudine alone (20); unpublished studies, however, have found no advantage over zidovudine alone, according to *Medical Letter* consultants. Used alone in one small study in patients with advanced infection previously treated with zidovudine, using DDC was at least as effective as continuing zidovudine (21). Peripheral neuropathy can limit dosage. Other adverse effects include rash, stomatitis, esophageal ulceration, fever, and possibly pancreatitis.

PNEUMOCYSTIS CARINII

Trimethoprim-Sulfamethoxazole

Oral or intravenous trimethoprim-sulfamethoxazole (Bactrim, Septra, and others) is the treatment of choice for *P. carinii* pneumonia (PCP) and extrapulmonary *P. carinii* infections, and oral trimethoprim-sulfamethoxazole prophylaxis can prevent PCP in most patients who take the drug (22). Adverse effects, particularly rash, nausea, and fever, are frequent in HIV-infected patients. Some episodes of toxicity respond to dosage reduction; others require discontinuation of the drug, but some of the patients who have to discontinue the drug may tolerate it subsequently.

Pentamidine Isethionate

Parenteral pentamidine (Pentam 300) is an alternative treatment for *P. carinii* infections (23). Adverse effects include hypo- and hyperglycemia, renal failure, leukopenia, cardiac arrhythmias, pancreatitis, and prolonged orthostatic hypotension. Sterile abscesses have been associated with intramuscular use, and hypotension with rapid intravenous injection. Aerosolized pentamidine (NebuPent) is generally well-tolerated but is much less effective for treatment of PCP than is giving the drug parenterally (24). For PCP prophylaxis, aerosolized pentamidine is less effective than oral trimethoprim-sulfamethoxazole (25, 26).

Dapsone

The antileprosy sulfone dapsone has been used successfully with oral trimethoprim (Trimpex and others) for treatment of mild or moderate PCP (27). Adverse effects of this combination include rash, nausea, methemoglobinemia, and hemolytic anemia. Hemolysis and methemoglobinemia are more common and can be severe in patients with glucose-6-phosphate dehydrogenase (G-6-PD) deficiency. Most patients who have rashes caused by trimethoprim-sulfamethoxazole can tolerate trimethoprim-dapsone. Dapsone alone and with pyrimethamine (Daraprim) has also been used as an alternative to trimethoprim-sulfamethoxazole for PCP prophylaxis (28, 29).

Atovaquone

For treatment of mild-to-moderate PCP, atovaquone (Mepron) has been less effective than trimethoprim-sulfamethoxazole but better tolerated (30, 31). It appears to be the safest of the alternatives to trimethoprim-sulfamethoxazole for treatment of PCP; no serious adverse effects have been reported. Absorption of atovaquone from the gastrointestinal tract can be a problem, however, and low serum concentrations of the drug can lead to treatment failure (32). Serum concentrations are two to three times higher when it is taken with food, especially fatty food. Atovaquone has not been evaluated as a prophylactic agent.

Clindamycin and Primaquine

Concurrent use of intravenous or oral clindamycin (Cleocin and others) with oral primaquine has been successful in treating patients with moderate-to-severe PCP (33). Adverse effects of this combination have included rash, leukopenia, nausea, and diarrhea. Primaquine can cause methemoglobinemia and hemolytic anemia in patients with G-6-PD deficiency.

Trimetrexate

The antifolate agent trimetrexate (34) has been used in PCP with variable success; response rates range from 10–20% in disease refractory to other agents to 60–90% in previously untreated patients (35, 36). The drug must be given with high-dose folinic acid (Leucovorin) to prevent bone marrow suppression; other adverse effects include rash and increased aminotransferase. Trimetrexate is available on a compassionate-use basis from U.S. BioScience (Telephone: (800) 537-9978 or (215) 832-4525)).

Prednisone

In PCP accompanied by moderate or severe hypoxia, treatment for 21 days or less with prednisone added to specific antimicrobial treatment has decreased the incidence of respiratory deterioration and death (37). Adverse effects have been uncommon but have included thrush and reactivation of herpes simplex infections.

TOXOPLASMOSIS

Pyrimethamine and Sulfadiazine

The antifolate agent pyrimethamine given with sulfadiazine is the treatment of choice for central nervous system (CNS) toxoplasmosis. A scarcity of sulfadiazine in the United States has prompted IND (investigational new drug) status for imported sulfadiazine, which is now available from the CDC (Telephone: (404) 488-4928) until a domestic source of the drug is reestablished (38). Folinic acid is given concurrently to attenuate leukopenia and thrombocytopenia due to pyrimethamine.

Alternatives

Clindamycin with pyrimethamine appears to be a reasonable alternative for treatment of cerebral toxoplasmosis (39). Atovaquone was well-tolerated and effective in a few patients, although several relapsed while still taking the drug (40). High-dose pyrimethamine is another alternative.

Prophylaxis

Prophylactic doses of trimethoprim-sulfamethoxazole used to prevent PCP also appear to prevent toxoplasmosis (41). A combination of daily dapsone and weekly pyrimethamine may also prevent first episodes of toxoplasmosis (42).

CRYPTOSPORIDIOSIS

Cryptosporidium can cause intractable diarrhea in patients with AIDS and has been difficult to treat; there is no good evidence that any drug is effective. Management has included fluid therapy, nutritional support, and use of antidiarrheal agents. Octreotide (Sandostatin), a somatostatin analog, may help control diarrhea (43). Paromomycin (Humatin) or azithromycin (Zithromax) may sometimes be helpful (44).

MUCOSAL CANDIDIASIS

Nystatin or Clotrimazole

Nystatin (Mycostatin and others) oral suspension or tablets or clotrimazole (Mycelex) troches are usually effective for oral thrush and can prevent recurrence.

Vaginal candidiasis often responds to suppository preparations of these agents. Esophageal candidiasis, however, is generally refractory to these drugs. Adverse effects are negligible.

Ketoconazole

Oral ketoconazole (Nizoral) is effective for treatment of severe oral thrush, severe vaginal candidiasis, and esophageal candidiasis. Normal gastric acidity is required for drug absorption and can be enhanced by taking the drug with a carbonated beverage or cranberry juice (45). Anorexia, nausea, and aminotransferase increases can occur.

Fluconazole

The oral triazole fluconazole (46) is effective for treatment of oral or esophageal candidiasis. One double-blind trial in 169 patients found it more effective than ketoconazole for treatment of esophageal candidiasis (47). In another study, it was effective in preventing recurrences of oral thrush (48). Fluconazole is well-absorbed even in the absence of gastric acidity. Nausea, skin rash, and aminotransferase increases occur infrequently; hepatic necrosis has occurred in a few patients.

Fluconazole-resistant candidiasis has been reported after prolonged use of the drug.

DRUGS FOR SYSTEMIC MYCOSES

Amphotericin B

Amphotericin B (Fungizone and others) is the standard treatment for systemic fungal infections in AIDS, including cryptococcosis, histoplasmosis, and coccidioidomycosis. Common adverse effects are fever, chills, and nausea during infusion, which can be attenuated by premedication with aspirin or other drugs (49). Renal insufficiency and anemia may develop after several weeks of treatment. Amphotericin B weekly, then twice monthly, can prevent recurrent histoplasmosis in AIDS patients (50).

Flucytosine

Recommended for concurrent use with amphotericin B for treatment of cryptococcal meningitis in patients who do not have AIDS, flucytosine (Ancobon) may also improve the outcome of this infection in patients with AIDS, but data from controlled trials are lacking. Preliminary data suggest that flucytosine might also enhance the response to fluconazole in patients with cryptococcal meningitis. Leukopenia can occur, however, especially when serum concentrations of flucytosine exceed 100 μg/ml.

Fluconazole

Oral fluconazole (Diflucan) achieves high concentrations in both cerebrospinal fluid (CSF) and urine. The drug was used successfully to treat patients with acute

Table 5.1. Drugs for AIDS and Associated Infections[a]

Condition	Standard Treatment		Alternative Treatment	
	Drug	Dosage	Drug	Dosage
HIV infection				
	Zidovudine[b]	100 mg p.o. 3–5 ×/day[c] or 200 mg q8h	DDI DDC	125–300 mg p.o. bid[d] 0.75 mg p.o. tid
P. carinii pneumonia				
	TMP-SMX	15–20 mg/kg/d[e] p.o. or i.v. in 3 or 4 doses × 21 days	Dapsone[f] + trimethoprim	100 mg p.o. daily × 21 days 5 mg/kg p.o. qid × 21 days
			Atovaquone	750 mg p.o. tid × 21 days
	or Pentamidine[g] ± prednisone[g]	3–4 mg/kg i.v. daily × 21 days 40 mg p.o. bid days 1–5 20 mg p.o. bid, days 6–10 20 mg p.o. daily, days 11–21	Primaquine[f] + clindamycin	15 mg base p.o. daily × 21 days 600 mg i.v. qid × 21 days, or 300–450 mg p.o. qid × 21 days
			Trimetrexate + folinic acid	45 mg/m² i.v. daily × 21 days 20 mg/m² p.o. or i.v. q6h × 21 days
Primary[h] and secondary prophylaxis				
	TMP-SMX	1 DS[i] tab p.o. daily or 3×/week	Dapsone[f]	50 mg p.o. daily, or 100 mg p.o. 2×/week
			Aerosol pentamidine	300 mg inhaled monthly via Respirgard II nebulizer
Toxoplasmosis				
	Pyrimethamine[j] + sulfadiazine	50–100 mg p.o. daily[k] 1–1.5 g p.o. q6h	Pyrimethamine[j] + clindamycin	50–100 mg p.o. daily[k] 450–600 mg p.o. or 600–1200 mg i.v. qid
			Atovaquone	750 mg p.o. qid
Chronic suppressive therapy				
	Pyrimethamine[j] + sulfadiazine	25–50 mg p.o. daily 500 mg–1 g p.o. q6h	Pyrimethamine[j] + clindamycin	50 mg p.o. daily 300 mg p.o. qid

Condition	Drug	Dosage	Drug	Dosage
Cryptosporidiosis	Paromomycin	500–750 mg p.o. qid	Azithromycin	500–1250 mg daily
Candidiasis				
Oral	Nystatin solution or tablets or clotrimazole troches	500,000–1,000,000 U p.o. 3–5 x/day; 10 mg p.o. 5x/day	Ketoconazole Fluconazole	200 mg p.o. daily; 50–100 mg p.o. daily
Esophageal	Fluconazole or ketoconazole	100–200 mg p.o. daily x 2–3 weeks; 200–400 mg p.o. daily x 2–3 weeks	Amphotericin B	0.3 mg/kg i.v. daily x 7 days[j]
Coccidioidomycosis	Amphotericin B	0.5–1 mg/kg i.v. daily[m]	Fluconazole	400–800 mg/day
Chronic suppressive therapy	Amphotericin B	1 mg/kg weekly	Ketoconazole Itraconazole Fluconazole	400 mg p.o. daily; 100–200 mg p.o. bid; 400 mg daily
Cryptococcosis	Amphotericin B ± flucytosine[p]	0.3–0.6 mg/kg i.v. daily[m]; 25–37.5 mg/kg p.o. q6h	Fluconazole Itraconazole	200–400 mg p.o. daily[o]; 200 mg p.o. bid
Chronic suppressive therapy	Fluconazole	200 mg p.o. daily	Amphotericin B	0.5–1 mg/kg i.v. weekly
Histoplasmosis	Amphotericin B	0.5–0.6 mg/kg i.v. daily[q]	Itraconazole	200 mg p.o. bid
Chronic suppressive therapy	Itraconazole	200 mg p.o. bid	Amphotericin B	0.5–0.8 mg/kg i.v. weekly
Cytomegalovirus				
Retinitis, colitis, esophagitis	Ganciclovir[r]	5 mg/kg i.v. q12h x 14–21 days	Foscarnet	60 mg/kg i.v. q8h x 14–21 days
Chronic suppressive therapy	Ganciclovir	5 mg/kg i.v. daily or 6 mg/kg 5x/week	Foscarnet	90–120 mg/kg i.v. daily

Table 5.1—continued

Condition	Standard Treatment		Alternative Treatment	
	Drug	Dosage	Drug	Dosage
Herpes Simplex Virus, Primary or Recurrent				
	Acyclovir	200 mg p.o. 5x/day[s]	Foscarnet	40 mg/kg i.v. q8h × 21 days
Secondary Prophylaxis				
	Acyclovir	400 mg p.o. bid	Foscarnet	40 mg/kg i.v. daily
Varicella-Zoster, primary or disseminated				
	Acyclovir	10–12 mg/kg i.v. q8h × 7–14 days	Foscarnet	40 mg/kg i.v. q8h[s]
Dermatomal zoster				
	Acyclovir	800 mg p.o. 5x/day × 7–10 days	Foscarnet	40 mg/kg i.v. q8h[s]
Syphilis				
Primary, secondary, latent	Benzathine penicillin	2.4 mil U i.m.	**For all stages:** Amoxicillin	2 gm p.o. tid × 14 days
	or doxycycline	100 mg p.o. bid × 14 days	+ probenecid	500 mg p.o. tid × 14 days
	or erythromycin	500 mg p.o. qid × 14 days	or doxycycline	200 mg p.o. bid × 21 days
			or ceftriaxone	1 qm i.m. daily × 5–14 days
Late latent	Benzathine penicillin	2.4 mil U i.m. weekly × 3	or benzathine penicillin	2.4 U i.m. weekly × 3 doses
	or doxycycline	100 mg p.o. bid × 28 day	+ doxycycline	200 mg p.o. bid × 21 days
Neurosyphilis	Aqueous penicillin or procaine penicillin	12 mil U/day i.v. × 10 days		
		2.4 mil U i.m. daily × 10 days		
	+ probenecid	500 mg p.o. bid × 10 days		
Tuberculosis,[t] Pulmonary or Extrapulmonary	Isoniazid	300 mg p.o. daily		
	+ rifampin	600 mg p.o. daily		

+ pyrazinamide	15–25 mg/kg p.o. daily
+ ethambutol	15–25 mg/kg p.o. daily
or streptomycin	15 mg/kg i.m. daily[u]

Primary[y] and Secondary[w] Prophylaxis

Isoniazid[x]	300 mg p.o. daily[v]

Disseminated *Mycobacterium avium complex*[z]

Clarithromycin	500–1000 mg p.o. bid
or azithromycin	500 mg p.o. daily
Rifabutin + one or more of the standard agents	450–600 mg p.o. daily
+ one or more of the following:	
ethambutol	15–25 mg/kg daily
clofazimine	100–200 mg daily
ciprofloxacin	750 mg bid
amikacin	7.5–15 mg/kg/daily

Prophylaxis

Rifabutin	300 mg daily

[a] Many of the choices in the table are based on limited studies.

[b] Recombinant erythropoietin given subcutaneously at a dose of 100 U/kg three times per week has been used to treat zidovudine-induced anemia if endogenous serum erythropoietin levels are ≤500 IU/L. Zidovudine-induced neutropenia can be treated with G-CSF (Neupogen) or GM-CSF (Leukin, Prokine) in doses of 1–2 µg/kg subcutaneously once a day or three times a week (Miles SA. Cancer Invest 1991;9:229.)

[c] At 4-hour intervals. The package insert recommends a dosage of 200 mg every 4 hours for the first month of therapy; most clinicians believe this is unnecessary or necessary only in suspected HIV encephalopathy. Low doses are generally better tolerated and may have clinical and virological effects similar to those of higher doses.

[d] With tablets: for patients 35–49 kg, 125 mg p.o. bid; 50–74 kg, 200 mg p.o. bid; ≥75 kg, 300 mg p.o. bid. With powder, dosage varies from 167 mg–375 mg bid. The drug can be suspended in water or juice for easier ingestion.

[e] Based on trimethoprim component.

[f] Assay for G-6-PD deficiency recommended before therapy.

[g] In moderate or severe PCP with room air $PO_2 \leq 70$ mm Hg or Aa gradient ≥35 mm Hg.

[h] Recommended for patients with a clinical diagnosis of AIDS, fewer than 200 circulating CD4 cells, or less than 20% circulating CD4 cells.

[i] Double strength.

[j] With folinic acid, 5–10 mg/day.

[k] After a 200-mg loading dose. Length of treatment determined by clinical response to therapy, usually 4–8 weeks.

[l] Used in severe disease refractory to oral agents.

Table 5.1—continued

[m] Length of treatment determined by clinical response, usually at least 8 weeks.

[n] Length of treatment is determined by clinical and serological response, but is usually at least 2 weeks.

[o] Often used to complete acute treatment courses in mild cryptococcal meningitis once the CSF has been sterilized by amphotericin B.

[p] Higher doses often poorly tolerated in HIV infection; determination of plasma drug concentrations essential in patients with renal insufficiency.

[q] Length of treatment is determined by clinical response, but generally is at least 4–8 weeks.

[r] G-CSF or GM-CSF administered subcutaneously, 1–8 μg/kg/day, has been used to treat ganciclovir-induced neutropenia.

[s] Duration of treatment is determined by clinical response.

[t] Treatment should be continued for at least 6 months after cultures become negative.

[u] For patients more than 40 years old, 500–750 mg/day or 20 mg twice/week.

[v] Tuberculin-negative HIV-infected patients with known exposure to active tuberculosis are usually treated prophylactically.

[w] For tuberculin reactions >5 mm to intermediate-strength PPD and anergic patients at high risk.

[x] A combined prophylactic regimen of daily rifampin and pyrazinamide for several months' duration has been advocated when exposure to isoniazid-resistant organisms is likely.

[y] Usually continued for at least 1 year; some authorities suggest longer duration.

[z] Some patients may not require treatment. The optimal duration of treatment is unknown; drugs have generally been continued indefinitely.

cryptococcal meningitis, although the time to sterilization of the CSF was often slower than with amphotericin B (51). In one small randomized trial, amphotericin B plus flucytosine was superior to fluconazole for acute treatment of cryptococcal meningitis (52). Subsequently, a large controlled trial found that a low dose of amphotericin B or a low dose of fluconazole were about equally effective in AIDS-associated cryptococcal meningitis in patients without altered mental status (53). Fluconazole may be used to complete a course of acute treatment for cryptococcal meningitis after the CSF has been sterilized by amphotericin B, particularly in patients with clinically mild disease. For prevention of recurrent cryptococcal meningitis, daily fluconazole appears to be more effective and is better tolerated than weekly amphotericin B (54). Fluconazole may also be effective in treating HIV-infected patients with coccidioidal meningitis (55).

Itraconazole

The oral azole itraconazole (Sporanox) has been used successfully to treat cryptococcosis, histoplasmosis, aspergillosis, and candidiasis in HIV infection and to prevent recurrence of histoplasmosis (56, 57). Adverse effects of itraconazole include nausea, epigastric pain, rash, headache, edema, and hypokalemia.

HERPES SIMPLEX AND VARICELLA-ZOSTER VIRUS

Acyclovir

Oral acyclovir (Zovirax) can decrease the duration and severity of mucocutaneous herpes simplex virus (HSV) infections in HIV-infected patients and can often prevent recurrences.

High-dose oral or intravenous acyclovir decreases the duration and severity of primary varicella or disseminated varicella-zoster virus (VZV) infection in HIV-infected adults. Adverse effects include nausea, headache, and reversible renal dysfunction with high doses. Emergence of resistance has occurred in both HSV and VZV strains from HIV-infected patients treated with acyclovir (58, 59).

Foscarnet

Foscarnet (Foscavir) demonstrates in vitro activity against all herpesviruses. It has been used successfully to treat HIV-infected patients with acyclovir-resistant HSV and VZV infections (60, 61). Adverse effects include renal toxicity, anemia, nausea, hypokalemia, hypocalcemia (sometimes with tetany and seizures), and hypo- and hyperphosphatemia.

CYTOMEGALOVIRUS

Ganciclovir

End-organ cytomegalovirus (CMV) infections in AIDS, most commonly, retinitis, colitis, and esophagitis, respond to intravenous ganciclovir (Cytovene) (62) in 80–90% of patients (83). In CMV retinitis, continued daily maintenance infusions can delay relapse. After CMV esophagitis or colitis, routine secondary prophylaxis may not be necessary (63).

Neutropenia is a frequent dose-limiting adverse effect of ganciclovir. If zidovudine treatment is continued, the incidence of dose-limiting hematological toxicity may increase (64). Neutropenia from ganciclovir has been successfully treated with the granulocyte colony-stimulating factors GM-CSF and G-CSF (65, 66). Ganciclovir-resistant CMV isolates have emerged in HIV-infected patients receiving chronic ganciclovir therapy (67).

Foscarnet

Foscarnet has been used to treat CMV infections in patients unable to tolerate ganciclovir and in those with ganciclovir-resistant disease (68). A randomized trial found the two drugs equally effective in the treatment of CMV retinitis, and patients treated with foscarnet survived longer (69). Foscarnet was associated, however, with more treatment-limiting toxicity and is more difficult to administer (70). Some patients who have failed to respond to either ganciclovir or foscarnet have benefited from concurrent use of both (71).

MYCOBACTERIUM TUBERCULOSIS

Because of the recent increase in multiple-drug-resistant tuberculosis, initial treatment of tuberculosis in HIV-infected patients should be with the four drugs, isoniazid, rifampin (Rimactane and others), pyrazinamide, and ethambutol (Myambutol or streptomycin), and should be continued for at least 6 months after cultures become negative (72). All HIV-infected patients with tuberculin reactions of 5 mm or more in duration, regardless of age, should take at least 1 year of isoniazid for prophylaxis. Anergic tuberculin-negative HIV-infected patients with a high risk of tuberculosis, such as known contact, should also be considered for isoniazid prophylaxis (73, 74).

MYCOBACTERIUM AVIUM COMPLEX

Mycobacterium avium complex (MAC) colonization of the respiratory tract or the gastrointestinal tract is common in HIV infection and is not generally treated; in patients with low CD4 counts, prophylaxis with rifabutin (Mycobutin) can prevent dissemination to the bloodstream, bone marrow, liver, or lymphatic system (75, 76). Clarithromycin (Biaxin) or azithromycin in combination with other antimycobacterial drugs has been helpful in suppressing MAC infection in some patients (77). Symptomatic improvement and suppression of mycobacteremia have been achieved in other patients with four- to five-drug regimens that may include rifampin or rifabutin, ethambutol, clofazimine (Lamprene), ciprofloxacin (Cipro), and amikacin (Amikin) (78, 79). Adverse effects of these regimens have included rash, nausea, anorexia, aminotransferase increases, and neutropenia.

SYPHILIS

Syphilis may have an accelerated clinical course, prominent neurological involvement, and relapse despite standard treatment regimens in HIV-infected patients (80). Some authorities now routinely use longer treatment courses for primary or secondary syphilis in HIV-infected patients and urge that HIV-infected patients with serological evidence of syphilis be evaluated for neurosyphilis and treated aggressively, if necessary (81, 82).

Recommendations for Evaluation and Treatment of Patients with Early HIV Infection

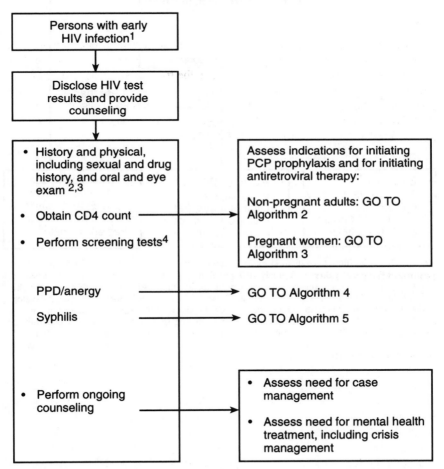

Figure 5.1. Algorithm 1. Selected elements of the initial and ongoing evaluation of adults with early HIV infection. [1]Provider should review and evaluate the adequacy of HIV diagnostic tests. [2]Appropriate immunizations should be provided. [3]Schedule follow-up appropriate for patient's condition. [4]Many other screening tests were not reviewed by this panel, including toxoplasmosis, hepatitis serology, and routine laboratory tests. (Reprinted with permission from U.S. Department of Health and Human Services clinical practice guideline number 7: evaluation and management of early HIV infection. January 1994.)

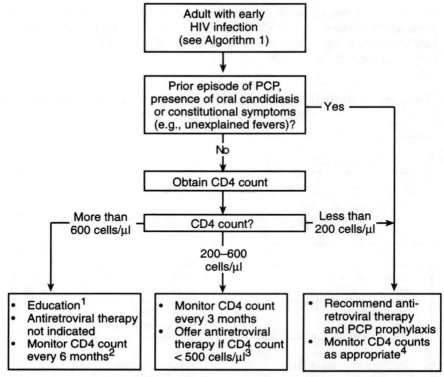

Figure 5.2. Algorithm 2. Evaluation for initiation of antiretroviral therapy and PCP prophylaxis; men and nonpregnant women with early HIV infection. [1]Education should include a discussion of enrollment into relevant investigational drug trials for asymptomatic persons. [2]If CD4 count has shown great variability or is rapidly declining, repeat the CD4 within 3 months. [3]If patient develops symptoms, recommend antiretroviral therapy. [4]If CD4 count is <200 cells/ml, continued monitoring of CD4 count may be needed to determine eligibility for clinical trials and prophylaxis for opportunistic infections other than PCP and to guide antiretroviral therapy. (Reprinted with permission from U.S. Department of Health and Human Services clinical practice guideline number 7: evaluation and management of early HIV infection. January 1994.)

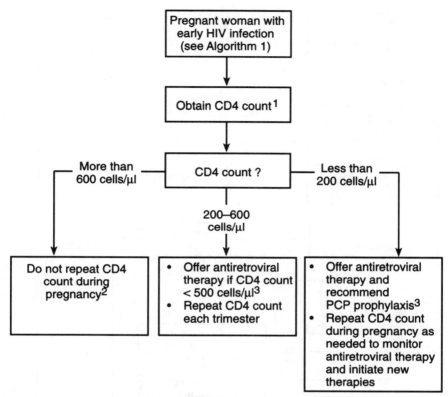

Figure 5.3. Algorithm 3. Evaluation for initiation of antiretroviral therapy and PCP prophylaxis; pregnant women with early HIV infection. [1]CD4 count should be obtained on presentation for prenatal care; women who have received no prenatal care should have CD4 counts taken at delivery. [2]Unless indicated by the presence of clinical symptoms. [3]The possible benefits and risks of antiretroviral therapy to both mother and fetus should be discussed fully with the patient. (Reprinted with permission from U.S. Department of Health and Human Services clinical practice guideline number 7: evaluation and management of early HIV infection. January 1994.)

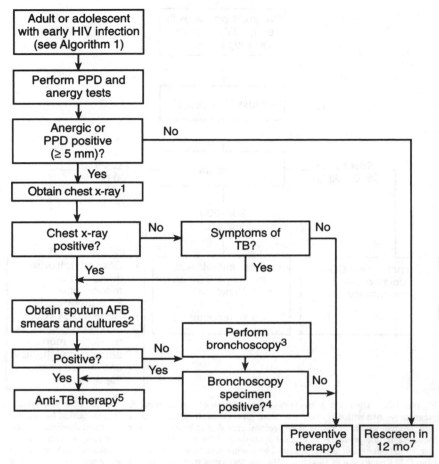

Figure 5.4.   Algorithm 4. Evaluation for *Mycobacterium tuberculosis* infection in adults and adolescents with early HIV infection. *TB*, tuberculosis; *AFB*, acid-fast bacilli. [1]Chest x-ray can be performed, using a lead apron shield, after the first trimester in pregnant women asymptomatic for TB or at any stage of pregnancy in women symptomatic for TB. [2]At least three sputum smears and cultures should be obtained. [3]If there is not other etiology for the abnormal chest x-ray. [4]Both AFB smears and cultures should be obtained at bronchoscopy. [5]Anti-TB therapy should be guided by local susceptibility patterns and modified appropriately when isolated susceptibilities become available. [6]Preventive therapy is indicated for PPD-positive patients and should be strongly considered for anergic patients who are known contacts of patients with tuberculosis and for anergic patients belonging to groups in which the prevalence of tuberculosis is at least 10% (e.g., injection drug users, prisoners, homeless persons, persons in congregate housing, migrant laborers, and persons born in foreign countries with high rates of TB). [7]Individuals who reside in settings where TB prevalence is high should be retested in 6 months; individuals who are exposed acutely to others with suspected or confirmed TB should be retested in 3 months; anergic individuals need not be retested, except in special circumstances. (Reprinted with permission from U.S. Department of Health and Human Services clinical practice guideline number 7: evaluation and management of early HIV infection. January 1994.)

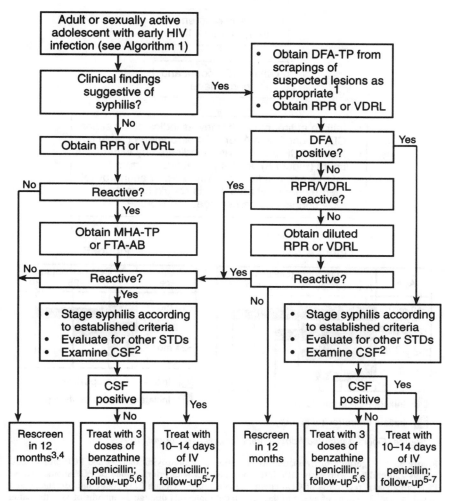

Figure 5.5. Algorithm 5. Evaluation for syphilis in adults and sexually active adolescents with early HIV infection. *STDs*, sexually transmitted diseases. [1]If Darkfield examination cannot be performed and primary syphilis is suspected, empiric treatment should be instituted. [2]Treatment for neurosyphilis recommended if the CSF cannot be evaluated. [3]Or after exposure to or diagnosis of any sexually transmitted disease. [4]Pregnant women should be screened for syphilis at entry to prenatal care, during the third trimester, or at delivery. [5]See recommended follow-up in U.S. Department of Health and Human Services Clinical Practice Guideline Number 7: Evaluation and Management of Early HIV Infection, January, 1994. [6]For issues specific to pregnant women, see recommended follow-up in U.S. Department of Health and Human Services Clinical Practice Guideline Number 7: Evaluation and Management of Early HIV Infection, January, 1994. [7]Alternative treatments include 10 days of intramuscular procaine penicillin or 10–14 days of 1–2 g of intramuscular ceftriaxome. (Reprinted with permission from U.S. Department of Health and Human Services clinical practice guideline number 7: evaluation and management of early HIV infection. January 1994.)

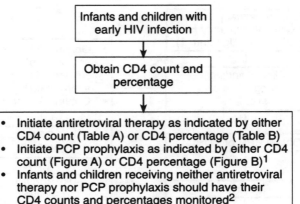

Infants and children with
early HIV infection

Obtain CD4 count and
percentage

- Initiate antiretroviral therapy as indicated by either
  CD4 count (Table A) or CD4 percentage (Table B)
- Initiate PCP prophylaxis as indicated by either CD4
  count (Figure A) or CD4 percentage (Figure B)[1]
- Infants and children receiving neither antiretroviral
  therapy nor PCP prophylaxis should have their
  CD4 counts and percentages monitored[2]

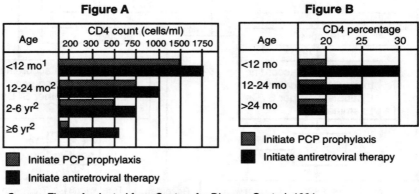

Figure A

Age	CD4 count (cells/ml) 200 300 500 750 1000 1500 1750
<12 mo[1]	
12-24 mo[2]	
2-6 yr[2]	
≥6 yr[2]	

Initiate PCP prophylaxis

Initiate antiretroviral therapy

Figure B

Age	CD4 percentage 20 25 30
<12 mo	
12-24 mo	
>24 mo	

Initiate PCP prophylaxis

Initiate antiretroviral therapy

Source: Figure A adapted from Centers for Disease Control, 1991

Figure 5.6. Algorithm 6. Evaluation for initiation of antiretroviral therapy and PCP prophylaxis; infants and children with early HIV infection. [1]Patients with prior episode of PCP should receive PCP prophylaxis regardless of CD4 count and percentage. [2]Obtain CD4 count and percentage at 1 month of age, 3 months of age, and then at 3 month intervals through 24 months of age; thereafter obtain CD4 count and percentage every 6 months, unless values reach an age-related threshold where testing should be repeated monthly. (Reprinted with permission from U.S. Department of Health and Human Services clinical practice guideline number 7: evaluation and management of early HIV infection. January 1994.)

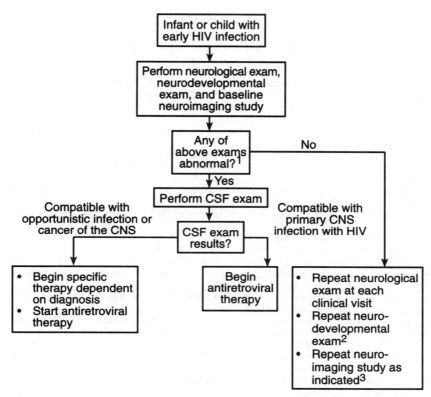

Figure 5.7. Algorithm 7. Neurologic evaluation of infants and children with early HIV infection. [1]Abnormal examination is defined as focal pathology, obstructive lesion, atypical CNS manifestations, or evidence of progressive neurologic disease. [2]Neurodevelopmental examination should be performed at 3-month intervals up to 24 months of age, then every 6 months thereafter. [3]Neuroimaging studies should be performed if CNS symptoms occur; such studies should be performed in conjunction with CSF analysis. (Reprinted with permission from U.S. Department of Health and Human Services clinical practice guideline number 7: evaluation and management of early HIV infection. January 1994.)

REFERENCES

1. Moore RD et al. Zidovudine and the natural history of the acquired immunodeficiency syndrome. N Engl J Med 1991;324:1412.
2. Fischl MA et al. The safety and efficacy of zidovudine (AZT) in the treatment of subjects with mildly symptomatic human immunodeficiency virus type 1 (HIV) infection. A double-blind, placebo-controlled trial. The AIDS Clinical Trials Group. Ann Intern Med 1990;112:727.
3. Graham NMH et al. The effects on survival of early treatment of human immunodeficiency virus infection. N Engl J Med 1992;326:1037.
4. Aboulker JP et al. Preliminary analysis of the Concorde trial. Concorde Coordinating Committee. Lancet 1993;341:889.
5. Cooper DA et al. Zidovudine in persons with asymptomatic HIV infection and CD4+ cell counts greater than 400 per cubic millimeter. The European-Australian Collaborative Group. N Engl J Med 1993;329:297.
6. Chattha G et al. Lactic acidosis complicating the acquired immunodeficiency syndrome. Ann Intern Med 1993;118:37.
7. Freiman JP et al. Hepatomegaly with severe steatosis in HIV-seropositive patients. AIDS 1993;7:379.
8. Erythropoietin for anemia. Med Lett 1989;31:85.   9. Henry DH et al. Recombinant human erythropoietan in the treatment of anemia associated with human immunodeficiency virus (HIV) infection and zidovudine therapy. Overview of four clinical trials. Ann Intern Med 1992;117:739.
10. Miles SA. The use of hematopoietic growth factors in HIV infection and AIDS-related malignancies. Cancer Invest 1991;9:229.
11. Sperling RS et al. A survey of zidovudine use in pregnant women with human immunodeficiency virus infection. N Engl J Med 1992;326:857.
12. Boucher CAB et al. Ordered appearance of zidovudine resistance mutations during treatment of 18 human immunodeficiency virus-positive subjects. J Infect Dis 1992;165:105.
13. Larder BA et al. Susceptibilities of zidovudine-susceptible and -resistant human immunodeficiency virus isolates to antiviral agents determined by using a quantitative plaque reduction assay. Antimicrob Agents Chemother 1990;34:436.
14. Yarchoan R et al. In vivo activity against HIV and favorable toxicity profile of 2',3'-dideoxyinosine. Science 1989;245:412.
15. Connolly KJ et al. Phase I study of 2',3'-dideoxyinosine administered orally twice daily to patients with AIDS or AIDS-related complex and hematologic intolerance to zidovudine. Am J Med 1991;91:471.
16. Butler KM et al. Dideoxyinosine in children with symptomatic human immunodeficiency virus infection. N Engl J Med 1991;324:137.
17. Kahn JO et al. Undiagnosed HIV infection in acute care hospitals (Letter). N Engl J Med 1992;327:1815.   18. Lai KK et al. Fulminant hepatic failure associated with 2',3'-dideoxyinosine (ddI). Ann Intern Med 1991;115:283.
19. Metroka CE et al. Failure of prophylaxis with dapsone in patients taking dideoxyinosine. N Engl J Med 1991;325:737.
20. Ruskin J, LaRiviere M. Low-dose co-trimoxazole for prevention of *Pneumocystis carinii* pneumonia in human immunodeficiency virus disease. Lancet 1991;337:468.
21. Fischl MA et al. Zalcitabine compared with zidovudine in patients with advanced HIV-1 infection who received previous zidovudine therapy. Ann Intern Med 1993;118:762.
22. Meng TC et al. Combination therapy with zidovudine and dideoxycytidine in patients with advanced human immunodeficiency virus infection. A phase I/II study. Ann Intern Med 1992;116:13.
23. Sattler FR et al. Trimethoprim-sulfamethoxazole compared with pentamidine for treatment of *Pneumocystis carinii* pneumonia in the acquired immunodeficiency syndrome. A prospective, noncrossover study. Ann Intern Med 1988;109:280.
24. Conte JE et al. Intraveneous or inhaled pentamidine for treating *Pneumocystis carinii* pneumonia in AIDS. A randomized trial. Ann Intern Med 1990;113:203.
25. Hardy WD et al. A controlled trial of trimethoprim-sulfamethoxazole or aerosolized pentamidine for secondary prophylaxis of *Pneumocystis carinii* pneumonia in patients with the acquired immunodeficiency syndrome. AIDS Clinical Trials Group Protocol 021. N Engl J Med 1992;327:1842.

26. Schneider MME et al. A controlled trial of aerosolized pentamidine or trimethoprim-sulfamethoxazole as primary prophylaxis against *Pneumocystis carinii* pneumonia in patients with human immunodeficiency virus infection. The Dutch AIDS Treatment Group. N Engl J Med 1992;327:1836.
27. Medina I et al. Oral therapy for *Pneumocystis carinii* pneumonia in the acquired immunodeficiency syndrome. A controlled trial of trimethoprim-sulfamethoxazole versus trimethoprim-dapsone. N Engl J Med 1990;323:776.
28. Hughes WT et al. Prevention of *Pneumocystis carinii* pneumonia in AIDS patients with weekly dapsone. Lancet 1990;336:1066.
29. Girard PM et al. Dapsone-pyrimethamine compared with aerosolized pentamidine as primary prophylaxis against *Pneumocystis carinii* pneumonia and toxoplasmosis in HIV infection. The PRIO Study Group. N Engl J Med 1993;328:1514.
30. Atovaquone for *Pneumocystis carinii* pneumonia. Med Lett 1993;35:28.
31. Hughes W et al. Comparison of atovaquone (566C80) with trimethoprim-sulfamethoxazole to treat *Pneumocystis carinii* pneumonia in patients with AIDS. N Engl J Med 1993;328:1521.
32. Hughes W et al. Safety and pharmacokinetics of 566C80—a hydroxynaphthoquinone with anti-*Pneumocystis carinii* activity. A phase I study in human immunodeficiency vius (HIV)-infected men. J Infect Dis 1991;163:843.
33. Toma E et al. Malaria in splenectomized patients (Letter). Clin Infect Dis 1993;17:936–937.
34. Trimetrexate for *Pneumocystis carinii* pneumonia. Med Lett 1989;31:5.
35. Allegra CJ et al. Trimetrexate for the treatment of *Pneumocystis carinii* pneumonia in patients with the acquired immunodeficiency syndrome. N Engl J Med 1987;317:978.
36. Sattler FR et al. Trimetrexate-leucovorin dosage evaluation study for treatment of *Pneumocystis carinii* pneumonia. J Infect Dis 1990;161:91.
37. NIH-University of California Expert Panel. Special report: consensus statement on the use of corticosteroids as adjunctive therapy for *Pneumocystis pneumonia* in the acquired immunodeficiency syndrome. N Engl J Med 1990;323:1500.
38. Update: availability of sulfadiazine—United States. MMWR 1993;42(5):105.
39. Dannemann B et al. Treatment of toxoplasmic encephalitis in patients with AIDS. A randomized trial comparing pyrimethamine plus clindamycin to pyrimethamine plus sulfadiazine. Ann Intern Med 1992;116:33.
40. Kovacs JA et al. Efficacy of atovaquone in treatment of toxoplasmosis in patients with AIDS. The NIAID-Clinical Center Intramural AIDS Program. Lancet 1992;340:637.
41. Carr A et al. Low-dose trimethoprim-sulfamethoxazole prophylaxis for toxoplasmic encephalitis in patients with AIDS. Ann Intern Med 1992;117:106.
42. Girard PM et al. Dapsone-pyrimethamine compared with aerosolized pentamidine as primary prophylaxis against *Pneumocystis carinii* pneumonia and toxoplasmosis in HIV infection. The PROI Study Group. N Engl J Med 1993;328:1514.
43. Cello JP et al. Effect of octreotide on refractory AIDS-associated diarrhea. A prospective, multicenter clinical trial. Ann Intern Med 1991;115:705.
44. Armitage K et al. Treatment of cryptosporidiosis with paromycin. A report of five cases. Arch Intern Med 1992;152:2497.
45. Sugar EF et al. Effect of various common beverages on the dissolution of ketoconazole tablets. AIDS 1992;6:1221.
46. Fluconazole. Med Lett 1990;32:50.
47. Laine L et al. Fluconazole compared with ketoconazole for the treatment of *Candida* esophagitis in AIDS. A randomized trial. Ann Intern Med 1992;117:655.
48. Stevens DA et al. Thrush can be prevented in patients with acquired immunodeficiency syndrome and the acquired immunodeficiency syndrome-related complex. Randomized, double-blind, placebo-controlled study of 100-mg oral fluconazole daily. Arch Intern Med 1991;151:2458.
49. Drugs for treatment of fungal infections. Med Lett 1992;34:14.
50. McKinsey DS et al. Histoplasmosis in patients with AIDS: efficacy of maintenance amphotericin B therapy. Am J Med 1992;92:225.
51. Sugar AM et al. Overview: treatment of cryptococcal meningitis. Rev Infect Dis 1990;12(suppl 3):S338.
52. Larsen RA et al. Fluconazole compared with amphotericin B plus flucytosine for cryptococcal meningitis in AIDS. A randomized trial. Ann Intern Med 1990;113:183.
53. Saag MS et al. Comparison of amphotericin B with fluconazole in the treatment of acute AIDS-associated cryptococcal meningitis. The NIAID Mycoses Study Group and the AIDS Clinical Trials Group. N Engl J Med 1992;326:83.

54. Powderly WG et al. A controlled trial of fluconazole or amphotericin B to prevent relapse of cryptococcal meningitis in patients with the acquired immunodeficiency syndrome. The NIAID AIDS Clinical Trials Group and Mycoses Study Group. N Engl J Med 1992;326:793.
55. Galgiani JN et al. Fluconazole therapy for coccidioidal meningitis. Ann Intern Med 1993;119:28.
56. Itraconazole. Med Lett 1993;35:7.
57. Wheat J et al. Prevention of relapse of histoplasmosis with itraconazole in patients with the acquired immunodeficiency syndrome. The National Institute of Allergy and Infectious Diseases Clinical Trials and Mycoses Study Group Collaborators. Ann Intern Med 1993;118:610.
58. Chatis PA et al. Successful treatment with foscarnet of an acyclovir-resistant mucocutaneous infection with herpes simplex virus in a patient with acquired immunodeficieny syndrome. N Engl J Med 1989;320:297.
59. Jacobson MA et al. Acyclovir-resistant varicella zoster virus infection after chronic oral acyclovir therapy in patients with the acquired immunodeficiency syndome (AIDS). Ann Intern Med 1990;112:187.
60. Safrin S et al. A controlled trial comparing foscarnet with vidarabine for acyclovir-resistant mucocutaneous herpes simplex in the acquired immunodeficiency syndrome. The AIDS Clinical Trial Group. N Engl J Med 1991;325:551.
61. Safrin S et al. Foscarnet therapy in five patients with AIDS and acyclovir-resistant varicella-zoster virus infection. Ann Intern Med 1991;115:19.
62. Ganciclovir. Med Lett 1989;31:79.
63. Dieterich DT et al. Concurrent use of ganciclovir and foscarnet to treat cytomegalovirus infection in AIDS patients. J Infect Dis 1993;167:278.
64. Hochster H et al. Toxicity of combined ganciclovir and zidovudine for cytomegalovirus disease associated with AIDS. An AIDS Clinical Trials Group Study. Ann Intern Med 1990;113:111.
65. Hardy WD. Combined ganciclovir and recombinant human granulocyte-macrophage colony-stimulating factor in the treatment of cytomegalovirus retinitis in AIDS patients. J Acquir Immune Defic Syndr 1991;4(suppl 1):S22.
66. Granulocyte colony-stimulating factors. Med Lett 1991;33:61.
67. Drew WL et al. Prevalence of resistance in patients receiving ganciclovir for serious cytomegalovirus infection. J Infect Dis 1991;163:716.
68. Jacobson MA et al. Foscarnet therapy for ganciclovir-resistant cytomegalovirus retinitis in patients with AIDS. J Infect Dis 1991;163:1348.
69. Studies of Ocular Complications of AIDS Research Group. Mortality in patients with the acquired immunodeficiency syndrome treated with either foscarnet or ganciclovir for cytomegalovirus retinitis. N Engl J Med 1992;326:213.
70. Foscarnet. Med Lett 1992;34:3.
71. Dieterich DT et al. Concurrent use of ganciclovir and foscarnet to treat cytomegalovirus infection in AIDS patients. J Infect Dis 1993;167:1184.
72. MMWR 1993;42,RR-7:1.
73. MMWR. Purified protein derivative (PPD)-tuberculin anergy and HIV infection. Guidelines for anergy testing and management of anergic persons at risk of tuberculosis. 1991;40,RR-5:27.
74. Moreno S et al. Risk for developing tuberculosis among anergic patients infected with HIV. Ann Intern Med 1993;119:194.
75. Rifabutin. Med Lett 1993;35:36.
76. Recommendations on prophylaxis and therapy for disseminated *Mycobacterium avium* complex for adults and adolescents infected with human immunodeficiency virus. MMWR 1993;42,RR-9:17.
77. Barradell LB et al. Clarithromycin, a review of its pharmacological properties and therapeutic use in *Mycobacterium avium-intracellulare* complex infection in patients with acquired immune deficiency syndrome. Drugs 1993;46:289.
78. Ellner JJ et al. *Mycobacterium avium* infection and AIDS: a therapeutic dilemma in rapid evolution. J Infect Dis 1991;163:1326.
79. Kemper CA et al. Treatment of *Mycobacterium avium* complex bacteremia in AIDS with a four-drug oral regimen. Rifampin, ethambutol, clofazimine, and ciprofloxacin. The California Collaborative Treatment Group. Ann Intern Med 1992;116:466.
80. Hook EW III, Marra CM. Acquired syphilis in adults. N Engl J Med 1992;326:1060.
81. Musher DM et al. Effect of human immunodeficiency virus (HIV) infection on the course of syphilis and on the response to treatment. Ann Intern Med 1990;113:872–881.
82. Tramont EC. In Volberding P, Jacobson M, eds. Controversies regarding the natural history and treatment of syphilis in HIV disease. AIDS Clin Rev 1991;97.
83. Schooley RT. Cytomegalovirus in the setting of infection with human immunodeficiency virus [Review]. Rev Infect Dis 1990;12:S811.

SECTION 6
Antibiotic Susceptibilities

Two standard methods are used for in vitro testing systems. The first uses antibiotic-impregnated discs (Kirby Bauer discs) and correlates sensitivity or resistance with zones of growth inhibition surrounding the disc; the other method involves either broth or agar dilution of antibiotics tested against standardized inoculums of microorganisms. The former method correlates inhibition zone size with sensitivity or resistance to a given antibiotic and roughly approximates zone size with concentration of antibiotic. The latter method (dilutional) more closely approximates specific antibiotic concentrations as the minimum inhibitory concentration (MIC). The MIC is the lowest concentration of a given antibiotic that inhibits growth of a standard inoculum of an organism (Fig. 6.1).

The treatment of certain infections, such as endocarditis and meningitis, requires killing the infecting organism. The efficacy with which an antibiotic kills is indicated by the minimum lethal concentration (MLC), also known as the minimum bactericidal concentration (MBC). The MLC is determined by serially

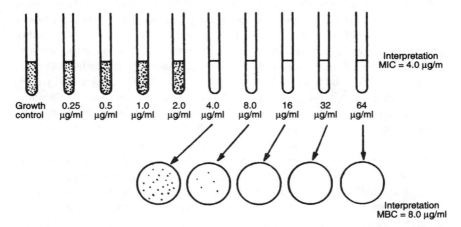

Figure 6.1. Determination of minimal inhibitory concentrations (*MIC*) and minimal bactericidal concentrations (*MBC*). The minimal inhibitory concentration is defined as the lowest concentration of antibiotic that results in no visible growth (turbidity). The minimal bactericidal (lethal) concentration is the lowest concentration of antibiotic that produces a 99.9% (10^3) reduction in organisms from the original inoculum of approximately 10^5.

subculturing apparently inhibited inocula and by determining that concentration of an antibiotic in which the organisms will not grow and, thus, have been killed (Fig. 6.1).

Bacteriostatic antibiotics (e.g., erythromycin, tetracycline) are those agents that inhibit the growth of microorganisms only in vitro. These agents may be capable of killing standardized inocula of bacteria at high concentrations; this killing cannot be achieved in vivo.

Bactericidal antibiotics (e.g., penicillins, cephalosporins, aminoglycosides) are lethal to standardized inocula at clinically achievable concentrations. These lethal concentrations are usually the same as or slightly higher than inhibitory concentrations. Certain antibiotics may be both bacteriostatic and bactericidal. Significant examples are chloramphenicol and certain penicillins. Chloramphenicol can be bactericidal against *Haemophilus influenzae*, *Neisseria meningitidis*, and *Streptococcus pneumoniae*. However, it inhibits growth of only staphylococci and susceptible Gram-negative bacilli. Penicillins inhibit the growth of only enterococci but are bactericidal for most other streptococci. Still other antibiotics are variably bactericidal against the same organism, as exemplified by clindamycin against *Staphylococcus aureus*.

Certain strains of microorganisms may manifest the so-called phenomenon of "tolerance." That is, antibiotics that are usually bactericidal at the same concentrations at which they are bacteriostatic may not kill the bacteria when tested in vitro. The most common example of this is tolerance of staphylococci when tested against penicillinase-resistant penicillins or cephalosporins. The clinical significance of this phenomenon is unclear because endocarditis produced by tolerant strains may respond to the agents. In some large hospitals, nearly 50% of isolates of *S. aureus* are resistant to methicillin (or nafcillin/oxacillin). Similarly, nearly 75% of isolates of coagulase-negative staphylococci are also resistant to these drugs. These isolates are reliably detected in the laboratory by incubation at 35°C; by use of fully potent methicillin, nafcillin, or oxacillin discs; and by careful reading of plates to detect light growth in the zone of inhibition. Despite apparent in vitro susceptibility to other drugs such as cephalosporins, these agents are not effective in treating infection due to methicillin-resistant staphylococci, and vancomycin remains the drug of choice.

The tables in this section (Tables 6.1 through 6.9) allow the clinician to compare the in vitro activity of various antibiotics for a given organism and to compare the spectrum of activity of various antibiotics. Knowledge of the pharmacology and clinical usefulness of the antibiotics, and a comparison of their in vitro activity, may help a clinician to choose one agent over another.

The tables in this section provide the concentrations of antibiotics that inhibit most strains (approximately 75–90%) of a given organism. An exception to this is the table on susceptibility of mycobacteria, which lists the percentage of susceptibility to a given concentration of drug.

The information was gathered, whenever possible, from large-scale trials using standardized in vitro methods. Cutoff points of susceptibility and resistance are often nebulous. Clinical efficacy depends largely on the pharmacology of the antibiotic and the site of infection, as well as on in vitro susceptibility. For example, in many cases, urinary tract infections due to *Enterobacteriaceae* that appear to be resistant to tetracycline respond to tetracycline therapy because urinary concentrations of the antibiotic are much higher than serum concentrations and may exceed the MIC. The criteria for susceptibility to the various antibiotics are given in Table 6.1 through 6.1D.[a]

---

[a] Permission to use portions of M2-A5 (Performance Standards for Antimicrobial Disk Susceptibility Tests, Fifth Edition; Approved Standard) and M11-A3 (Methods for Antimicrobial Susceptibility Testing of Anaerobic Bacteria, Third Edition; Approved Standard) has been granted by NCCLS. The interpretive data are valid only if the methodology in M2-A5 and M11-A3 is followed. NCCLS frequently updates the interpretive tables through new editions of the standards and supplements to them. Users should refer to the most recent editions. The current standards and supplements to them may be obtained from NCCLS, 771 E. Lancaster Avenue, Villanova, PA 19085.

Table 6.1. Zone Diameter Interpretive Standards and Equivalent Minimum Inhibitory Concentration (MIC) Breakpoints for Organisms Other Than *Haemophilus*, *Neisseria gonorrhoeae*, and *Streptococcus pneumoniae* (Disk Diffusion)

Antimicrobial Agent	Zone Diameter (Nearest Whole mm)			Equivalent MIC Breakpoints[p] (μg/ml)	
	Resistant	Intermediate[m]	Susceptible[o]	Resistant	Susceptible
β-Lactams					
Penicillins					
Ampicillin[a]					
When testing Gram-negative enteric organisms	≤13	14–16	≥17	≥32	≤8
When testing enterococci[d]	≤16		≥17[d]	≥16	
When testing streptococci (not *S. pneumoniae*)[e]	≤21	22–29	≥30	≥4	≤0.12
Nafcillin when testing staphylococci[g]	≤10	11–12	≥13		≤1
Penicillin					
When testing staphylococci[b,c]	≤28		≥29	β-Lactamase[b]	≤0.1
When testing enterococci[d]	≤14		≥15[d]	≥16	
When testing streptococci (not *S. pneumoniae*)[e]	≤19	20–27	≥28	≥4	≤0.12
When testing *L. monocytogenes*	≤19		≥20	≥4	≤2
Piperacillin[b]					
When testing *P. aeruginosa*[f]	≤17		≥18	≥128	≤64
When testing other Gram-negative organisms	≤17	18–20	≥21	≥128	≤16
β-Lactam/β-Lactamase Inhibitor Combinations					
Amoxicillin/clavulanic acid[h]					
When testing staphylococci[c]	≤19		≥20	≥8/4	≤4/2
When testing other organisms	≤13	14–17	≥18	≥16/8	≤8/4
Ampicillin/sulbactam[h]					
When testing Gram-negative enterics and staphylococci[c]	≤11	12–14	≥15	≥32/16	≤8/4
Ticarcillin/clavulanic acid					
When testing *P. aeruginosa*[f]	≤14		≥15	≥128/2	≤64/2
When testing other Gram-negative organisms	≤14	15–19	≥20	≥128/2	≤16/2
Cephalosporins and other Cephems					
Cefazolin[c]	≤14	15–17	≥18	≥32	≤8
Cefixime[c,j]	≤15	16–18	≥19	≥4	≤1
Cefoperazone[e]	≤15	16–20	≥21	≥64	≤16

Cefoxitin[a]	≤14	15–17	≥18	≥32	≤8
Ceftazidime[c,f]	≤14	15–17	≥18	≥32	≤8
Ceftizoxime[c]	≤14	15–19	≥20	≥32	≤8
Ceftriaxone[c]	≤13	14–20	≥21	≥64	≤8
Cefuroxime sodium (parenteral)[c]	≤14	15–17	≥18	≥32	≤8
Carbapenems					
Imipenem[c]	≤13	14–15	≥16	≥16	≤4
Glycopeptides					
Vancomycin					
When testing enterococci[d,j]	≤14	15–16	≥17	≥32	≤4
When testing other Gram-positive organisms	≤9	10–11	≥12	≥32	≤4
Aminoglycosides					
Amikacin	≤14	15–16	≥17	≥32	≤16
Gentamicin					
When testing enterococci for high-level resistance	6	7–9[h]	≥10	>500	≤500
When testing other organisms	≤12	13–14	≥15	≥8	≤4
Streptomycin					
When testing enterococci for high-level resistance	6	7–9[h]	≥10	—[g]	—[g]
When testing other organisms	≤11	12–14	≥15	—	—
Tobramycin	≤12	13–14	≥15	≥8	≤4
Macrolides					
Azithromycin	≤13	14–17	≥18	≥8	≤2
Clarithromycin	≤13	14–17	≥18	≥8	≤2
Erythromycin	≤13	14–22	≥23	≥8	≤0.5
Tetracyclines					
Doxycycline[k]	≤12	13–15	≥16	≥16	≤4
Tetracycline[k]	≤14	15–18	≥19	≥16	≤4
Quinolones					
Ciprofloxacin	≤15	16–20	≥21	≥4	≤1
Ofloxacin	≤12	13–15	≥16	≥8	≤2
Others					
Chloramphenicol	≤12	13–17	≥18	≥32	≤8
Clindamycin	≤14	15–20	≥21	≥4	≤0.5
Trimethoprim/sulfamethoxazole[l]	≤10	11–15	≥16	≥8/152	≤2/38

NOTE: Information in boldface type is considered tentative for 1 year.

[a] Class disk for ampicillin, amoxicillin, bacampicillin, cyclacillin, and hetacillin.

[b] Resistant strains of S. aureus produce β-lactamase, and the testing of the 10-unit penicillin disk is preferred. Penicillin should be used to test the susceptibility of all penicillinase-sensitive penicillins, such as ampicillin, amoxicillin, azlocillin, bacampicillin, hetacillin, cerbenicillin, mezlocillin, piperacillin, and ticarcillin. Results may also be applied to phenoxymethyl penicillin or phenethicillin.

Table 6.1—continued

Staphylococci exhibiting resistance to methicillin, oxacillin, or nafcillin should be reported as also resistant to other penicillins, cephalosporins, carbacephems, carbapenems, and β-lactamase inhibitor combinations despite apparent in vitro susceptibility of some strains to the latter agents. This is because infections with methicillin-resistant staphylococci have not responded favorably to therapy with β-lactam antibiotics.

The "Susceptible" category for penicillin or ampicillin implies the need for high-dose therapy for serious enterococcal infections. If possible, this should be denoted by a footnote on the susceptibility report form. Enterococcal endocarditis requires combined therapy with high-dose penicillin or high-dose ampicillin, or vancomycin, or teicoplanin plus gentamicin or streptomycin for bactericidal action. **Since ampicillin or penicillin resistance among enterococci due to β-lactamase production is not reliably detected using routine disk or dilution methods, a direct nitrocefin-based β-lactamase test is recommended. Synergy between ampicillin, penicillin, or vancomycin and an aminoglycoside can be predicted for enterococci by using a high-level aminoglycoside screening test.**

A penicillin MIC should be determined on isolates of viridans *Streptococcus* from patients with infective endocarditis.

P. aeruginosa infections in granulocytopenic patients and serious infections in other patients should be treated with maximum doses of the selected antipseudomonal penicillins (carboxypenicillin or acylaminocillins) or ceftazidime in combination with an aminoglycoside.

Of the antistaphylococcal, β-lactamase-resistant penicillins, either oxacillin, methicillin, or nafcillin could be tested, and results can be applied to the other penicillinase-resistant penicillins, cloxacillin and dicloxacillin. Oxacillin is preferred due to more resistance to degradation in storage and its application to pneumococcal testing and because it is more likely to detect heteroresistant staphylococcal strains. Do not use nafcillin on blood-containing media. Cloxacillin disks should not be used because they may not detect methicillin-resistant *S. aureus.* If intermediate results are obtained **when testing penicillinase-resistant penicillins with staphylococci, the disk test should be repeated, or one of the testing methods described in NCCLS document M7 should be used alternatively.**

The ampicillin test results may be used for determining susceptibility to amoxicillin/clavulanic acid and ampicillin/sulbactam among streptococci and non-β-lactamase-producing enterococci.

Not applicable for testing *Moranella.*

When testing vancomycin against enterococci, plates should be held a full 24 hr and examined using transmitted light; the presence of a haze or any growth within the zone of inhibition indicates resistance. If vancomycin is being considered for treatment of serious enterococcal infection, those organisms with intermediate zones should be tested by an MIC method **as described in NCCLS document M7.**

Tetracycline is the class disk for all tetracyclines, and the results can be applied to chlortetracycline, demeclocycline, doxycycline, methacycline, minocycline, and oxytetracycline. However, certain organisms may be more susceptible to doxycycline and minocycline than to tetracycline **(e.g., some staphylococci and *Acinetobacter*).**

The sulfisoxazole disk can be used to represent any of the currently available sulfonamide preparations. Blood-containing media except for lysed horse blood) are **generally not suitable for testing sulfonamides or trimethoprim.** Mueller-Hinton agar should be checked for excessive levels of thymidine.

The category "Intermediate" should be reported. MICs for these isolates approach usually attainable blood and tissue levels, and response rates may be lower than for susceptible isolates. The "Intermediate" category implies clinical applicability in body sites where the drugs are physiologically concentrated (e.g., quinolones and β-lactams in urine), or when a high dosage of a drug can be used (e.g. β-lactams). The "Intermediate" category also indicates a "buffer zone," which should prevent small uncontrolled technical factors from causing major discrepancies in interpretation, especially for drugs with narrow pharmacotoxicity margins.

If the zone is 7 to 9 mm, the test is inconclusive, and an agar dilution or broth microdilution screen test should be performed to confirm resistance.

Policies regarding generation of cumulative antibiograms should be developed in concert with the infectious disease service, infection control personnel, and the pharmacy and therapeutics committee. Under most circumstances, **the percentage of susceptible and intermediate results should not be combined into the same statistic.**

These values represent MIC breakpoints used in determining approximate zone size interpretive criteria. They relate to MICs determined by M7 methodology. Occasional discrepancies may exist between M2 and M7 due to methodological limitations.

MIC correlates for streptomycin broth microdilution are resistant >1000 μg/ml and for agar >2000 μg/ml.

Table 6.1A. Some Examples of Zone Diameter Interpretive Standards and Equivalent Minimum Inhibitory Concentration (MIC) Breakpoints for *Haemophilus*[a] (Disk Diffusion)

Antimicrobial Agent	Zone Diameter (Nearest Whole mm)			Equivalent MIC Breakpoints[e] (μg/ml)	
	Resistant	Intermediate[d]	Susceptible	Resistant	Susceptible
Ampicillin	≤18	19–21	≥22	≥4	≤1
Azithromycin[b]			≥12		≤4
Ceftizoxime[b]			≥26		≤2
Cefuroxime[c]	≤16	17–19	≥20	≥16	≤4
Ciprofloxacin[b]			≥21		≤1
Clarithromycin	≤10	11–12	≥13	≤32	≤8
Imipenem[b]			≥16		≤4
Ofloxacin[b]			≥16		≤2
Trimethoprim/sulfamethoxazole	≤10	11–15	≥16	≥4/76	≤0.5/9.5

NOTE 1: These zone diameter standards and MIC breakpoints apply only to tests with *Haemophilus* species using *Haemophilus* Test Medium (HTM).

NOTE 2: Information in boldface type is considered tentative for 1 year.

[a] Amoxicillin/clavulanic acid and ampicillin/sulbactam may be of use in the management of *Haemophilus* infections; however, a reliable disk diffusion test method for assessing the activity of these agents against *Haemophilus* does not currently exist. Their in vitro activity is best determined by a broth microdilution method.

[b] For these antimicrobial agents, the current absence of resistant strains precludes defining any results categories other than "Susceptible." Strains yielding results suggestive of a "Nonsusceptible" category should be submitted to a reference laboratory for further testing.

[c] Rare β-lactamase-negative, ampicillin-resistant (BLNAR) strains of *Haemophilus influenzae* should be considered resistant at this time to amoxicillin/clavulanic acid, ampicillin/sulbactam, cefaclor, cefonicid, cefprozil, cefuroxime, and loracarbef despite apparent in vitro susceptibility of some BLNAR strains to these agents.

[d] The category "Intermediate" should be reported. It generally indicates that the result be considered equivocal or indeterminate.

[e] These values represent MIC breakpoints used in determining approximate zone size interpretive criteria. In all cases, they correspond to the MIC interpretive criteria published in the M7 document.

Table 6.1B. Some Examples of Zone Diameter Interpretive Standards and Equivalent Minimum Inhibitory Concentration (MIC) Breakpoints for *Neisseria gonorrhoeae* (Disk Diffusion)

Antimicrobial Agent	Zone Diameter (Nearest Whole mm)			Equivalent MIC Breakpoints[d] (µg/ml)	
	Resistant	Intermediate[c]	Susceptible	Resistant	Susceptible
Ceftriaxone[a]			≥35		≤0.25
Ciprofloxacin[a]			≥36		≤0.06
Ofloxacin[a]			≥31		≤0.25
Penicillin[b]	≤26	27–46	≥47	≥2	≤0.06
Spectinomycin	≤14	15–17	≥18	≥128	≤32

NOTE 1: Information in boldface type is considered tentative for 1 year.

NOTE 2: The use of a cysteine-free supplement is required for agar dilution tests with carbapenems and clavulanate. Cysteine-containing defined growth supplements *do not* significantly alter dilution test results with other drugs, or disk diffusion tests with carbapenems or clavulanic acid combinations.

[a] For these antimicrobial agents, the current absence of resistant strains precludes defining any results categories other than "Susceptible." Strains yielding results suggestive of a "Nonsusceptible" category should be submitted to a reference laboratory for further testing.

[b] Gonococci with 10 U-penicillin disk zone diameters of ≤19 mm are likely to be β-lactamase-producing strains. However, the β-lactamase test remains preferable to other susceptibility methods for rapid, accurate recognition of this plasmid-mediated penicillin resistance.

[c] An intermediate or indeterminate result for an antimicrobial agent indicates either a technical problem that should be resolved by repeating testing or a lack of clinical experience in treating organisms with these zones or MICs. The latter seems to be the case for cefotetan, cefmetazole, cefoxitin, and spectinomycin (see text). **Strains with intermediate zones to the other agents have a documented lower clinical cure rate (85 to 95%) compared with >95% for susceptible strains.**

[d] These values represent MIC breakpoints used in determining approximate zone size interpretive criteria. They relate to MICs determined by M7 methodology. Occasional discrepancies may exist between M2 and M7 due to methodological limitations.

Table 6.1C. Some Examples of Zone Diameter Interpretive Standards and Equivalent Minimum Inhibitory Concentration (MIC) Breakpoints for *Streptococcus pneumoniae* (Disk Diffusion)[a]

Antimicrobial Agent	Zone Diameter (Nearest Whole mm)			Equivalent MIC Breakpoints[e] (µg/ml)	
	Resistant	Intermediate	Susceptible	Resistant	Susceptible
Erythromycin	≤15	16–20	≥21	≥4	≤0.5
Penicillin[b]			≥20		≤0.06
Vancomycin[c]			≥16		≤4

NOTE 1: All information in this table is considered tentative for 1 year.

NOTE 2: These zone diameter standards apply only to tests performed using Mueller-Hinton agar supplemented with 5% sheep blood; equivalent MIC breakpoints relate to tests performed by broth microdilution using CAMHB-LHB.

[a] Cefepime, cefotaxime, ceftriaxone, cefuroxime sodium (parenteral), cefuroxime axetil (oral), and imipenem may be used to treat pneumococcal infections; however, reliable disk diffusion susceptibility tests with these agents do not yet exist. Their in vitro activity is best assessed using a broth microdilution MIC method.

[b] Isolates of *S. pneumoniae* with oxacillin zone sizes of ≥20 mm are susceptible (MIC ≤0.06 µg/ml) to penicillin. The disk test does not, however, distinguish penicillin intermediate strains (i.e., MICs = 0.12 to 1.0 µg/ml) from strains that are penicillin-resistant (i.e., MICs ≥2.0 µg/ml). A penicillin MIC should be determined on isolates of *S. pneumoniae* with oxacillin zone sizes of ≤19 mm. The results of the oxacillin disk test also predict the activity of ampicillin, amoxicillin, amoxicillin/clavulanic acid, and ampicillin/sulbactam. Penicillin-susceptible strains of *S. pneumoniae* may be considered susceptible to other β-lactam antimicrobials described in this table (including those in footnote a) and need not be tested against these agents.

[c] The absence of resistant strains precludes defining any results categories other than "Susceptible." Strains yielding results suggestive of a "Nonsusceptible" category should be submitted to a reference laboratory for further testing.

[d] These values represent MIC breakpoints used in determining approximate zone size interpretive criteria. They relate to MICs determined by M7 methodology.

Table 6.1D. Some Examples of Tentative Interpretive Categories and Correlative Minimum Inhibitory Concentrations (MICs) (Anaerobic Dilution)[a]

Antimicrobial Agent	MIC (μg/ml)		
	Susceptible	Intermediate	Resistant
Ampicillin/ sulbactam	≤8/4	16/8	≥32/16
Cefoxitin	≤16	32	≥64
Clindamycin	≤2	4	≥8
Imipenem	≤4	8	≥16
Metronidazole	≤8	16	≥32
Piperacillin/ tazobactam	≤32/4	64/4	≥128/4

NOTE 1: The interpretations and correlative breakpoint values in this table are new and should be considered tentative for 1 year after publication of this document.

[a] The previous NCCLS recommendations did not include an "Intermediate" category for anaerobes. The intermediate range has been established because of the difficulty in reading end-points and the clustering of MICs at breakpoint concentrations. Where data are available, the interpretation guidelines are based on pharmacokinetic data, population distribution of MICs, and studies of clinical efficacy. To achieve the best possible levels of a drug in abscesses and necrotic, or poorly perfused, tissues, which are encountered commonly in these infections, maximum dosages of antimicrobial agents are recommended for therapy of anaerobic infections. With such dosages, it is believed that organisms with susceptible or intermediate end-points are generally amenable to therapy. Ancillary therapy, such as drainage procedures and debridement, are obviously of great importance for the proper management of anaerobic infections.

Table 6.2. Minimum Inhibitory Concentrations for Susceptible Organisms (µg/ml)—Gram-Positive Bacteria

Organism	Penicillin G or Penicillin V	Ampicillin	Nafcillin/oxacillin	Cephalosporin[a]	Cephalosporin[b]	Cefixime	Erythromycin	Clindamycin	Cefmetazole	Vancomycin	Chloramphenicol	Sulfonamides	Trimethoprim/ Sulfamethoxazole (T-1/S-19)[g]	Gentamicin[c]
Streptococci														
group A (S. pyogenes)	0.01	0.04	0.03	0.06	0.4	0.12	0.04	0.1	0.5	2.5	3.0	R[i]	1	R
group B	0.03	0.08	0.32	0.16	6	0.25	0.08	0.08	2	2	0.8			
group D (S. bovis)	0.1	0.2	0.5-1.0	0.1	R	R	0.05	0.1	R	1.6	1.6-3.2			R
enterococci	3.2	1.6	8-64	R	4	R	R	R	R	3.2	R	100	0.5	1.6-12
viridans type	0.01-0.1[d]	0.02-0.8	0.03-2.0	0.05-0.8	4	0.12	0.01-0.05	0.01-0.1	8	1.6	6	80.25	3-25	R
S. pneumoniae	0.01[e]	0.05	0.03-0.5	0.06-0.12		0.25	0.1	0.01-0.04		0.3	2.0	32	2	
Staphylococci														
S. aureus[h] (penicillinase +)	R	R	0.25	1-2	4-8	16	0.5	0.04-0.8	2	0.2-0.8	12.5	4.0	0.3	1.0
(penicillinase −)	0.03	0.05												
S. epidermidis (nafcillin-resistant)	R	R	R	R	R	R	25	25	R	3.12	2.5	50	3	
C. diphtheriae	0.1	0.2		0.2			0.03	0.05		1	2	25	0.4	
Diphtheroids	1.6	3.2	R	3.2			3.2			1.6	1.6			
L. monocytogenes	0.2-0.6	0.1-0.3		4.0	R	R	0.2	2	R	5.0	4.0		0.5-1.0	4.0[f]

[a] Parenteral (cefazolin, cephalothin, cephapirin, cefamandole, cefuroxime).

[b] Oral (cephalexin, cephradine, cefadroxil, cefaclor).

[c] Streptococci are resistant to aminoglycosides in vitro, but combinations of penicillins and aminoglycosides are bactericidal. Although nearly all staphylococci are sensitive to aminoglycosides in vitro, the clinical role of these agents used alone is uncertain. Combinations of penicillinase-resistant penicillins and aminoglycosides have not been demonstrated to improve outcome of staphylococcal endocarditis.

[d] Strains of S. viridans with MICs as high as 4 µg/ml have been isolated from patients with endocarditis.

[e] Strains of pneumococci with MICs as high as 0.5 µg/ml have been occasionally isolated. Rare strains have emerged with MIC of 4 µg/ml.

[f] Listeria is killed more rapidly in vitro by combinations of penicillin and gentamicin.

[g] Denotes total concentration trimethoprim and sulfamethoxazole in a fixed ratio of 1:19.

[h] S. aureus resistant to semisynthetic penicillins such as methicillin, nafcillin, or oxacillin has been reported. Although some strains may be susceptible to cephalosporins, the drug of choice of the treatment of infection is vancomycin.

[i] R, resistant.

Table 6.3. Minimum Inhibitory Concentration for Susceptible Organisms (μg/ml)—Gram-Negative Bacteria

Antimicrobial Agents

Organisms	Penicillin G	Ampicillin	Carbenicillin/Ticarcillin	Cephalosporin[a]	Cephalosporin[b]	Cefmetazole	Cefotoxin	Cefuroxime	Cefotetan	Cefixime	Chloramphenicol	Tobramycin/Gentamicin	Netilmicin	Amikacin	Mezlocillin	Piperacillin	Trimethoprim/Sulfamethoxazole[c] (T-1/S-19)	Aztreonam	Imipenem
N. gonorrhoeae	0.01-2.0[f]	0.02-0.6	0.3	2	8	1	1	0.1	2-4	≤0.01	1.0	1			0.1	0.1	10	0.2	0.1
N. meningitidis	0.03	0.05	0.1	2	16	0.12	1	1		<0.1	1.5	R[i]	R				1	0.2	0.06
E. coli	64	2-8	4-16	6-8	8-32*	1-32	6	4	0.5	0.5	4-8	0.5-1.0	0.4	1-4	8-16	8-16	3	12.5-50	0.5
Enterobacter	R	R	50	R	8	1-32	R	R	R	R	0.5-12	0.5-4	0.4	1-4	8-16	32	4	0.3	2
Klebsiella	R	R	R	8	8	2	6	4	0.5	≤0.25	3.1	0.06-2.0	0.1-0.4	1-6	32-64			0.05	0.5
Proteus (indole-negative)	32	1-4	3-6	4-8	16	4	4	1	0.25	≤0.25	8-16	1-2	1.6	1-6	1-2	1-8	1	0.1-0.8	4
(indole-positive)	R	R	1-25	R	R	2-4	8	R	0.5	≤0.25	8-16	2-6	1.6	1-6	2-64	2-64	3		4
Providencia	R	R	5	R	R	2-16	2	R	4	0.5-R	2.5	6	6	6-12	16	8	3	0.1	2
Serratia	4	R	3-25	R	R	R	8-32	R	16	16	1.6	1-5[j]	2-12	1-6	8	4	4	0.4-1.6	4
Salmonella	16	0.25-5.0	25	4-8	12	2	6	6	1	0.5	5.0	0.25-1.0	0.4	2-6	8	4	1	0.3	0.5
Shigella	R	1.0		12	12	2	6	25	0.1		5.0	1-2	0.8	4			1	6	0.5
Acinetobacter	R	R	32	R	R	R	R	R	32	R	2.0	1-4	2-6		32	16	2	R	0.5
Brucella	R	0.25-0.8																	
H. influenzae	1.0	0.5[g]	0.5	4	8-32	2-4	4	0.5	1.0	<0.1		3			4	1	0.6	0.2	0.5
Pseudomonas																			
P. aeruginosa	R	R	32-64	R	R	R	R	R	R	R	R	0.5-2[j]	2	4-8	32-128	8-64	R	12.5-25	2
P. cepacia	R	R	R	R	R	R		R	R	R	≤8	R	R	R	R	10	10	8-16	8
C. jejuni[h]	R	2.5	10	R	R		R	R			6.2	0.4		1.6					

[a] Parenteral (cefazolin, cephalothin/cephapirin).
[b] Oral (cephalexin/cephradine).

Table 6.3—continued

[d] β-lactamase-producing strains (PPNG) have MIC >2 μg/ml; 35% of PPNG have MCl > 1 μg/ml to erythromycin, and 50% are sensitive to ≤1 μg/ml of tetracycline.

[e] Concentrations that are reliably achieved only in urine.

[f] Tobramycin is two to four times as active as gentamicin against *P. aeruginosa*. Gentamicin is two to four times as active as tobramycin against *Serratia*.

[g] β-lactamase-producing strains of *H. influenzae* are resistant to penicillins. These strains are sensitive to cefamandole and chloramphenicol.

[h] MIC of clindamycin is 0.4 μg/ml.

[i] R, resistant.

Table 6.4A. In Vitro Activity of Third-Generation Cephalosporins against Gram-Positive Organisms[a]

	Moxalactam	Cefotaxime	Ceftizoxime	Ceftriaxone	Cefoperazone	Ceftazidime
			MIC_{90} in µg/ml (% Strains Susceptible)			
S. aureus	8 (90)	2 (>90)	3 (99)	4 (100)	4 (90)	16 (89)
S. epidermidis	32 (64)	8 (90)	25 (75)	16 (70)	8 (90)	32 (83)
Streptococcus species						
pyogenes	2 (>90)	<0.03 (100)	<0.03 (100)	0.03 (100)	0.12 (100)	0.25 (100)
viridans group	>32 (50)	0.4 (100)	8 (90)	1 (>90)	1 (>90)	8 (90)
pneumoniae	2 (>90)	0.03 (100)	0.1 (100)	<0.03 (100)	0.25 (100)	0.25 (100)
faecalis	>32 (0)	>32 (50)	>32 (50)	>32 (0)	>32 (<50)	>32 (0)

Reprinted by permission of the New England Journal of Medicine from Donowitz GR, Mandell GL. 1988; 318:490–500.
[a] MIC_{90} denotes the lowest concentration of an antibiotic inhibiting growth in 90% of the strains tested. The susceptibility break point is ≤8 µg/ml for all agents except cefoperazone, for which a value of ≤16 µg/ml is used.

Table 6.4B. In Vitro Activity of Third-Generation Cephalosporins against Gram-Negative Organisms and Anaerobes[a]

	Moxalactam	Cefotaxime	Ceftizoxime	Ceftriaxone	Cefoperazone	Ceftazidime
			(MIC$_{90}$ in μg/ml (% Strains Susceptible))			
Gram-negative organisms						
N. meningitidis	0.05 (100)	<0.01 (100)	<0.01 (100)	0.025 (100)	0.01 (100)	0.01 (100)
N. gonorrhoeae	0.06 (100)	0.05 (100)	0.03 (100)	0.025 (100)	0.06 (100)	0.06 (100)
H. influenzae	0.1 (100)	0.03 (100)	<0.01 (100)	0.1 (100)	0.06 (100)	0.1 (100)
E. coli	0.25 (100)	0.25 (100)	0.13 (100)	0.1 (100)	2 (100)	0.5 (100)
K. pneumoniae	0.25 (100)	0.25 (100)	0.25 (100)	0.1 (100)	4 (100)	0.5 (100)
E. cloacae	4 (>98)	32 (>64)	16 (<89)	16 (<89)	8 (>93)	16 (89)
S. marcescens	4 (>99)	2 (>90)	2 (>96)	4 (>90)	16 (>93)	1 (100)
Proteus						
Indole-positive	0.25 (100)	0.5 (100)	0.12 (100)	0.12 (100)	4 (100)	0.12 (100)
Indole-negative	0.12 (100)	0.12 (100)	<0.03 (99)	0.008 (100)	0.5 (100)	0.06 (100)
P. aeruginosa	64 (40)	>32 (<5)	>32 (5)	32 (50)	32 (60)	4 (99)
Other Pseudomonas species	64 (50)	>32 (<5)	>32 (50)	>32 (50)	>32 (65)	32 (>50)
Anaerobes[b]						
Fusobacterium	4 (77)	0.5 (90)	0.5 (90)	2.0 (90)	4 (77)	64 (54)
B. fragilis	16 (85)	64 (60)	32 (70)	>64 (45)	>64 (40)	>64 (30)
B. fragilis group	>32 (72)	>32 (54)	>32 (30)	>32 (50)	>32 (74)	>32 (57)
Peptococcus/peptostreptococcus	4 (100)	2 (100)	1 (100)	4 (90)	1 (100)	8 (96)
	32 (100)			8 (90)	2 (100)	16 (96)
C. perfringens	0.5 (100)	4 (100)	2 (100)	2 (100)	2 (100)	8 (100)
Clostridium species	16 (79)	16 (57)	>32 (50)	16 (<50)	16 (64)	>32 (21)

Reprinted by permission of The New England Journal of Medicine from Donowitz GR, Mandell GL. Drug therapy. Beta-lactam antibiotics. N. Engl J Med 318:490–500, 1988.

[a] MIC$_{90}$ denotes the lowest concentration of an antibiotic inhibiting growth in 90% of the strains tested. The susceptibility break point is ≤8 μg/ml for all agents, except cefoperazone, for which a value of ≤16 μg/ml is used.

[b] Data on minimal inhibitory concentrations for anaerobes depend on the medium and the assay conditions and therefore vary widely between studies.

Table 6.5A. Antimicrobial Activity of the Fluoroquinolones

Bacterial Species	MIC_{50}/MIC_{90} (μg/ml)		
	Norfloxacin	Ciprofloxacin	Ofloxacin
Gram-positive			
S. aureus	0.8/6.3	0.5/1.0	0.4/0.4
Staphylococcus spp., coagulase negative	1.6/3.1	0.25/0.25	0.4/0.8
S. saphrophyticus	2.0/4.0	0.5/0.5	1.0/1.0
S. pyogenes	1.6/6.3	0.5/2.0	1.6/3.1
S. agalactiae	2.0/4.0	0.5/1.0	2.0/2.0
Streptococcus spp., group C	4.0/8.0	0.5/2.0	1.0/2.0
S. bovis	4.0/1.6	2.0/2.0	2.0/4.0
Streptococcus spp., group F	2.0/2.0	1.0/2.0	
Streptococcus spp., group G	2.0/4.0	0.25/1.0	1.0/2.0
Streptococcus, viridans group	4.0/16	1.0/2.0	2.0/2.0
S. pneumoniae	8.0/16	1.0/2.0	2.0/2.0
E. faecalis	4.0/8.0	2.0/4.0	2.0/2.4
E. faecium	4.0/8.0	1.0/2.0	3.1/6.2
L. monocytogenes	2.0/4.0	0.5/0.5	0.5/1.0
Corynebacterium JK	1.0/4.0	0.25/1.0	0.25/1.0
Corynebacterium D2	1.0/8.0	<0.3/1.0	0.5/0.5
Enterobacteriaceae			
E. coli	0.06/0.12	0.02/0.03	0.06/0.12
K. pneumoniae	0.12/0.5	0.03/0.06	0.1/0.2
K. oxytocia	0.12/0.25	0.03/0.13	
E. aerogenes	0.1/0.4	0.03/0.06	0.1/0.8
E. cloacae	0.1/0.4	0.02/0.13	0.05/0.1
E. agglomerans	0.2/0.2	0.03/0.13	0.6/2.0
C. freundii	0.06/0.5	0.02/0.13	0.6/2.0
C. diversus	0.02/0.2	0.02/0.13	0.1/04
P. mirabilia	0.01/0.5	0.06/0.13	0.1/0.2
P. vulgaris	0.1/0.4	0.02/0.06	0.1/1.6
P. stuartii	0.12/1.0	0.03/0.5	0.4/1.6
P. rettgeri	0.5/1.0	0.13/0.25	0.4/1.6
M. morganii	0.02/0.06	0.02/0.03	0.01/0.02
S. typhi	0.03/0.06	0.01/0.02	0.03/0.06
Salmonella spp.	0.06/0.06	0.01/0.02	0.06/0.06
Shigella spp.	0.03/0.06	0.01/0.02	0.06/0.12
Y. enterocolitica	0.06/0.06	0.02/0.02	0.06/0.12
S. marcescens	0.8/3.1	<0.1/1.0	0.4/1.6
Other Gram-negative			
P. aeruginosa	1.0/2.0	0.12/0.5	1.0/2.0
P. maltophilia	1.0/4.0	1.0/2.0	0.8/3.1
P. cepacia	4.0/8.0	1.0/2.0	0.8/3.1
P. pseudomallei	4.0/8.0	2.0/8.0	8.0/32
P. shigelloides	0.02/0.02	0.01/0.01	0.02/0.02
A. hydrophila	0.02/0.03	0.01/0.02	0.02/0.03
A. calcoaceticus subsp. anitratum	8.0/64	0.13/0.25	1.0/4.0
A. calcoaceticus subsp. lwoffi	4.0/8.0	0.06/0.13	0.25/0.5
H. alvei	0.12/0.12	0.03/0.03	0.06/0.06
N. meningitidis	0.02/0.03	0.01/0.01	0.02/0.02
N. gonorrhoeae	0.03/0.06	0.01/0.01	0.02/0.06
C. jejuni	0.25/0.5	0.06/0.12	0.12/0.25
C. coli	0.4/0.8	0.2/0.4	0.4/0.8
C. pylori	2.0/2.0	0.25/0.25	1.0/1.0

Table 6.5A—*continued*

V. cholerae	0.01/0.02	0.005/0.01	0.01/0.01
V. parahaemolyticus	0.03/0.06	0.06/0.06	0.06/0.12
H. influenzae	0.06/0.06	0.01/0.01	0.03/0.03
H. parainfluenzae	0.03/0.13	0.02/0.03	0.06/0.25
H. ducreyi	0.06/0.12	0.02/0.02	0.03/0.03
G. vaginalis	16/16	1.0/1.0	2.0/2.0
B. catarrhalis	0.5/0.4	0.02/0.03	0.05/0.1
L. pneumophila	2.0/2.0	0.5/0.5	0.25/0.5
Legionella spp.	0.08/0.2	0.01/0.02	0.01/0.02
P. multocida	0.06/0.13	0.01/0.02	<0.06/0.06
E. corrodens	0.03/0.06	0.01/0.02	0.02/0.03
B. pertussis	0.25/0.25	<0.1/<0.1	0.12/0.12
Moraxella spp.	0.13/1.0	<0.3/0.5	0.5/1.0
Anaerobic			
Peptococci	8.0/64	0.25/2.0	0.5/4.0
Peptostreptococci	4.0/16	0.5/8.0	2.0/8.0
C. perfringens	1.0/8.0	0.25/1.0	1.0/2.0
Clostridium spp.	1.0/2.0	1.0/4.0	1.0/16
C. difficile	64/128	8.0/16	8.0/16
B. fragilis	32/>128	4.0/8.0	4.0/8.0
Bacteroides spp., non-*B. fragilis*	8.0/128	1.0/4.0	1.0/2.0
Fusobacterium spp.	8.0/16	2.0/2.0	2.0/4.0
Eubacterium spp.	4.0/32	8.0/16	2.0/4.0
Capnocytophaga spp.	1.0/2.0	0.12/0.25	0.12/0.5
Mobiluncus spp.	32/32	0.5/1.0	
Other			
M. tuberculosis	4.0/8.0	0.5/1.0	0.6/1.3
M. avium complex	16/>16	2.0/16	2.5/10
M. chelonei	16/>16	1.0/8.0	10/>20
M. fortuitum	0.5/2.0	0.3/0.3	1.3/1.3
M. kansasii	4.0/8.0	1.0/1.0	0.5/1.0
M. xenopi	2.0/4.0	0.5/1.0	1.0/2.0
N. asteroides	32/64	4.0/8.0	4.0/16
M. pneumoniae	6.3/12	2.0/2.0	1.0/2.0
M. hominis	4.0/16	1.0/1.0	0.4/0.8
C. trachomatis	25/25	1.6/1.6	0.8/0.8
U. urealyticum	16/32	2.0/4.0	0.8/1.6
C. albicans		>100/>100	>100/>100

Adapted from Wolfson JS, Hooper DC. Fluoroquinolone antimicrobial agents. Clin Microbiol Rev 1989; 2:384–385.
[a] MIC_{50}/MIC_{90}, concentrations of drug that inhibited 50 and 90%, respectively, of ≥10 isolates.

Table 6.5B. Activity of Fleroxacin and Lomefloxacin in Vitro

Bacterial Species	MIC_{50}/MIC_{90} (μg/ml)[a]	
	Flerfloxacin	Lomefloxacin
Gram-positive		
S. aureus	0.5/1.0	1.0/2.0
Staphylococcus spp., coagulase negative	0.5/1.0	0.5/1.0
S. saprophyticus	2.0/2.0	2.0/2.0
S. pyogenes	4.0/16	4.0/8.0
S. agalactiae	8.0/16	16/16
Streptococcus, viridans group	16/>16	8.0/8.0
S. pneumoniae	4.0/8.0	4.0/8.0
E. faecalis	4.0/8.0	8.0/16
L. monocytogenes	2.0/4.0	2.0/4.0
Corynebacterium JK	2.0/2.0	
Enterobacteriaceae		
E. coli	0.06/1.0	0.03/0.25
K. pneumoniae	0.12/0.5	0.5/0.5
K. oxytoca	0.12/0.5	0.25/0.6
E. aerogenes	0.25/0.5	0.25/0.5
E. cloacae	0.25/0.5	0.5/0.5
C. freundii	0.12/0.25	0.25/1.0
C. diversus	0.12/0.25	0.12/0.12
P. mirabilia	0.12/0.5	0.5/1.0
P. vulgaris	0.06/0.12	0.12/0.5
P. stuartii	0.12/0.5	1.0/4.0
P. rettgeri	0.25/4.0	0.5/4.0
Morganella morganii	0.06/0.12	0.06/0.25
Salmonella spp.	0.12/0.12	0.25/0.25
Shigella spp.	0.12/0.12	0.12/0.25
Y. enterocolitica	0.03/0.06	0.12/0.12
Serratia spp.	1.6/12	0.5/2.0
Other Gram-negative		
P. aeruginosa	0.5/2.0	2.0/4.0
P. maltophilia	1.6/3.1	8.0/8.0
P. cepacia	0.5/4.0	8.0/16
A. hydrophila	0.02/0.03	0.06/0.12
A. calcoaceticus	0.5/1.0	0.5/4.0
H. alvei		0.12/0.12
N. gonorrhoeae	0.02/0.2	0.02/0.12
C. jejuni	0.4/0.8	
C. pylori	2.0/2.0	2.0/2.0
H. influenzae	0.06/0.12	0.06/0.12
H. ducreyi	0.03/0.06	
G. vaginalis	4.0/8.0	
B. catarrhalis	0.12/0.25	0.25/0.25
L. pneumophila	0.13/0.25	
Anaerobic		
Peptococcus-peptostreptococcus spp.		
Clostridium spp.	4.0/16	2.0/16
C. difficile		25/50
B. fragilis	8.0/32	16/32
Bacteroides spp., non-B. fragilis	6.3/6.3	
Fusobacterium spp.		

Table 6.5B—*continued*

Gram-positive		
Other		
N. asteroides	16/64	
M. hominis	1.6/1.6	0.5/2.0
C. trachomatis	3.1/3.1	3.1/3.1
U. urealyticum	1.6/3.2	2.0/4.0

Adapted from Wolfson JS, Hooper DC. Fluoroquinolone antimicrobial agents. Clin Microbiol Rev 1989; 2:386.
[a] MIC_{50}/MIC_{90}, concentrations of drug that inhibited 50 and 90%, respectively, of ≥10 isolates.

Table 6.6. Minimum Inhibitory Concentrations for Susceptible Organisms (µg/ml)—Anaerobic Bacteria

Organism	Antimicrobial Agents												
	Penicillin G	Mezlocillin[a]	Cephalosporins[b]	Cefoxitin	Cefotetan	Cefmetazole	Chloramphenicol	Clindamycin	Erythromycin	Tetracycline	Metronidazole	Cefotaxime/Ceftizoxime	Imipenem
Bacteroides													
B. fragilis	32–64	32–64	R[c]	4–16	16	8–128	1–8	0.1–0.5	R[c]	1–16	0.5–0.8	8–64[d]	0.1
B. melaninogenicus	0.1–4	2	8	1	0.5	4	1–2	0.1–0.5	0.5–1.0	0.25	0.5	2–8	0.1
Other	0.5–8	16–32	8–64	2–4	8–R	2–128	1–2	0.1–0.5	1–2	0.5	1–4	8–64	0.5
Fusobacteria	0.1–1.0	0.25–1.0	0.5–1.0	1.0	0.1	<0.1	0.5–1.0	0.1–0.5	1–8	0.5	0.5	0.5	0.25
Peptococcus	0.5	0.1–0.5	0.1–1.0	0.25–1.0	2	0.1–8	1–2	0.1	1–4	0.5	0.5	2–8	0.1
Peptostreptococcus	0.5	0.5–2.0	0.4–3.0	0.5–2.0	2	0.1–8	1–2	0.1	0.4	0.5	0.5	0.5	0.1
Streptococci	0.25	1–2	0.25	1–2	1	0.1–8	0.5–2	0.5	0.5	0.5	4	2	0.1
Clostridia													
C. perfringens	0.1–1.0	0.5	1.0	1–4	8	32	1–2	0.5–1	1.6	0.25–2.0	1.0	2	0.5
Other	0.25–4.0	1–8	1–8	4–64	8	32	1–8	1–4	0.4–1.6	0.5	1.0	4–8	0.5
Veillonella	0.25	2–4	4–8	0.5–1.0		8	0.25–2	0.1	1–4	0.25	1.0	0.5	

[a] Also reflects activity of piperacillin.
[b] Cephalosporins are cefazolin, cephalothin/cephapirin, and cefamandole.
[c] R, resistant.
[d] Ceftizoxime is approximately twice as active as cefotaxime versus B. fragilis.

Table 6.7. Minimum Inhibitory Concentrations for Susceptible Organisms (μg/ml)—Miscellaneous Organisms

Organism	Antimicrobial Agents												
	Penicillin G	Chloramphenicol	Tetracycline	Erythromycin	Rifampin	Ampicillin	Minocycline	Sulfonamides	Clindamycin	Co-trimoxazole	Amikacin	Ciprofloxacin	Ofloxacin
Rickettsia[a]	R[b]	1.0	0.1	0.06	0.01		0.1						
Chlamydia	0.06	4	0.1–1.0	0.1–1.0	0.05–0.25	0.25		0.5–4				1–4	0.5–2
Actinomyces	R	R	2.0	0.25				32	0.125				
Nocardia	R	R	R	6.3	R	12.5	3.1	25[c]	R	50–100[d]	12.5	R	R
Treponema pallidum	0.018		1.0	0.05		0.02							
Legionella pneumophila[e]		0.5	4.0	0.5	0.25	1.0				0.125		1	0.5

[a] C. burnetti and other rickettsial organisms have not been tested in vitro in order to determine a minimum inhibitory concentration. The available data are expressed as amounts of drug required to cure mice or chick embryos of infection.
[b] R, resistant.
[c] Sulfonamides in combination with ampicillin are synergistic in vitro.
[d] The in vitro activity of co-trimoxazole varies according to the ratio of the two drugs. Increasing the amount of trimethoprim enhances activity.
[e] In vitro susceptibility does not equate with clinical efficacy. Only erythromycin and rifampin have been shown to be effective.

Table 6.8. Minimum Inhibitory Concentrations for Susceptible Organisms (µg/ml)—Mycobacteria

Organism	Antimicrobial Agents														
	Isoniazid	Ethambutol	Rifampin	Streptomycin	Cycloserine	Kanamycin	Viomycin	Capreomycin	Pyrazinamide	Ethionamide	Para-aminosalicylic Acid	Amikacin	Imipenem	Ciprofloxacin	Ofloxacin
M. tuberculosis	0.2	1–2	0.5	2.5	25	2.5	2.5	2.5	12	1.2–2.5	1		1	1	1
Atypicals															
M. kanasasi (I)	1/40[a]	5/65	1.25/100	10/86	25/80	R[b]	10/63	R		1.2/92	25/47			3–6	2
M. scrofulaceum (II)	1/20		R	10/93	R	10/87	10/80	10/40	R	2.5/47	25/67			>6	>6
M. avium-intracellulare	5/48	R	5/30	10/31	R	10/27	10/25	R	R	5/44	25/14	1		>6	>6
M. fortuitum (IV)[c]	R	R	R	10/14	R	10/21	10/24	10/21		5/28	R	2		1	1

[a] Denotes concentration of drug percent sensitive.
[b] R, resistant.
[c] Gentamicin 6.2/30.

Table 6.9. Runyon Classification of Atypical Mycobacteria

Group	Pigment Production	Growth Rate (days)	Species
I	Photochromogenic	14–21	*M. kansasii*
II	Photochromogenic	10–14	*M. marinum*
III	Nonphotochromogenic	14–21	*M. avium-intracellulare*
IV	Variable	5–7	*M. fortuitum*

SECTION 7

Bacterial Resistance

Epidemiology and Susceptibility of Resistant Organisms to Antimicrobial Agents

In a review entitled "Resistance to Antimicrobial Drugs—A Worldwide Calamity," Kunin (1) outlined the global problem of bacterial resistance to antibiotics. The extent and importance of this problem has been addressed by numerous authors (2–8). Clinically important resistance has been observed in staphylococci (methicillin-resistant *Staphylococcus aureus* (MRSA)), enterococci, pneumococci, meningococci, enterobacteriaceae, anaerobes, gonococci, intestinal pathogens, and *Mycobacterium tuberculosis*.

The following tables and figures summarize some of the more important aspects of the epidemiology, microbiology, and clinical features of bacterial resistance to antibiotics.

174

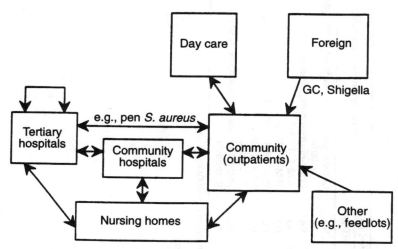

Figure 7.1. Environmental influences important in the development and spread of bacterial resistance. (Reprinted with permission from Murray BE. New aspects of antimicrobial resistance and the resulting therapeutic dilemmas. J Infect Dis 1991;163:1185–1194.)

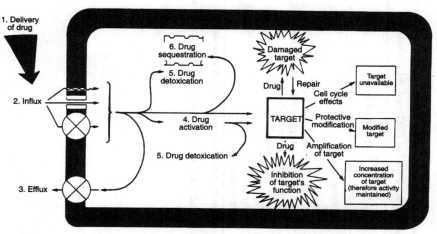

Figure 7.2. Mechanisms of resistance. (Reprinted with permission from Hayes JD, Wolf RC. Molecular mechanisms of drug resistance. Biochem J 1990;272:281–295.)

Table 7.1. Classification Scheme for Bacterial β-Lactamases

Group	Subtitle	Preferred Substrates	Inhibited by CA[a]	Inhibited by EDTA	Representative Enzyme(s)
1	CEP-N	Cephalosporins	No	No	Chromosomal enzymes from Gram-negative bacteria
2a	PEN-Y	Penicillins	Yes	No	Gram-positive penicillinases
2b	BDS-Y	Cephalosporins, penicillins	Yes	No	TEM-1, TEM-2
2b'	EBS-Y	Cephalosporins, penicillins, cefotaxime	Yes	No	TEM-3, TEM-5
2c	CAR-Y	Penicillins, carbenicillin	Yes	No	PSE-1, PSE-3, PSE-4
2d	CLX-Y	Penicillins, cloxacillin	Yes[b]	No	OXA-1, PSE-2
2e	CEP-Y	Cephalosporins	Yes	No	P. vulgaris
3	MET-N	Variable	No	Yes	Bacillus cereus II, Pseudomonas maltophilia L1
4	PEN-N	Penicillins	No	?[c]	P. cepacia

Reprinted with permission from Bush K. Characterization of β-lactamases. Antimicrob Agents Chemother 1989;33(3):259–263.
[a] 10 μM clavulanic acid.
[b] Inhibition by clavulanic acid may occur at higher concentrations for some members of the group.
[c] Variable.

Table 7.2 Resistance Patterns in *E. coli* and *Klebsiella* spp.

β-Lactam Class	Agent	Plasmid-medicated Penicillinase	Hyperproduction	Mutation to Broaden Spectrum
Penicillins Ureidopenicillins	Ampicillin Piperacillin	■ (common) ■ (common)	■ (common) ■ (common)	■ (common) ■ (common)
Penicillinase inhibitor combinations	Pip./Tazob. mp./Sulb. Amox./Clav.		■ (common) ■ (common) ■ (common)	▨ (variable) ▨ (variable) ▨ (variable)
1st & 2nd Gen. cephalosporins	Cefazolin Cefuroxime		■ (common) ■ (common)	■ (common) ■ (common)
3rd Gen. cephalosporins	Cefotaxime Ceftriaxone Ceftazidime			▨ (variable) ▨ (variable) ▨ (variable)
Monobactams	Aztreonam			▨ (variable)
Carbapenems	Imipenem			

Resistance
  Common ■
  Variable ▨

Table 7.3 Resistance Patterns in the Inducible *Enterobacteriaceae* due to Chromosomal Class I Cephalosporinase

β-Lactam Class	Agent	Wild-type Strains	Constitutive "Derepressed" Mutants
Penicillins Ureidopenicillins	Ampicillin Piperacillin	■ ■ ±	■ ▨ ■
Penicillinase inhibitor combinations	Amox./Clav. Pip./Tazob. Ticar./Clav.	■	▨ ▨ ■ ■
1st & 2nd Gen. cephalosporins	Cefazolin Cefuroxime	■ ■	■ ■
3rd Gen. cephalosporins	Cefotaxime Ceftriaxone Ceftazidime		▨ ▨ ▨
Monobactams	Aztreonam		▨
Carbapenems	Imipenem	⬚	

Resistance
  Common ■
  Variable ▨

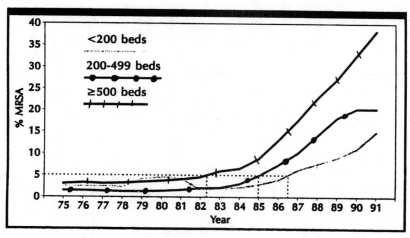

Figure 7.3.   Temporal trends in percent of *S. aureus* resistant to methicillin (*MRSA*), oxacillin, or nafcillin by number of hospital beds. (Reprinted with permission from Panlilio AL, Culver DH, et al. Methicillin-resistant *S. aureus* in U.S. hospitals, 1975–1991. Infect Control Hosp Epidemiol 1992;13(10):582–586.)

Table 7.4. Activity of Twenty-One Antimicrobial Agents against S. aureus Strains

Antimicrobial Agent	MRSA[a]			MRSA[b]			MSSA[c]		
	MIC$_{50}$[d]	MIC$_{90}$	MIC$_{100}$	MIC$_{50}$	MIC$_{90}$	MIC$_{100}$	MIC$_{50}$	MIC$_{90}$	MIC$_{100}$
Amikacin	8	32	>32	8/≤8	32	>32	≤2	≤8/≤2	>32
Amoxicillin/clavulanic acid	>8	>8	>8	>8/NT	>8/NT	>8/NT	≤2/NT	≤2/NT	≤8/NT
Ampicillin/sulbactam	16	32	32	16	32/>16	32/>16	2/1	4/≤8	8/16
Cefazolin	>32	>32	>32	>32/>8	>32/>8	>32/>8	0.5/≤1	1/≤1	2/8
Ceftizoxime	>16	>16	>16	>16/>64	>16/>64	>16/>64	≤4	≤16	>16/16
Chloramphenicol	≤16	≤16	≤16	≤16	≤16	≤16	≤16	≤16	≤16
Ciprofloxacin	16	64	>64	16/>2	32/>2	>64/>2	0.5	1/0.5	>64/>2
Clarithromycin	NT	NT	NT	NT/>8	NT/>8	NT/>8	NT/≤2	NT/8	NT/>8
Clindamycin	>4	>4	>4	>4	>4	>4	≤1	≤1	>4
Gentamicin	>16	>16	>16	>16/>8	>16/>8	>16/>8	≤1/≤0.5	≤1/≤0.5	>16/>8
Imipenem	≤1	>8	>8	8/4	>8	>8	≤1	≤1	≤1
Norfloxacin	64	>64	>64	64/NT	>64/NT	>64/NT	1/NT	4/NT	>64/NT
Ofloxacin	16	16	32	16/>4	32/>4	>128/>4	>0.5/≤2	2/≤2	>128/>4
L-Ofloxacin	NT	NT	NT	NT/8	NT/16	NT/>16	NT/≤0.5	NT/≤0.5	NT/16
Oxacillin	>32	>32	>32	>32/>8	>32/>8	>32/>8	≤0.5/0.5	1	4
Penicillin G	>8	>8	>8	>8/NT	>8/NT	>8/NT	>8/NT	>8/NT	>8/NT
Rifampin	≤0.5	≤0.5	>2	≤0.5	≤0.5/>2	>2	0.5	0.5	>2
Temafloxacin	4	≤32	≤32	8/NT	≤32/NT	≤32/NT	≤125/NT	0.5/NT	>32/NT
Ticarcillin/clavulanic acid	>32	>32	>32	>32/NT	>32/NT	>32/NT	≤8/NT	≤8/NT	≤8/NT
Trimethoprim/ sulfamethoxazole	>4	>4	>4	>4/2	>4	>4	≤2/≤0.5	≤2/≤0.5	>4
Vancomycin	1	1	2	1/2	1/2	2/6	1/2	1/2	2

Reprinted with permission from Peterson LR, Cooper I, Willard KE, et al. Activity of twenty-one antimicrobial agents including l-ofloxacin against quinolone-sensitive and -resistant, methicillin-sensitive and -resistant Staphylococcus aureus. Chemotherapy 1994;40:21–25.

[a] Banked isolates (n = 520) were from freezer storage.

[b] Nonstored fresh isolates from the Minneapolis VA Medical Center (248) and Northwestern Memoral Hospital (150). When the results from the two locations differ, those from the former are given first.

[c] Nonstored fresh isolates from the Minneapolis VA Medical Center (375) and Northwestern Hospital (450). When the results from the two locations differ, those from the former are given first.

[d] MICS are given in μg/ml. NT, not tested.

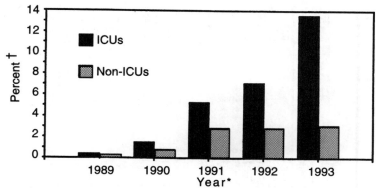

* For 1989–1992, N>1000 isolates for each year; for first quarter 1993, N=291 isolates.
† $p < 0.0001$, chi-square test for linear trend.

Figure 7.4.   Percentage of nosocomial enterococci reported as resistant to vancomycin isolated from infections in patients in intensive care units (*ICUs*) and non-ICUs by year*—National Nosocomial Infections Surveillance System, 1989—March 31, 1993. (Reprinted with permission from Nosocomial enterococci resistant to vancomycin—United States, 1989–1993. MMWR 1993;42(30):597– 599.)

Table 7.5. Antimicrobial Susceptibilities of Recent Isolates of *E. faecalis* and *E. faecium*

Species (No. of Isolates)	Antibiotic	MIC (μg/ml)[a]		Range	No. of Isolates with HLR[b]
		50%	90%		
E. faecalis (75)	Ampicillin	1	4	0.5–8	0
	Imipenem	1	4	0.26–8	0
	Ciprofloxacin	1	16	0.25–≥128	7
	Vancomycin	2	4	0.25–≥128	1
	Teicoplanin	0.06	0.25	≤0.03–≥128	1
	Mideplanin	0.12	0.25	≤0.03–≥128	1
	Ramoplanin	1	2	≤0.03–4	0
	Gentamicin	NE	NE		22
	Streptomycin	NE	NE		36
E. faecium (22)	Ampicillin	64	≥128	2–≥128	16
	Imipenem	64	≥128	1–≥128	16
	Ciprofloxacin	2	64	1–64	2
	Vancomycin	2	8	0.5–8	0
	Teicoplanin	0.12	0.5	≤0.03–1	0
	Mideplanin	0.12	1	≤0.03–1	0
	Ramoplanin	0.5	2	≤0.03–2	0
	Gentamicin	NE	NE		5
	Streptomycin	NE	NE		13

Reprinted with permission from Venditti M, Agapito T, et al. Antimicrobial susceptibilities of enterococci isolated from hospitalized patients. Antimicrob Agents Chemother 1993;37(5):1190–1192.
[a] 50% and 90%, MICs for 50 and 90% of isolates tested, respectively. NE, not evaluated.
[b] For details about HLR, see the text.

Table 7.6. Susceptibility of 1936 Enterococcal Isolates

Antibiotic	Percent Susceptible		
	E. faecalis (n = 1428)	E. faecium (n = 306)	Other Species (n = 202)
Ampicillin	99.4	41.3	81.0
Gentamicin	74.0	69.2	72.5
Streptomycin	68.5	44.3	65.0

Reprinted with permission from Jones RN, Helio SS. The clinical impact of enterococcal resistance (Abstract 1052). Challenges Infect Dis 1993;1(3):4. (ICAAC, New Orleans, LA.)

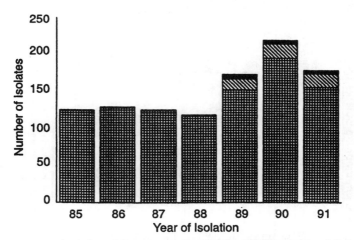

Isolation of *S. pneumoniae* at Texas Children's Hospital between 1985 and 1991. Symbols: ▦, susceptible to penicillin (MIC, ≤ 0.1 μg/ml); ▨, intermediate in resistance to penicillin (0.1 μg/ml ≤ MIC, < 2 μg/ml); ■, highly resistant to penicillin (MIC, ≥ 2 mg/ml).

Figure 7.5. Isolation of *S. pneumoniae*. (Reprinted with permission from Mason EO, Kaplan SL, Lamberth LB, et al. Increased rate of isolation of penicillin-resistant *Streptococcus pneumoniae* in a children's hospital and in vitro susceptibilities to antibiotics of potential therapeutic use. Antimicrobial Agents Chemother 1992;36(8):1703–1707.)

Table 7.7. Susceptibilities to Selected Antibiotics of _S. pneumoniae_ Isolates That Were Susceptible to Penicillin, Intermediate in Resistance to Penicillin, and Highly Resistant to Penicillin

Antimicrobial Agent	MIC Breakpoint (μg/ml)	Susceptible to Penicillin (n = 34)			Intermediate in Resistance to Penicillin (n = 42)			Highly Resistant to Penicillin (n = 19)		
		MIC$_{50}$	MIC$_{90}$	% Susceptible	MIC$_{50}$	MIC$_{90}$	% Susceptible	MIC$_{50}$	MIC$_{90}$	% Susceptible
Amoxicillin-clavulanate[b]	0.125[a]	0.06	0.25	85	0.25	2	48	2	4	0
Amoxicillin-clavulanate[b]	8[c]	0.06	0.25	100	0.25	2	100	2	4	100
Cefaclor	8	1	4	100	2	32	67	64	64	7
Cefixime	1	0.5	2	88	1	8	55	8	16	7
Cefotaxime	8	0.06	0.25	100	0.125	1	100	0.5	2	100
Cefpirome	8	0.015	0.25	100	0.125	0.25	100	0.5	1	100
Cefpodoxime	2	0.125	0.5	100	0.25	2	100	2	8	61
Cefuroxime	8	0.25	2	100	0.5	2	100	4	8	93
Chloramphenicol	8	2	2	96	1	2	100	2	2	100
Ciprofloxacin	1	1	2	87	1	2	89	1	2	82
Clarithromycin	2	0.008	0.03	100	0.015	2	100	1	2	100
Clindamycin	0.5	0.008	0.03	97	0.008	0.03	100	0.03	1	83
Erythromycin	0.5	0.015	0.5	94	0.03	2	69	1	4	21
Imipenem	4	0.008	0.03	100	0.03	0.25	100	0.5	1	100
Rifampin	1	0.06	0.125	100	0.06	0.125	100	0.06	0.125	100
Trimethoprim-sulfamethoxazole[d]	2	0.25/5	2/38	100	0.5/10	1/19	100	1/19	4/76	73
Vancomycin	4	0.25	1	100	0.25	2	100	0.25	0.5	100

Reprinted with permission from Mason EO, Kaplan SL, Lamberth LB, et al. Increased rate of isolation of penicillin-resistant _Streptococcus pneumoniae_ in a children's hospital and in vitro susceptibilities to antibiotics of potential therapeutic use. Antimicrob Agents Chemother. 1992;36(8):1703–1707.
[a] Interpretive standard for the ampicillin class (amoxicillin) in tests of "other streptococci."
[b] Ratio, 2:1; amoxicillin component reported.
[c] Interpretive standard for amoxicillin-clavulanate in tests of "other organisms."
[d] Ratio, 1:19.

Table 7.8. Enterobacteriaceae Susceptibility Patterns: Antibiograms for 28,569 Isolates (Data from 286 ICUs in the United States in 1989)

Species	No. of Patients	Antibiogram for Selected Agents vs. Principal Species in a Pool of 286 Hospital ICUs[a] Percent Fully Susceptible at NCCLS Breakpoint							
		Ceftazidime	Aztreonam	Cefotaxime	Ticar. Clav.	Mezlocillin	Imipanem	Ciprofloxacin	bNetilmicin
Pseudomonas aeruginosa	6861	77	70	16	80	67	83	90	59
E. coli	5536	97	94	97	88	68	97	99	98
K. pneumoniae	2994	95	94	95	87	33	96	98	96
E. cloacae	2708	61	63	59	49	54	94	97	94
E. aerogenes	1702	68	78	71	57	58	95	98	97
P. mirabilis	1536	94	89	95	90	82	85	97	97
S. marcescens	1379	84	84	79	75	67	92	91	90
Acinetobacter spp.	1377	77	33	53	76	38	93	74	64
X. maltophilia	1095	42	5	7	54	15	6	27	17
K. oxytoca	694	98	89	96	87	26	96	99	98
C. freundii	562	52	60	55	44	43	95	97	95
M. morganii	397	74	83	78	84	58	88	99	96
C. diversus	300	96	92	95	89	30	96	97	97
All isolates	28569	81	75	63	76	57	88	91	81

Provided courtesy of Fred M. Kahan. The publishing costs were supported by an unrestricted grant from Merck, Co.
[a]Included, for reference, are all studies in the data base. Repeat isolates have not been excluded.

REFERENCES

1. Kunin CM. Resistance to antimicrobial drugs—a worldwide calamity. Ann Intern Med 1993;118(7):557–561.
2. Tauxe RV, Puhr ND, Wells JG, Hargrett-Bean N, Blake PA. Antimicrobial resistance of *Shigella* isolates in the USA: the importance of international travelers. J Infect Dis 1990;162:1107–1111.
3. Appelbaum PC. Antimicrobial resistance in *Streptococcus pneumoniae*: an overview. Clin Infect Dis 1992;15:77–83.
4. Seppala H, Nissinen A, Jarvinen H, Houvinen S, Henriksson T, Herva E, et al. Resistance to erythromycin in group A streptococci. N Engl J Med 1992;326:292–297.
5. Burke JP, Levy SB. Summary report of worldwide antibiotic resistance: international task forces on antibiotic use. Rev Infect Dis 1985;7:560–564.
6. Cohen ML. Epidemiology of drug resistance: implications for a post-antimicrobial era. Science 1992;257:1050–1055.
7. Neu HC. The crisis in antibiotic resistance. Science 1992;257:1064–1073.
8. O'Brien TF. Global surveillance of antibiotic resistance. N Engl J Med 1992;326:339–340.

SECTION 8
Clinical Use of Immunobiologic Agents

Availability and Use of Immunobiologic Agents

AGENTS AVAILABLE FROM THE CENTERS FOR DISEASE CONTROL AND PREVENTION (1)

The Centers for Disease Control and Prevention (CDC) distributes 13 special immunobiologic materials and drugs through the Drug Service, Division of Host Factors, Center for Infectious Diseases, and the Quarantine Branch of the Center for Preventive Services. This summary reviews these agents, describing their sources, licensure, investigational new drug (IND) application and status, distribution, and storage (Table 8.1). An updated listing of products (2) can be obtained from the CDC Drug Service and from the publications *Facts and Comparisons* (3) and *American Hospital Formulary Service Drug Information 88* (4). In the United States, it is illegal to administer a drug not licensed by the U.S. Food and Drug Administration (FDA). The FDA issues an exemption known as an IND to allow treatment of patients with unlicensed drugs. To obtain an IND, a protocol for the clinical use of the unlicensed drug or biologic must be submitted to and approved by the FDA before any drugs are released.

There are two main categories of INDs: research and treatment (1). Research INDs are used mainly by manufacturers as part of the process for the development of new licensed drugs. Treatment INDs are used for immediate life-threatening or serious disease conditions when no other satisfactory drug or alternative therapy is available (1). Many of the products carried by the Drug Service at the CDC are treatment INDs. They are generally manufactured by foreign drug companies and commercially available in various countries overseas. Their demand in this country is so limited that commercial licensure is not practical or remunerative. IND status is maintained by the CDC so that these products can be available in the United States.

The CDC dispenses immunobiologics or drugs to physicians requesting them for patients with approved indications for their use. Physicians requesting an investigational drug stocked at the CDC must register as coinvestigators and provide the CDC Drug Service with data on product efficacy and adverse reactions. FDA requirements for IND products released in this country are as follows (5):

187

Table 8.1. Immunobiologics and Drugs Distributed by the Centers for Disease Control and Prevention

Product	Producer	Licensed or IND	Distributed to	Release	Storage Conditions
Immunobiologics, therapeutic use					
Botulism equine trivalent antitoxin (ABE)	Connaught Laboratories	Licensed	M.D. as required	Emergency	4–8°C
Diphtheria equine antitoxin	Sclavo, Connaught Laboratories	Licensed	M.D. as required	Emergency	4–8°C
Vaccinia immune globulin (VIG)	Hyland Laboratories	Licensed	M.D. as required	Emergency	4–8°C
Immunobiologics, prophylactic use					
Botulinum toxoid pentavalent (ABCDE)[a]	Michigan State Health Laboratory	IND[b]	Clinical investigators	Prophylaxis	4–8°C
Smallpox vaccine	Wyeth Laboratories	Licensed	M.D. as required	Prophylaxis	4–8°C
Drugs					
Bithionol	Tanabe	IND	Clinical investigators	Compassionate treatment IND	15–30°C
Dehydroemetine	Hoffmann-La Roche	IND	Clinical investigators	Compassionate treatment IND	15–30°C
Diloxanide furoate	Boots	IND	Clinical investigators	Compassionate treatment IND	15–30°C
Ivermectin	Merck	IND	Clinical investigators	Compassionate treatment IND	15–30°C
Melarsoprol	Specia	IND	Clinical investigators	Compassionate treatment IND	15–30°C

Nifurtimox	FBA	IND	Clinical investigators	Compassionate treatment IND	15–30°C
Pentostam	Wellcome	IND	Clinical investigators	Compassionate treatment IND	4–8°C
Suramin	FBA	IND	Clinical investigators	Compassionate treatment IND	15–30°C

Modified and reprinted with permission from Becher JA, Parvin M, Van Assendelh OW. J Pharm Tech 1989;5:181–186.

[a] These products are not expected to be produced again by these manufacturers.

[b] IND, investigational new drug; FBA, Farbenfabr. Bayer AG.

1. The requesting physician is required to complete form FDA-1572, Statement of Investigator.
2. The physician must fill out and return a specific Patient Report Form, with results of therapy and any adverse reactions. This information is used in IND annual reports required by the FDA. Severe reactions must be reported immediately to the CDC by telephone.
3. A patient Informed Consent Form signed by both the clinical investigator and the patient is required.

Information about indication, contraindication, dosage, routes and frequency of administration, reported adverse reactions, toxicity, and other data are sent to the physician with the investigational drug or immunobiologic. Physicians who wish to use these products in clinical situations for unapproved indications or to alter dosing schedules or drug dosage must register with the FDA as clinical investigators under a separate Investigational New Drug application, obtained directly from the FDA.

Some drugs and immunobiologics dispensed by the CDC are licensed by the FDA but their use is restricted. Restrictions are outlined under each section in this summary.

1. Modified and reprinted with permission from Becher JA, Parvin M, Van Assendelft OW. J Pharm Tech 1989;5:181–186.
2. Immunobiologic agents and drugs available from the Centers for Disease Control. Atlanta: Department of Health and Human Services, Centers for Disease Control, 1987.
3. Drug Facts and Comparisons. Philadelphia: JB Lippincott, 1989.
4. McEvoy GK, ed. American hospital formulary service drug information 88. Bethesda, MD: American Society of Hospital Pharmacists, 1988.
5. New drug, antibiotic, and biologic drug product regulations; final rule. Federal Register 1987;52(March 19):8798–8847.

Botulism Equine Trivalent Antitoxin (ABE) (1, 2)

Botulism antitoxin for patients with signs and symptoms of human food-borne or wound botulism is released to physicians by the CDC from its quarantine stations located throughout the United States. Any health-care provider requesting botulism antitoxin should first contact his/her state health department. Daytime and 24-hour telephone numbers are listed in Table 8.2. if the state health department is unreachable during nights or on weekends, the CDC may be called at (404) 639-3670 (24-hour number). This allows the CDC and the state health departments to maintain effective botulinum surveillance and to detect outbreaks as quickly as possible. In the United States, the antitoxin is available only from the CDC because of its limited use and its relatively short supply.

When botulism is suspected, a careful food history, especially for home-canned vegetables or fruits, should be sought and the suspected food items saved. Stool and serum should be obtained from patients with possible botulism and refrigerated.

Table 8.2. Telephone Numbers for Requesting Botulism Antitoxin

State	Daytime No.	24-Hour or Night No.
Alabama	(205) 261-5131	(205) 277-8660
Alaska	(907) 561-4406	
Arizona	(602) 255-1280	
Arkansas	(501) 661-2597	(501) 661-2136
California	(415) 540-2566	(415) 540-2308
Colorado	(303) 331-8330	(303) 370-9395
Connecticut	(203) 566-2540	(203) 566-4800
Delaware	(302) 856-5152	(302) 736-4714
District of Columbia	(202) 673-6757	(202) 727-1000
Florida	(904) 487-2905	
Georgia	(404) 894-6527	
Hawaii	(808) 548-4580	(808) 247-2191
Idaho	(208) 334-5941	(208) 334-2241 (out of state)
		(800) 632-8000 (in state)
Illinois	(217) 782-2016	(217) 782-7860
Indiana	(317) 633-8414	(317) 633-0144
Iowa	(515) 281-5643	(515) 281-3561
Kansas	(913) 862-9360	(913) 862-9360
Kentucky	(502) 564-3418	(502) 564-7078
Louisiana	(504) 568-5005	
Maine	(207) 289-3591	(800) 821-5821
Maryland	(301) 225-6677	(301) 243-8700
Massachusetts	(617) 522-3700	(617) 522-3700
Michigan	(517) 335-8165	(517) 335-9030
Minnesota	(612) 623-5414	(612) 623-5414
Mississippi	(601) 354-6660	(601) 354-6612
Missouri	(314) 751-8129	(314) 751-2335
Montana	(406) 444-4740	(406) 444-4740
Nebraska	(401) 471-2937	(402) 471-2927
Nevada	(702) 885-4988	
New Hampshire	(603) 271-4477	(800) 852-3345
New Jersey	(609) 292-7300	(609) 392-2020
New Mexico	(505) 827-0006	(505) 827-0006
New York City	(212) 566-7160	(212) 340-4494
New York State	(518) 474-3186	(518) 465-9720
North Carolina	(919) 733-3421	(919) 733-4646
North Dakota	(701) 224-2378	(701) 224-2398 (out of state)
		(800) 472-2180 (in state)
Ohio	(614) 466-0265	
Oklahoma	(405) 271-4060	(405) 271-4060
Oregon	(503) 229-5792	(503) 229-5599
Pennsylvania	(717) 787-3350	(717) 737-5349
Rhode Island	(401) 277-2362	(401) 277-2840
South Carolina	(803) 758-7970	
South Dakota	(605) 773-3357	
Tennessee	(615) 741-7247	(615) 741-3011
Texas	(512) 458-7207	(512) 458-7111
Utah	(801) 538-6191	
Vermont	(802) 863-7240	(802) 863-7240
Virginia	(804) 786-6261	(804) 786-4000
Washington	(206) 361-2914	(206) 464-6289
West Virginia	(304) 348-3530	(304) 744-2678
Wisconsin	(608) 267-9003	(608) 238-5064
Wyoming	(307) 777-6018	

Botulism equine trivalent antitoxin, types A, B, and E, is a refined concentrated preparation of horse globulins modified by enzymatic digestion. It is a licensed product and is supplied in 10 ml multidose vials, each of which contains the following:

Type A—7500 IU, equivalent to 2381 U.S. Units
Type B—5500 IU, equivalent to 1839 U.S. Units
Type E—8500 IU, equivalent to 8500 U.S. Units

DOSAGE

Treatment for botulism includes optimum respiratory care and use of antitoxin early in the disease. Because allergic reactions occur in about 9% of all persons treated with botulinal antitoxin, the risk of treatment should be weighed carefully in each instance. If one decides to use antitoxin to ensure rapid neutralization of all unbound toxin in tissue and fluids, it is advisable, after appropriate skin testing, to give 1 vial intravenously. To provide a reservoir of antitoxin, an additional vial should be given by intramuscular injection. One additional vial may be given intravenously in 4 hours if signs and symptoms worsen. The patient must be queried and tested for hypersensitivity to horse serum, and, if necessary, initial intravenous dosages must be small and well diluted. Serum is warmed to body temperature and is injected slowly.

Antitoxin prophylaxis is necessary only when a person is definitely known to have eaten food contaminated with toxin of *Clostridium botulinum*. That person should receive a rapid-acting purgative, such as magnesium sulfate, as soon as possible after suspected exposure. Prophylaxis is accomplished, after appropriate sensitivity testing, by the intramuscular injection of $\frac{1}{5}$ to 1 vial. If signs or symptoms of botulism subsequently appear, additional antitoxin may be given.

REFERENCES

1. Modified and abstracted from Centers for Disease Control. Immunobiologic agents and drugs available from the Centers for Disease Control—descriptions, recommendations, and adverse reactions. 2nd ed. Atlanta: Centers for Disease Control, 1979.
2. Modified from CDC. Release of botulism antitoxin. MMWR 1988;35(30):490–491.
3. Modified and reprinted with permission from Becher JA, Parvin RM, Van Assendelft OW. Immunobiologics and drugs available from the Centers for Disease Control. Harvey Whitney Books, P.O. Box 42696, Cincinnati, OH 45242, 1989.

Diphtheria Equine Antitoxin (1)

PREPARATION

Diphtheria equine antitoxin is a sterile aqueous solution of enzyme refined and concentrated immunoglobulin obtained from the blood of horses immunized against diphtheria toxin. Each vial contains 20,000 U. The antitoxin is used to treat or prevent diphtheria by neutralizing the toxins produced by *Corynebacterium diphtheriae*. Diphtheria antitoxin is a licensed product and is available from Connaught Laboratories and from Sclavo. The CDC drug service keeps a limited supply in Atlanta and at various quarantine stations.

TREATMENT

Treatment for diphtheria should begin as early as the clinical diagnosis becomes reasonably established; it should not be delayed until the diagnosis is bacteriologically confirmed, because each hour's delay increases the required dosage and decreases the beneficial effect. Adequate dosage (20,000 to 80,000 U or more) should be intravenously or intramuscularly depending upon the site, severity, and duration of the infection. The antitoxin should be administered immediately after sensitivity testing is completed. The dose for children is the same as that recommended for adults. Early treatment with appropriate antimicrobial therapy is also recommended (see Section 2).

Treatment should be continued until all local and general symptoms are controlled or until another etiologic agent has been identified. There is no contraindication to administration of antitoxin to a patient with acute, diagnosed diphtheria; antitoxin must be given.

PROPHYLAXIS FOR CASE CONTACTS

All close contacts, household and other, with less than three doses of diphtheria toxoid should receive an immediate dose of diphtheria toxoid-containing preparation and should complete the series according to schedule. Close contacts with three or more doses who have not received a dose of a preparation containing diphtheria toxoid within the previous 5 years should receive a booster dose of a diphtheria toxoid-containing preparation appropriate for their age.

All close contacts should be examined daily for 7 days for evidence of disease. Any symptomatic unimmunized or inadequately immunized close contacts should receive prompt chemoprophylaxis with either an intramuscular injection of benzathine penicillin (600,000 U for persons under 6 years old and 1.2 million U for those 6 years old or older) or a 7- to 10-day course of oral erythromycin (children: 40 mg/kg/day; adults: 1 gm/day). Erythromycin may be slightly more effective, but intramuscular benzathine penicillin may be preferred, since it avoids possible problems of noncompliance with an oral drug regimen. Bacteriologic cultures before and after antibiotic prophylaxis may be useful in the follow-up and management of contacts. Identified untreated carriers of toxigenic *C. diphtheriae* should receive antibiotics as recommended above for unimmunized household contacts. Those who continue to harbor the organism after either penicillin or erythromycin should receive an additional 10-day course of oral erythromycin.

Even when close surveillance of unimmunized close contacts is impossible, the use of equine diphtheria antitoxin is not generally recommended because of the risks of allergic reaction to horse serum. Immediate hypersensitivity reactions occur in about 7%, and serum sickness, in 5% of adults receiving the recommended prophylactic dose of equine antitoxin. The risk of adverse reactions to equine antitoxin must be weighed against the small risk of diphtheria occurring in an unimmunized household contact who receives chemoprophylaxis. If antitoxin is to be used, the usually recommended dose is 5,000 to 10,000 U intramuscularly—after appropriate testing for sensitivity—at a site different from that of toxoid injection. The immune response to simultaneous diphtheria antitoxin and toxoid inoculation is unlikely to be impaired, but this has not been adequately studied.

Cases of cutaneous diphtheria generally are caused by infections with nontoxigenic strains of *C. diphtheriae*. However, a lesion suspected of being cutaneous diphtheria should be considered to be caused by a toxigenic strain until proven otherwise. Recommendations for prophylaxis of close case contacts are the same as for respiratory diphtheria, since cutaneous diphtheria may be more contagious than respiratory infection for close contacts. If a cutaneous case is known to be due to a nontoxigenic strain, routine investigation or prophylaxis of contacts is not necessary.

REFERENCES

1. Modified and abstracted from Centers for Disease Control. Immunobiologic agents and drugs available from the Centers for Disease Control—descriptions, recommendations, and adverse reactions. 2nd ed. Atlanta: Centers for Disease Control, 1979.
2. Modified and reprinted with permission from Becher JA, Parvin RM, Van Assendelft OW. Immunobiologics and drugs available from the Centers for Disease Control. Harvey Whitney Books, P.O. Box 42696, Cincinnati, OH 45242, 1989.

General Recommendations on Immunization[a]

Recommendations of the Advisory Committee on Immunization Practices (ACIP)

This revision of the General Recommendations on Immunization updates the 1989 statement (1). Changes in the immunization schedule for infants and children include recommendations that the third dose of oral polio vaccine be administered routinely at 6 months of age rather than at age 15 months and that measles-mumps-rubella vaccine be administered routinely to all children at 12 to 15 months of age. Other updated or new sections include (1) a listing of vaccines and other immunobiologics available in the United States by type and recommended routes, advice on the proper storage and handling of immunobiologics, a section on the recommended routes for administration of vaccines, and discussion of the use of jet injectors; (2) revisions in the guidelines for spacing administration of immune globulin preparations and live virus vaccines, a discussion of vaccine interactions and recommendations for the simultaneous administration of multiple vaccines, a section on the interchangeability of vaccines from different manufacturers, and a discussion of hypersensitivity to vaccine components; (3) a discussion of vaccination during pregnancy, a section on breast-feeding and vaccination, recommendations for the vaccination of premature infants, and updated schedules for immunizing infants and children (including recommendations for the use of *Haemophilus influenzae* type b conjugate vaccines); (4) sections

[a] Modified and reprinted from General recommendations on immunization. Recommendations of the Advisory Committee on Immunization Practices (ACIP). MMWR January 28, 1994;43(No. RR-1).

on the immunization of hemophiliacs and immunocompromised persons; (5) discussion of the Standards for Pediatric Immunization Practices (including a new table of contraindications and precautions to vaccination), information on the National Vaccine Injury Compensation Program, the Vaccine Adverse Events Reporting System, and Vaccine Information Pamphlets; and (6) guidelines for vaccinating persons without documentation of immunization, a section on vaccinations received outside the United States, and a section on reporting of vaccine-preventable diseases. These recommendations are based on information available before publishing and are not comprehensive for each vaccine. The most recent ACIP recommendations for each specific vaccine should be consulted for more details.

Additional copies of this document and other ACIP statements can be purchased from Superintendent of Documents, U.S. Government Printing Office, Washington, DC 20202-9325. Telephone: (202) 783-3238.

Introduction

Recommendations for vaccinating infants, children, and adults are based on characteristics of immunobiologics, scientific knowledge about the principles of active and passive immunization and the epidemiology of diseases, and judgments by public health officials and specialists in clinical and preventive medicine. Benefits and risks are associated with the use of all immunobiologics: no vaccine is completely safe or completely effective. Benefits of vaccination range from partial to complete protection against the consequences of infection, ranging from asymptomatic or mild infection to severe consequences, such as paralysis or death. Risks of vaccination range from common, minor, and inconvenient side effects to rare, severe, and life-threatening conditions. Thus, recommendations for immunization practices balance scientific evidence of benefits, costs, and risks to achieve optimal levels of protection against infectious disease. These recommendations describe this balance and attempt to minimize risk by providing information regarding dose, route, and spacing of immunobiologics and delineating situations that warrant precautions or contraindicate the use of these immunobiologics. These recommendations are for use only in the United States because vaccines and epidemiologic circumstances often differ in other countries. Individual circumstances may warrant deviations from these recommendations. The relative balance of benefits and risks can change as diseases are controlled or eradicated. For example, because smallpox has been eradicated throughout the world, the risk of complications associated with smallpox vaccine (vaccinia virus) now outweighs any theoretical risk of contracting smallpox or related viruses for the general population. Consequently, smallpox vaccine is no longer recommended routinely for civilians or most military personnel. Smallpox vaccine is now recommended only for selected laboratory and health-care workers with certain defined exposures to these viruses (2).

Immunobiologics

The specific nature and content of immunobiologics can differ. When immunobiologics against the same infectious agents are produced by different manufacturers, active and inert ingredients in the various products are not always the same. Practitioners are urged to become familiar with the constituents of the products they use.

SUSPENDING FLUIDS

These may be sterile water, saline, or complex fluids containing protein or other constituents derived from the medium or biologic system in which the vaccine is produced (e.g., serum proteins, egg antigens, and cell-culture-derived antigens).

PRESERVATIVES, STABILIZERS, ANTIBIOTICS

These components of vaccines, antitoxins, and globulins are used to inhibit or prevent bacterial growth in viral cultures or the final product, or to stabilize the antigens or antibodies. Allergic reactions can occur if the recipient is sensitive to one of these additives (e.g., mercurials (thimerosal), phenols, albumin, glycine, and neomycin).

ADJUVANTS

Many antigens evoke suboptimal immunologic responses. Efforts to enhance immunogenicity include mixing antigens with a variety of substances or adjuvants (e.g., aluminum adjuvants such as aluminum phosphate or aluminum hydroxide).

STORAGE AND HANDLING OF IMMUNOBIOLOGICS

Failure to adhere to recommended specifications for storage and handling of immunobiologics can make these products impotent (3). Recommendations included in a product's package inserts, including reconstitution of vaccines, should be followed closely to assure maximum potency of vaccines. Vaccine quality is the shared responsibility of all parties from the time the vaccine is manufactured until administration. In general, all vaccines should be inspected and monitored to assure that the cold chain has been maintained during shipment and storage. Vaccines should be stored at recommended temperatures immediately upon receipt. Certain vaccines, such as oral polio vaccine (OPV) and yellow fever vaccine, are very sensitive to increased temperature. Other vaccines are sensitive to freezing, including diphtheria and tetanus toxoids and pertussis vaccine, adsorbed (DTP), diphtheria and tetanus toxoids and acellular pertussis vaccine, adsorbed (DEP), diphtheria and tetanus toxoids for pediatric use (DT), tetanus and diphtheria toxoids for adult use (Td), inactivated poliovirus vaccine (IPV), *Haemophilus influenzae* type b conjugate vaccine (Hib), hepatitis B vaccine, pneumococcal vaccine, and influenza vaccine. Mishandled vaccine may not be easily distinguished from potent vaccine. When in doubt about the appropriate handling of a vaccine, contact the manufacturer.

Administration of Vaccines

GENERAL INSTRUCTIONS

Persons administering vaccines should take the necessary precautions to minimize risk for spreading disease. They should be adequately immunized against hepatitis B, measles, mumps, rubella, and influenza. Tetanus and diphtheria toxoids are recommended for all persons. Hands should be washed before each new patient is seen. Gloves are not required when administering vaccinations, unless the persons who administer the vaccine will come into contact with potentially infectious body fluids or have open lesions on their hands. Syringes and needles used for injections must be sterile and preferably disposable to minimize the risk of contamination. A separate needle and syringe should be used for each injection. Different vaccines should not be mixed in the same syringe unless specifically licensed for such use. The only vaccines currently licensed to be mixed in the same syringe by the person administering the vaccine are PRP-T *Haemophilus influenzae* type b conjugate vaccine, lyophilized, which can be reconstituted with DTP vaccine produced by Connaught. This PRP-T/ DTP combination was licensed by the FDA on November 18, 1993. Disposable needles and syringes should be discarded in labeled, puncture-proof containers to prevent inadvertent needlestick injury or reuse.

Routes of administration are recommended for each immunobiologic (Tables 8.3 and 8.4). to avoid unnecessary local or systemic effects and to ensure optimal efficacy, the practitioner should not deviate from the recommended routes. Injectable immunobiologics should be administered where there is little likelihood of local, neural, vascular, or tissue injury. In general, vaccines containing adjuvants should be injected into the muscle mass; when administered subcutaneously or intradermally they can cause local irritation, induration, skin discoloration, inflammation, and granuloma formation. Before the vaccine is expelled into the body, the needle should be inserted into the injection site and the syringe plunger should be pulled back—if blood appears in the needle hub, the needle should be withdrawn and a new site selected. The process should be repeated until no blood appears.

SUBCUTANEOUS INJECTIONS

Subcutaneous injections are usually administered into the thigh of infants and in the deltoid area of older children and adults. A $\frac{5}{8}$- to $\frac{3}{4}$-inch, 23- to 25-gauge needle should be inserted into the tissues below the dermal layer of the skin.

INTRAMUSCULAR INJECTIONS

The preferred sites for intramuscular injections are the anterolateral aspect of the upper thigh and the deltoid muscle of the upper arm. *The buttock should not*

Table 8.3. Licensed Vaccines and Toxoids Available in the United States by Type and Recommended Routes of Administration

Vaccine	Type	Route
Adenovirus[a]	Live virus	Oral
Anthrax[b]	Inactivated bacteria	Subcutaneous
Bacillus of Calmette and Guérin (BCG)	Live bacteria	Intradermal/percutaneous
Cholera	Inactivated bacteria	Subcutaneous or intradermal[c]
Diphtheria-tetanus-pertussis (DTP)	Toxoids and inactivated whole bacteria	Intramuscular
DTP-*Haemophilus influenzae* type b conjugate (DTP-Hib)	Toxoids, inactivated whole bacteria, and bacterial polysaccharide conjugated to protein	Intramuscular
Diphtheria-tetanus-acellular pertussis (DTaP)	Toxoids and inactivated bacterial components	Intramuscular
Hepatitis B	Inactive viral antigen	Intramuscular
Haemophilus influenzae type b conjugate (Hib)[d]	Bacterial polysaccharide conjugated to protein	Intramuscular
Influenza	Inactivated virus or viral components	Intramuscular
Japanese encephalitis	Inactivated virus	Subcutaneous
Measles	Live virus	Subcutaneous
Measles-mumps-rubella (MMR)	Live virus	Subcutaneous
Meningococcal	Bacterial polysaccharides of serotypes A/C/Y/W-135	Subcutaneous
Mumps	Live virus	Subcutaneous
Pertussis[b]	Inactivated whole bacteria	Intramuscular
Plague	Inactivated bacteria	Intramuscular
Pneumococcal	Bacterial polysaccharides of 23 pneumococcal types	Intramuscular or subcutaneous
Poliovirus vaccine, inactivated (IPV)	Inactivated viruses of all 3 serotypes	Subcutaneous
Poliovirus vaccine, oral (OPV)	Live viruses of all 3 serotypes	Oral
Rabies	Inactivated virus	Intramuscular or intradermal[e]
Rubella	Live virus	Subcutaneous
Tetanus	Inactivated toxin (toxoid)	Intramuscular[f]
Tetanus-diphtheria (Td or DT)[g]	Inactivated toxins (toxoids)	Intramuscular[f]
Typhoid (parenteral) (Ty21a oral)	Inactivated bacteria Live bacteria	Subcutaneous[h] Oral
Varicella[i]	Live virus	Subcutaneous
Yellow fever	Live virus	Subcutaneous

[a] Available only to the U.S. Armed Forces.
[b] Distributed by the Division of Biologic Products, Michigan Department of Public Health.
[c] The intradermal dose is lower than the subcutaneous dose.
[d] The recommended schedule for infants depends on the vaccine manufacturer; consult the package insert and ACIP recommendations for specific products.

Table 8.3—*continued*

e The intradermal dose of rabies vaccine, human diploid cell (HDCV), is lower than the intramuscular dose and is used only for preexposure vaccination. *Rabies vaccine, adsorbed (RVA) should not be used intradermally.*
f Preparations with adjuvants should be administered intramuscularly.
g Td, tetanus and diphtheria toxoids for use among persons ≥ 7 years of age. Td contains the same amount of tetanus toxoid as DTP or DT, but contains a smaller dose of diphtheria toxoid. DT, tetanus and diphtheria toxoids for use among children <7 years of age.
h Booster doses may be administered intradermally unless vaccine that is acetone-killed and dried is used.
i A live, attenuated varicella vaccine is currently under consideration for licensure. This vaccine may be available for use through a special study protocol to any physician requesting it for certain pediatric patients with acute lymphocytic leukemia. Additional information about eligibility criteria and vaccine administration is available from the Varivax Coordinating Center; Telephone: (215) 283-0897 (4).

be used routinely for active vaccination of infants, children, or adults because of the potential risk of injury to the sciatic nerve (5). In addition, injection into the buttock has been associated with decreased immunogenicity of hepatitis B and rabies vaccines in adults, presumably because of inadvertent subcutaneous injection or injection into deep fat tissue (6). If the buttock is used for passive immunization when large volumes are to be injected or multiple doses are necessary (e.g., large doses of immune globulin (IG)), the central region should be avoided; only the upper, outer quadrant should be used, and the needle should be directed anteriorly (i.e., not interiorly or perpendicular to the skin) to minimize the possibility of involvement with the sciatic nerve (7).

For all intramuscular injections, the needle should be long enough to reach the muscle mass and prevent vaccine from seeping into subcutaneous tissue, but not so long as to endanger underlying neurovascular structures or bone. Vaccinators should be familiar with the structural anatomy of the area into which they are injecting vaccine. An individual decision on needle size and site of injection must be made for each person based on age, the volume of the material to be administered, the size of the muscle, and the depth below the muscle surface into which the material is to be injected.

Infants (<12 Months of Age)

Among most infants, the anterolateral aspect of the thigh provides the largest muscle mass and is therefore the recommended site. However, the deltoid can also be used with the thigh, for example, when multiple vaccines must be administered at the same visit. In most cases, a ⅞- to 1-inch, 22- to 25-gauge needle is sufficient to penetrate muscle in the thigh of a 4-month-old infant. The free hand should bunch the muscle, and the needle should be directed interiorly along the long axis of the leg at an angle appropriate to reach the muscle while avoiding nearby neurovascular structures and bone.

Toddlers and Older Children

The deltoid may be used if the muscle mass is adequate. The needle size can range from 22 to 25 gauge and from ⅝ to 1¼ inches, based on the size of the

Table 8.4. Indications for Immune Globulin for the Prevention of Specific Infectious Diseases

Infection	Indication	Preparation	Dose
Botulism	Treatment and prophylaxis of ingestor of botulinus toxin	Specific equine antibodies	Consult CDC[a] (404-639-3670)
Cytomegalovirus	Prophylaxis and treatment of CMV infections in organ transplant recipients	CMV-IVIG	See package insert, intravenous preparation
Diphtheria	Treatment of respiratory diphtheria	Specific equine antibody	Consult manufacturer (800-822-2463)
Hepatitis A	Family contacts; sexual contacts; institutional or day-care outbreaks	IG	0.02 ml/kg up to 2 ml
	Travelers to developing countries	IG	0.02 ml/kg up to 2 ml for short-term (less than 3 months) travel
			0.06 ml/kg up to 5 ml for long-term (3 months or longer) travel; repeat at 4- to 6-month intervals
Hepatitis B	Percutaneous or mucosal exposure	HBIG	0.06 ml/kg, vaccinate with hepatitis B vaccine if at risk for repeated exposure (for example, health care workers)
	Newborns of HB₅Ag-positive mothers	HBIG	0.5 ml at birth, vaccinate with hepatitis B vaccine
	Sexual contacts of persons with acute or chronic hepatitis B	HBIG	0.06 ml/kg vaccinate with hepatitis B vaccine
Measles	Nonimmune contacts of acute cases exposed fewer than 6 days previously	IG	0.25 ml/kg up to 15 ml for normal hosts
			0.5 ml/kg up to 15 ml for immunocompromised persons
Rabies	Persons exposed to rabid or potentially rabid animals	HRIG	20 IU/kg

Tetanus	Following significant exposure of an unimmunized person	TIG	250 units for prophylaxis
Vaccinia	Immediately on diagnosis of disease	TIG	3000–6000 units for therapy
	Severe reactions to vaccinia vaccination	VIG	Available only from CDC's Drug Service (404-639-3670)
Varicella zoster	Immunosuppressed or newborn contacts	VZIG	125 units per 10 kg, up to 625 units. Fractional doses are not recommended

Reprinted with permission from ACP Task Force on Adult Immunization and Infectious Diseases Society of America, Guide for Adult Immunization. 3rd ed. Philadelphia: American College of Physicians, United States of America, 1994:86.

[a] CDC, Centers for Disease Control and Prevention; IG, immune globulin; HBIG, hepatitis B immune globulin; TIC, tetanus immune globulin; VZIG, varicella zoster immune globulin; HRIG, human rabies immune globulin; CMV-IVIG, cytomegalovirus-intravenous immune globulin; VIG, vaccinia immune globulin. Immune globulin should be administered intramuscularly, except if clearly labeled for intravenous use. See text for details.

muscle. As with infants, the anterolateral thigh may be used, but the needle should be longer—generally ranging from $\frac{7}{8}$ to $1\frac{1}{4}$ inches.

Adults

The deltoid is recommended for routine intramuscular vaccination among adults, particularly for hepatitis B vaccine. The suggested needle size is 1 to $1\frac{1}{2}$ inches and 20 to 25 gauge.

INTRADERMAL INJECTIONS

Intradermal injections are generally administered on the volar surface of the forearm, except for human diploid cell rabies vaccine (HDCV) for which reactions are less severe when administered in the deltoid area. With the bevel facing upward, a $\frac{3}{8}$- to $\frac{3}{4}$-inch, 25- or 27-gauge needle can be inserted into the epidermis at an angle parallel to the long axis of the forearm. The needle should be inserted so the entire bevel penetrates the skin and the injected solution raises a small bleb. Because of the small amounts of antigen used in intradermal injections, care must be taken not to inject the vaccine subcutaneously because it can result in a suboptimal immunologic response.

MULTIPLE VACCINATIONS

If more than one vaccine preparation is administered or if vaccine and an immune globulin preparation are administered simultaneously, it is preferable to administer each at a different anatomic site. It is also preferable to avoid administering two intramuscular injections in the same limb, especially if DTP is one of the products administered. However, if more than one injection must be administered in a single limb, the thigh is usually the preferred site because of the greater muscle mass; the injections should be sufficiently separated (i.e., 1 to 2 inches apart) so that any local reactions are unlikely to overlap (8, 9).

JET INJECTORS

Jet injectors that use the same nozzle tip to vaccinate more than one person (multiple-use nozzle jet injectors) have been used worldwide since 1952 to administer vaccines when many persons must be vaccinated with the same vaccine within a short time period. These jet injectors have been generally considered safe and effective for delivering vaccine if used properly by trained personnel; the safety and efficacy of vaccine administered by these jet injectors are considered comparable to vaccine administered by needle and syringe.

The multiple-use nozzle jet injector most widely used in the United States (Ped-o-Jet) has never been implicated in transmission of blood-borne diseases. However, the report of an outbreak of hepatitis B virus (HBV) transmission following use of one type of multiple-use nozzle jet injector in a weight loss clinic and laboratory studies in which blood contamination of jet injectors has been simulated have caused concern that the use of multiple-use nozzle jet injectors may pose a potential hazard of blood-borne-disease transmission to vaccine recipients (10). This potential risk for disease transmission would exist if the jet injector nozzle became contaminated with blood during an injection and was not properly cleaned and disinfected before subsequent injections. The potential risk of blood-borne-disease transmission would be greater when vaccinating persons at increased risk for blood-borne diseases such as HBV or human immunodeficiency virus (HIV) infection because of behavioral or other risk factors (11, 12).

Multiple-use nozzle jet injectors can be used in certain situations in which large numbers of persons must be rapidly vaccinated with the same vaccine, the use of needles and syringes is not practical and state and/or local health authorities judge that the public health benefit from the use of the jet injector outweighs the small potential risk of blood-borne-disease transmission. This potential risk can be minimized by training health-care workers before the vaccine campaign on the proper use of jet injectors and by changing the injector tip or removing the jet injector from use if there is evidence of contamination with blood or other body fluid. In addition, mathematical and animal models suggest that the potential risk for blood-borne-disease transmission can be substantially reduced by swabbing the stationary injector tip with alcohol or acetone after each injection. It is advisable to consult sources experienced in the use of jet injectors (e.g., state or local health departments) before beginning a vaccination program in which these injectors will be used. Manufacturer's directions for use and maintenance of the jet injector devices should be followed closely.

Newer models of jet injectors that employ single-use disposable nozzle tips should not pose a potential risk of blood-borne-disease transmission if used appropriately.

REGURGITATED ORAL VACCINE

Infants may sometimes fail to swallow oral preparations (e.g., OPV) after administration. If, in the judgment of the person administering the vaccine, a substantial amount of vaccine is spit out, regurgitated, or vomited shortly after administration (i.e., within 5 to 10 minutes), another dose can be administered at the same visit. If this repeat dose is not retained, neither dose should be counted, and the vaccine should be readministered at the next visit.

NONSTANDARD VACCINATION PRACTICES

The recommendations on route, site, and dosages of immunobiologics are derived from theoretical considerations, experimental trials, and clinical experience. The ACIP strongly discourages any variations from the recommended route, site, volume, or number of doses of any vaccine.

Varying from the recommended route and site can result in (1) inadequate protection (e.g., when hepatitis B vaccine is administered in the gluteal area rather than the deltoid muscle or when vaccines are administered intradermally rather than intramuscularly) and (2) increased risk for reactions (e.g., when DTP is administered subcutaneously rather than intramuscularly). Administration of volumes smaller than those recommended, such as split doses, can result in inadequate protection. Use of larger than the recommended dose can be hazardous because of excessive local or systemic concentrations of antigens or other vaccine constituents. The use of multiple reduced doses that together equal a full immunizing dose or the use of smaller divided doses is not endorsed or recommended. The serologic response, clinical efficacy, and frequency and severity of adverse reactions with such schedules have not been adequately studied. Any vaccination using less than the standard dose or a nonstandard route or site of administration should not be counted, and the person should be revaccinated according to age. If a medically documented concern exists that revaccination may result in an increased risk of adverse effects because of repeated prior exposure from nonstandard vaccinations, immunity to most relevant antigens can be tested serologically to assess the need for revaccination.

Age at Which Immunobiologics Are Administered

Recommendations for the age at which vaccines are administered (Tables 8.5–8.7) are influenced by several factors: age-specific risks of disease, age-specific risks of complications, ability of persons of a given age to respond to the vaccine(s), and potential interference with the immune response by passively transferred maternal antibody. In general, vaccines are recommended for the youngest age group at risk for developing the disease whose members are known to develop an adequate antibody response to vaccination.

Spacing of Immunobiologics

INTERVAL BETWEEN MULTIPLE DOSES OF SAME ANTIGEN

Some products require administration of more than one dose for development of an adequate antibody response. In addition, some products require periodic reinforcement or booster doses to maintain protection. In recommending the ages and intervals for multiple doses, the ACIP considers risks from disease and the need to induce or maintain satisfactory protection (Tables 8.5–8.7).

Longer-than-recommended intervals between doses do not reduce final antibody concentrations. Therefore, an interruption in the immunization schedule does not require reinstitution of the entire series of an immunobiologic or the addition of extra doses. However, administering doses of a vaccine or toxoid at less than the recommended minimum intervals may decrease the antibody response and therefore should be avoided. Doses administered at less than the recommended minimum intervals should not be considered part of a primary series.

Some vaccines produce increased rates of local or systemic reactions in certain recipients when administered too frequently (e.g., adult Td, pediatric DT, tetanus toxoid, and rabies vaccines). Such reactions are thought to result from the formation of antigen-antibody complexes. Good record keeping, maintaining careful

Table 8.5. Recommended Schedule for Routine Active Vaccination of Infants and Children[a]

Vaccine	At Birth (before Hospital Discharge)	1-2 months	2 months[b]	4 months	6 months	6-18 months	12-15 months	15 months	4-6 Years (before School Entry)
Diphtheria-tetanus-pertussis[c]			DTP	DTP	DTP			DTaP/DTP[d]	DTaP/DTP
Polio, live oral			OPV	OPV	OPV[e]				OPV
Measles-mumps-rubella							MMR		MMR[f]
Haemophilus influenzae type b conjugate									
HbOC/PRP-T[c, g]			Hib	Hib	Hib		Hib[h]		
PRP-OMP[g]			Hib	Hib			Hib[h]		
Hepatitis B[i]									
Option 1	HepB	HepB[j]				HepB[j]			
Option 2		HepB[j]		HepB[j]		HepB[j]			

[a] See Table 8.6 for the recommended immunization schedule for infants and children up to their 7th birthday who do not begin the vaccination series at the recommended times or who are >1 month behind in the immunization schedule.

[b] Can be administered as early as 6 weeks of age.

[c] Two DTP and Hib combination vaccines are available (DTP/HbOC (TETRAMUNE™); and PRP-T (ActHIB™, OmniHIB™), which can be reconstituted with DTP vaccine produced by Connaught).

[d] This dose of DTP can be administered as early as 12 months of age provided that the interval since the previous dose of DTP is at least 6 months. *Diphtheria and tetanus toxoids and acellular pertussis vaccine (DTaP) are currently recommended only for use as the fourth and/or fifth doses of the DTP series among children aged 15 months through 6 years (before the seventh birthday).* Some experts prefer to administer these vaccines at 18 months of age.

[e] The American Academy of Pediatrics (AAP) recommends this dose of vaccine at 6-18 months of age.

[f] The AAP recommends that two doses of MMR should be administered by 12 years of age, with the second dose being administered preferentially at entry to middle school or junior high school.

[g] HbOC, HibTITER® (Lederle Praxis); PRP-T, ActHIB™, OmniHIB™ (Pasteur Merieux); PRP-OMP, PedvaxHIB® (Merck, Sharp, and Dohme). A DTP/Hib combination vaccine can be used in place of HbOC/PRP-T.

[h] After the primary infant Hib conjugate vaccine series is completed, any of the licensed Hib conjugate vaccines may be used as a booster dose at age 12-15 months.

[i] For use among infants born to HB₅Ag-negative mothers. The first dose should be administered during the newborn period, preferably before hospital discharge, but no later than age 2 months. Premature infants of HB₅Ag-negative mothers should receive the first dose of the hepatitis B vaccine series at the time of hospital discharge or when the other routine childhood vaccines are initiated. (All infants born to HB₅Ag-positive mothers should receive immunoprophylaxis for hepatitis B as soon as possible after birth.)

[j] Hepatitis B vaccine can be administered simultaneously at the same visit with DTP (or DTaP), OPV, Hib, and/or MMR.

Table 8.6. Recommended Accelerated Immunization Schedule for Infants and Children <7 Years of Age Who Start the Series Late[a] or Who Are >1 Month Behind in the Immunization Schedule[b] (i.e., Children for Whom Compliance with Scheduled Return Visits Cannot Be Assured)

Timing	Vaccine(s)	Comments
First visit (≥ 4 months of age)	DTP,[c, d] OPV, Hib,[d, e] hepatitis B, MMR (should be given as soon as child is age 12–15 months)	All vaccines should be administered simultaneously at the appropriate visit.
Second visit (1 month after first visit)	DTP,[d] Hib,[d, e] hepatitis B	
Third visit (1 month after second visit)	DTP,[d] OPV, Hib[d, e]	
Fourth visit (6 weeks after third visit)	OPV	
Fifth visit (≥6 months after third visit)	DTaP[d] or DTP, Hib,[d, e] hepatitis B	
Additional visits (Age 4–6 years)	DTaP[d] or DTP, OPV, MMR	Preferably at or before school entry.
(Age 14–16 years)	Td	Repeat every 10 years throughout life.

[a] If initiated in the first year of life, administer DTP doses 1, 2, and 3 and OPV doses 1, 2, and 3 according to this schedule; administer MMR when the child reaches 12–15 months of age.

[b] See individual ACIP recommendations for detailed information on specific vaccines.

[c] DTP, diphtheria-tetanus-pertussis; DTaP, diphtheria-tetanus-acellular pertussis; Hib, *Haemophilus influenzae* type b conjugate; MMR, measles-mumps-rubella; OPV, poliovirus vaccine, live oral, trivalent; Td, tetanus and diphtheria toxoids (for use among persons ≥7 years of age).

[d] Two DTP and Hib combination vaccines are available (DTP/HbOC (TETRAMUNE™) and PRP-T (ActHIB™, OmniHIB™), which can be reconstituted with DTP vaccine produced by Connaught). DTaP preparations are currently recommended only for use as the fourth and/or fifth doses of the DTP series among children 15 months through 6 years of age (before the seventh birthday). DTP and DTaP should not be used on or after the seventh birthday.

[e] The recommended schedule varies by vaccine manufacturer. For information specific to the vaccine being used, consult the package insert and ACIP recommendations. Children beginning the Hib vaccine series at age 2–6 months should receive a primary series of three doses of HbOC (HibTITER® (Lederle-Praxis)), PRP-T (ActHIB™, OmniHIB™ (Pasteur Merieux; SmithKline Beecham; Connaught)), or a licensed DTP-Hib combination vaccine; or two doses of PRP-OMP [PedvaxHIB®] (Merck, Sharp, and Dohme). An additional booster dose of any licensed Hib conjugate vaccine should be administered at 12–15 months of age and at least 2 months after the previous dose. Children beginning the Hib vaccine series at 7–11 months of age should receive a primary series of two doses of an HbOC, PRP-T, or PRP-OMP-containing vaccine. An additional booster dose of any licensed Hib conjugate vaccine should be administered at 12–18 months of age and at least 2 months after the previous dose. Children beginning the Hib vaccine series at ages 12–14 months should receive a primary series of one dose of an HbOC, PRP-T, or PRP-OMP-containing vaccine. An additional booster dose of any licensed Hib conjugate vaccine should be administered 2 months after the previous dose. Children beginning the Hib vaccine series at ages 15–59 months should receive one dose of any licensed Hib vaccine. Hib vaccine should not be administered after the fifth birthday, except for special circumstances as noted in the specific ACIP recommendations for the use of Hib vaccine.

Table 8.7. Recommended Immunization Schedule for Persons ≥7 Years of Age Not Vaccinated at the Recommended Time in Early Infancy[a]

Timing	Vaccine(s)	Comments
First visit	Td,[b, c] OPV[d] MMR,[e] and hepatitis B[f]	Primary poliovirus vaccination is not routinely recommended for persons ≥18 years of age.
Second visit (6–8 weeks after first visit)	Td, OPV, MMR,[d, g] hepatitis B[e]	
Third visit (6 months after second visit)	Td, OPV, hepatitis B[e]	
Additional visits	Td	Repeat every 10 years throughout life.

[a] See Individual ACIP recommendations for details.
[b] Td, tetanus and diphtheria toxoids (for use among persons ≥7 years of age); MMR, measles-mumps-rubella; OPV, poliovirus vaccine, live oral, trivalent.
[c] The DTP and DTaP doses administered to children <7 years of age who remain incompletely vaccinated at age ≥7 years should be counted as having prior exposure to tetanus and diphtheria toxoids (e.g., a child who previously received two doses of DTP needs only one dose of Td to complete a primary series for tetanus and diphtheria).
[d] When polio vaccine is administered to previously unvaccinated persons ≥18 years of age, inactivated poliovirus vaccine (IPV) is preferred. For the immunization schedule for IPV, see specific ACIP statement on the use of polio vaccine.
[e] Persons born before 1957 can generally be considered immune to measles and mumps and need not be vaccinated. Rubella (or MMR) vaccine can be administered to persons of any age, particularly to nonpregnant women of childbearing age.
[f] Hepatitis B vaccine, recombinant. Selected high-risk groups for whom vaccination is recommended include persons with occupational risk, such as health-care and public-safety workers who have occupational exposure to blood, clients and staff of institutions for the developmentally disabled, hemodialysis patients, recipients of certain blood products (e.g., clotting factor concentrates), household contacts and sex partners of hepatitis B virus carriers, injecting drug users, sexually active homosexual and bisexual men, certain sexually active heterosexual men and women, inmates of long-term correctional facilities, certain international travelers, and families of HB₅Ag-positive adoptees from countries where HBV infection is endemic. Because risk factors are often not identified directly among adolescents, universal hepatitis B vaccination of teenagers should be implemented in communities where injecting drug use, pregnancy among teenagers, and/or sexually transmitted diseases are common.
[g] The ACIP recommends a second dose of measles-containing vaccine (preferably MMR to assure immunity to mumps and rubella) for certain groups. Children with no documentation of live measles vaccination after the first birthday should receive two doses of live measles-containing vaccine not less than 1 month apart. In addition, the following persons born in 1957 or later should have documentation of measles immunity (i.e., two doses of measles-containing vaccine [at least one of which being MMR], physician-diagnosed measles, or laboratory evidence of measles immunity): (1) those entering post-high school educational settings; (2) those beginning employment in health-care settings who will have direct patient contact; and (3) travelers to areas with endemic measles.

patient histories, and adherence to recommended schedules can decrease the incidence of such reactions without sacrificing immunity.

SIMULTANEOUS ADMINISTRATION

Experimental evidence and extensive clinical experience have strengthened the scientific basis for administering certain vaccines simultaneously (13–16). Many of the commonly used vaccines can safely and effectively be administered simultaneously (i.e., on the same day, *not* at the same anatomic site). Simultaneous administration is important in certain situations, including (1) imminent exposure to several infectious diseases, (2) preparation for foreign travel, and (3) uncertainty that the person will return for further doses of vaccine.

Killed Vaccines

In general, inactivated vaccines can be administered simultaneously at separate sites. However, when vaccines commonly associated with local or systemic reactions (e.g., cholera, parenteral typhoid, and plague) are administered simultaneously, the reactions might be accentuated. When feasible, it is preferable to administer these vaccines on separate occasions.

Live Vaccines

The simultaneous administration of the most widely used live and inactivated vaccines has not resulted in impaired antibody responses or increased rates of adverse reactions. Administration of combined measles-mumps-rubella (MMR) vaccine yields results similar to administration of individual measles, mumps, and rubella vaccines at different sites. Therefore, there is no medical basis for administering these vaccines separately for routine vaccination instead of the preferred MMR combined vaccine.

Concern has been raised that oral live attenuated typhoid (Ty21a) vaccine theoretically might interfere with the immune response to OPV when OPV is administered simultaneously or soon after live oral typhoid vaccine (17). However, no published data exist to support this theory. Therefore, if OPV and oral live typhoid vaccine are needed at the same time (e.g., when international travel is undertaken on short notice), both vaccines may be administered simultaneously or at any interval before or after each other.

Routine Childhood Vaccines

Simultaneous administration of all indicated vaccines is important in childhood vaccination programs because it increases the probability that a child will be fully immunized at the appropriate age. During a recent measles outbreak, one study indicated that about one-third of measles cases among unvaccinated preschool children could have been prevented if MMR had been administered at the same time another vaccine had been received (18).

The simultaneous administration of routine childhood vaccines does not interfere with the immune response to these vaccines. When administered at the same time and at separate sites, DTP, OPV, and MMR have produced seroconversion rates and rates of side effects similar to those observed when the vaccines are administered separately (13). Simultaneous vaccination of infants with DTP, OPV (or IPV), and either Hib vaccine or hepatitis B vaccine has resulted in acceptable response to all antigens (14, 16). Routine simultaneous administration of DTP (or DTaP), OPV (or IPV), Hib vaccine, MMR, and hepatitis B vaccine is encouraged for children who are the recommended age to receive these vaccines and for whom no specific contraindications exist at the time of the visit, unless, in the judgment of the provider, complete vaccination of the child will not be compromised by administering different vaccines at different visits. Simultaneous administration is particularly important if the child might not return for subsequent vaccinations. Administration of MMR and Hib vaccine at 12–15 months of age, followed by DTP (or DTaP, if indicated) at age 18 months remains an acceptable alternative for children with caregivers known to be compliant with other health-care recommendations and who are likely to return for future visits; hepatitis B vaccine can be administered at either of these two visits. DTaP may be used instead of DTP only for the fourth and fifth dose for children 15 months of age through 6 years (i.e., before the seventh birthday). Individual vaccines should not be mixed in the same syringe unless they are licensed for mixing by the FDA. The only vaccines currently licensed to be mixed in the same syringe by the person administering the vaccine are PRP-T *Haemophilus influenzae* type b conjugate vaccine, lyophilized, which can be reconstituted with DTP vaccine produced by Connaught. This PRP-T/DTP combination was licensed by the FDA on November 18, 1993.

Other Vaccines

The simultaneous administration of pneumococcal polysaccharide vaccine and whole-virus influenza vaccine elicits a satisfactory antibody response without increasing the incidence or severity of adverse reactions in adults (19). Simultaneous administration of pneumococcal vaccine and split-virus influenza vaccine can be expected to yield satisfactory results in both children and adults.

Hepatitis B vaccine administered with yellow fever vaccine is as safe and efficacious as when these vaccines are administered separately (20). Measles and yellow fever vaccines have been administered together safely and with full efficacy of each of the components (21).

The antibody response of yellow fever and cholera vaccines is decreased if administered simultaneously or within a short time of each other. If possible, yellow fever and cholera vaccinations should be separated by at least 3 weeks. If time constraints exist and both vaccines are necessary, the injections can be administered simultaneously or within a 3-week period with the understanding that antibody response may not be optimal. Yellow fever vaccine is required by many countries and is highly effective in protecting against a disease with substantial mortality and for which no therapy exists. The currently used cholera vaccine provides limited protection of brief duration; few indications exist for its use.

Antimalarials and Vaccination

The antimalarial mefloquine (Lariam™) could potentially affect the immune response to oral live attenuated typhoid (Ty21a) vaccine if both are taken simultaneously (17, 22, 23). To minimize this effect it may be prudent to administer Ty21a typhoid vaccine at least 24 hours before or after a dose of mefloquine. Because chloroquine phosphate (and possibly other structurally related antimalarials such as mefloquine) may interfere with the antibody response to HDCV when HDCV is administered by the intradermal dose/route, HDCV should not be

Table 8.8. Guidelines for Spacing the Administration of Live and Killed Antigens

Antigen Combination	Recommended Minimum Interval between Doses
≥2 killed antigens	None. May be administered simultaneously or at any interval between doses.[a]
Killed and live antigens	None. May be administered simultaneously or at any interval between doses.[b]
≥2 live antigens	4-Week minimum interval if not administered simultaneously.[c] However, oral polio vaccine can be administered at any time before, with, or after measles-mumps-rubella, if indicated.

[a] If possible, vaccines associated with local or systemic side effects (e.g., cholera, parenteral typhoid, and plague vaccines) should be administered on separate occasions to avoid accentuated reactions.
[b] Cholera vaccine with yellow fever vaccine is the exception. If time permits, there antigens should not be administered simultaneously, and at least 3 weeks should elapse between administration of yellow fever vaccine and cholera vaccine. If the vaccines must be administered simultaneously or within 3 weeks of each other, the antibody response may not be optimal.
[c] If oral live typhoid vaccine is indicated (e.g., for international travel undertaken on short notice), it can be administered before, simultaneously with, or after OPV.

administered by the intradermal dose/route when chloroquine, mefloquine, or other structurally related antimalarials are used (24–26).

NONSIMULTANEOUS ADMINISTRATION

Inactivated vaccines generally do not interfere with the immune response to other inactivated vaccines or to live vaccines except in certain instances (e.g., yellow fever and cholera vaccines). In general an inactivated vaccine can be administered either simultaneously or at any time before or after a different inactivated vaccine or live vaccine. However, limited data have indicated that prior or concurrent administration of DTP vaccine may enhance anti-PRP antibody response following vaccination with certain *Haemophilus influenzae* type b conjugate vaccines (i.e., PRP-T, PRP-D, and HbOC) (27–29). For infants the immunogenicity of PRP-OMP appears to be unaffected by the absence of prior or concurrent DTP vaccination (28, 30).

Theoretically, the immune response to one live-virus vaccine might be impaired if administered within 30 days of another live-virus vaccine; however, no evidence exists for currently available vaccines to support this concern (31). Whenever possible, live-virus vaccines administered on different days should be administered at least 30 days apart (Table 8.8). However, OPV and MMR vaccines can be administered at any time before, with, or after each other, if indicated. Live-virus vaccines can interfere with the response to a tuberculin test (32–34). Tuberculin testing, if otherwise indicated, can be done either on the same day that live-virus vaccines are administered or 4 to 6 weeks later.

IMMUNE GLOBULIN

Live Vaccines

OPV and yellow fever vaccines can be administered at any time before, with, or after the administration of immune globulin or specific immune globulins (e.g., hepatitis B immune globulin (HBIG) and rabies immune globulin (RIG)) (Table 8.7) (35). The concurrent administration of immune globulin should not interfere with the immune response to oral Ty21a typhoid vaccine.

Previous recommendations, based on data from persons who received low doses of immune globulin, have stated that MMR and its individual component vaccines can be administered as early as 6 weeks to 3 months after administration of immune globulin (1, 36). However, recent evidence suggests that high doses of immune globulin can inhibit the immune response to measles vaccine for more than 3 months (37, 38). Administration of immune globulin can also inhibit the response to rubella vaccine (37). The effect of immune globulin preparations on the response to mumps and varicella vaccines is unknown, but commercial immune globulin preparations contain antibodies to these viruses.

Blood (e.g., whole blood, packed red blood cells, and plasma) and other antibody-containing blood products (e.g., immune globulin; specific immune globulins; and immune globulin, intravenous (IVIG)) can diminish the immune response to MMR or its individual component vaccines. Therefore, after an immune globulin preparation is received, these vaccines should not be administered before the recommended interval (Tables 8.9 and 8.10). However, the postpartum vaccination of rubella-susceptible women with rubella or MMR vaccine should not be delayed because anti-Rho(D) IG (human) or any other blood product was received during the last trimester of pregnancy or at delivery. These women should be vaccinated immediately after delivery and, if possible, tested at least 3 months later to ensure immunity to rubella and, if necessary, to measles.

If administration of an immune globulin preparation becomes necessary because of imminent exposure to disease, MMR or its component vaccines can be administered simultaneously with the immune globulin preparation, although vaccine-induced immunity might be compromised. The vaccine should be administered at a site remote from that chosen for the immune globulin inoculation. Unless serologic testing indicates that specific antibodies have been produced, vaccination should be repeated after the recommended interval (Tables 8.9 and 8.10).

If administration of an immune globulin preparation becomes necessary after MMR or its individual component vaccines have been administered, interference can occur. Usually, vaccine virus replication and stimulation of immunity will occur 1 to 2 weeks after vaccination. Thus, if the interval between administration of any of these vaccines and subsequent administration of an immune globulin preparation is <14 days, vaccination should be repeated after the recommended interval (Tables 8.9 and 8.10), unless serologic testing indicates that antibodies were produced.

Killed Vaccines

Immune globulin preparations interact less with inactivated vaccines and toxoids than with live vaccines (39). Therefore, administration of inactivated vaccines and toxoids either simultaneously with or at any interval before or after receipt of immune globulins should not substantially impair the development of a protective

Table 8.9. Guidelines for Spacing the Administration of Immune Globulin Preparations[a] and Vaccines

Simultaneous Administration	
Immunobiologic Combination	Recommended Minimum Interval between Doses
Immune globulin and killed antigen	None. May be given simultaneously at different sites or at any time between doses.
Immune globulin and live antigen	Should generally not be administered simultaneously.[b] If simultaneous administration of measles-mumps-rubella [MMR], measles-rubella, and monovalent measles vaccine is unavoidable, administer at different sites and revaccinate or test for seroconversion after the recommended interval (Table 8.8)

Nonsimultaneous Administration		
Immunobiologic Administered		Recommended Minimum Interval between Doses
First	Second	
Immune globulin	Killed antigen	None
Killed antigen	Immune globulin	None
Immune globulin	Live antigen	Dose related[b, c]
Live antigen	Immune globulin	2 weeks

[a] Blood products containing large amounts of immune globulin (such as serum immune globulin, specific immune globulins (e.g., TIG and HBIG), intravenous immune globulin (IGIV), whole blood, packed red cells, plasma, and platelet products).
[b] Oral polio virus, yellow fever, and oral typhoid (Ty21a) vaccines are exceptions to these recommendations. These vaccines may be administered at any time before, after, or simultaneously with an immune globulin-containing product without substantially decreasing the antibody response (35).
[c] The duration of interference of immune globulin preparations with the immune response to the measles component of the MMR, measles-rubella, and monovalent measles vaccine is dose-related (Table 8.8).

antibody response. The vaccine or toxoid and immune globulin preparation should be administered at different sites using the standard recommended dose of corresponding vaccine. Increasing the vaccine dose volume or number of vaccinations is not indicated or recommended.

INTERCHANGEABILITY OF VACCINES FROM DIFFERENT MANUFACTURERS

When at least one dose of a hepatitis B vaccine produced by one manufacturer is followed by subsequent doses from a different manufacturer, the immune response has been shown to be comparable with that resulting from a full course of vaccination with a single vaccine (11, 40).

Both HDCV and rabies vaccine, adsorbed (RVA) are considered equally efficacious and safe and, when used as licensed and recommended, are considered interchangeable during the vaccine series. RVA should not be used intradermally. The full 1.0-ml dose of either product, administered by intramuscular injection, can be used for both preexposure and postexposure prophylaxis (25).

When administered according to their licensed indications, different diphtheria and tetanus toxoids and pertussis vaccines as single antigens or various combina-

Table 8.10. Suggested Intervals between Administration of Immune Globulin Preparations for Various Indications and Vaccines Containing Live Measles Virus[a]

Indication	Dose (including mg IgG/kg)	Suggested Interval before Measles Vaccination (months)
Tetanus (TIG)	250 units (10 mg IgG/kg) i.m.	3
Hepatitis A (IG)		
Contact prophylaxis	0.02 ml/kg (3.3 mg IgG/kg) i.m.	3
International travel	0.06 ml/kg (10 mg IgG/kg) i.m.	3
Hepatitis B prophylaxis (HBIG)	0.06 ml/kg (10 mg IgG/kg) i.m.	3
Rabies prophylaxis (HRIG)	20 IU/kg (22 mg IgG/kg) i.m.	4
Varicella prophylaxis (VZIG)	125 units/10 kg (20–40 mg IgG/kg) i.m. (maximum 625 units)	5
Measles prophylaxis (IG)		
Normal contact	0.25 ml/kg (40 mg IgG/kg) i.m.	5
Immunocompromised contact	0.50 ml/kg (80 mg IgG/kg) i.m.	6
Blood transfusion		
Red blood cells (RBCs), washed	10 ml/kg (negligible IgG/kg) i.v.	0
RBCs, adenine-saline added	10 ml/kg (10 mg IgG/kg i.v.)	3
Packed RBCs (Hct 65%)[b]	10 ml/kg (60 mg IgG/kg) i.v.	6
Whole blood (Hct 35–50%)[b]	10 ml/kg (80–100 mg IgG/kg) i.v.	6
Plasma/platelet products	10 ml/kg (160 mg IgG/kg) i.v.	7
Replacement of humoral immune deficiencies	300–400 mg/kg i.v.[c] (as IGIV)	8
Treatment of:		
ITP[d]	400 mg/kg i.v. (as IGIV)	8
ITP[d]	1000 mg/kg i.v. (as IGIV)	10
Kawasaki disease	2 gm/kg i.v. (as IGIV)	11

[a] This table is not intended for determining the correct indications and dosage for the use of immune globulin preparations. Unvaccinated persons may not be fully protected against measles during the entire suggested interval, and additional doses of immune globulin and/or measles vaccine may be indicated following measles exposure. The concentration of measles antibody in a particular immune globulin preparation can vary by lot. The rate of antibody clearance following receipt of an immune globulin preparation can also vary. The recommended intervals are extrapolated from an estimated half-life of 30 days for passively acquired antibody and an observed interference with the immune response to measles vaccine for 5 months following a dose of 80 mg IgG/kg (37).
[b] Assumes a serum IgG concentration of 16 mg/ml.
[c] Measles vaccination is recommended for children with HIV infection but is contraindicated in patients with congenital disorders of the immune system.
[d] Immune (formally, idiopathic) thrombocytopenic purpura.

tions, as well as the live and inactivated polio vaccines, also can be used interchangeably. However, published data supporting this recommendation are generally limited (41).

Currently licensed *Haemophilus influenzae* type b conjugate vaccines have been shown to induce different temporal patterns of immunologic response in infants (42). Limited data suggest that infants who receive sequential doses of different vaccines produce a satisfactory antibody response after a complete primary series (43–45). The primary vaccine series should be completed with the same Hib vaccine, if feasible. However, if different vaccines are administered, a total of three doses of Hib vaccine is considered adequate for the primary series among infants, and any combination of Hib conjugate vaccines licensed for use among infants (i.e., PRP-OMP, PRP-T, HbOC and combination DTP-Hib vaccines) may be used to complete the primary series. Any of the licensed conjugate vaccines can be used for the recommended booster dose at 12–18 months of age (Tables 8.5 and 8.6).

Hypersensitivity to Vaccine Components

Vaccine components can cause allergic reactions in some recipients. These reactions can be local or systemic and can include mild to severe anaphylaxis or anaphylactic-like responses (e.g., generalized urticaria or hives, wheezing, swelling of the mouth and throat, difficulty breathing, hypotension, and shock). The responsible vaccine components can derive from (1) vaccine antigen, (2) animal protein, (3) antibiotics, (4) preservatives, and (5) stabilizers. The most common animal protein allergen is egg protein found in vaccines prepared using embryonated chicken eggs (e.g., influenza and yellow fever vaccines) or chicken embryo cell cultures (e.g., measles and mumps vaccines). Ordinarily, persons who are able to eat eggs or egg products safely can receive these vaccines; persons with histories of anaphylactic or anaphylactic-like allergy to eggs or egg proteins should not. Asking persons if they can eat eggs without adverse effects is a reasonable way to determine who might be at risk for allergic reactions from receiving measles, mumps, yellow fever, and influenza vaccines. Protocols requiring caution have been developed for testing and vaccinating with measles, mumps, and MMR vaccines those persons with anaphylactic reactions to egg ingestion (46–49). A regimen for administering influenza vaccine to children with egg hypersensitivity and severe asthma has also been developed (50). Rubella vaccine is grown in human diploid cell cultures and can safely be administered to persons with histories of severe allergy to eggs or egg proteins.

Some vaccines contain trace amounts of antibiotics (e.g., neomycin) to which patients may be hypersensitive. The information provided in the vaccine package insert should be carefully reviewed before deciding if the uncommon patient with such hypersensitivity should receive the vaccine(s). No currently recommended vaccine contains penicillin or penicillin derivatives.

MMR and its individual component vaccines contain trace amounts of neomycin. Although the amount present is less than would usually be used for the skin test to determine hypersensitivity, persons who have experienced anaphylactic reactions to neomycin should not receive these vaccines. Most often, neomycin allergy is a contact dermatitis—a manifestation of a delayed-type (cell-mediated) immune response rather than anaphylaxis. A history of delayed-type reactions to neomycin is not a contraindication for these vaccines.

Certain parenteral bacterial vaccines such as cholera, DTP, plague, and typhoid are frequently associated with local or systemic adverse effects, such as redness, soreness, and fever. These reactions are difficult to link with a specific sensitivity to vaccine components and appear to be toxic rather than hypersensitive. Urticarial or anaphylactic reactions in DTP, DT, Td, or tetanus toxoid recipients have been reported rarely. When these reactions are reported, appropriate skin tests can be performed to determine sensitivity to tetanus toxoid before its use is discontinued (51). Alternatively, serologic testing to determine immunity to tetanus can be performed to evaluate the need for a booster dose of tetanus toxoid.

Exposure to vaccines containing the preservative thimerosal (e.g., DTP, DTaP, DT, Td, Hib, hepatitis B, influenza, and Japanese encephalitis) can lead to induction of hypersensitivity. However, most patients do not develop reactions to thimerosal given as a component of vaccines even when patch or intradermal tests for thimerosal indicate hypersensitivity. Hypersensitivity to thimerosal usually consists of local delayed-type hypersensitivity reactions (52, 53).

Vaccination of Preterm Infants

Infants born prematurely, regardless of birthweight, should be vaccinated at the same chronological age and according to the same schedule and precautions as full-term infants and children (Tables 8.5 and 8.6). Birthweight and size generally are not factors in deciding whether to postpone routine vaccination of a clinically stable premature infant (54–56). The full recommended dose of each vaccine should be used. Divided or reduced doses are not recommended (57). To prevent the theoretical risk of poliovirus transmission in the hospital, the administration of OPV should be deferred until discharge.

Any premature infant born to a hepatitis B surface antigen (HB$_s$Ag)-positive mother should receive immunoprophylaxis with hepatitis B vaccine and HBIG beginning at or shortly after birth. For premature infants of HB$_s$Ag-negative mothers, the optimal timing of hepatitis B vaccination has not been determined. Some studies suggest that decreased seroconversion rates might occur in some premature infants with low birthweights (i.e., <2000 gm) following administration of hepatitis B vaccine at birth (58). Such low birthweight premature infants of HB$_s$Ag-negative mothers should receive the hepatitis B vaccine series, which can be initiated at discharge from the nursery if the infant weighs at least 2000 gm or at 2 months of age along with DTP, OPV, and Hib vaccine.

Breast-feeding and Vaccination

Neither killed nor live vaccines affect the safety of breast-feeding for mothers or infants. Breast-feeding does not adversely affect immunization and is not a contraindication for any vaccine. Breast-fed infants should be vaccinated according to routine recommended schedules (59–61).

Inactivated or killed vaccines do not multiply within the body. Therefore they should pose no special risk for mothers who are breast-feeding or for their infants. Although live vaccines do multiply within the mother's body, most have not been demonstrated to be excreted in breast milk. Although rubella vaccine virus may be transmitted in breast milk, the virus usually does not infect the infant, and if it does, the infection is well tolerated. There is no contraindication for vaccinating breast-feeding mothers with yellow fever vaccine. Breast-feeding mothers can receive OPV without any interruption in the feeding schedule.

Vaccination During Pregnancy

Risk from vaccination during pregnancy is largely theoretical. The benefit of vaccination among pregnant women usually outweighs the potential risk when (1) the risk for disease exposure is high, (2) infection would pose a special risk to the mother or fetus, and (3) the vaccine is unlikely to cause harm.

Combined tetanus and diphtheria toxoids are the only immunobiologic agents routinely indicated for susceptible pregnant women. Previously vaccinated pregnant women who have not received a Td vaccination within the last 10 years should receive a booster dose. Pregnant women who are unimmunized or only partially immunized against tetanus should complete the primary series. Depending on when a woman seeks prenatal care and the required interval between doses, one or two doses of Td can be administered before delivery. Women for whom the vaccine is indicated but who have not completed the required three-dose series during pregnancy should be followed up after delivery to assure they receive the doses necessary for protection.

There is no convincing evidence of risk from vaccinating pregnant women with other inactivated virus or bacteria vaccines or toxoids. Hepatitis B vaccine is recommended for women at risk for hepatitis B infection, and influenza and pneumococcal vaccines are recommended for women at risk for infection and for complications of influenza and pneumococcal disease.

OPV can be administered to pregnant women who are at substantial risk of imminent exposure to natural infection (62). Although OPV is preferred, IPV may be considered if the complete vaccination series can be administered before the anticipated exposure. Pregnant women who must travel to areas where the risk for yellow fever is high should receive yellow fever vaccine. In these circumstances, the small theoretical risk from vaccination is far outweighed by the risk of yellow fever infection (21, 63). Known pregnancy is a contraindication for rubella, measles, and mumps vaccines. Although of theoretical concern, no cases of congenital rubella syndrome or abnormalities attributable to a rubella vaccine virus infection have been observed in infants born to susceptible mothers who received rubella vaccine during pregnancy.

Persons who receive measles, mumps, or rubella vaccines can shed these viruses but generally do not transmit them. These vaccines can be administered safely to the children of pregnant women. Although live polio virus is shed by persons recently vaccinated with OPV (particularly after the first dose), this vaccine can also be administered to the children of pregnant women because experience has not revealed any risk of polio vaccine virus to the fetus.

All pregnant women should be evaluated for immunity to rubella and tested for the presence of HB$_s$Ag. Women susceptible to rubella should be vaccinated immediately after delivery. A woman infected with HBV should be followed carefully to ensure that the infant receives HBIG and begins the hepatitis B vaccine series shortly after birth.

There is no known risk to the fetus from passive immunization of pregnant women with immune globulin preparations. Further information regarding immunization of pregnant women is available in the American College of Obstetricians and Gynecologists Technical Bulletin Number 160, October 1991. This publication is available from the American College of Obstetricians and Gynecologists, Attention: Resource Center, 409 12th Street SW, Washington, DC 20024-2188.

Altered Immunocompetence

The ACIP statement on vaccinating immunocompromised persons summarizes recommendations regarding the efficacy, safety, and use of specific vaccines and immune globulin preparations for immunocompromised persons (64). ACIP statements on individual vaccines or immune globulins also contain additional information regarding these issues.

Severe immunosuppression can be the result of congenital immunodeficiency, HIV infection, leukemia, lymphoma, generalized malignancy or therapy with alkylating agents, antimetabolites, radiation, or large amounts of corticosteroids. Severe complications have followed vaccination with live, attenuated virus vaccines and live bacterial vaccines among immunocompromised patients (65–71). In general, these patients should not receive live vaccines except in certain circumstances that are noted below. In addition, OPV should not be administered to any household contact of a severely immunocompromised person. If polio immunization is indicated for immunocompromised patients, their household members, or other close contacts, IPV should be administered. MMR vaccine is not contraindicated in the close contacts of immunocompromised patients. The degree to which a person is immunocompromised should be determined by a physician.

Limited studies of MMR vaccination in HIV-infected patients have not documented serious or unusual adverse events. Because measles may cause severe illness in persons with HIV infection, MMR vaccine is recommended for all asymptomatic HIV-infected persons and should be considered for all symptomatic HIV-infected persons. HIV-infected persons on regular IVIG therapy may not respond to MMR or its individual component vaccines because of the continued presence of passively acquired antibody. However, because of the potential benefit, measles vaccination should be considered approximately 2 weeks before the next monthly dose of IVIG (if not otherwise contraindicated), although an optimal immune response is unlikely to occur. Unless serologic testing indicates that specific antibodies have been produced, vaccination should be repeated (if not otherwise contraindicated) after the recommended interval (Table 8.10).

An additional dose of IVIG should be considered for persons on routine IVIG therapy who are exposed to measles 23 weeks after administration of a standard dose (100 to 400 mg/kg) of IVIG.

Killed or inactivated vaccines can be administered to all immunocompromised patients, although response to such vaccines may be suboptimal. All such childhood vaccines are recommended for immunocompromised persons in usual doses and schedules; in addition, certain vaccines such as pneumococcal vaccine or Hib vaccine are recommended specifically for certain groups of immunocompromised patients, including those with functional or anatomic asplenia.

Vaccination during chemotherapy or radiation therapy should be avoided because antibody response is poor. Patients vaccinated while on immunosuppressive therapy or in the 2 weeks before starting therapy should be considered unimmunized and should be revaccinated at least 3 months after therapy is discontinued. Patients with leukemia in remission whose chemotherapy has been terminated for 3 months may receive live-virus vaccines.

The exact amount of systemically absorbed corticosteroids and the duration of administration needed to suppress the immune system of an otherwise healthy child are not well defined. Most experts agree that steroid therapy usually does not contraindicate administration of live virus vaccine when it is short term (i.e., <2 weeks); low to moderate dose; long-term, alternate-day treatment with short-acting preparations; maintenance physiologic doses (replacement therapy); or administered topically (skin or eyes), by aerosol, or by intraarticular, bursal, or tendon injection (64). Although of recent theoretical concern, no evidence of increased severe reactions to live vaccines has been reported among persons receiving steroid therapy by aerosol, and such therapy is not in itself a reason to delay vaccination. The immunosuppressive effects of steroid treatment vary, but many clinicians consider a dose equivalent to either 2 mg/kg of body weight or a total of 20 mg/day of prednisone as sufficiently immunosuppressive to raise concern about the safety of vaccination with live-virus vaccines (64). Corticosteroids used in greater than physiologic doses also can reduce the immune response to vaccines. Physicians should wait at least 3 months after discontinuation of therapy before administering a live-virus vaccine to patients who have received high systemically absorbed doses of corticosteroids for 22 weeks.

Vaccination of Persons with Hemophilia

Persons with bleeding disorders such as hemophilia have an increased risk of acquiring hepatitis B and at least the same risk as the general population of acquiring other vaccine-preventable diseases. However, because of the risk of hematomas, intramuscular injections are often avoided among persons with bleeding disorders by using the subcutaneous or intradermal routes for vaccines that are normally administered by the intramuscular route. Hepatitis B vaccine administered intramuscularly to 153 hemophiliacs using a 23-gauge needle, followed by steady pressure to the site for 1 to 2 minutes, has resulted in a 4% bruising rate with no patients requiring factor supplementation (72). Whether an antigen that produces more local reactions, such as pertussis, would produce an equally low rate of bruising is unknown.

When hepatitis B or any other intramuscular vaccine is indicated for a patient with a bleeding disorder, it should be administered intramuscularly if, in the opinion of a physician familiar with the patient's bleeding risk, the vaccine can be administered with reasonable safety by this route. If the patient receives antihemophilic or other similar therapy, intramuscular vaccination can be scheduled shortly after such therapy is administered. A fine needle (<23 gauge) can be used for the vaccination and firm pressure applied to the site (without rubbing) for at least 2 minutes. The patient or family should be instructed concerning the risk of hematoma from the injection.

Misconceptions Concerning True Contraindications and Precautions to Vaccination

Some health-care providers inappropriately consider certain conditions or circumstances to be true contraindications or precautions to vaccination. This misconception results in missed opportunities to administer needed vaccines. Likewise, providers may fail to understand what constitutes a true contraindication or precaution and may administer a vaccine when it should be withheld. This practice can result in an increased risk of an adverse reaction to the vaccine.

STANDARDS FOR PEDIATRIC IMMUNIZATION PRACTICE

National standards for pediatric immunization practices have been established and include true contraindications and precautions to vaccination (Table 8.11) (73). True contraindications, applicable to all vaccines, include a history of anaphylactic or anaphylactic-like reactions to the vaccine or a vaccine constituent (unless the recipient has been desensitized) and the presence of a moderate or severe illness with or without a fever. Except as noted previously, severely immunocompromised persons should not receive live vaccines. Persons who developed an encephalopathy within 7 days of administration of a previous dose of DTP or DTaP should not receive further doses of DTP or DTaP. Persons infected with HIV, with household contacts infected with HIV, or with known altered immunodeficiency should receive IPV rather than OPV. Because of the theoretical risk to the fetus, women known to be pregnant should not receive MMR.

Certain conditions are considered precautions rather than true contraindications for vaccination. When faced with these conditions, some providers may elect to administer vaccine if they believe that the benefits outweigh the risks for the patient. For example, caution should be exercised in vaccinating a child with DTP who, within 48 hours of receipt of a prior dose of DTP, developed fever ≥40.5°C (105°F); had persistent, inconsolable crying for ≥3 hours; collapsed or

Table 8.11. Guide to Contraindications and Precautions to Vaccinations[a]

True Contraindications and Precautions	Not Contraindications (Vaccines May Be Administered)
General for All Vaccines (DTP/DTaP, OPV, IPV, MMR, Hib, Hepatitis B)	
Contraindications Anaphylactic reaction to a vaccine contraindicates further doses of that vaccine Anaphylactic reaction to a vaccine constituent contraindicates the use of vaccines containing that substance Moderate or severe illness with or without a fever	*Not contraindications* Mild to moderate local reaction (soreness, redness, swelling) following a dose of an injectable antigen Mild acute illness with or without low-grade fever Current antimicrobial therapy Convalescent phase of illnesses Prematurity (same dosage and indications as for normal, full-term infants) Recent exposure to an infectious disease History of penicillin or other nonspecific allergies or family history of such allergies
DTP/DTaP	
Contraindications Encephalopathy within 7 days of administration of previous dose of DTP *Precautions[b]* Fever of ≥40.5°C (105°F) within 48 hr after vaccination with a prior dose of DTP Collapse or shocklike state (hypotonic-hyporesponsive episode) within 48 hr of receiving a prior dose of DTP Seizures within 3 days of receiving a prior dose of DTP[c] Persistent, inconsolable crying lasting ≥3 hr within 48 hr of receiving a prior dose of DTP	*Not contraindications* Temperature of <40.5°C (105°F) following a previous dose of DTP Family history of convulsions[c] Family history of sudden infant death syndrome Family history of an adverse event following DTP administration
OPV[d]	
Contraindications Infection with HIV or a household contact with HIV Known altered immunodeficiency (hematologic and solid tumors; congenital immunodeficiency; and long-term immunosuppressive therapy) Immunodeficient household contact	*Not contraindications* Breast-feeding Current antimicrobial therapy Diarrhea

Table 8.11—*continued*

Precaution[b]
Pregnancy

IPV

Contraindication
Anaphylactic reaction to neomycin or
   streptomycin
Precaution[b]
Pregnancy

MMR[d]

Contraindications	*Not contraindications*
Anaphylactic reactions to egg ingestion and to neomycin[e]	Tuberculosis or positive PPD skin test
	Simultaneous TB skin testing[f]
Pregnancy	Breast-feeding
Known altered immunodeficiency (hematologic and solid tumors; congenital immunodeficiency; and long-term immunosuppressive therapy)	Pregnancy of mother of recipient
	Immunodeficient family member or household contact
	Infection with HIV
Precaution[b]	Nonanaphylactic reactions to eggs or neomycin
Recent immune globulin administration (see Table 8.8)	

Hib

Contraindication	*Not a contraindication*
None identified	History of Hib disease

Hepatitis B

Contraindication	*Not a contraindication*
Anaphylactic reaction to common baker's yeast	Pregnancy

[a] This information is based on the recommendations of the Advisory Committee on Immunization Practices (ACIP) and those of the Committee on Infectious Diseases (Red Book Committee) of the American Academy of Pediatrics (AAP). Sometimes these recommendations vary from those contained in the manufacturer's package inserts. For more detailed information, providers should consult the published recommendations of the ACIP, AAP, and the manufacturer's package inserts.

[b] The events or conditions listed as precautions, although not contraindications, should be carefully reviewed. The benefits and risks of administering a specific vaccine to an individual under the circumstances should be considered. If the risks are believed to outweigh the benefits, the vaccination should be withheld; if the benefits are believed to outweigh the risks (for example, during an outbreak or foreign travel), the vaccination should be administered. Whether and when to administer DTP to children with proven or suspected underlying neurologic disorders should be decided on an individual basis. It is prudent on theoretical grounds to avoid vaccinating pregnant women. However, if immediate protection against poliomyelitis is needed, OPV is preferred, although IPV may be considered if full vaccination can be completed before the anticipated imminent exposure.

[c] Acetaminophen given before administering DTP and thereafter every 4 hr for 24 hr should be considered for children with a personal or family history of convulsions in siblings or parents.

[d] No data exist to substantiate the theoretical risk of a suboptimal immune response from the administration of OPV and MMR within 30 days of each other.

[e] Persons with a history of anaphylactic reactions following egg ingestion should be vaccinated only with caution. Protocols have been developed for vaccinating such persons and should be consulted. (J Pediatr 1983;102:196–199, J Pediatr 1988;113:504–506).

[f] Measles vaccination may temporarily suppress tuberculin reactivity. If testing can not be done the day of MMR vaccination, the test should be postponed for 4–6 weeks.

developed a shock-like state; or had a seizure within 3 days of receiving the previous dose of DTP.

Conditions often inappropriately regarded as contraindications to vaccination are also noted (Table 8.11). Among the most important are diarrhea and minor upper-respiratory illnesses with or without fever, mild to moderate local reactions to a previous dose of vaccine, current antimicrobial therapy, and the convalescent phase of an acute illness. Diarrhea is not a contraindication to OPV.

FEBRILE ILLNESS

The decision to administer or delay vaccination because of a current or recent febrile illness depends on the severity of symptoms and on the etiology of the disease.

All vaccines can be administered to persons with minor illness such as diarrhea, mild upper-respiratory infection with or without low-grade fever, or other low-grade febrile illness. Studies suggest that failure to vaccinate children with minor illness can seriously impede vaccination efforts (74–76). Among persons whose compliance with medical care cannot be assured, it is particularly important to take every opportunity to provide appropriate vaccinations.

Most studies from developed and developing countries support the safety and efficacy of vaccinating persons who have mild illness (77–79). One large ongoing study in the United States has indicated that more than 97% of children with mild illnesses develop measles antibody after vaccination (80). Only one study has reported a somewhat lower rate of seroconversion (79%) to the measles component of MMR vaccine among children with minor, afebrile upper-respiratory infection (81). Therefore, vaccination should not be delayed because of the presence of mild respiratory illness or other illness with or without fever.

Persons with moderate or severe febrile illness should be vaccinated as soon as they have recovered from the acute phase of the illness. This precaution avoids superimposing adverse effects of the vaccine on the underlying illness or mistakenly attributing a manifestation of the underlying illness to the vaccine.

Routine physical examinations and measuring temperatures are not prerequisites for vaccinating infants and children who appear to be healthy. Asking the parent or guardian if the child is ill and then postponing vaccination for those with moderate to severe illness, or proceeding with vaccination if no contraindications exist, are appropriate procedures in childhood immunization programs.

Reporting of Adverse Events Following Vaccination

Modern vaccines are safe and effective. However, some adverse events have been reported following the administration of all vaccines. These events range from frequent, minor, local reactions to extremely rare, severe, systemic illness, such as paralysis associated with OPV. It is often impossible to establish evidence for cause-and-effect relationships on the basis of case reports alone because temporal association alone does not necessarily indicate causation. Unless the syndrome following vaccination is clinically or pathologically distinctive, more detailed epidemiologic studies to compare the incidence rates of the event in vaccinees with the incidence rates among unvaccinated persons may be necessary. Reporting of serious adverse events is extremely important to stimulate studies to confirm a causal association and to study risk factors for adverse events. More complete information on adverse reactions to a specific vaccine may be found in the ACIP recommendations for that vaccine.

Health-care providers are required to report selected events occurring after vaccination to the Vaccine Adverse Events Reporting System (VAERS). Persons other than health-care workers can also report adverse events to VAERS. Adverse events other than those that must be reported or that occur after administration of other vaccines, especially events that are serious or unusual, should also be reported to VAERS regardless of whether the provider thinks they are causally associated. VAERS forms and instructions are available in the *FDA Drug Bulletin* and the *Physicians' Desk Reference*, or by calling the 24-hour VAERS information recording at (800) 822-7967.

Vaccine Injury Compensation

The National Vaccine Injury Compensation Program (NVICP), established by the National Childhood Vaccine Injury Act of 1986, is a system under which compensation can be paid on behalf of a person who was injured or died as a result of receiving a vaccine. The program, which became effective on October 1, 1988, is intended as an alternative to civil litigation under the traditional tort system in that negligence need not be proven.

The law establishing the program also created a vaccine injury table, which lists the vaccines covered by the program and the injuries, disabilities, illnesses, and conditions (including death) for which compensation may be paid. The table also defines the period of time during which the first symptom or substantial aggravation of the injury must appear. Persons may be compensated for an injury listed in the established table or one that can be demonstrated to result from administration of a listed vaccine. Injuries following administration of vaccines not listed in the legislation authorizing the program are not eligible for compensation through the program. Additional information about the program is available from

National Vaccine Injury Compensation Program
Health Resources and Services Administration
Parklawn Building, Room 8-05
5600 Fishers Lane
Rockville, MD 20857
Telephone: (800) 338-2382 (24-hour recording)

Persons wishing to file a claim for vaccine injury should call or write to

U.S. Court of Federal Claims
717 Madison Place, NW

Washington, DC 20005
Telephone: (202) 219-9657

Patient Information

Parents, guardians, legal representatives, and adolescent and adult patients should be informed about the benefits and risks of vaccine in understandable language. Opportunity for questions and answers should be provided before each vaccination.

VACCINE INFORMATION PAMPHLETS

The National Childhood Vaccine Injury Act (NCVIA) requires that vaccine information materials be developed for each vaccine covered by the Act (DTP or component antigens, MMR or component antigens, IPV, and OPV). The resulting Vaccine Information Pamphlets must be used by *all public and private* providers of vaccines, although private providers may elect to develop their own materials. Such materials must contain the specific, detailed elements required by law. Copies of these pamphlets are available from individual providers and from state health authorities responsible for immunization (82).

IMPORTANT INFORMATION STATEMENTS

CDC has developed Important Information Statements for the vaccines not covered by the NCVIA. These statements must be used in public health clinics and other settings where federally purchased vaccines are used. Copies can be obtained from state health authorities responsible for immunization. The use of similar statements in the private sector is encouraged.

Immunization Records

PROVIDER RECORDS

Documentation of patient vaccinations helps ensure that persons in need of vaccine receive it and that adequately vaccinated patients are not overimmunized, increasing the risk for hypersensitivity (e.g., tetanus toxoid hypersensitivity). Serologic test results for vaccine-preventable diseases (such as those for rubella screening) as well as documented episodes of adverse events also should be recorded in the permanent medical record of the vaccine recipient.

Health-care providers who administer one or more of the vaccines covered by NVICP are required to ensure that the permanent medical record of the recipient (or a permanent office log or file) states the *date the vaccine was administered, the vaccine manufacturer, the vaccine lot number, and the name, address, and title of the person administering the vaccine.* The term *health-care provider* is defined as any licensed health-care professional, organization, or institution, whether private or public (including federal, state, and local departments and agencies), under whose authority a specified vaccine is administered.

The ACIP recommends that the above information be kept for all vaccines and not only for those required by the National Vaccine Injury Act.

PATIENT'S PERSONAL RECORD

Official immunization cards have been adopted by every state and the District of Columbia to encourage uniformity of records and to facilitate the assessment of immunization status by schools and child care centers. The records are also important tools in immunization education programs aimed at increasing parental and patient awareness of the need for vaccines. A permanent immunization record card should be established for each newborn infant and maintained by the parent. In many states, these cards are distributed to new mothers before discharge from the hospital. Some states are developing computerized immunization record systems.

PERSONS WITHOUT DOCUMENTATION OF VACCINATIONS

Health-care providers frequently encounter persons who have no adequate documentation of vaccinations. Although vaccinations should not be postponed if records cannot be found, an attempt to locate missing records should be made by contacting previous health-care providers. If records cannot be located, such persons should be considered susceptible and should be started on the age-appropriate immunization schedule (Tables 8.6 and 8.7). The following guidelines are recommended:

MMR, OPV (or IPV, if indicated), Hib, hepatitis B, and influenza vaccines can be administered because no adverse effects of repeated vaccination have been demonstrated with these vaccines. Persons who develop a serious adverse reaction after administration of DTP, DTaP, DT, Td, or tetanus toxoid should be individually assessed before the administration of further doses of these vaccines (see the ACIP recommendations for use of diphtheria, tetanus, and pertussis vaccines) (14, 83, 84). Pneumococcal vaccine should be administered, if indicated. In most studies, local reactions in adults after revaccination were similar compared with initial vaccination (see the ACIP recommendations for the use of Pneumococcal Polysaccharide Vaccine for further details) (85).

ACCEPTABILITY OF VACCINATIONS RECEIVED OUTSIDE THE UNITED STATES

The acceptability of vaccines received in other countries for meeting vaccination requirements in the United States depends on vaccine potency, adequate documentation of receipt of the vaccine, and the vaccination schedule used. Although problems with vaccine potency have occasionally been detected (most notably with tetanus toxoid and OPV), the majority of vaccine used worldwide is from reliable local or international manufacturers. It is reasonable to assume that vaccine received in other countries was of adequate potency.

Thus, the acceptability of vaccinations received outside the United States depends primarily on whether receipt of the vaccine was adequately documented and whether the immunization schedule (i.e., age at vaccination and spacing of vaccine doses) was comparable with that recommended in the United States (Tables 8.5–8.7 and 8.12). The following recommendations are derived from current immunization guidelines in the United States. They are based on minimum acceptable standards and may not represent optimal recommended ages and intervals.

Only doses of vaccine with written documentation of the date of receipt should be accepted as valid. Self-reported doses of vaccine without written documentation should not be accepted.

Because childhood vaccination schedules vary in different countries, the age at vaccination and the spacing of doses may differ from that recommended in the United States. The age at vaccination is particularly important for measles vaccine. In most developing countries, measles vaccine is administered at 9 months of age when seroconversion rates are lower than at ages 12 to 15 months. For this reason, children vaccinated against measles before their first birthday should be revaccinated at 12 to 15 months of age and again, depending on state or local policy, upon entry to primary, middle, or junior high school. Doses of MMR or other measles-containing vaccines should be separated by at least 1 month. Combined MMR vaccine is preferred. Children who received monovalent measles vaccine rather than MMR on or after their first birthday also should receive a primary dose of mumps and rubella vaccines.

In most countries, including the United States, the first of three regularly scheduled doses of OPV is administered at 6 weeks of age at the same time as DTP vaccine. However, in polio-endemic countries, an extra dose of OPV is often administered at birth or at ≤2 weeks of age. For acceptability in the United States, doses of OPV and IPV administered at ≥6 weeks (42 days) of age can be counted as a valid part of the vaccination series. For the primary vaccination series, each of the three doses of OPV should have been separated by a minimum of 6 weeks (42 days). If enhanced-potency IPV (available in the United States beginning in 1988) was received, the first two doses should have been separated by at least 4 weeks with at least 6 months between the second and third dose. If conventional inactivated poliovirus vaccine (available in the United States until 1988 and still used routinely in some countries (e.g., the Netherlands)) was used for the primary series, the first three doses should have been separated by at least 4 weeks with at least 6 months between the third and fourth dose. If both OPV and an inactivated poliovirus vaccine were received, the primary vaccination series should consist of a combined total of four doses of polio vaccine, unless the use of enhanced-potency IPV can be verified. If OPV and enhanced-potency IPV were received, the primary series consists of a combined total of three doses of polio vaccine. Any dose of polio vaccine administered at the above recommended minimum intervals can be considered valid. Because the recommended polio vaccination schedule in many countries differs from that used in the United States, persons vaccinated outside the United States may need one or more additional doses of OPV (or enhanced-potency IPV) to meet current immunization guidelines in the United States.

Table 8.12. Minimum Age for Initial Vaccination and Minimum Interval between Vaccine Doses by Type of Vaccine

Vaccine	Minimum Age for First Dose[a]	Minimum Interval from Dose 1 to 2[a]	Minimum Interval from Dose 2 to 3[a]	Minimum Interval from Dose 3 to 4[a]
DTP[b] (DT)[c]	6 weeks[d]	4 weeks	4 weeks	6 months
Combined DTP-Hib	6 weeks	1 month	1 month	6 months
DTaP[b]	15 months			6 months
Hib (primary series)				
HbOC	6 weeks	1 month	1 month	—[e]
PRP-T	6 weeks	1 month	1 month	—[e]
PRP-OMP	6 weeks	1 month	—[e]	
OPV	6 weeks[d]	6 weeks	6 weeks	
IPV[f]	6 weeks	4 weeks	6 months[g]	
MMR	12 months[h]	1 month		
Hepatitis B	Birth	1 month	2 months[i]	

[a] These minimum acceptable ages and intervals may not correspond with the optimal recommended ages and intervals for vaccination. See Tables 8.3–8.5 for the current recommended routine and accelerated vaccination schedules.
[b] DTP, diphtheria-tetanus-pertussis; DTaP, diphtheria-tetanus-acellular pertussis; Hib, Haemophilus influenza type b conjugate; IPV, inactivated poliovirus vaccine; MMR, measles-mumps-rubella; OPV, live oral polio vaccine.
[c] DTaP can be used in place of the fourth (and fifth) dose of DTP for children who are at least 15 months of age. Children who have received all four primary vaccination doses before their fourth birthday should receive a fifth dose of DTP (DT) or DTaP at 4–6 years of age before entering kindergarten or elementary school and at least 6 months after the fourth dose. The total number of doses of diphtheria and tetanus toxoids should not exceed six each before the seventh birthday (14).
[d] The American Academy of Pediatrics permits DTP and OPV to be administered as early as 4 weeks of age in areas with high endemicity and during outbreaks.
[e] The booster dose of Hib vaccine, which is recommended following the primary vaccination series, should be administered no earlier than 12 months of age and at least 2 months after the previous dose of Hib vaccine (Tables 8.3 and 8.4).
[f] See text to differentiate conventional inactivated poliovirus vaccine from enhanced-potency IPV.
[g] For unvaccinated adults at increased risk of exposure to poliovirus with <3 months but >2 months available before protection is needed, three doses of IPV should be administered at least 1 month apart.
[h] Although the age for measles vaccination may be as young as 6 months in outbreak areas where cases are occurring in children <1 year of age, children initially vaccinated before the first birthday should be revaccinated at 12–15 months of age, and an additional dose of vaccine should be administered at the time of school entry or according to local policy. Doses of MMR or other measles-containing vaccines should be separated by at least 1 month.
[i] This final dose is recommended for no earlier than 4 months of age.

Any dose of DTP vaccine or Hib vaccine administered at ≥6 weeks of age can be considered valid. The "booster" dose of Hib vaccine should not have been administered before age 12 months. The first three doses of DTP vaccine should have been separated by a minimum of 4 weeks, and the fourth dose should have been administered no less than 6 months after the third dose. Doses of Hib vaccine in the primary series should have been administered no less than 1 month apart. The booster dose of Hib vaccine should have been administered at least 2 months after the previous dose.

The first dose of hepatitis B vaccine can be administered as early as at birth and should have been separated from the second dose by at least 1 month. The final (third or fourth) dose should have been administered no sooner than 4 months of age and at least 2 months after the previous dose, although an interval of at least 4 months is preferable.

Any dose of vaccine administered at the recommended minimum intervals can be considered valid. Intervals longer than those recommended do not affect antibody titers and may be counted.

Immunization requirements for school entry vary by state. Specific state requirements should be consulted if vaccinations have been administered by schedules substantially different from those routinely recommended in the United States.

Vaccine Programs

The best way to reduce vaccine-preventable diseases is to have a highly immune population. Universal immunization is an important part of good health care and should be accomplished through routine and intensive programs carried out in physicians' offices and in public-health clinics. Programs should be established and maintained in all communities with the goal to ensure vaccination of all children at the recommended age. In addition, appropriate vaccinations should be available for all adults.

Providers should strive to adhere to the *Standards for Pediatric Immunization Practices* (74). These Standards define appropriate immunization practices for both the public and private sectors. The Standards provide guidance on how to make immunization services more conducive to the needs of children through implementation of practices that will result in eliminating barriers to vaccination. These include practices aimed at eliminating unnecessary prerequisites for receiving vaccines, eliminating missed opportunities to vaccinate, improving procedures to assess a child's need for vaccines, enhancing knowledge about vaccinations among both parents and providers, and improving the management and reporting of adverse events. In addition, the Standards address the importance of tracking systems and the use of audits to monitor clinic/office immunization coverage levels among clients. The Standards are the goal to which all providers should strive to attain appropriate vaccination of all children.

Standards of practice have also been published to increase vaccination levels among adults (86). All adults should complete a primary series of tetanus and diphtheria toxoids and receive a booster dose every 10 years. Persons ≥65 years of age and all adults with medical conditions that place them at risk for pneumococcal disease or serious complications of influenza should receive pneumococcal polysaccharide vaccine and annual injections of influenza vaccine. Adult immunization programs should also provide MMR vaccine whenever possible to anyone susceptible to measles, mumps, or rubella. Persons born after 1956 who are attending college (or other post-high school educational institutions), who are newly employed in situations that place them at high risk for measles transmission (e.g., health-care facilities), or who are traveling to areas with endemic measles should have documentation of having received two doses of live MMR on or after their first birthday or other evidence of immunity. All other young adults in this age group should have documentation of a single dose of live MMR vaccine on or after their first birthday or have other evidence of immunity. Use of MMR causes no harm if the vaccinee is already immune to one or more of its components and its use ensures that the vaccinee has been immunized against three different diseases. In addition, widespread use of hepatitis B vaccine is encouraged for all persons who are or may be at increased risk (e.g., adolescents and adults who are either in a high-risk group or reside in areas with high rates of injecting drug use, teenage pregnancy, and/or sexually transmitted disease).

Every visit to a health-care provider is an opportunity to update a patient's immunization status with needed vaccines. Official health agencies should take necessary steps, including developing and enforcing school immunization requirements, to ensure that students at all grade levels (including college students) and those in child care centers are protected against vaccine-preventable diseases. Agencies should also encourage institutions such as hospitals and long-term care facilities to adopt policies regarding the appropriate vaccination of patients, residents, and employees.

Dates of vaccination (day, month, and year) should be recorded on institutional immunization records, such as those kept in schools and child care centers. This will facilitate assessments that a primary vaccine series has been completed according to an appropriate schedule and that needed boosters have been obtained at the correct time.

The ACIP recommends the use of "tickler" or recall systems by all health-care providers. Such systems should also be used by health-care providers who treat adults to ensure that at-risk persons receive influenza vaccine annually and that other vaccinations, such as Td, are administered as needed.

Reporting Vaccine-Preventable Diseases

Public health officials depend on the prompt reporting of vaccine-preventable diseases to local or state health departments by health-care providers to effectively monitor the occurrence of vaccine-preventable diseases for prevention and control efforts.

Nearly all vaccine-preventable diseases in the United States are notifiable; individual cases should be reported to local or state health departments. State health departments report these diseases each week to CDC. The local and state health departments and CDC use these surveillance data to determine whether outbreaks or other unusual events are occurring and to evaluate prevention and control strategies. In addition, CDC uses these data to evaluate the impact of national policies, practices, and strategies for vaccine programs.

Sources of Vaccine Information

In addition to these general recommendations, other sources are available that contain specific and updated vaccine information. These sources include the following:

Official Vaccine Package Circulars.   These are manufacturer-provided product-specific information circulars approved by the FDA and provided with each vaccine. Some of these materials are reproduced in the *Physicians' Desk Reference* (*PDR*).

Morbidity and Mortality Weekly Report (MMWR).   Published weekly by CDC, *MMWR* contains regular and special ACIP recommendations on vaccine use and statements of vaccine policy as they are developed and reports of specific disease activity. Subscriptions are available through Superintendent of Documents, U.S. Government Printing Office, Washington, DC 20402-9235; Telephone: (202) 783-3238. Also available through MMS Publications, C.S.P.O. Box 9120, Waltham, MA 02254-9120; Telephone: (800) 843-6356.

Health Information for International Travel.   This booklet is published annually by CDC as a guide to national requirements and contains recommendations for specific immunizations and health practices for travel to foreign countries. Purchase from the Superintendent of Documents (address above).

Advisory Memoranda.   Published as needed by CDC, these memoranda advise international travelers or persons who provide information to travelers about specific outbreaks of communicable diseases abroad. They include health information for prevention and specific recommendations for immunization. Memoranda and/or placement on mailing list are available from: Travelers' Health Section, Division of Quarantine MS-E03, National Center for Prevention Services (NCPS), CDC, Atlanta, GA 30333. The Division of Quarantine also maintains a 24-hour Travelers' Health Hotline voice information system that can be reached by dialing: (404) 332-4559.

The Report of the Committee on Infectious Diseases of the American Academy of Pediatrics (Red Book).   This report, which contains recommendations on all licensed vaccines, is updated every 2 to 3 years—most recently in 1994. Policy changes for individual recommendations for immunization practices are published as needed by the American Academy of Pediatrics in the journal *Pediatrics*. They are available from the American Academy of Pediatrics, Publications Division, 141 Northwest Point Boulevard, P.O. Box 927, Elk Grove Village, IL 60009-0927; Telephone: (708) 228-5005.

Control of Communicable Diseases in Man.   This manual is published by the American Public Health Association every 5 years—most recently in 1990 (15th ed.). The manual contains information about infectious diseases, their occurrence worldwide, diagnoses and therapy, and up-to-date recommendations on isolation and other control measures for each disease presented. It is available from the American Public Health Association, 1015 Fifteenth Street, NW, Washington, DC 20005; Telephone: (202) 789-5600.

Guide for Adult Immunization (1994).   Produced by the American College of Physicians for physicians caring for adults, this guide emphasizes use of vaccines in healthy adults and adults with specific disease problems. It is available from Subscriber Services, American College of Physicians, Independence Mall West, Sixth Street at Race, Philadelphia, PA 19106-1572; Telephone: (215) 351-2600 or (800) 523-1546.

Technical Bulletins of the American College of Obstetricians and Gynecologists.   These bulletins contain important information on immunization of pregnant women and are updated periodically. They are available from the American College of Obstetricians and Gynecologists, Attention: Resource Center, 409 12th Street, SW, Washington, DC 20024-2188.

State and Many Local Health Departments.   These departments frequently provide technical advice, printed information on vaccines and immunization schedules, posters, and other educational materials.

National Immunization Program, CDC.   This program maintains a 24-hour voice information hotline that provides technical advice on vaccine recommendations, disease outbreak control, and sources of immunobiologics. In addition, a course on the epidemiology, prevention, and control of vaccine-preventable diseases is offered each year in Atlanta and in various states. For further information, contact CDC, National Immunization Program, Atlanta, GA 30333; Telephone: (404) 332-4553.

Definitions

IMMUNOBIOLOGICS

Immunobiologics include antigenic substances, such as vaccines and toxoids, or antibody-containing preparations, such as globulins and antitoxins, from human or animal donors. These products are used for active or passive immunization or therapy. The following are examples of immunobiologics:

Vaccine.   A suspension of live (usually attenuated) or inactivated microorganisms (e.g., bacteria, viruses, or rickettsiae) or fractions thereof administered to induce immunity and prevent infectious disease or its sequelae. Some vaccines contain highly defined antigens (e.g., the polysaccharide of *Haemophilus influenzae* type b or the surface antigen of hepatitis B); others have antigens that are complex or incompletely defined (e.g., killed *Bordetella pertussis* or live attenuated viruses). For a list of licensed vaccines, see Table 8.1.

Toxoid.   A modified bacterial toxin that has been made nontoxic, but retains the ability to stimulate the formation of antitoxin. For a list of licensed toxoids, see Table 8.3.

Immune Globulin (IG).   A sterile solution containing antibodies from human blood. It is obtained by cold ethanol fractionation of large pools of blood plasma and contains 15 to 18% protein. Intended for intramuscular administration, IG is primarily indicated for routine maintenance of immunity of certain immunodeficient persons and for passive immunization against measles and hepatitis A. IG does not transmit hepatitis B virus, human immunodeficiency virus (HIV), or other infectious diseases. An intravenous preparation, IVIG, has been reported to transmit hepatitis C. For a list of immune globulins, see Table 8.4.

Intravenous Immune Globulin (IVIG).   A product derived from blood plasma from a donor pool similar to the IG pool, but prepared so it is suitable for intravenous use. IVIG does not transmit infectious diseases. It is primarily used for replacement therapy in primary antibody-deficiency disorders, for the treatment of Kawasaki disease, immune thrombocytopenic purpura, hypogammaglobulinemia in chronic lymphocytic leukemia, and some cases of HIV infection. For a list of intravenous immune globulins, see Table 8.4.

Specific Immune Globulin.   Special preparations obtained from blood plasma from donor pools preselected for a high antibody content against a specific antigen (e.g., hepatitis B immune globulin, varicella-zoster immune globulin, rabies immune globulin, tetanus immune globulin, vaccinia immune globulin, and cytomegalovirus immune globulin). Like IG and IVIG, these preparations do not transmit infectious diseases. For a list of specific immune globulins, see Table 8.4.

Antitoxin.   A solution of antibodies (e.g., diphtheria antitoxin and botulinum antitoxin) derived from the serum of animals immunized with specific antigens. Antitoxins are used to confer passive immunity and for treatment. For a list of antitoxins, see Table 8.4.

Vaccination and Immunization

The words vaccination and vaccine derive from vaccinia, the virus once used as smallpox vaccine. Thus, vaccination originally meant inoculation with vaccinia virus to make a person immune to smallpox. Vaccination currently denotes the physical act of administering any vaccine or toxoid.

Immunization is a more inclusive term denoting the process of inducing or providing immunity artificially by administering an immunobiologic. Immunization can be active or passive.

Active immunization is the production of antibody or other immune responses through the administration of a vaccine or toxoid. Passive immunization means the provision of temporary immunity by the administration of preformed antibodies. Three types of immunobiologics are administered for passive immunization: (1) pooled human IG or IVIG, (2) specific immune globulin preparations, and (3) antitoxins.

Although persons often use vaccination and immunization interchangeably in reference to active immunization, the terms are not synonymous because the administration of an immunobiologic cannot mean automatically adequate immunity.

REFERENCES

 1. CDC. General recommendations on immunization: recommendations of the Immunization Practices Advisory Committee (ACIP). MMWR 1989;38:205–214, 219–227.
 2. CDC. Vaccinia (smallpox) vaccine: recommendations of the Immunization Practices Advisory Committee. MMWR 1991;40(No. RR-14):1–10.
 3. U.S. Department of Health and Human Services, Public Health Service, CDC. Vaccine management: recommendations for handling and storage of selected biologicals. Atlanta: CDC, March 1991.
 4. CDC. Change in source of information: availability of varicella vaccine for children with acute lymphocytic leukemia. MMWR 1993;42:499.
 5. Gilles FH, French JH. Postinjection sciatic nerve palsies in infants and children. J Pediatr 1961;58:195–204.
 6. Shaw FE Jr, Guess HA, Roets JM, et al. Effect of anatomic injection site, age, and smoking on the immune response to hepatitis B vaccination. Vaccine 1989;7:425–430.
 7. Bergeson PS, Singer SA, Kaplan AM. Intramuscular injections in children. Pediatrics 1982;70:944–948.
 8. Scheifele D, Bjornson G, Barreto L, Meekison W, Guasparini R. Controlled trial of *Haemophilus influenzae* type B diphtheria, tetanus and pertussis vaccines, in 18-month-old children, including comparison of arm versus thigh injection. Vaccine 1992;10:455–460.
 9. Ipp MM, Gold R, Goldback M, et al. Adverse reactions to diphtheria, tetanus, pertussis-polio vaccination at 18 months of age: effect of injection site and needle length. Pediatrics 1989;83:679–682.
10. Canter J, Mackay K, Good LS, et al. An outbreak of hepatitis B associated with jet injections in a weight reduction clinic. Arch Intern Med 1990;150:1923–1927.
11. CDC. Hepatitis B virus: a comprehensive strategy for eliminating transmission in the United States through universal childhood vaccination. Recommendations of the Immunization Practices Advisory Committee (ACIP). MMWR 1991;40(No. RR-13):1–25.
12. CDC. Publicly funded HIV counseling and testing—United States, 1991. MMWR 1992;41:613–617.
13. Deforest A, Long SS, Lischner HW, et al. Simultaneous administration of measles-mumps-rubella vaccine with booster doses of diphtheria-tetanus-pertussis and poliovirus vaccines. Pediatrics 1988;81:237–246.
14. CDC. Diphtheria, tetanus, and pertussis: recommendations for vaccine use and other preventive measures. Immunization Practices Advisory Committee (ACIP). MMWR 1991;40(No. RR-10):1–28.
15. Dashefsky B, Wald E, Guerra N, Byers C. Safety, tolerability, and immunogenicity of concurrent administration of *Haemophilus influenzae* type B conjugate vaccine (meningococcal protein conjugate) with either measles-mumps-rubella vaccine or diphtheria-tetanus-pertussis and oral poliovirus vaccines in 14- to 23-month-old infants. Pediatrics 1990;85(suppl):682–689.
16. Giammanco G, LiVolti S, Mauro L. Immune response to simultaneous administration of a recombinant DNA hepatitis B vaccine and multiple compulsory vaccines in infancy. Vaccine 1991;9:747–750.
17. Cryz SJ. Post-marketing experience with live oral Ty21a vaccine [Letter]. Lancet 1993;341:49–50.
18. Hutchins SS, Escolan J, Markowitz LE, et al. Measles outbreak among unvaccinated preschool-age children: opportunities missed by health care providers to administer measles vaccine. Pediatrics 1989;83:369–374.
19. DeStefano F, Goodman RA, Noble GR, et al. Simultaneous administration of influenza and pneumococcal vaccines. JAMA 1982;247:2551–2554.
20. Yvonnet B, Coursaget P, Deubel V, et al. Simultaneous administration of hepatitis B and yellow fever vaccinations. Bull WHO 1986;19:307–311.
21. CDC. Yellow fever vaccine: recommendations of the Immunization Practices Advisory Committee (ACIP). MMWR 1990;39(No. RR-6):1–6.

22. Ambrosch F, Hirschl A, Kollaritsch H, et al. Immunologic investigations with oral live typhoid vaccine Ty21a strain. In: Steffen R, Lobel HO, Bradley DJ, eds. Travel Medicine: Proceedings of the First Conference on International Travel Medicine. Berlin: Springer-Verlag, 1989:248–253.

23. Horowitz H, Carbonaro CA. Inhibition of the *Salmonella typhi* oral vaccine strain Ty21a, by mefloquine and chloroquine. J Infect Dis 1992;166:1462–1464.

24. Pappaioanou M, Fishbein DB, Dreeson DW, et al. Antibody response to pre-exposure human diploid-cell rabies vaccine given concurrently with chloroquine. N Engl J Med 1986;314:280–284.

25. CDC. Rabies prevention—1991: recommendations of the Immunization Practices Advisory Committee (ACIP). MMWR 1991;40(No. RR-3):1–19.

26. Bernard KW, Fishbein DB, Miller KD, et al. Pre-exposure rabies immunization with human diploid cell vaccine: decreased antibody responses in persons immunized in developing countries. Am J Trop Med Hyg 1985;34:633–647.

27. Schneerson R, Robbins JB, Chu C, et al. Serum antibody responses of juvenile and infant rhesus monkeys injected with *Haemophilus influenzae* type b and pneumococcus type 6A capsular polysaccharide-protein conjugates. Infect Immun 1984;45:582–591.

28. Vella PA, Ellis RW. Immunogenicity of *Haemophilus influenzae* type b conjugate vaccines in infant rhesus monkeys. Pediatr Res 1991;29:10–13.

29. Granoff DM, Rathore MH, Holmes SJ, Granoff PD, Lucas AH. Effect of immunity to the carrier protein on antibody responses to *Haemophilus influenzae* type b conjugate vaccines. Vaccine 1993;11:S46–51.

30. CDC. Recommendations for use of *Haemophilus* b conjugate vaccines and a combined diphtheria, tetanus, pertussis, and *Haemophilus* b vaccine. MMWR 1993;42(No. RR-13):1–15.

31. Petralli JK, Merigan TC, Wilbur JR. Action of endogenous interferon against vaccinia infection in children. Lancet 1965;2:401–405.

32. Starr S, Berkovich S. The effects of measles, gamma globulin modified measles and vaccine measles on the tuberculin test. N Engl J Med 1964;270:386–391.

33. Brickman HF, Beaudry PH, Marks ML. The timing of tuberculin tests in relation to immunization with live viral vaccines. Pediatrics 1975;55:392–396.

34. Berkovich S, Starr S. Effects of live type 1 poliovirus vaccine and other viruses on the tuberculin test. N Engl J Med 1966;274:67–72.

35. Kaplan JE, Nelson DB, Schonberger LB, et al. The effect of immune globulin on the response to trivalent oral poliovirus and yellow fever vaccinations. Bull WHO 1984;62:585–590.

36. CDC. Measles prevention: recommendations of the Immunization Practices Advisory Committee. MMWR 1989;38(S-9):1–18.

37. Siber GR, Werner BC, Halsey NA. Interference of immune globulin with measles and rubella immunization. J Pediatr 1993;122:204–211.

38. Mason W, Takahashi M, Schneider T. Persisting passively acquired measles antibody following gamma globulin therapy for Kawasaki disease and response to live virus vaccination. Presented at the 32nd meeting of the Interscience Conference on Antimicrobial Agents and Chemotherapy [Abstract 311]. Los Angeles, October 1992.

39. Siber GR, Snydman DR. Use of immune globulin in the prevention and treatment of infections. In: Remington J, Swartz M, eds. Current clinical topics in infectious diseases. vol 12. Oxford: Blackwell Scientific, 1992.

40. Bush LM, Moonsammy GL, Boscia JA. Evaluation of initiating a hepatitis B vaccination schedule with one vaccine and completing it with another. Vaccine 1991;9:807–809.

41. Faden H, Modlin JF, Thoms ML, McBean AM, Ferdon MB, Ogra PL. Comparative evaluation of immunization with live attenuated and enhanced-potency inactivated trivalent poliovirus vaccines in childhood: systemic and local immune responses. J Infect Dis 1990;162:1291–1297.

42. Granoff DM, Anderson EL, Osterholm MT, et al. Differences in the immunogenicity of three *Haemophilus influenzae* type b conjugate vaccines in infants. J Pediatr 1992;121:187–194.

43. Greenberg DP, Leiberman JM, Marcy SM, et al. Safety and immunogenicity of mixed sequences of *Haemophilus influenzae* type B (HIB) conjugate vaccines in infants [Abstract 997]. Pediatr Res 1993;33:169A.

44. Daum RS, Milewski WM, Ballanco GA. Interchangeability of *H. influenzae* type B vaccines for the primary series ("mix and match")—a preliminary analysis [Abstract 976]. Pediatr Res 1993;33:166A.

45. Anderson EL, Decker MD, Edwards KM, England JA, Belshe RB. Interchangeability of conjugated *Haemophilus influenzae* type B (HIB) vaccines in infants [Abstract 493]. Pediatr Res 1993;33:85A.
46. Peter G, Lepow ML, McCracken GH Jr, Phillips CF, eds. 1991 Redbook—Report of the Committee on Infectious Diseases. Elk Grove Village, IL: American Academy of Pediatrics, 1991.
47. Lavi S, Zimmerman B, Koren G, Gold R. Administration of measles, mumps, and rubella virus vaccine (live) to egg-allergic children. JAMA 1990;263:269–271.
48. Greenberg MA, Birx DL. Safe administration of mumps-measles-rubella vaccine in egg-allergic children. J Pediatr 1988;13:504–506.
49. Herman JJ, Radin R, Schneiderman R. Allergic reactions to measles (rubeola) vaccine in patients hypersensitive to egg protein. J Pediatr 1983;102:196–199.
50. Murphy KR, Strunk RC. Safe administration of influenza vaccine in asthmatic children hypersensitive to egg proteins. J Pediatr 1985;106:931–933.
51. Jacobs RL, Lowe RS, Lanier BQ. Adverse reactions to tetanus toxoid. JAMA 1982;247:40–42.
52. Kirkland LR. Ocular sensitivity to thimerosal: a problem with hepatitis vaccine? South Med J 1990;83:497–499.
53. Aberer W. Vaccination despite thimerosal sensitivity. Contact Dermatitis 1991;24:6–10.
54. Bernbaum JC, Daft A, Anolik R, et al. Response of preterm infants to diphtheria-tetanus-pertussis immunizations. J Pediatr 1985;107:184–188.
55. Koblin BA, Townsend TR, Munoz A, Onorato I, Wilson M, Polk BE. Response of preterm infants to diphtheria-tetanus-pertussis vaccine. Pediatr Infect Dis J 1988;7:704–711.
56. Smolen P, Bland R, Heiligenstein E, Lawless MR, Dillard R, Abramson J. Antibody response to oral polio vaccine in premature infants. J Pediatr 1983;103:917–919.
57. Bernbaum J, Daft A, Samuelson J, Poiin RA. Half-dose immunization for diphtheria, tetanus, pertussis: response of pre-term infants. Pediatrics 1989;83:471–476.
58. Lau YL, Tam AYC, Ng KW, et al. Response of preterm infants to hepatitis B vaccine. J Pediatr 1992;121:962–965.
59. Kim-Farley R, Brink E, Orenstein W, Bart K. Vaccination and breast-feeding [Letter]. JAMA 1982;248:2451–2452.
60. Patriarca PA, Wright PF, John TJ. Factors affecting the immunogenicity of oral polio vaccine in developing countries: review. Rev Infect Dis 1991;13:926–939.
61. Hahn-Zoric M, Fulconis F, Minoli I, et al. Antibody response to parenteral and oral vaccines are impaired by conventional and low-protein formulas as compared to breast-feeding. Acta Paediatr Scand 1990;79:1137–1142.
62. CDC. Poliomyelitis prevention: enhanced-potency inactivated poliomyelitis vaccine—supplementary statement. MMWR 1987;36:795–798.
63. Tsai TF, Paul R, Lynberg MC, Letson GW. Congenital yellow fever virus infection after immunization in pregnancy. J Infect Dis 1993;168:1520–1523.
64. CDC. Recommendations of the Advisory Committee on Immunization Practices (ACIP): use of vaccines and immune globulins in persons with altered immunocompetence. MMWR 1993;42(No. RR-4):1–18.
65. Sixby JW. Routine immunization of the immunocompromised child. Adv Pediatr Infect Dis 1987;2:79–114.
66. Wright PF, Hatch MH, Kasselberg AG, et al. Vaccine-associated poliomyelitis in a child with sex-linked agammaglobulinemia. J Pediatr 1977;91:408–412.
67. Wyatt HV. Poliomyelitis in hypogammaglobulinemics. J Infect Dis 1973;128:802–806.
68. Davis LE, Bodian D, Price D, et al. Chronic progressive poliomyelitis secondary to vaccination of an immunodeficient child. N Engl J Med 1977;297:241–245.
69. CDC. Disseminated mycobacterium bovis infection from BCG vaccination of a patient with acquired immunodeficiency syndrome. MMWR 1985;34:227–228.
70. Ninane J, Grymonprez A, Burtonboy G, et al. Disseminated BCG in HIV infection. Arch Dis Child 1988;63:1268–1269.
71. Redfield RR, Wright DC, James WD, et al. Disseminated vaccinia in a military recruit with human immunodeficiency virus (HIV) disease. N Engl J Med 1987;316:673–676.
72. Evans DIK, Shaw A. Safety of intramuscular injection of hepatitis B vaccine in hemophiliacs. Br Med J 1990;300:1694–1695.
73. CDC. Standards for pediatric immunization practices recommended by the National Vaccine Advisory Committee. MMWR 1993;42:1–13.
74. Wald ER, Dashefsky B, Byers C, et al. Frequency and severity of infections in day care. J Pediatr 1988;112:540–546.

75. Lewis T, Osborn LM, Lewis K, et al. Influence of parental knowledge and opinions on 12-month diphtheria, tetanus, and pertussis vaccination rates. Am J Dis Child 1988;142:283–286.
76. Farizo KM, Stehr-Green PA, Markowitz LE, Patriarca PA. Vaccination levels and missed opportunities for measles vaccination: a record audit in a public pediatric clinic. Pediatrics 1992;89:589–592.
77. Halsey NA, Boulos R, Mode F, et al. Response to measles vaccine in Haitian infants 6 to 12 months old. Influence of maternal antibodies, malnutrition, and concurrent illnesses. N Engl J Med 1985;313:544–549.
78. Ndikuyeze A, Munoz A, Stewart S, et al. Immunogenicity and safety of measles vaccine in ill African children. Int J Epidemiol 1988;17:448–455.
79. Lindegren ML, Reynolds S, Atkinson W, Davis A, Falter K, Patriarca P. Adverse events following measles vaccination of ill preschool-aged children [Abstract 270]. Abstracts of the 1991 Interscience Conference on Antimicrobial Agents and Chemotherapy (ICAAC), Washington, DC: American Society for Microbiology, 1991:144.
80. Atkinson W, Markowitz L, Baughman A, et al. Serologic response to measles vaccination among ill children [Abstract 422]. Abstracts of the 1992 Interscience Conference on Antimicrobial Agents and Chemotherapy, Washington, DC: American Society for Microbiology, 1992:181.
81. Krober MS, Stracener LE, Bass JW. Decreased measles antibody response after measles-mumps-rubella vaccine in infants with colds. JAMA 1991;265:2095–2096.
82. CDC. Publication of vaccine information pamphlets. MMWR 1991;40:726–727.
83. CDC. Pertussis vaccination: acellular pertussis vaccine for reinforcing and booster use—supplementary ACIP statement: recommendations of the Immunization Practices Advisory Committee (ACIP). MMWR 1992;41(No. RR- 1):1–10.
84. CDC. Pertussis vaccination: acellular pertussis vaccine for the fourth and fifth doses of the DTP series: update to the supplementary ACIP statement: recommendations of the Advisory Committee on Immunization Practices. MMWR 1992;41(No. RR-15):1–5.
85. CDC. Pneumococcal polysaccharide vaccine: recommendations of the Immunization Practices Advisory Committee. MMWR 1989;38:64–68, 73–76.
86. CDC. The public health burden of vaccine preventable diseases among adults: standards for adult immunization practice. MMWR 1990;39:725–729.

Prevention and Control of Influenza: Vaccines (1)

SUMMARY

These recommendations update information on the vaccine available for controlling influenza during the 1994–1995 influenza season. The recommendations supersede MMWR 1993;42(No. RR-6):1–13.

Antiviral agents also have an important role in the control of influenza.

Introduction

Influenza A viruses are classified into subtypes on the basis of two surface antigens: hemagglutinin (H) and neuraminidase (N). Three subtypes of hemagglutinin (H1, H2, and H3) and two subtypes of neuraminidase (N1 and N2) are recognized among influenza A viruses that have caused widespread human disease. Immunity to these antigens—especially to the hemagglutinin—reduces the likelihood of infection and lessens the severity of disease if infection occurs. Infection with a virus of one subtype confers little or no protection against viruses of other subtypes. Furthermore, over time, antigenic variation (antigenic drift) within a subtype may be so marked that infection or vaccination with one strain may not induce immunity to distantly related strains of the same subtype. Although influenza B viruses have shown more antigenic stability than influenza A viruses, antigenic variation does occur. For these reasons, major epidemics of respiratory disease caused by new variants of influenza continue to occur. The antigenic characteristics of circulating strains provide the basis for selecting the virus strains included in each year's vaccine.

Typical influenza illness is characterized by abrupt onset of fever, myalgia, sore throat, and nonproductive cough. Unlike other common respiratory illnesses, influenza can cause severe malaise lasting several days. More severe illness can result if either primary influenza pneumonia or secondary bacterial pneumonia occurs. During influenza epidemics, high attack rates of acute illness result in both increased numbers of visits to physicians' offices, walk-in clinics, and emergency rooms and increased hospitalizations for management of lower respiratory tract complications.

Elderly persons and persons with underlying health problems are at increased risk for complications of influenza. If they become ill with influenza, such members of high-risk groups (see Groups at Increased Risk for Influenza-Related Complications under Target Groups for Special Vaccination Programs) are more likely than the general population to require hospitalization. During major epidemics, hospitalization rates for persons at high risk may increase 2- to 5-fold, depending on the age group. Previously healthy children and younger adults may also require hospitalization for influenza-related complications, but the relative increase in their hospitalization rates is less than for persons who belong to high-risk groups.

An increase in mortality further indicates the impact of influenza epidemics. Increased mortality results not only from influenza and pneumonia but also from cardiopulmonary and other chronic diseases that can be exacerbated by influenza. It is estimated that >10,000 influenza-associated deaths occurred during each of seven different U.S. epidemics from 1977 to 1988, and >40,000 influenza-associated deaths occurred during each of two of these epidemics. Approximately 90% of the deaths attributed to pneumonia and influenza occurred among persons ≥65 years of age.

Because the proportion of elderly persons in the U.S. population is increasing and because age and its associated chronic diseases are risk factors for severe influenza illness, the number of deaths from influenza can be expected to increase unless control measures are implemented more vigorously. The number of persons <65 years of age at increased risk for influenza-related complications is also increasing. Better survival rates for organ-transplant recipients, the success of neonatal intensive-care units, and better management of diseases such as cystic fibrosis and acquired immunodeficiency syndrome (AIDS) result in a higher survival rate for younger persons at high risk.

Options for the Control of Influenza

In the United States, two measures are available that can reduce the impact of influenza: immunoprophylaxis with inactivated (killed-virus) vaccine and chemoprophylaxis or therapy with an influenza-specific antiviral drug (amantadine or rimantadine). Vaccination of persons at high risk each year before the influenza season is currently the most effective measure for reducing the impact of influenza. Vaccination can be highly cost effective when (1) it is directed at persons who are most likely to experience complications or who are at increased risk for exposure and (2) it is administered to persons at high risk during hospitalizations or routine health-care visits before the influenza season, thus making special visits to physicians' offices or clinics unnecessary. When vaccine and epidemic strains of virus are well matched, achieving high vaccination rates among persons living in closed settings (e.g., nursing homes and other chronic-care facilities) can reduce the risk for outbreaks by inducing herd immunity.

Inactivated Vaccine for Influenza A and B

Each year's influenza vaccine contains three virus strains (usually two type A and one type B) representing the influenza viruses that are likely to circulate in the United States in the upcoming winter. The vaccine is made from highly purified, egg-grown viruses that have been made noninfectious (inactivated). Influenza vaccine rarely causes systemic or febrile reactions. Whole-virus, subvirion, and purified-surface-antigen preparations are available. To minimize febrile reactions, only subvirion or purified-surface-antigen preparations should be used for children; any of the preparations may be used for adults.

Most vaccinated children and young adults develop high postvaccination hemagglutination-inhibition antibody titers. These antibody titers are protective against illness caused by strains similar to those in the vaccine or the related variants that may emerge during outbreak periods. Elderly persons and persons with certain chronic diseases may develop lower postvaccination antibody titers than healthy young adults and thus may remain susceptible to influenza-related upper respiratory tract infection. However, even if such persons develop influenza illness despite vaccination, the vaccine has been shown to be effective in preventing lower respiratory tract involvement or other secondary complications, thereby reducing the risk for hospitalization and death.

The effectiveness of influenza vaccine in preventing or attenuating illness varies, depending primarily on the age and immunocompetence of the vaccine recipient and the degree of similarity between the virus strains included in the vaccine and those that circulate during the influenza season. When there is a good match between vaccine and circulating viruses, influenza vaccine has been shown to prevent illness in approximately 70% of healthy persons <65 years of age. In these circumstances, studies have also indicated that influenza vaccine is approximately 70% effective in preventing hospitalization for pneumonia and influenza among elderly persons living in settings other than nursing homes or similar chronic-care facilities.

Among elderly persons residing in nursing homes, influenza vaccine is most effective in preventing severe illness, secondary complications, and death. Studies of this population have shown the vaccine to be 50 to 60% effective in preventing

Table 8.13. Influenza Vaccine[a] Dosage by Age Group—United States, 1994–1995 Season

Age Group	Product[b]	Dosage (ml)	No. Doses	Routes[c]
6–35 months	Split virus only	0.25	1 or 2[d]	i.m.
3–8 years	Split virus only	0.50	1 or 2[d]	i.m.
9–12 years	Split virus only	0.50	1	i.m.
>12 years	Whole or split virus	0.50	1	i.m.

[a] Contains 15 μg each of A/Texas/36/91-like (H1N1), A/Shangdong/9/93-like (H3N2), and B/Panama/45/90-like hemagglutinin antigens in each 0.5 ml. Manufacturers include: Connaught Laboratories, Inc. (Fluzone® whole or split); Evans Medical Ltd. (distributed by Adams Laboratories, Inc.) (Fluviron™ purified surface antigen vaccine); Parke-Davis (Fluogen® split); and Wyeth-Ayerst Laboratories (Flu-shield™ split). For further product information call Connaught, (800) 822-2463; Adams, (800) 932-1950; Parke-Davis, (800) 223-0432; Wyeth-Ayerst, (800) FLU-SHIELD.
[b] Because of the lower potential for causing febrile reactions, only split-virus vaccines should be used for children. They may be labeled as "split," "subvirion," or "purified-surface-antigen" vaccine. Immunogenicity and side effects of split- and whole-virus vaccines are similar among adults when vaccines are administered at the recommended dosage.
[c] The recommended site of vaccination is the deltoid muscle for adults and older children. The preferred site for infants and young children is the anterolateral aspect of the thigh.
[d] Two doses administered at least 1 month apart are recommended for children <9 years of age who are receiving influenza vaccine for the first time.

hospitalization and pneumonia and 80% effective in preventing death, even though efficacy in preventing influenza illness may often be in the range of 30 to 40% among the frail elderly. Achieving a high rate of vaccination among nursing home residents has been shown to reduce the spread of infection in a facility, thus preventing disease through herd immunity.

Recommendations for Use of Influenza Vaccine

Influenza vaccine is strongly recommended for any person ≥6 months of age who—because of age or underlying medical condition—is at increased risk for complications of influenza. Health-care workers and others (including household members) in close contact with persons in high-risk groups should also be vaccinated. In addition, influenza vaccine may be administered to any person who wishes to reduce the chance of becoming infected with influenza. The trivalent influenza vaccine prepared for the 1994–1995 season will include A/Texas/36/91-like(H1N1), A/Shangdong/9/93-like(H3N2), and B/Panama/45/90-like hemagglutinin antigens. Recommended doses are listed in Table 8.13. Guidelines for the use of vaccine among different groups follow.

Although the current influenza vaccine can contain one or more of the antigens administered in previous years, annual vaccination with the current vaccine is necessary because immunity declines in the year following vaccination. Because the 1994–1995 vaccine differs from the 1993–1994 vaccine, supplies of 1993–1994 vaccine should not be administered to provide protection for the 1994–1995 influenza season.

Two doses administered at least 1 month apart may be required for satisfactory antibody responses among previously unvaccinated children <9 years of age;

however, studies with vaccines similar to those in current use have shown little or no improvement in antibody responses when a second dose is administered to adults during the same season.

During the past decade, data on influenza vaccine immunogenicity and side effects have been obtained for intramuscularly administered vaccine. Because there has been no adequate evaluation of recent influenza vaccines administered by other routes, the intramuscular route is recommended. Adults and older children should be vaccinated in the deltoid muscle and infants and young children in the anterolateral aspect of the thigh.

Target Groups for Special Vaccination Programs

To maximize protection of high-risk persons, they and their close contacts should be targeted for organized vaccination programs.

GROUPS AT INCREASED RISK FOR INFLUENZA-RELATED COMPLICATIONS

Groups at increased risk are: persons ≥65 years of age; residents of nursing homes and other chronic-care facilities that house persons of any age with chronic medical conditions; adults and children with chronic disorders of the pulmonary or cardiovascular systems, including children with asthma; adults and children who have required regular medical follow-up or hospitalization during the preceding year because of chronic metabolic diseases (including diabetes mellitus), renal dysfunction, hemoglobinopathies, or immunosuppression (including immunosuppression caused by medications); and children and teenagers (6 months to 18 years of age) who are receiving long-term aspirin therapy and therefore may be at risk for developing Reye syndrome after influenza.

GROUPS THAT CAN TRANSMIT INFLUENZA TO PERSONS AT HIGH RISK

Persons who are clinically or subclinically infected and who care for or live with members of high-risk groups can transmit influenza virus to them. Some persons at high risk (e.g., the elderly, transplant recipients, and persons with AIDS) can have low antibody responses to influenza vaccine. Efforts to protect these members of high-risk groups against influenza may be improved by reducing the likelihood of influenza exposure from their caregivers. Therefore, the following groups should be vaccinated: physicians, nurses, and other personnel in both hospital and outpatient-care settings; employees of nursing homes and chronic-care facilities who have contact with patients or residents; providers of home care to persons at high risk (e.g., visiting nurses and volunteer workers); and household members (including children) of persons in high-risk groups.

Vaccination of Other Groups

GENERAL POPULATION

Physicians should administer influenza vaccine to any person who wishes to reduce the likelihood of becoming ill with influenza. Persons who provide essential community services may be considered for vaccination to minimize disruption of essential activities during influenza outbreaks. Students or other persons in institutional settings, such as those who reside in dormitories, should be encouraged to receive vaccine to minimize the disruption of routine activities during epidemics.

PREGNANT WOMEN

Influenza-associated excess mortality among pregnant women has not been documented except in the pandemic of 1918–1919 and 1957–1958. However, pregnant women who have other medical conditions that increase their risks for complications from influenza should be vaccinated because the vaccine is considered safe for pregnant women, regardless of the stage of pregnancy. Thus, it is undesirable to delay vaccination of pregnant women who have high-risk conditions and who will still be in the first trimester of pregnancy when the influenza season begins.

PERSONS INFECTED WITH HUMAN IMMUNODEFICIENCY VIRUS (HIV)

Limited information exists regarding the frequency and severity for influenza illness among HIV-infected persons, but reports suggest that symptoms may be prolonged and the risk for complications increased for some HIV-infected persons. Because influenza can result in serious illness and complications, vaccination is a prudent precaution and will result in protective antibody levels in many recipients. However, the antibody response to vaccine may be low in persons with advanced HIV-related illnesses; a booster dose of vaccine does not improve the immune response for these persons.

FOREIGN TRAVELERS

The risk for exposure to influenza during foreign travel varies, depending on season and destination. In the tropics, influenza can occur throughout the year; in the southern hemisphere, the season of greatest activity is April to September. Because of the short incubation period for influenza, exposure to the virus during travel can result in clinical illness that begins while traveling, an inconvenience or potential danger, especially for persons at increased risk for complications. Persons preparing to travel to the tropics at any time of year or to the southern hemisphere during April to September should review their influenza vaccination histories. If they were not vaccinated the previous fall or winter, they should consider influenza vaccination before travel. Persons in the high-risk categories should be especially encouraged to receive the most current vaccine. Persons at high risk who received the previous season's vaccine before travel should be revaccinated in the fall or winter with the current vaccine.

Persons Who Should Not Be Vaccinated

Inactivated influenza vaccine should not be administered to persons known to have anaphylactic hypersensitivity to eggs or to other components of the influenza vaccine without first consulting a physician (see Side Effects and Adverse Reactions). Use of an antiviral agent (amantadine or rimantadine) is an option for prevention of influenza A in such persons. However, persons who have a history of anaphylactic hypersensitivity to vaccine components but who are also at higher risk for complications of influenza may benefit from vaccine after appropriate allergy evaluation and desensitization. Specific information about vaccine components can be found in package inserts for each manufacturer.

Adults with acute febrile illness usually should not be vaccinated until their symptoms have abated. However, minor illnesses with or without fever should not contraindicate the use of influenza vaccine, particularly among children with mild upper respiratory tract infection or allergic rhinitis.

Side Effects and Adverse Reactions

Because influenza vaccine contains only noninfectious viruses, it cannot cause influenza. Respiratory disease after vaccination represents coincidental illness unrelated to influenza vaccination. The most frequent side effect of vaccination reported by fewer than one-third of vaccinees is soreness at the vaccination site that lasts for up to 2 days. In addition, two types of systemic reactions have occurred:

Fever, malaise, myalgia, and other systemic symptoms occur infrequently and most often affect persons who have had no exposure to the influenza virus antigens in the vaccine (e.g., young children). These reactions begin 6 to 12 hours after vaccination and can persist for 1 or 2 days;

Immediate—presumably allergic—reactions (e.g., hives, angioedema, allergic asthma, and systemic anaphylaxis) occur rarely after influenza vaccination. These reactions probably result from hypersensitivity to some vaccine component; the majority of reactions are most likely related to residual egg protein. Although current influenza vaccines contain only a small quantity of egg protein, this protein may induce immediate hypersensitivity reactions among persons with severe egg allergy. Persons who have developed hives, have had swelling of the lips or tongue, or have experienced acute respiratory distress or collapse after eating eggs should consult a physician for appropriate evaluation to help determine if vaccine should be administered. Persons with documented IgE-mediated hypersensitivity to eggs—including those who have had occupational asthma or other allergic responses due to exposure to egg protein—may also be at increased risk for reactions from influenza vaccine, and similar consultation should be considered. The protocol for influenza vaccination developed by Murphy and Strunk may be considered for patients who have egg allergies and medical conditions that place them at increased risk for influenza-associated complications (Murphy and Strunk, 1985).

Hypersensitivity reactions to any vaccine component can occur. Although exposure to vaccines containing thimerosal can lead to induction of hypersensitivity, most patients do not develop reactions to thimerosal when administered as a component of vaccines even when patch or intradermal tests for thimerosal indicate hypersensitivity. When reported, hypersensitivity to thimerosal has usually consisted of local, delayed-type hypersensitivity reactions.

Unlike the 1976–1977 swine influenza vaccine, subsequent vaccines prepared from other virus strains have not been associated clearly with an increased frequency of Guillain-Barré syndrome (GBS). However, it is difficult to make a precise estimate of risk for a rare condition such as GBS. In 1990–1991, although there was no overall increase in frequency of GBS among vaccine recipients, there may have been a small increase in GBS cases in vaccinated persons 18 to 64 years of age, but not in those ≥65 years old. In contrast to the swine influenza vaccine, the epidemiologic features of the possible association of the 1990–1991 vaccine with GBS were not as convincing. Even if GBS were a true side effect, the very low estimated risk for GBS is less than that of severe influenza that could be prevented by vaccine.

Simultaneous Administration of Other Vaccines, Including Childhood Vaccines

The target groups for influenza and pneumococcal vaccination overlap considerably. Both vaccines can be administered at the same time at different sites without increasing side effects. However, influenza vaccine must be administered each year, whereas pneumococcal vaccine is not. Children at high risk for influenza-related complications may receive influenza vaccine at the same time they receive other routine vaccinations, including pertussis vaccine (DTP or DTaP). Because influenza vaccine can cause fever when administered to young children, DTaP may be preferable in those children ≥15 months of age who are receiving the fourth or fifth dose of pertussis vaccine. DTaP is not licensed for the initial three-dose series of pertussis vaccine.

Timing of Influenza Vaccination Activities

Beginning each September (when vaccine for the upcoming influenza season becomes available) persons at high risk who are seen by health-care providers for routine care or as a result of hospitalization should be offered influenza vaccine. Opportunities to vaccinate persons at high risk for complications of influenza should not be missed.

The optimal time for organized vaccination campaigns for persons in high-risk groups is usually the period from mid-October through mid-November. In the United States, influenza activity generally peaks between late December and early March. High levels of influenza activity infrequently occur in the contiguous 48 states before December. It is particularly important to avoid administering vaccine too far in advance of the influenza season in facilities such as nursing homes because antibody levels may begin to decline within a few months of vaccination. Vaccination programs can be undertaken as soon as current vaccine is available if regional influenza activity is expected to begin earlier than December.

Children <9 years of age who have not been vaccinated previously should receive two doses of vaccine at least 1 month apart to maximize the likelihood of a satisfactory antibody response to all three vaccine antigens. The second dose should be administered before December, if possible. Vaccine should be offered to both children and adults up to and even after influenza virus activity is documented in a community.

Strategies for Implementing Influenza Vaccine Recommendations

Although rates of influenza vaccination have increased in recent years, surveys indicate that less than half of the high-risk population receives influenza vaccine each year. More effective strategies are needed for delivering vaccine to persons at high risk and to their health-care providers and household contacts.

In general, successful vaccination programs have combined education for health-care workers, publicity and education targeted toward potential recipients, a plan for identifying (usually by medical-record review) persons at high risk, and efforts to remove administrative and financial barriers that prevent persons from receiving the vaccine. Persons for whom influenza vaccine is recommended can be identified and vaccinated in the settings described in the following paragraphs.

OUTPATIENT CLINICS AND PHYSICIANS' OFFICES

Staff in physicians' offices, clinics, health-maintenance organizations, and employee health clinics should be instructed to identify and label the medical records of patients who should receive vaccine. Vaccine should be offered during visits beginning in September and throughout the influenza season. The offer of vaccine and its receipt or refusal should be documented in the medical record. Patients among high-risk groups who do not have regularly scheduled visits during the fall should be reminded by mail or telephone of the need for vaccine. If possible, arrangements should be made to provide vaccine with minimal waiting time and at the lowest possible cost.

FACILITIES PROVIDING EPISODIC OR ACUTE CARE

Health-care providers in these settings (e.g., emergency rooms and walk-in clinics) should be familiar with influenza vaccine recommendations. They should offer vaccine to persons in high-risk groups or should provide written information on why, where, and how to obtain the vaccine. Written information should be available in language(s) appropriate for the population served by the facility.

NURSING HOMES AND OTHER RESIDENTIAL LONG-TERM CARE FACILITIES

Vaccination should be routinely provided to all residents of chronic-care facilities with the concurrence of attending physicians rather than by obtaining individual vaccination orders for each patient. Consent for vaccination should be obtained from the resident or a family member at the time of admission to the facility and all residents should be vaccinated at one time, immediately preceding the influenza season. Residents admitted during the winter months after completion of the vaccination program should be vaccinated when they are admitted.

ACUTE-CARE HOSPITALS

All persons ≥65 years of age and younger persons (including children) with high-risk conditions who are hospitalized from September through March should be offered and strongly encouraged to receive influenza vaccine before they are discharged. Household members and others with whom they have contact should receive written information about why and where to obtain influenza vaccine.

OUTPATIENT FACILITIES PROVIDING CONTINUING CARE TO PATIENTS AT HIGH RISK

All patients should be offered vaccine before the beginning of the influenza season. Patients admitted to such programs (e.g., hemodialysis centers, hospital specialty-care clinics, outpatient rehabilitation programs) during the winter months after the earlier vaccination program has been conducted should be vaccinated at the time of admission. Household members should receive written information regarding the need for vaccination and the places to obtain influenza vaccine.

VISITING NURSES AND OTHERS PROVIDING HOME CARE TO PERSONS AT HIGH RISK

Nursing-care plans should identify patients in high-risk groups, and vaccine should be provided in the home if necessary. Caregivers and others in the household (including children) should be referred for vaccination.

FACILITIES PROVIDING SERVICES TO PERSONS ≥65 YEARS OF AGE

In these facilities (e.g., retirement communities and recreation centers), all unvaccinated residents/attendees should be offered vaccine on site before the influenza season. Education/publicity programs should also be provided; these programs should emphasize the need for influenza vaccine and provide specific information on how, where, and when to obtain it.

CLINICS AND OTHERS PROVIDING HEALTH CARE FOR TRAVELERS

Indications for influenza vaccination should be reviewed before travel, and vaccine should be offered if appropriate (see Foreign Travelers).

HEALTH-CARE WORKERS

Administrators of all health-care facilities should arrange for influenza vaccine to be offered to all personnel before the influenza season. Personnel should be provided with appropriate educational materials and strongly encouraged to receive vaccine. Particular emphasis should be placed on vaccination of persons who care for members of high-risk groups (e.g., staff of intensive-care units (including newborn intensive-care units), staff of medical/surgical units, and employees of nursing homes and chronic-care facilities). Using a mobile cart to take vaccine to hospital wards or other work sites and making vaccine available during night and weekend work shifts may enhance compliance, as may a follow-up campaign early in the course of community outbreak.

Sources of Information on Influenza-Control Programs

Information regarding influenza surveillance is available through the CDC Voice Information System (influenza update), telephone (404) 332-4551, or through the CDC Information Service on the Public Health Network electronic bulletin board. From October through May, the information is updated at least every other week. In addition, periodic updates about influenza are published in *MMWR*. State and local health departments should also be consulted regarding availability of vaccine, access to vaccination programs, and information about state or local influenza activity.

REFERENCES

1. Reprinted from Morbidity and Mortality Weekly Report (MMWR), Prevention and control of influenza: Part 1, Vaccines. Recommendations of the Advisory Committee on Immunization Practices (ACIP). May 27, 1994;43(No. RR-9).

SUGGESTED READINGS

General

Douglas RG. Drug therapy: prophylaxis and treatment of influenza. N Engl J Med 1990;322:443–450.
Kendal AP, Patriarca PA, eds. Options for the control of influenza. New York: Alan R Liss, 1986.
Kilbourne ED. Influenza. New York: Plenum, 1987.
Noble GR. Epidemiological and clinical aspects of influenza. In: Beare AS, ed. Basic and applied influenza research. Boca Raton, FL: CRC Press, 1982:11–50.

Surveillance, Morbidity, and Mortality

Barker WH. Excess pneumonia and influenza associated hospitalization during influenza epidemics in the United States, 1970–78. Am J Public Health 1986;76:761–765.
Barker WH, Mullooly JR. Impact of epidemic type A influenza in a defined adult population. Am J Epidemiol 1980;112:798–813.

Barker WH, Mullooly JP. Pneumonia and influenza deaths during epidemics: implications for prevention. Arch Intern Med 1982;142:85–89.

Baron RC, Dicker RC, Bussell KE, Herndon JL. Assessing trends in mortality in 121 U.S. cities, 1970–79, from all causes and from pneumonia and influenza. Public Health Rep 1988;103:120–128.

Couch RB, Kasel WP, Glezen TR, et al. Influenza: its control in persons and populations. J Infect Dis 1986;153:431–440.

Glezen WP. Serious morbidity and mortality associated with influenza epidemics. Epidemiol Rev 1982;4:25–44.

Glezen WP, Six HR, Frank AL, Taber LH, Perrotta DM, Decker M. Impact of epidemics upon communities and families. In: Kendal AP, Patriarca PA, eds. Options for the control of influenza. New York: Alan R Liss, 1986:63–73.

Lui KJ, Kendal AP. Impact of influenza epidemics on mortality in the United States from October 1972 to May 1985. Am J Public Health 1987;77:712–716.

Mullooly JP, Barker WH, Nolan TF, Jr. Risk of acute respiratory disease among pregnant women during influenza A epidemics. Public Health Rep 1986;101:205–211.

Perrotta DM, Decker M, Glezen WP. Acute respiratory disease hospitalizations as a measure of impact of epidemic influenza. Am J Epidemiol 1985;122:468–476.

Thacker SB. The persistence of influenza A in human populations. Epidemiol Rev 1986;8:129–142.

Vaccines

SAFETY, IMMUNOGENICITY, EFFICACY

ACIP. General recommendations on immunization. MMWR 1989;38:205–214, 219–227.

Arden NH, Patriarca PA, Kendal AP. Experiences in the use and efficacy of inactivated influenza vaccine in nursing homes. In: Kendal AP, Patriarca PA, eds. Options for the control of influenza. New York: Alan R Liss, 1986:155–168.

Barker WH, Mullooly JP. Effectiveness of inactivated influenza vaccine among non-institutionalized elderly persons. In: Kendal AP, Patriarca PA, eds. Options for the control of influenza. New York: Alan R Liss, 1986:169–182.

Beyer WEP, Palache AM, Baljet M, Masurel N. Antibody induction by influenza vaccines in the elderly: a review of the literature. Vaccine 1989;7:385–394.

Cate TR, Couch RB, Parker D, Baxter B. Reactogenicity, immunogenicity, and antibody persistence in adults given inactivated influenza virus vaccines—1978. Rev Infect Dis 1983;5:737–747.

CDC. Influenza vaccination levels in selected states—Behavioral Risk Factor Surveillance System, 1987. MMWR 1989;38:124, 129–133.

Dowdle WR. Influenza immunoprophylaxis after 30 years' experience. In: Nayak DP, ed. Genetic variation among influenza viruses. New York: Academic Press, 1981:525– 534.

Foster DA, Talsma AN, Furumoto-Dawson A, et al. Influenza vaccine effectiveness in preventing hospitalization for pneumonia in the elderly. Am J Epidemiol 1992;136:296–307.

Glezen WP, Glezen LS, Alcorn R. Trivalent, inactivated influenza virus vaccine in children with sickle cell disease. Am J Dis Child 1983;137:1095–1097.

Gross PA, Quinnan GV, Rodstein M, et al. Association of influenza immunization with reduction in mortality in an elderly population: a prospective study. Arch Intern Med 1988;148:562–565.

Gross PA, Weksler ME, Quinnan GV Jr, Douglas RG Jr, Gaerlan PF, Denning CR. Immunization of elderly people with two doses of influenza vaccine. J Clin Microbiol 1987;25:1763–1765.

Gruber WC, Taber LH, Glezen WP, et al. Live attenuated and inactivated influenza vaccine in school-aged children. Am J Dis Child 1990;144:595–600.

Helliwell BE, Drummond MF. The costs and benefits of preventing influenza in Ontario's elderly. Can J Public Health 1988;79:175–180.

La Montagne JR, Noble GR, Quinnan GB, et al. Summary of clinical trials of inactivated influenza vaccine—1978. Rev Infect Dis 1983;5:723–736.

Patriarca PA, Weber JA, Parker RA, et al. Efficacy of influenza vaccine in nursing homes: reduction in illness and complications during an influenza A(H3N2) epidemic. JAMA 1985;253:1136–1139.

Quinnan GV, Schooley R, Dolin R, Ennis FA, Gross P, Gwaltney JM. Serologic responses and systemic reactions in adults after vaccination with monovalent A/USSR/77 and trivalent A/USSR/77, A/Texas/77, B/Hong Kong/72 influenza vaccines. Rev Infect Dis 1983;5:748–757.

Wright PF, Cherry JD, Foy HM, et al. Antigenicity and reactogenicity of influenza A/ USSR/77 virus vaccine in children—a multicentered evaluation of dosage and safety. Rev Infect Dis 1983;5:758–764.

SIDE EFFECTS, ADVERSE REACTIONS, INTERACTIONS

Aberer W. Vaccination despite thimerosal sensitivity. Contact Dermatitis 1991;24:6–10.
American Academy of Pediatrics Committee on Infectious Diseases. The Red Book: Report of the
    Committee on Infectious Disease. 22nd ed. Elk Grove, IL: American Academy of Pediatrics,
    1991.
Bierman CW, Shapiro GG, Pierson WE, Taylor JW, Foy HM, Fox JP. Safety of influenza vaccination
    in allergic children. J Infect Dis 1977;136:S652–655.
Chen R, Kent J, Rhodes P, Simon P, Schonberger L: Investigation of a possible association between
    influenza vaccination and Guillain-Barré syndrome in the United States, 1990–1991 [Abstract].
    Post Marketing Surveillance 1992;6:5–6.
Govaet TME, Aretz K, Masurel N, et al. Adverse reactions to influenza vaccine in elderly people:
    a randomized double blind placebo controlled trial. Br Med J 1993;307:988– 990.
Kaplan JE, Katona P, Hurwitz ES, Schonberger LB. Guillain-Barré syndrome in the United States,
    1979–1980 and 1980–1981: lack of an association with influenza vaccination. JAMA
    1982;248:698–700.
Margolis KL, Nichols KL, Poland GA, et al. Frequency of adverse reactions to influenza vaccine
    in the elderly: a randomized, placebo-controlled trial. JAMA 1990;307:988– 990.
Margolis KL, Poland GA, Nichol KL, et al. Frequency of adverse reactions after influenza vaccination.
    Am J Med 1990;88:27–30.
Murphy KR, Strunk RC. Safe administration of influenza vaccine in asthmatic children hypersensitive
    to egg proteins. J Pediatr 1985;106:931–933.

SIMULTANEOUS ADMINISTRATION OF OTHER VACCINES

CDC. Recommendations of the ACIP: pneumococcal polysaccharide vaccine. MMWR 1989;38:64–
    68, 73–76.
DeStefano F, Goodman RA, Noble GR, McClary GD, Smith J, Broome CV. Simultaneous administra-
    tion of influenza and pneumococcal vaccines. JAMA 1982;247:2551–2554.
Peter G, ed. Summaries of infectious diseases: influenza. In: Report of the Committee on Infectious
    Diseases. 21st ed. Elk Grove Village, IL: American Academy of Pediatrics, 1988:243–251.

VACCINATION OF PERSONS INFECTED WITH HIV

Huang KL, Ruben FL, Rinaldo CR Jr, Kingsley L, Lyter DW, Ho M. Antibody responses after
    influenza and pneumococcal immunization in HIV-infected homosexual men. JAMA
    1987;257:2047–2050.
Miotti PG, Nelson KE, Dallabetta GA, Farzadegan H, Margolick J, Clements ML. The influence
    of HIV infection on antibody responses to a two-dose regimen of influenza vaccine. JAMA
    1989;262:779–783.
Nelson KE, Clements ML, Miotti P, Cohn S, Polk BF. The influence of human immunodeficiency virus
    (HIV) infection on antibody responses to influenza vaccines. Ann Intern Med 1988;109:383–388.
Safrin S, Rush JD, Mills J. Influenza in patients with human immunodeficiency virus infection. Chest
    1990;98:33–37.
Thurn JR, Henry K. Influenza A pneumonitis in a patient infected with the human immunodeficiency
    virus (HIV). Chest 1989;95:807–810.

VACCINATION OF FOREIGN TRAVELERS

CDC. Update: influenza activity-worldwide and recommendations for influenza vaccine composition
    for the 1990–91 influenza season. MMWR 1990;39:293–296.
CDC. Acute respiratory illness among cruise-ship passengers—Asia. MMWR 1988;37:63– 66.

INFLUENZA IN THE HOSPITAL SETTING

Bean B, Rhame FS, Hughes RS, Weiler MD, Peterson LR, Gerding DN. Influenza B: hospital activity
    during a community epidemic. Diagn Microbiol Infect Dis 1983;1:177–183.
Pachucki CT, Walsh Pappas SA, Fuller GF, Krause SL, Lentino JR, Schaaff DM. Influenza A among
    hospital personnel and patients: implications for recognition, prevention, and control. Arch Intern
    Med 1989;149:77–80.

STRATEGIES FOR VACCINATION OF HIGH-RISK GROUPS

CDC. Arm with the facts: a guidebook for promotion of adult immunization. Atlanta: U.S. Department of Health and Human Services, Public Health Service, 1987.

Fedson DS. Immunizations for health care workers and patients in hospitals. In: Wenzel RP, ed. Prevention and control of nosocomial infections. Baltimore: Williams & Wilkins, 1987:116–174.

Fedson DS, Kessler HA. A hospital–based influenza immunization program, 1977–78. Am J Public Health 1983;73:442–445.

Margolis KL, Lofgren RP, Korn JE. Organizational strategies to improve influenza vaccine delivery: a standing order in a general medical clinic. Arch Intern Med 1988;148:2205–2207.

Nichol KL, Korn JE, Margolis KL, Poland GA, Petzel RA, Lofgren RP. Achieving the national health objective for influenza immunization: success of an institution-wide vaccination program. Am J Med 1990;89:156–160.

Weingarten S, Riedinger M, Bolton LB, Miles P, Ault M. Barriers to influenza vaccine acceptance: a survey of physicians and nurses. Am J Infect Control 1989;17:202– 207.

Williams WW, Garner JS. Personnel health services. In: Bennett JV, Brachman PS, eds. Hospital infections. 2nd ed. Boston: Little, Brown & Co, 1986:17–38.

Williams WW, Hickson MA, Kane MA, Kendal AP, Spika JS, Hinman AR. Immunization policies and vaccine coverage among adults: the risk for missed opportunities. Ann Intern Med 1988;108:616–625.

Diagnostic Methods

Harmon MW. Influenza viruses. In: Lennette EH, ed. Laboratory diagnosis of viral infections. 2nd ed. New York: Marcel Dekker, 1992:515–534.

Prevention and Control of Influenza: Antiviral Agents for Influenza A[b]

SUMMARY

These recommendations provide information about the antiviral agents amantadine hydrochloride and rimantadine hydrochloride. These recommendations supersede MMWR 1992;41(No. RR-9). The primary changes include information about the recently licensed drug rimantadine and expanded information on the potential for adverse reactions to amantadine and rimantadine and guidelines for the use of these drugs in certain patient populations.

Introduction

The two antiviral agents with specific activity against influenza A viruses are amantadine hydrochloride and rimantadine hydrochloride. These chemically related drugs interfere with the replication cycle of type A (but not type B) influenza viruses. When administered prophylactically to healthy adults or children in advance of and throughout the epidemic period, both drugs are approximately 70 to 90% effective in preventing illnesses caused by naturally occurring strains of type A influenza viruses. Since antiviral agents taken prophylactically may prevent illness but not subclinical infection, some persons who take these

---

[b]Modified and reprinted from Prevention and control of influenza: part II, antiviral agents. Recommendations of the Advisory Committee on Immunization Practices (ACIP). MMWR, in press.

drugs may still develop immune responses that will protect them when exposed to antigenically related viruses in later years.

In otherwise healthy adults, amantadine and rimantadine have been shown to reduce the severity and duration of signs and symptoms of influenza A illness when administered within 48 hours of illness onset. Studies evaluating the efficacy of treatment with either amantadine or rimantadine in children are limited. Amantadine has been approved by the FDA for treatment and prophylaxis of all influenza type A virus infections since 1978, when rimantadine was approved for marketing in September 1993. By present FDA standards, there are insufficient data to support the efficacy of rimantadine treatment in children. Thus, rimantadine is currently approved only for prophylaxis in children, not for treatment. Further studies of rimantadine treatment in children were conducted during the 1993-1994 influenza season and may provide data to support future FDA approval of rimantadine treatment for children.

As with all drugs, amantadine and rimantadine may cause adverse reactions in some persons. Such adverse reactions are rarely severe, but may be important for some categories of patients. Amantadine has been associated with a higher incidence of adverse central nervous system (CNS) reactions than rimantadine.

Recommendations for the Use of Amantadine and Rimantadine

USE AS PROPHYLAXIS

Chemoprophylaxis is not a substitute for vaccination. Recommendations for chemoprophylaxis are provided primarily to help health-care providers make decisions regarding persons who are at greatest risk of severe illness and complications if infected with influenza A virus.

When amantadine or rimantadine are administered as prophylaxis, factors such as cost, compliance and potential side effects should be taken into consideration when determining the period of prophylaxis. To be maximally effective as prophylaxis, the drug must be taken each day for the duration of influenza activity in the community. However, amantadine or rimantadine prophylaxis is likely to be most beneficial during the period of peak influenza activity in a community.

FOR HIGH-RISK PERSONS VACCINATED AFTER INFLUENZA A ACTIVITY HAS BEGUN

High-risk persons can still be vaccinated after an outbreak of influenza A has begun in a community. However, the development of antibodies in adults after vaccination can take up to 2 weeks, during which time chemoprophylaxis should be considered. Children who receive influenza vaccine for the first time may require up to 6 weeks of prophylaxis or until 2 weeks after the second dose of vaccine has been received. Amantadine and rimantadine do not interfere with the antibody response to the vaccine.

PERSONS PROVIDING CARE TO HIGH-RISK PERSONS

To reduce the spread of virus and to maintain care for high-risk persons in the home, hospital, or institutional setting, chemoprophylaxis may be considered during community outbreaks for unvaccinated persons who have frequent contact with high-risk persons in the home setting (e.g., household members, visiting nurses, volunteer workers) and unvaccinated employees of hospitals, clinics, and chronic-care facilities. For employees who cannot be vaccinated, chemoprophylaxis during the period of peak influenza activity may be considered. For those who receive vaccine at a time when influenza A is present in the community, chemoprophylaxis can be administered for 2 weeks after vaccination. Prophylaxis should be considered for all employees, regardless of their vaccination status, if the outbreak is caused by a variant strain of influenza A that is not covered by the vaccine.

IMMUNODEFICIENT PERSONS

Chemoprophylaxis may be indicated for high-risk persons who are expected to have a poor antibody response to influenza vaccine. This includes many persons with HIV infection, especially those with advanced disease. No data are available on possible interactions with other drugs used in the management of patients with HIV infection. Such patients should be monitored closely if amantadine or rimantadine chemoprophylaxis is administered.

PERSONS FOR WHOM INFLUENZA VACCINE IS CONTRAINDICATED

Chemoprophylaxis throughout the influenza season during peak influenza activity may be appropriate for high-risk persons for whom influenza vaccine is contraindicated because of anaphylactic hypersensitivity to egg protein or other vaccine components.

OTHER PERSONS

Amantadine or rimantadine can also be administered prophylactically to anyone who wishes to avoid influenza A illness. This decision should be made by the physician and patient on an individual basis.

USE AS THERAPY

Amantadine and rimantadine have been shown to reduce the severity and shorten the duration of influenza A illness among healthy adults when taken within 48 hours after onset of illness. It is not known whether antiviral therapy will prevent complications of influenza type A among high-risk persons. Because there are insufficient data on the efficacy of rimantadine therapy in children based on current FDA standards, rimantadine is not approved for treatment of influenza A in children.

Amantadine- and rimantadine-resistant influenza A viruses can emerge when either of these drugs are administered for treatment; amantadine-resistant strains are cross-resistant to rimantadine. The frequency with which resistant viruses emerge and the extent of their transmission are unknown, but there is no evidence that amantadine- or rimantadine-resistant viruses are more virulent or more transmissible than amantadine or rimantadine-sensitive viruses.

Screening of naturally occurring epidemic strains of influenza type A has rarely detected amantadine- or rimantadine-resistant viruses. Resistant viruses have most frequently been isolated from persons taking one of these drugs as therapy for influenza infection. Resistant viruses have sometimes been isolated from people who live in residential or institutional settings where other residents are taking or have recently taken amantadine or rimantadine as therapy. Persons with influenza-like illness should, to the extent possible, avoid contact with uninfected persons, whether or not they are taking amantadine or rimantadine as treatment. Persons with influenza type A infection treated with either drug may shed amantadine- or rimantadine-sensitive viruses early in the course of treatment, but may later shed drug-resistant viruses, especially after 3 to 7 days of therapy. Such persons may benefit from therapy even when resistant viruses emerge, but they may also transmit infection to contacts. Because of possible induction of amantadine or rimantadine resistance, it is advisable to discontinue treatment of persons who have influenza-like illness as soon as clinically warranted, generally after 3 to 5 days of treatment or within 24 to 48 hours after the disappearance of signs and symptoms. Laboratory isolation of influenza viruses from persons who are receiving amantadine or rimantadine should be reported through state health departments to CDC and the isolates saved for antiviral sensitivity testing.

OUTBREAK CONTROL IN INSTITUTIONS

When confirmed or suspected outbreaks of influenza A occur in institutions that house high-risk persons, chemoprophylaxis should begin as early as possible to reduce the spread of the infection. Contingency planning is needed to ensure rapid administration of amantadine or rimantadine to residents. This should include preapproved medication orders or plans to obtain physician's orders on short notice. When amantadine or rimantadine is used for outbreak control, drug should be administered to all residents of the institution regardless of whether they received influenza vaccine the previous fall. The drug should be continued for at least 2 weeks or until approximately 1 week after the outbreak has stopped. The dose for each resident should be determined after consulting the dosage recommendations and precautions that follow in this document and those listed in the manufacturer's package insert. To reduce spread of virus and to minimize disruption of patient care, chemoprophylaxis may also be offered to unvaccinated staff who provide care to high-risk persons. Prophylaxis should be considered for all employees, regardless of their vaccination status, if the outbreak is caused by a variant strain of influenza A that is not covered by the vaccine.

Chemoprophylaxis may also be considered for controlling influenza A outbreaks in other closed or semiclosed settings, such as dormitories or other settings where person live in close proximity to one another. In order to decrease spread of infection and reduce the chances of prophylaxis failure due to transmission of drug-resistant virus, measures should be taken to reduce contact between persons on chemoprophylaxis and those taking the drug for treatment to the extent that this is possible.

Considerations for the Selection of Amantadine or Rimantadine for Chemoprophylaxis or Treatment

SIDE EFFECTS/TOXICITY

Despite the similarities between the two drugs, amantadine and rimantadine differ in their pharmacokinetic properties. More than 90% of amantadine is excreted unchanged, while approximately 90% of rimantadine is metabolized by the liver. However, both drugs and their metabolites are excreted by the kidney.

The pharmacokinetic differences between amantadine and rimantadine may in part explain differences in side effects. Although side effects associated with both drugs are qualitatively similar, when administered to young, healthy adults at equivalent dosages of 200 mg daily, the incidence of (CNS) side effects, such as nervousness, anxiety, difficulty concentrating, and light-headedness is higher among persons taking amantadine compared with those taking rimantadine. In a 6-week study of prophylaxis in healthy adults, approximately 6% of participants taking rimantadine at a dose of 200 mg/day experienced at least one CNS symptom, compared with approximately 14% of those taking the same dose of amantadine and 4% of those taking placebo. The incidence of gastrointestinal side effects, such as nausea and anorexia, is about 3% in persons taking either drug, compared with that in 1 to 2% of placebo recipients. Side effects associated with both drugs are usually mild and cease soon after discontinuing the drug. Side effects associated with amantadine may diminish or disappear after the first week despite continued drug ingestion. However, serious side effects such as marked behavioral changes, delirium, hallucinations, agitation, and seizures have been observed. These more severe side effects have been associated with high plasma drug concentrations and have been observed most often in elderly persons and in persons with renal insufficiency, seizure disorders, or certain psychiatric disorders who have been taking amantadine at a dose of 200 mg/day. Clinical observations and studies have provided evidence that lowering the dosage of amantadine in these persons will reduce the incidence and severity of such side effects, and recommendations for reduced dosages for these groups of patients have been made. Because rimantadine has only recently been approved for marketing, there have been fewer observations of its safety in certain patient populations, such as chronically ill and elderly persons, who have been included in clinical trials of rimantadine less often than have young, healthy persons.

The package insert should be reviewed before use of amantadine or rimantadine for any patient. The patient's age, weight, renal function, other medications, presence of other medical conditions and indications for use of amantadine or rimantadine (prophylaxis or therapy) must be considered, and the dosage and duration of treatment adjusted appropriately. Modifications in dosage may be required for persons with impaired renal or hepatic function, the elderly, children,

MANUAL OF ANTIBIOTICS AND INFECTIOUS DISEASES

and persons with a history of seizures. Following are guidelines for the use of
amantadine and rimantadine in certain patient populations. Dosage recommendations for these drugs are summarized in Table 1.3.

PERSONS WITH IMPAIRED RENAL FUNCTION

Amantadine

Amantadine is excreted unchanged in the urine by glomerular filtration and
tubular secretion. Compared with that in healthy younger persons, clearance of
amantadine is significantly reduced in those with renal insufficiency. A reduction
in dosage is recommended for patients with creatinine clearance ≤50 ml/min.
Guidelines for amantadine dosage based on creatinine clearance can be found in
the packet insert. However, because recommended dosages based on creatinine
clearance may provide only an approximation of the optimal dose for a given
patient, such individuals should be carefully observed so that adverse reactions
can be recognized promptly and the dose further reduced or the drug discontinued
if necessary. Hemodialysis contributes little to drug clearance.

Rimantadine

The safety and pharmacokinetics of rimantadine in patients with renal insufficiency have been evaluated only after single-dose administration. Further studies
are needed to determine the multiple-dose pharmacokinetic in these patients and
the most appropriate dosages.

In a single-dose study of patients with anuric renal failure, the apparent
clearance of rimantadine was approximately 40% lower and the elimination half-
life was approximately 1.6-fold greater than that in healthy age-matched controls.
Hemodialysis did not contribute to drug clearance. In studies of patients with
less severe renal disease, drug clearance was also reduced and plasma concentrations were higher compared with weight-, age-, and sex-matched healthy controls.

A reduction in dosage to 100 mg daily has been recommended for patients
with creatinine clearance ≤10 ml/min. Because of the potential for accumulation
of rimantadine and its metabolites, patients with any degree of renal insufficiency,
including elderly persons, should be monitored for adverse effects and the dosage
reduced or the drug discontinued as necessary.

ELDERLY PERSONS

Amantadine

Because renal function declines with aging, the daily dose for persons ≥65
years of age should not exceed 100 mg for prophylaxis or treatment. For some
elderly persons, the dose should be further reduced. Studies suggest that because
of their smaller average body size, elderly women are more likely than elderly
men to experience side effects at a daily dose of 100 mg.

Rimantadine

The incidence and severity of CNS side effects appear to be substantially lower
among elderly persons taking rimantadine at a dose of 200 mg/day compared with

that in elderly persons taking the same dose of amantadine. However, when rimantadine has been administered at a dose of 200 mg/day to chronically ill elderly persons, they have had a higher incidence of CNS and gastrointestinal symptoms compared with that in healthy, younger persons taking rimantadine at the same dose. After long-term administration of rimantadine at a dose of 200 mg daily, serum rimantadine concentrations among elderly nursing home residents have been found to be two to four times higher than those reported in younger adults.

It is recommended that the dose of rimantadine be reduced to 100 mg daily for treatment or prophylaxis of elderly nursing home residents. Although further studies are needed to determine the optimal dose for other elderly persons, a reduction in dose to 100 mg daily should be considered for all persons ≥65 years of age if they experience signs and symptoms that may represent side effects when taking a dose of 200 mg daily.

PERSONS WITH LIVER DISEASE

Amantadine

There has been no increase in adverse reactions to amantadine observed among patients with liver disease.

Rimantadine

The safety and pharmacokinetics of rimantadine have been evaluated only after single-dose administration. In a study of patients with chronic liver disease (most with stabilized cirrhosis), no alterations were observed after a single dose. However, in patients with severe liver dysfunction, the apparent clearance of rimantadine was 50% lower than that reported for healthy persons. A dose reduction to 100 mg/day is recommended for persons with severe hepatic dysfunction.

PERSONS WITH SEIZURE DISORDERS

Amantadine

An increased incidence of seizures has been reported in patients with a history of seizure disorders who have received amantadine. Patients with seizure disorders should be observed closely for possible increased seizure activity when taking amantadine.

Rimantadine

In clinical trials, seizures or seizure-like activity have been observed in a small number of patients with a history of seizures who were not receiving anticonvulsant medication while taking rimantadine. The extent to which rimantadine may increase the incidence of seizures in persons with seizure disorders has not been adequately evaluated, since such persons have usually been excluded from participating in clinical trials of rimantadine.

CHILDREN

Amantadine

The use of amantadine in children <1 year of age has not been adequately evaluated. The FDA-approved dosage for children 1 to 9 years of age is 4.4 to 8.8 mg/kg/day, not to exceed 150 mg/day. Although further studies to determine the optimal dosage for children would be desirable, physicians should consider prescribing only 5 mg/kg/day (not to exceed 150 mg/day) to reduce the risk of toxicity. The approved dosage for children ≥10 years of age is 200 mg daily, however, for children weighing <40 kg, it is also advisable to prescribe 5 mg/kg/day regardless of age.

Rimantadine

The use of rimantadine in children 1 year of age has not been adequately evaluated. In children 1-9 years of age, rimantadine should be administered in one or two divided doses at a dose of 5 mg/kg/day, not to exceed 150 mg/day. The approved dosage for children 10 years of age is 200 mg daily (100 mg twice a day); however, for children weighing 40 kg, it is also advisable to prescribe 5 mg/kg/day regardless of age.

DRUG INTERACTIONS

Amantadine

Careful observation is advised when amantadine is administered concurrently with drugs having CNS effects, especially CNS stimulants.

Rimantadine

No clinically significant drug interactions have been identified.

For more detailed information concerning potential drug interactions for either drug, the package should be consulted.

SOURCES OF INFORMATION ON INFLUENZA-CONTROL PROGRAMS

Information regarding influenza surveillance is available through the CDC Voice Information System (influenza update), telephone (404) 332-4551, or through the CDC Information Service on the Public Health Network electronic bulletin board. From October through May, the information is updated at least every other week. In addition, periodic updates about influenza are published in *MMWR*. State and local health departments should also be consulted regarding availability of vaccine, access to vaccination programs, and information about state and local activity.

SUGGESTED READINGS

Aoki FY, Sitar DS. Amantadine kinetics in healthy elderly men: implications for influenza prevention. Clin Pharmacol Ther 1985;37:137–144.

Aoki FY, Sitar DS. Clinical pharmacokinetics of amantadine hydrochloride. Clin Pharmacokinet 1988;14:35–51.

Atkinson WL, Arden NH, Patriarca PA, Leslie N, Lui KI, Gohd R. Amantadine prophylaxis during an institutional outbreak of type A (H1N1) influenza. Arch Intern Med 1986;146:1751–1756.

Balfour HH Jr, Englund JA. Antiviral drugs in pediatrics. Am J Dis Child 1989;143:1307– 1316.

Belshe RB, Burk B, Newman F, Cerruti RL, Sim IS. Resistance of influenza A virus to amantadine and rimantadine: results of one decade of surveillance. J Infect Dis 1989;159:430–435.

Dolin R. Antiviral chemotherapy and chemoprophylaxis. Science 1985;227:1296–303.

Dolin R, Reichman RC, Madore HP, Maynard R, Linton PN, Webber-Jones J. A controlled trial of amantadine and rimantadine in the prophylaxis of influenza A infection. N Engl J Med 1982;307:580–583.

Douglas RG. Drug therapy: prophylaxis and treatment of influenza. N Engl J Med 1990;322:443– 450.

Hall CB, Dolin R, Gala CL, et al. Children with influenza A infection: treatment with rimantadine. Pediatrics 1987;80:275–282.

Hayden FG, Belshe RB, Clover RD, Hay AJ, Oakes MG, Soo W. Emergence and apparent transmission of rimantadine-resistant influenza A in families. N Engl J Med 1989;321:1696–1702.

Hayden FG, Couch RB. Clinical and epidemiological importance of influenza A viruses resistant to amantadine and rimantadine. Rev Med Virol 1992;2:89–96.

Hayden FG, Hay AJ. Emergence and transmission of influenza A viruses resistant to amantadine and rimantadine. Curr Top Microbiol Immunol 1992;176:120–130.

Horadam VW, Sharp JG, Smilack JD, et al. Emergence and possible transmission of amantadine-resistant viruses during nursing home outbreaks of influenza A(H3N2). Am J Epidemiol 1991;13:988–997.

Monto AS, Arden NH. Implications of viral resistance to amantadine in control of influenza A. Clin Infect Dis 1992;15:362–367.

Mostow SR. Prevention, management, and control of influenza: role of amantadine. Am J Med 1987;82(suppl 6A):35–41.

Pettersson RF, Hellstrom PE, Penttinen K, et al. Evaluation of amantadine in the prophylaxis of influenza A (H1N1) virus infection: a controlled field trial among young adults and high-risk patients. J Infect Dis 1980;142:377–383.

Sears SD, Clements ML. Protective efficacy of low-dose amantadine in adults challenged with wild-type influenza A virus. Antimicrob Agents Chemother 1987;31:1470– 1473.

Somani SK, Degelau J, Cooper SL, et al. Comparison of pharmacokinetic and safety profiles of amantadine 50 and 100 mg daily doses in elderly nursing home residents. Pharmacotherapy 1991;11(6):460–466.

Strange KC, Little DW, Blatnik B. Adverse reactions to amantadine prophylaxis of influenza in a retirement home. J Am Geriatr Soc 1991;39:700–705.

Tominack RL, Hayden FG. Rimantadine hydrochloride and amantadine hydrochloride use in influenza A virus infections. Infect Dis Clin North Am 1987;1:459–478.

Pneumococcal Polysaccharide Vaccine[c]

SUMMARY

These recommendations update the last statement by the Immunization Practices Advisory Committee (ACIP) on pneumococcal polysaccharide vaccine (MMWR 1984;33:273–276, 281) and include new information regarding (1) vaccine efficacy, (2) use in persons with human immunodeficiency virus (HIV)

---

[c] Modified from Advisory Committee on Immunization Practices. Pneumococcal polysaccharide vaccine [Review]. MMWR 1989;38(5):64–76.

infection and in other groups at increased risk of pneumococcal disease, and (3) guidelines for revaccination.

Introduction

Disease caused by *Streptococcus pneumoniae* (pneumococcus) remains an important cause of morbidity and mortality in the United States, particularly in the very young, the elderly, and persons with certain high-risk conditions. Pneumococcal pneumonia accounts for 10 to 25% of all pneumonias and an estimated 40,000 deaths annually (1). Although no recent data from the United States exist, in the United Kingdom pneumococcal infections may account for 34% of pneumonias in adults who require hospitalization (2). The best estimates of the incidence of serious pneumococcal disease in the United States are based on surveys and community-based studies of pneumococcal bacteremia. Recent studies suggest annual rates of bacteremia of 15–19/100,000 for all persons, 50/100,000 for persons ≥65 years old, and 160/100,000 for children ≤2 years old (3, 4). These rates are two to three times those previously documented in the United States. The overall rate for pneumococcal bacteremia in some Native American populations can be six times the rate of the general population (5). The incidence of pneumococcal pneumonia can be three to five times that of the detected rates of bacteremia. The estimated incidence of pneumococcal meningitis is 1–2/100,000 persons.

Mortality from pneumococcal disease is highest in patients with bacteremia or meningitis, patients with underlying medical conditions, and older persons. In some high-risk patients, mortality has been reported to be >40% for bacteremia disease and 55% for meningitis, despite appropriate antimicrobial therapy. Over 90% of pneumococci remain very sensitive to penicillin.

In addition to the very young and persons ≥65 years old, patients with certain chronic conditions are at increased risk of developing pneumococcal infection and severe pneumococcal illness. Patients with chronic cardiovascular diseases, chronic pulmonary disease, diabetes mellitus, alcoholism, and cirrhosis are generally immunocompetent but have increased risk. Other patients at greater risk because of decreased responsiveness to polysaccharide antigens or more rapid decline in serum antibody include those with functional or anatomic splenia (e.g., sickle cell disease or splenectomy), Hodgkin's disease, lymphoma, multiple myeloma, chronic renal failure, nephrotic syndrome, and organ transplantation. In a recent population-based study, all persons 55 to 64 years old with pneumococcal bacteremia had at least one of these chronic conditions (4). Studies indicate that patients with acquired immunodeficiency syndrome (AIDS) are also at increased risk of pneumococcal disease, with an annual attack rate of pneumococcal pneumonia as high as 17.9/1000 (6–8). This observation is consistent with the B-cell dysfunction noted in patients with AIDS (9, 10). Recurrent pneumococcal meningitis may occur in patients with cerebrospinal fluid leakage complicating skull fractures or neurologic procedures.

Pneumococcal Polysaccharide Vaccine

The current pneumococcal vaccine (Pneumovax™23, Merck Sharp & Dohme, and Pnu-Imune™23, Lederle Laboratories) is composed of purified capsular polysaccharide antigens of 23 types of *S. pneumoniae* (Danish types 1, 2, 3, 4, 5, 6B, 7F, 8, 9N, 9V, 10A, 11A, 12F, 14, 15B, 17F, 18C, 19F, 19A, 20, 22F, 23F, 33F). It was licensed in the United States in 1983, replacing a 14-valent vaccine licensed in 1977. Each vaccine dose (0.5 ml) contains 25 µg of each polysaccharide antigen. The 23 capsular types in the vaccine cause 88% of the bacteremia pneumococcal disease in the United States. In addition, studies of the human antibody response indicate that cross-reactivity occurs for several types (e.g., 6A and 6B) that cause an additional 8% of bacteremia disease (11).

Most healthy adults, including the elderly, show a 2-fold or greater rise in type-specific antibody, as measured by radioimmunoassay, within 2 to 3 weeks of vaccination. Similar antibody responses have been reported in patients with alcoholic cirrhosis and diabetes mellitus requiring insulin. In immunocompromised patients, the response to vaccination may be less. In children <2 years old, antibody response to most capsular types is generally poor. In addition, response to some important pediatric pneumococcal types (e.g., 6A and 14) is decreased in children <5 years old (12, 13).

Following vaccination of healthy adults with polyvalent pneumococcal vaccine, antibody levels for most pneumococcal vaccine types remain elevated at least 5 years; in some persons, they fall to prevaccination levels within 10 years (14, 15). A more rapid decline in antibody levels may occur in children. In children who have undergone splenectomy following trauma and in those with sickle cell disease, antibody titers for some types can fall to prevaccination levels 3 to 5 years after vaccination (16, 17). Similar rates of decline can occur in children with nephrotic syndrome (18).

Patients with AIDS have been shown to have an impaired antibody response to pneumococcal vaccine (10, 19). However, asymptomatic HIV-infected men or those with persistent generalized lymphadenopathy respond to the 23-valent pneumococcal vaccine (20).

VACCINE EFFICACY

In the 1970s, pneumococcal vaccine was shown to reduce significantly the occurrence of pneumonia in young, healthy populations in South Africa and Papua New Guinea, where incidence of pneumonia is high (21, 22). It was also demonstrated to protect against systemic pneumococcal infection in hyposplenic patients in the United States (23). Since then, studies have attempted to assess vaccine efficacy in other U.S. populations (24–30) (CDC, unpublished data) (Table 8.14). A prospective, ongoing case-control study in Connecticut has shown an overall protective efficacy of 61% against pneumococcal bacteremia caused

Table 8.14. Clinical Effectiveness of Pneumococcal Vaccination in U.S. Populations

Location	Method	No. Persons	Type Infection	Vaccine Efficacy (%)	95% C.I.
Connecticut (25, 26)	Case-control[a]	543 cases 543 controls	VT,[b] VT-related	61	42, 73
Philadelphia (27)	Case-control[a]	122 cases 244 controls	All serotypes	70	37, 86
Denver (28)	Case-control[a]	89 cases 89 controls	All serotypes	-21	-221, 55
CDC-1 (29)	Epidemiologic[a]	249 vaccinated 1638 unvaccinated	VT	64	47, 76
CDC-2 (unpublished)	Epidemiologic[a]	240 vaccinated 1527 unvaccinated	VT	60	45, 70
VA cooperative study (30)	Randomized controlled trial[c]	1145 vaccinated 1150 controls	All serotypes VT	-34[d] -19[d]	-119, 18[d] -164, 47[d]

[a] Only patients with isolates from normally sterile body sites were included.
[b] Vaccine-type pneumococcal infection.
[c] Pneumococcal pneumonia and bronchitis were diagnosed primarily by culture of respiratory secretions.
[d] Values calculated from the published data.

by vaccine- and vaccine-related serotypes. The protective efficacy was 60% for patients with alcoholism or chronic pulmonary, cardiac, or renal disease and 64% for patients ≥55 years old without other high-risk chronic conditions (25, 26). In another multicenter case-control study, vaccine efficacy in immunocompetent persons ≥55 years old was 70% (27). A smaller case-control study of veterans failed to show efficacy in preventing pneumococcal bacteremia (28), but determination of the vaccination status was judged to be inadequate and the selection of controls was considered to be potentially biased.

Studies based on CDC's pneumococcal surveillance system suggest an efficacy of 60 to 64% for vaccine-type strains in patients with bacteremia disease. For all persons ≥65 years of age (including persons with chronic heart disease, pulmonary disease, or diabetes mellitus), vaccine efficacy was 44 to 61% (29) (CDC, unpublished data). In addition, estimates of vaccine efficacy for serologically related types were 29 to 66% (29). Limited data suggest that clinical efficacy may decline ≥6 years after vaccination (CDC, unpublished data).

A randomized, double-blind, placebo-controlled trial among high-risk veterans showed no vaccine efficacy against pneumococcal pneumonia or bronchitis (30); however, case definitions used were judged to have uncertain specificity. In addition, this study had only a 6% ability to detect a vaccine efficacy of 65% for pneumococcal bacteremia (31). In contrast, a French clinical trial found pneumococcal vaccine to be 77% effective in reducing the incidence of pneumonia in nursing home residents (32).

Despite conflicting findings, the data continue to support the use of the pneumococcal vaccine for certain well-defined groups at risk.

RECOMMENDATIONS FOR VACCINE USE

Adults

1. Immunocompetent adults who are at increased risk of pneumococcal disease or its complications because of chronic illnesses (e.g., cardiovascular disease, pulmonary disease, diabetes mellitus, alcoholism, cirrhosis, or cerebrospinal fluid leaks) or who are ≥65 years old.
2. Immunocompromised adults at increased risk of pneumococcal disease or its complications (e.g., persons with splenic dysfunction or anatomic splenia, Hodgkin's disease, lymphoma, multiple myeloma, chronic renal failure, nephrotic syndrome, or conditions such as organ transplantation associated with immunosuppression).
3. Adults with asymptomatic or symptomatic HIV infection.

Children

1. Children ≥2 years old with chronic illnesses specifically associated with increased risk of pneumococcal disease or its complications (e.g., anatomic or functional splenia (including sickle cell disease), nephrotic syndrome, cerebrospinal fluid leaks, and conditions associated with immunosuppression).
2. Children ≥2 years old with asymptomatic or symptomatic HIV infection.

3. The currently available 23-valent vaccine is not indicated for patients having only recurrent upper respiratory tract disease, including otitis media and sinusitis.

SPECIAL GROUPS

Persons living in special environments or social settings with an identified increased risk of pneumococcal disease or its complications (e.g., certain Native American populations).

ADVERSE REACTIONS

Approximately 50% of persons given pneumococcal vaccine develop mild side effects, such as erythema and pain at the injection site. Fever, myalgia, and severe local reactions have been reported in <1% of those vaccinated. Severe systemic reactions, such as anaphylaxis, rarely have been reported.

PRECAUTIONS

The safety of pneumococcal vaccine for pregnant women has not been evaluated. Ideally, women at high risk of pneumococcal disease should be vaccinated before pregnancy.

TIMING OF VACCINATION

When elective splenectomy is being considered, pneumococcal vaccine should be given at least 2 weeks before the operation, if possible. Similarly, for planning cancer chemotherapy or immunosuppressive therapy, as in patients who undergo organ transplantation, the interval between vaccination and initiation of chemotherapy or immunosuppression should also be at least 2 weeks.

REVACCINATION

In one study, local reactions after revaccination in adults were more severe than after initial vaccination when the interval between vaccinations was 13 months (33) (Table 8.15). Reports of revaccination after longer intervals in children and adults, including a large group of elderly persons revaccinated at least 4 years after primary vaccination, suggest a similar incidence of such reactions after primary vaccination and revaccination (unpublished data) (17, 34–38).

Without more information, persons who received the 14-valent pneumococcal vaccine should not be routinely revaccinated with the 23-valent vaccine, as increased coverage is modest and duration of protection is not well defined. However, revaccination with the 23-valent vaccine should be strongly considered for persons who received the 14-valent vaccine if they are at highest risk of fatal pneumococcal infection (e.g., asplenic patients). Revaccination should also be considered for adults at highest risk who received the 23-valent vaccine ≥6 years before and for those shown to have rapid decline in pneumococcal antibody levels (e.g., patients with nephrotic syndrome or renal failure, or transplant

Table 8.15. Reactions to Revaccination with Pneumococcal Vaccine

Study	Vaccinees			Revaccination Period	Reactions
	Condition	Age	No.		
Borgono et al., 1978 (33)	Normal	Adults	7	13 months	Increase in local reactions
Carlson et al., 1979 (34)	Normal	21–62 years	23	12–18 months	Increase in local reactions
Rigau-Perez et al., 1983 (35)	Sickle cell disease	≥3 years	28	28–35 months	No increase in reactions compared with primary vaccination
Lawrence et al., 1983 (36)	Normal	2–5 years	52	35 months (mean)	Increase in local reactions
Mufson et al., 1984 (37)	Normal	23–40 years	12	24–48 months	No increase in reactions compared with primary vaccination
Weintrub et al., 1984 (17)	Sickle cell disease	10–27 years	17	8–9 years	No "serious" local reactions
Kaplan et al., 1986 (38)	Sickle cell disease	4–23 years	86	37–53 months	Four "severe" reactions[a]

[a] Severe reaction was defined as presence of local pain, redness, swelling, and axillary temperature >100°F (37.8°C); two patients, 21 and 23 years old, had temperatures of 102°F (38.9°C).

recipients). Revaccination after 3 to 5 years should be considered for children with nephrotic syndrome, splenia, or sickle cell anemia who would be ≤10 years old at revaccination.

STRATEGIES FOR VACCINE DELIVERY

Recommendations for pneumococcal vaccination have been made by the ACIP, the American Academy of Pediatrics, the American College of Physicians, and the American Academy of Family Physicians. Recent analysis indicates that pneumococcal vaccination of elderly persons is cost-effective (39). The vaccine is targeted for approximately 27 million persons aged ≥65 years and 21 million persons aged ≤65 years with high-risk conditions (1). Despite Medicare reimbursement for costs of the vaccine and its administration, which began in 1981, annual use of pneumococcal vaccine has not increased above levels observed in earlier years (40) (Fig. 8.1). In 1985, <10% of the 48 million persons considered to be at increased risk of serious pneumococcal infection were estimated to have ever received pneumococcal vaccine (1).

Opportunities to vaccinate high-risk persons are missed both at time of hospital discharge and during visits to clinicians' offices. Two thirds or more of patients with serious pneumococcal disease had been hospitalized at least once within 5 years before their pneumococcal illness, yet few had received pneumococcal vaccine (40). More effective programs for vaccine delivery are needed, including offering pneumococcal vaccine in hospitals (at the time of discharge), clinicians'

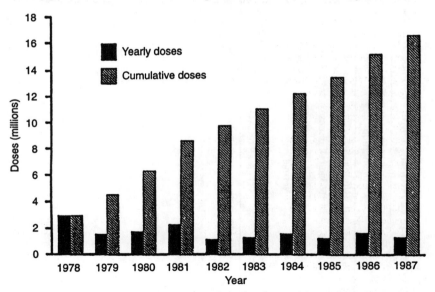

Figure 8.1. Pneumococcal vaccine distribution—United States, 1978–1987. Data for 1978–1985 were obtained from Bush LM, Moonsammy GL, Boscia JA. Evaluation of initiating a hepatitis B vaccination schedule with one vaccine and completing it with another. Vaccine 1991;9:807–809. Data for 1986 and 1987 were obtained from Lederle Laboratories and Merck, Sharp & Dohme (net doses distributed).

offices, nursing homes, and other chronic-care facilities. Many patients who receive pneumococcal vaccine should also be immunized with influenza vaccine (41), which can be given simultaneously at a different site. In contrast to pneumococcal vaccine, influenza vaccine is given annually.

VACCINE DEVELOPMENT

A more immunogenic pneumococcal vaccine preparation is needed, particularly for children <2 years old. The development of a protein-polysaccharide conjugate vaccine for selected capsular types holds promise.

REFERENCES

1. Williams WW, Hickson MA, Kane MA, Kendal AP, Spika JS, Hinman AR. Immunization policies and vaccine coverage among adults: the risk for missed opportunities. Ann Intern Med 1988;108:616–625.
2. Research Committee of the British Thoracic Society and the Public Health Laboratory Service. Community-acquired pneumonia in adults in British hospitals in 1982–1983: a survey of aetiology, mortality, prognostic factors and outcome. Q J Med 1987;62:195–220.
3. Istre GR, Tarpay M, Anderson M, Pryor A, Welch D. Pneumococcus Study Group. Invasive disease due to *Streptococcus pneumoniae* in an area with a high rate of relative penicillin resistance. J Infect Dis 1987;156:732–735.
4. Breiman RF, Navarro VJ, Darden PM, Darby CP, Spika JS. *Streptococcus pneumoniae* bacteremia in residents of Charleston County, South Carolina, a decade later [Abstract]. In: Program and abstracts of the 28th Interscience Conference on Antimicrobial Agents and Chemotherapy. Washington DC: American Society for Microbiology, 1988:343.
5. Davidson M, Schraer CD, Parkinson AJ, et al. Invasive pneumococcal disease in an Alaska Native population, 1980 through 1986. JAMA 1989;261:715–718.
6. Polsky B, Gold JWM, Whimbey E, et al. Bacterial pneumonia in patients with the acquired immunodeficiency syndrome. Ann Intern Med 1986;104:38–41.
7. Simberkoff MS, Sadr WE, Schiffman G, Rahal JJ. *Streptococcus pneumoniae* infections and bacteremia in patients with acquired immune deficiency syndrome, with report of a pneumococcal vaccine failure. Am Rev Respir Dis 1984;130:1174–1176.
8. Stover DE, White DA, Romano PA, Gellene RA, Robeson WA. Spectrum of pulmonary diseases associated with the acquired immune deficiency syndrome. Am J Med 1985;78:429–437.
9. Lane CH, Masur H, Edgar LC, Whalen G, Rook AH, Fauci AS. Abnormalities of B-cell activation and immunoregulation in patients with the acquired immunodeficiency syndrome. N Engl J Med 1983;309:453–458.
10. Ammann AJ, Schiffman G, Abrams D, Volberding P, Ziegler J, Conant M. B-cell immunodeficiency in acquired immune deficiency svndrome. JAMA 1984;251:1447–1449.
11. Robbins JB, Austrian R, Lee C-J, et al. Considerations for formulating the second-generation pneumococcal capsular polysaccharide vaccine with emphasis on the cross-relative types within groups. J Infect Dis 1983;148:1136–1159.
12. Douglas RM, Paton JC, Duncan SJ, Hansman DJ. Antibody response to pneumococcal vaccination in children younger than five years of age. J Infect Dis 1983;148:131–137.
13. Leinonen M, Sakkinen A, Kalliokoski R, Luotenen J, Timonen M, Makela PH. Antibody response to 14-valent pneumococcal capsular polysaccharide vaccine in pre-school age children. Pediatr Infect Dis 1986;5:39–44.
14. Mufson MA, Krause HE, Schiffman G. Long-term persistence of antibody following immunization with pneumococcal polysaccharide vaccine. Proc Soc Exp Biol Med 1983;173:270–275.
15. Mufson MA, Krause HE, Schiffman G, Hughey DF. Pneumococcal antibody levels one decade after immunization of healthy adults. Am J Med Sci 1987;293:279–284.
16. Giebink GS, Le CT, Schiffman G. Decline of serum antibody in splenectomized children after vaccination with pneumococcal capsular polysaccharides. J Pediatr 1984;105:576–584.
17. Weintrub PS, Schiffman G, Addiego JE Jr, et al. Long-term follow-up and booster immunization with polyvalent pneumococcal polysaccharide in patients with sickle cell anemia. J Pediatr 1984;105:261–263.

18. Spika JS, Halsey NA, Le CT, et al. Decline of vaccine-induced anti-pneumococcal antibody in children with nephrotic syndrome. Am J Kidney Dis 1986;7:466–470.
19. Ballet J-J, Sulcebe G, Couderc L-J, et al. Impaired anti-pneumococcal antibody response in patients with AIDS-related persistent generalized lymphadenopathy. Clin Exp Immunol 1987;68:479–487.
20. Huang K-L, Ruben FL, Rinaldo CR Jr, Kingsley L, Lyter DW, Ho M. Antibody responses after influenza and pneumococcal immunization in HIV-infected homosexual men. JAMA 1987;257:2047–2050.
21. Austrian R, Douglas RM, Schiffman G, et al. Prevention of pneumococcal pneumonia by vaccination. Trans Assoc Am Physicians 1976;89:184–194.
22. Riley ID, Tarr PI, Andrews M, et al. Immunisation with a polyvalent pneumococcal vaccine: reduction of adult respiratory mortality in a New Guinea Highlands community. Lancet 1977;1:1338–1341.
23. Ammann AJ, Addiego J, Wara DW, Lubin B, Smith WB, Mentzer WC. Polyvalent pneumococcal-polysaccharide immunization of patients with sickle-cell anemia and patients with splenectomy. N Engl J Med 1977;297:897–900.
24. Austrian R: Surveillance of pneumococcal infection for field trials of polyvalent pneumococcal vaccines. Bethesda, MD: National Institutes of Health, National Institute of Allergy and Infectious Diseases, 1980; report no. DAB-VDP-12-84.
25. Shapiro ED, Clemens JD. A controlled evaluation of the protective efficacy of pneumococcal vaccine for patients at high risk of serious pneumococcal infections. Ann Intern Med 1984:101:325–330.
26. Shapiro ED, Austrian R, Adair RK, Clemens JD. The protective efficacy of pneumococcal vaccine [Abstract]. Clin Res 1988;36:470A.
27. Sims RV, Steinmann WC, McConville JH, King LR, Zwick WC, Schwartz JS. The clinical effectiveness of pneumococcal vaccine in the elderly. Ann Intern Med 1988;108:653–657.
28. Forrester HL, Jahnigen DW, LaForce FM. Inefficacy of pneumococcal vaccine in a high-risk population. Am J Med 1987;83:425–430.
29. Bolan G, Broome CV, Facklam RR, Plikaytis BD, Fraser DW, Schlech WF III. Pneumococcal vaccine efficacy in selected populations in the United States. Ann Intern Med 1986;104:1–6.
30. Simberkoff MS, Cross AP, Al-Ibrahim M, et al. Efficacy of pneumococcal vaccine in high-risk patients: results of a Veterans Administration cooperative study. N Engl J Med 1986;315:1318–1327.
31. Shapiro ED. Pneumococcal vaccine failure [Letter]. N Engl J Med 1987;316:1272–1273.
32. Gaillat J, Zmirou D, Mallaret MR, et al. Essai clinique du vaccin anti-pneumococcique chez des personnes agees vivant en institution. Rev Epidemiol Sante Publique 1985;33;437–444.
33. Borgono JM, McLean AA, Vella PP, et al. Vaccination and revaccination with polyvalent pneumococcal polysaccharide vaccines in adults and infants. Proc Soc Exp Biol Med 1978;157:148–154.
34. Carlson AJ, Davidson WL, McLean AA, et al. Pneumococcal vaccine: dose, revaccination, and coadministration with influenza vaccine. Proc Soc Exp Biol Med 1979;161:558–563.
35. Rigau-Perez JG, Overturf GD, Chan LS, Weiss J, Powars D. Reactions to booster pneumococcal vaccination in patients with sickle cell disease. Pediatr Infect Dis 1983;2:199–202.
36. Lawrence EM, Edwards KM, Schiffman G, Thompson JM, Vaughn WK, Wright PF. Pneumococcal vaccine in normal children. Am J Dis Child 1983;137:846–850.
37. Mufson MA, Krause HE, Schiffman G. Reactivity and antibody responses of volunteers given two or three doses of pneumococcal vaccine. Proc Soc Exp Biol Med 1984;177:220–225.
38. Kaplan J, Sarnaik S, Schiffman G. Revaccination with polyvalent pneumococcal vaccine in children with sickle cell anemia. Am J Pediatr Hematol Oncol 1986;8:80–82.
39. Sisk JE, Riegelman RK. Cost effectiveness of vaccination against pneumococcal pneumonia: an update. Ann Intern Med 1986;104:79–86.
40. Fedson DS. Influenza and pneumococcal immunization strategies for physicians. Chest 1987;91:436–443.
41. ACIP. Prevention and control of influenza. MMWR 1988;37:361–364, 369–373.

Rabies Prevention[d]

Introduction

Following the marked decrease of rabies cases among domestic animals in the United States in the 1940s and 1950s, indigenously acquired rabies among humans decreased to fewer than two cases per year in the 1960s and 1970s and fewer than one case per year during the 1980s (1). In 1950, for example, 4979 cases of rabies were reported among dogs and 18 were reported among human populations; in 1989, 160 cases were reported among dogs and one was reported among humans. Thus, the likelihood of human exposure to a rabid domestic animal has decreased greatly; however, the many possible exposures that result from frequent contact between domestic dogs and humans continue to be the basis of most antirabies treatments (2).

Rabies among wild animals—especially skunks, raccoons, and bats—has become more prevalent since the 1950s, accounting for >85% of all reported cases of animal rabies every year since 1976 (1). Rabies among animals occurs throughout the continental United States; only Hawaii remains consistently rabies-free. Wild animals now constitute the most important potential source of infection for both humans and domestic animals in the United States. In much of the rest of the world, including most of Asia, Africa, and Latin America, the dog remains the major species with rabies and the major source of rabies among humans. Nine of the 13 human rabies deaths reported to CDC from 1980 through 1990 appear to have been related to exposure to rabid animals outside of the United States (3–9).

Although rabies among humans is rare in the United States, every year approximately 18,000 persons receive rabies preexposure prophylaxis and an additional 10,000 receive postexposure prophylaxis. Appropriate management of persons possibly exposed to rabies depends on the interpretation of the risk of infection. Decisions about management must be made immediately. All available methods of systemic prophylactic treatment are complicated by occasional adverse reactions, but these are rarely severe (10–14).

Data on the efficacy of active and passive rabies immunization have come from both human and animal studies. Evidence from laboratory and field experience in many areas of the world indicates that postexposure prophylaxis combining local wound treatment, passive immunization, and vaccination is uniformly effective when appropriately applied (15–20). However, rabies has occasionally developed among humans when key elements of the rabies postexposure prophylaxis treatment regimens were omitted or incorrectly administered (see Postexposure Treatment Outside the United States).

---

[d]From Advisory Committee on Immunization Practices. Rabies prevention—United States, 1991. MMWR 1991;40(No. RR- 3):1–19.

Rabies Immunizing Products

There are two types of rabies immunizing products.

1. Rabies vaccines induce an active immune response that includes the production of neutralizing antibodies. This antibody response requires approximately 7 to 10 days to develop and usually persists for ≥2 years.
2. Rabies immune globulins (RIG) provide rapid, passive immune protection that persists for only a short time (half-life of approximately 21 days) (21, 22).

In almost all postexposure prophylaxis regimens, both products should be used concurrently.

RABIES IMMUNIZING PRODUCTS, UNITED STATES, 1991

Human Rabies Vaccine

Rabies Vaccine, Human Diploid Cell (HDCV)
Intramuscular   Imovax™ Rabies
Intradermal   Imovax™ Rabies I.D.
Rabies Vaccine Adsorbed (RVA)

Rabies Immune Globulin

Rabies Immune Globulin, Human (HRIG):
Hyperab™
Imogram™ Rabies

VACCINES LICENSED FOR USE IN THE UNITED STATES

Two inactivated rabies vaccines are currently licensed for preexposure and postexposure prophylaxis in the United States.

Rabies Vaccine, Human Diploid Cell (HDCV)

HDCV is prepared from the Pitman-Moore strain of rabies virus grown in MRC-5 human diploid cell culture and concentrated by ultrafiltration (23). The vaccine is inactivated with β-propiolactone (18) and is supplied in forms for

1. Intramuscular administration, a single-dose vial containing lyophilized vaccine (Pasteur-Merieux Serum et Vaccins, Imovax™ Rabies, distributed by Connaught Laboratories, Inc., Telephone: (800) VACCINE) that is reconstituted in the vial with the accompanying diluent to a final volume of 1.0 ml just before administration.
2. Intradermal administration, a single-dose syringe containing lyophilized vaccine (Pasteur-Merieux Serum et Vaccins, Imovax™ Rabies I.D., distributed by Connaught Laboratories, Inc.) that is reconstituted in the syringe to a volume of 0.1 ml just before administration (24).

A human diploid cell-derived rabies vaccine developed in the United States (Wyeth Laboratories, Wyvac™) was recalled by the manufacturer from the market in 1985 and is no longer available (25).

Rabies Vaccine, Adsorbed (RVA)

RVA (Michigan Department of Public Health) was licensed on March 19, 1988; it was developed and is currently distributed by the Biologics Products Program, Michigan Department of Public Health. The vaccine is prepared from the Kissling strain of Challenge Virus Standard (CVS) rabies virus adapted to fetal rhesus lung diploid cell culture (26–32). The vaccine virus is inactivated with β-propiolactone and concentrated by adsorption to aluminum phosphate. Because RVA is adsorbed to aluminum phosphate, it is liquid rather than lyophilized. RVA is currently available only from the Biologics Products Program, Michigan Department of Public Health. Telephone: (517) 335–8050.

Both types of rabies vaccines are considered equally efficacious and safe when used as indicated. The full 1.0-ml dose of either product can be used for both preexposure and postexposure prophylaxis. Only the Imovax™ Rabies I.D. vaccine (HDCV) has been evaluated by the intradermal dose/route for preexposure vaccination (33–36); the antibody response and side effects after intradermal administration of RVA have not been studied (24). *Therefore, RVA should not be used intradermally.*

RABIES IMMUNE GLOBULINS LICENSED FOR USE IN THE UNITED STATES

HRIG (Cutter Biological (a division of Miles Inc.), Hyperab™; and Pasteur-Merieux Serum et Vaccins, Imogam™ Rabies, distributed by Connaught Laboratories, Inc.) is an antirabies γ-globulin concentrated by cold ethanol fractionation from plasma of hyperimmunized human donors. Rabies neutralizing antibody content, standardized to contain 150 international units (IU) per ml, is supplied in 2-ml (300 IU) and 10-ml (1500 IU) vials for pediatric and adult use, respectively.

Both HRIG preparations are considered equally efficacious and safe when used as described in this document.

Postexposure Prophylaxis: Rationale for Treatment

Physicians should evaluate each possible exposure to rabies and if necessary consult with local or state public health officials regarding the need for rabies prophylaxis (Table 8.16). In the United States, the following factors should be considered before specific antirabies treatment is initiated.

TYPE OF EXPOSURE

Rabies is transmitted only when the virus is introduced into open cuts or wounds in skin or mucous membranes. If there has been no exposure (as described in this section), postexposure treatment is not necessary. The likelihood of rabies

Table 8.16. Rabies Postexposure Prophylaxis Guide, United States, 1991

Animal Type	Evaluation and Disposition of Animal	Postexposure Prophylaxis Recommendations
Dogs and cats	Healthy and available for 10 days observation	Should not begin prophylaxis unless animal develops symptoms of rabies[a]
	Rabid or suspected rabid	Immediate vaccination
	Unknown (escaped)	Consult public health officials
Skunks, raccoons, bats, foxes, and most other carnivores; woodchucks	Regarded as rabid unless geographic area is known to be free of rabies or until animal proven negative by laboratory tests[b]	Immediate vaccination
Livestock, rodents, and lagomorphs (rabbits and hares)	Consider individually	Consult public health officials. Bites of squirrels, hamsters, guinea pigs, gerbils, chipmunks, rats, mice, other rodents, rabbits, and hares almost never require antirabies treatment

[a] During the 10-day holding period, begin treatment with HRIG and HDCV or RVA at first sign of rabies in a dog or cat that has bitten someone. The symptomatic animal should be killed immediately and tested.
[b] The animal should be killed and tested as soon as possible. Holding for observation is not recommended. Discontinue vaccine if immunofluorescence test results of the animal are negative.

infection varies with the nature and extent of exposure. Two categories of exposure (bite and nonbite) should be considered.

Bite

Any penetration of the skin by teeth constitutes a bite exposure. Bites to the face and hands carry the highest risk, but the site of the bite should not influence the decision to begin treatment (17).

Nonbite

Scratches, abrasions, open wounds, or mucous membranes contaminated with saliva or other potentially infectious material (such as brain tissue) from a rabid animal constitute nonbite exposures. If the material containing the virus is dry, the virus can be considered noninfectious.

Other contact by itself, such as petting a rabid animal and contact with the blood, urine, or feces (e.g., guano) of a rabid animal, does not constitute an exposure and is not an indication for prophylaxis.

Although occasional reports of transmission by nonbite exposure suggest that such exposures constitute sufficient reason to initiate postexposure prophylaxis under some circumstances, nonbite exposures rarely cause rabies (37). The nonbite exposures of highest risk appear to be exposures to large amounts of aerosol-ized rabies virus, organs (i.e., corneas) transplanted from patients who died of rabies, and scratches by rabid animals. Two cases of rabies have been attributed to airborne exposures in laboratories, and two cases of rabies have been attributed to probable airborne exposures in a bat-infested cave in Texas (38, 39).

The only documented cases of rabies caused by human-to-human transmission occurred among six recipients of transplanted corneas. Investigations revealed each of the donors had died of an illness compatible with or proven to be rabies (40–43). The six cases occurred in four countries: Thailand (two cases), India (two cases), the United States (one case), and France (one case). Stringent guidelines for acceptance of donor corneas have reduced this risk.

Apart from corneal transplants, bite and nonbite exposures inflicted by infected humans could theoretically transmit rabies, but no such cases have been docu-mented (44). Adherence to respiratory precautions will minimize the risk of airborne exposure (45).

ANIMAL RABIES EPIDEMIOLOGY AND EVALUATION OF INVOLVED SPECIES

Wild Animals

Carnivorous wild animals (especially skunks, raccoons, and foxes) and bats are the animals most often infected with rabies and the cause of most indigenous cases of human rabies in the United States since 1960 (1). All bites by wild carnivores and bats must be considered possible exposures to the disease. Postex-posure prophylaxis should be initiated when patients are exposed to wild carni-vores unless (1) the exposure occurred in a part of the continental United States known to be free of terrestrial rabies and the results of immunofluorescence antibody testing will be available within 48 hours or (2) the animal has already been tested and shown not to be rabid. If treatment has been initiated and subsequent immunofluorescence testing shows that the exposing animal was not rabid, treatment can be discontinued.

Signs of rabies among carnivorous wild animals cannot be interpreted reliably; therefore, any such animal that bites or scratches a person should be killed at once (without unnecessary damage to the head) and the brain submitted for rabies testing. If the results of testing are negative by immunofluorescence, the saliva can be assumed to contain no virus, and the person bitten does not require treatment.

If the biting animal is a particularly rare or valuable specimen and the risk of rabies small, public health authorities may choose to administer postexposure treatment to the bite victim in lieu of killing the animal for rabies testing (46). Such animals should be quarantined for 30 days.

Rodents (such as squirrels, hamsters, guinea pigs, gerbils, chipmunks, rats, and mice) and lagomorphs (including rabbits and hares) are almost never found to be infected with rabies and have not been known to cause rabies among humans in the United States. However, from 1971 through 1988, woodchucks accounted for 70% of the 179 cases of rabies among rodents reported to CDC

(47). In all cases involving rodents, the state or local health department should be consulted before a decision is made to initiate postexposure antirabies prophylaxis.

Exotic pets (including ferrets) and domestic animals crossbred with wild animals are considered wild animals by the National Association of State Public Health Veterinarians (NASPHV) and the Conference of State and Territorial Epidemiologists (CSTE) because they may be highly susceptible to rabies and could transmit the disease. Because the period of rabies virus shedding in these animals is unknown, these animals should be killed and tested rather than confined and observed when they bite humans (46). Wild animals (skunks, raccoons, and bats) and wild animals crossbred with dogs should not be kept as pets (46).

Domestic Animals

The likelihood that a domestic animal is infected with rabies varies by region; hence, the need for postexposure prophylaxis also varies. In the continental United States, rabies among dogs is reported most commonly along the U.S.-Mexico border and sporadically from the areas of the United States with enzootic wildlife rabies, especially the Midwest. During most of the 1980s in the United States, more cats than dogs were reported rabid; the majority of these cases were associated with the mid-Atlantic epizootic of rabies among raccoons. The large number of rabies-infected cats may be attributed to fewer cat vaccination laws, fewer leash laws, and the roaming habits of cats. Cattle tend to be most often exposed to rabies via rabid skunks.

In areas where canine rabies is not enzootic (including virtually all of the United States and its territories), a healthy domestic dog or cat that bites a person should be confined and observed for 10 days. Any illness in the animal during confinement or before release should be evaluated by a veterinarian and reported immediately to the local health department. If signs suggestive of rabies develop, the animal should be humanely killed and its head removed and shipped, under refrigeration, for examination by a qualified laboratory. Any stray or unwanted dog or cat that bites a person should be killed immediately and the head submitted as described for rabies examination (46).

In most developing countries of Asia, Africa, and Central and South America, dogs are the major vector of rabies; exposures to dogs in such countries represent a special threat. Travelers to these countries should be aware that >50% of the rabies cases among humans in the United States result from exposure to dogs outside the United States. Although dogs are the main reservoir of rabies in these countries, the epizootiology of the disease among animals differs sufficiently by region or country to warrant the evaluation of the animal bites.

Exposures to dogs in canine rabies-enzootic areas outside the United States carry a high risk; some authorities therefore recommend that postexposure rabies treatment be initiated immediately after such exposures. Treatment can be discontinued if the dog or cat remains healthy during the 10-day observation period.

CIRCUMSTANCES OF BITING INCIDENT AND VACCINATION STATUS OF EXPOSING ANIMAL

An unprovoked attack by a domestic animal is more likely than a provoked attack to indicate that the animal is rabid. Bites inflicted on a person attempting to feed or handle an apparently healthy animal should generally be regarded as provoked.

A fully vaccinated dog or cat is unlikely to become infected with rabies, although rare cases have been reported (48). In a nationwide study of rabies among dogs and cats in 1988, only one dog and two cats that were vaccinated contracted rabies (49). All three of these animals had received only single doses of vaccine; no documented vaccine failures occurred among dogs or cats that had received two vaccinations.

Postexposure Prophylaxis: Local Treatment of Wounds and Vaccination

The essential components of rabies postexposure prophylaxis are local wound treatment and the administration, in most instances, of both HRIG and vaccine (Table 8.17). Persons who have been bitten by animals suspected or proven rabid should begin treatment within 24 hours. However, there have been instances when the decision to begin treatment was not made until many months after the exposure because of a delay in recognition that an exposure had occurred and awareness that incubation periods of >1 year have been reported.

In 1977, the World Health Organization (WHO) recommended a regimen of RIG and six doses of HDCV over a 90-day period. This recommendation was based on studies in Germany and Iran (16, 20). When used this way, the vaccine was found to be safe and effective in protecting persons bitten by proven rabid animals and induced an excellent antibody response in all recipients (16). Studies conducted in the United States by CDC have shown that a regimen of one dose of HRIG and five doses of HDCV over a 28-day period was safe and induced an excellent antibody response in all recipients (15).

LOCAL TREATMENT OF WOUNDS

Immediate and thorough washing of all bite wounds and scratches with soap and water is an important measure for preventing rabies. In studies of animals, simple local wound cleansing has been shown to reduce markedly the likelihood of rabies (50, 51). Tetanus prophylaxis and measures to control bacterial infection should be given as indicated. The decision to suture large wounds should take into account cosmetic factors and the potential for bacterial infections.

IMMUNIZATION

Vaccine Usage

Two rabies vaccines are currently available in the United States; either is administered in conjunction with HRIG at the beginning of postexposure therapy.

Table 8.17. Rabies Postexposure Prophylaxis Schedule, United States, 1991

Vaccination Status	Treatment	Regimen[a]
Not previously vaccinated	Local wound cleansing	All postexposure treatment should begin with immediate thorough cleansing of all wounds with soap and water.
	HRIG	20 IU/kg body weight. If anatomically feasible, up to one-half the dose should be infiltrated around the wound(s) and the rest should be administered i.m. in the gluteal area. HRIG should not be administered in the same syringe or into the same anatomical site as vaccine. Because HRIG may partially suppress active production of antibody, no more than the recommended dose should be given.
	Vaccine	HDCV or RVA, 1.0 ml, i.m. (deltoid area[b]), one each on days 0, 3, 7, 14, and 28.
Previously vaccinated[c]	Local wound cleansing	All postexposure treatment should begin with immediate thorough cleansing of all wounds with soap and water.
	HRIG	HRIG should not be administered.
	Vaccine	HDCV or RVA, 1.0 ml, i.m. (deltoid area[b]), one each on days 0 and 3.

[a] These regimens are applicable for all age groups, including children.
[b] The deltoid area is the only acceptable site of vaccination for adults and older children. For younger children, the outer aspect of the thigh may be used. Vaccine should never be administered in the gluteal area.
[c] Any person with a history of preexposure vaccination with HDCV or RVA; prior postexposure prophylaxis with HDCV or RVA; or previous vaccination with any other type of rabies vaccine and a documented history of antibody response to the prior vaccination.

A regimen of five 1-ml doses of HDCV or RVA should be given intramuscularly. The first dose of the five-dose course should be given as soon as possible after exposure. Additional doses should be given on days 3, 7, 14, and 28 after the first vaccination. For adults, the vaccine should always be administered intramuscularly in the deltoid area. For children, the anterolateral aspect of the thigh is also acceptable. The gluteal area should never be used for HDCV or RVA injections, since administration in this area results in lower neutralizing antibody titers (52).

Postexposure antirabies vaccination should always include administration of both passive antibody and vaccine, with the exception of persons who have previously received complete vaccination regimens (preexposure or postexposure) with a cell culture vaccine, or persons who have been vaccinated with other types of vaccines and have had documented rabies antibody titers. These persons should receive only vaccine (see Postexposure Therapy of Previously Vaccinated Persons). The combination of HRIG (local and systemic) and vaccine is recommended for both bite and nonbite exposures (see Postexposure Prophylaxis: Rationale for Treatment), regardless of the interval between exposure and initiation of treatment.

Because the antibody response after the recommended postexposure vaccination regimen with HDCV or RVA has been satisfactory, routine postvaccination serologic testing is not recommended. Serologic testing is indicated only in unusual instances, as when the patient is known to be immunosuppressed. The state health department may be contacted for recommendations on this matter.

HRIG Usage

HRIG is administered only once (i.e., at the beginning of antirabies prophylaxis) to provide immediate antibodies until the patient responds to HDCV or RVA by actively producing antibodies. If HRIG was not given when vaccination was begun, it can be given through the seventh day after administration of the first dose of vaccine. Beyond the seventh day, HRIG is not indicated since an antibody response to cell culture vaccine is presumed to have occurred. The recommended dose of HRIG is 20 IU/kg body weight. This formula is applicable for all age groups, including children. If anatomically feasible, up to one half the dose of HRIG should be thoroughly infiltrated in the area around the wound and the rest should be administered intramuscularly in the gluteal area. *HRIG should never be administered in the same syringe or into the same anatomical site as vaccine.* Because HRIG may partially suppress active production of antibody, no more than the recommended dose should be given (53).

Vaccination and Serologic Testing

The effectiveness of rabies vaccines is primarily measured by their ability to protect persons exposed to rabies. HDCV has been used effectively with HRIG or equine antirabies serum (ARS) worldwide to treat persons bitten by various rabid animals (15, 16). An estimated 1 million people worldwide have received rabies postexposure prophylaxis with HDCV since its introduction 12 years ago (54).

In studies of animals, antibody titers have been shown to be markers of protection. Antibody titers will vary with time since the last vaccination. Differences among laboratories that test blood samples may also influence the results.

SEROLOGIC RESPONSE SHORTLY AFTER VACCINATION

All persons tested at CDC 2 to 4 weeks after completion of preexposure and postexposure rabies prophylaxis according to ACIP guidelines have demonstrated an antibody response to rabies (15, 55, 56). Therefore, it is not necessary to test serum samples from patients completing preexposure or postexposure prophylaxis to document seroconversion unless the person is immunosuppressed (see Precautions and Contraindications). If titers are obtained, specimens collected 2 to 4 weeks after preexposure or postexposure prophylaxis should completely neutralize challenge virus at a 1:25 serum dilution by the rapid fluorescent focus inhibition test (RFFIT). (This dilution is approximately equivalent to the minimum titer of 0.5 IU recommended by the WHO.)

SEROLOGIC RESPONSE AND PREEXPOSURE BOOSTER DOSES OF VACCINE

Two years after primary preexposure vaccination, a 1:5 serum dilution will fail to neutralize challenge virus completely (by RFFIT) among 2 to 7% of persons who received the three-dose preexposure series intramuscularly and 5 to 17% of persons who received the three-dose series intradermally (57). If the titer falls below 1:5, a preexposure booster dose of vaccine is recommended for a person at continuous or frequent risk (Table 8.18) of exposure to rabies. The following guidelines are recommended for determining when serum testing should be performed after primary preexposure vaccination:

1. A person in the continuous risk category (Table 8.18) should have a serum sample tested for rabies antibody every 6 months (58).
2. A person in the frequent risk category (Table 8.18) should have a serum sample tested for rabies antibody every 2 years.

State or local health departments may provide the names and addresses of laboratories performing rabies serologic testing.

Postexposure Treatment Outside the United States

U.S. citizens and residents who are exposed to rabies while traveling outside the United States in countries where rabies is endemic may sometimes receive postexposure therapy with regimens or biologics that are not used in the United States. The following information is provided to familiarize physicians with some of the regimens used more widely abroad. These schedules have not been submitted for approval by the FDA for use in the United States. If postexposure treatment is begun outside the United States using one of these regimens or biologics of nerve tissue origin, it may be necessary to provide additional treatment when the patient reaches the United States. State or local health departments should be contacted for specific advice in such cases.

Modifications to the postexposure vaccine regimen approved for use in the United States have been made to reduce the cost of postexposure prophylaxis and hasten the development of active immunity (59). Costs are reduced primarily by substituting various schedules of ID injections (0.1 ml each) of HDCV (or newer tissue culture-derived rabies vaccines for humans) for intramuscular injection of HDCV. Two such regimens are efficacious among persons bitten by rabid

Table 8.18. Rabies Preexposure Prophylaxis Guide, United States, 1991

Risk Category	Nature of Risk	Typical Populations	Preexposure Recommendations
Continuous	Virus present continuously, often in high concentrations. Aerosol, mucous membrane, bite, or nonbite exposure. Specific exposures may go unrecognized.	Rabies research lab workers,[a] rabies biologics production workers.	Primary course. Serologic testing every 6 months; booster vaccination when antibody level falls below acceptable level.[b]
Frequent	Exposure usually episodic, with source recognized, but exposure may also be unrecognized. Aerosol, mucous membrane, bite, or nonbite exposure.	Rabies diagnostic lab workers,[a] spelunkers, veterinarians and staff, and animal-control and wildlife workers in rabies enzootic areas. Travelers visiting foreign areas of enzootic rabies for more than 30 days.	Primary course. Serologic testing or booster vaccination every 2 years.[b]
Infrequent (greater than population at large)	Exposure nearly always episodic with source recognized. Mucous membrane, bite, or nonbite exposure.	Veterinarians and animal-control and wildlife workers in areas of low rabies enzooticity. Veterinary students.	Primary course; no serologic testing or booster vaccination.
Rare (population at large)	Exposures always episodic. Mucous membrane, or bite with source unrecognized.	U.S. population at large, including persons in rabies epizootic areas.	No vaccination necessary.

[a] Judgment of relative risk and extra monitoring of vaccination status of laboratory workers is the responsibility of the laboratory supervisor (58).
[b] Minimum acceptable antibody level is complete virus neutralization at a 1:5 serum dilution by RFFIT. Booster dose should be administered if the titer falls below this level.

animals (60). One of these regimens consists of 0.1-ml intradermal doses of HDCV given at eight different sites (deltoid, suprascapular, thigh, and abdominal wall) on day 0; four intradermal 0.1-ml doses given at four sites on day 7 (deltoid, thigh); and one intradermal 0.1-ml dose given in the deltoid on both day 28 and 91. Another intradermal regimen shown to be efficacious and now widely used in Thailand employs Purified VERO Cell Rabies Vaccine (Pasteur-Merieux), with 0.1-ml doses given at two different sites on days 0, 3, and 7, followed by one 0.1-ml booster on days 30 and 90 (61).

Strategies designed to hasten the development of active immunity have concentrated on administering more intramuscular or intradermal doses at the time postexposure prophylaxis is initiated with fewer doses thereafter (62). The most extensively evaluated regimen in this category, developed in Yugoslavia, has been the 2-1-1 regimen (two 1.0-ml intramuscular doses on day 0, and one each on days 7 and 21) (63–65). However, when using HRIG in conjunction with this schedule, there may be some suppression of the neutralizing antibody response (65).

Purified antirabies sera of equine origin (Sclavo; Pasteur-Merieux; Swiss Serum and Vaccine Institute, Bern) have been used effectively in developing countries where HRIC may not be available. The incidence of adverse reactions has been low (0.8 to 6.0%) and most of those that occurred were minor (66–68).

Although no postexposure vaccine failures have occurred in the United States during the 10 years that HDCV has been licensed, seven persons have contracted rabies after receiving postexposure treatment with both HRIG and HDCV outside the United States. An additional six persons have contracted the disease after receiving postexposure prophylaxis with other cell culture-derived vaccines and HRIG or ARS. However, in each of these cases, there was some deviation from the recommended postexposure treatment protocol (69–71). Specifically, patients who contracted rabies after postexposure prophylaxis did not have their wounds cleansed with soap and water or other antiviral agents, did not receive their rabies vaccine injections in the deltoid area (i.e., vaccine was administered in the gluteal area), or did not receive passive vaccination around the wound site.

Preexposure Vaccination and Postexposure Therapy of Previously Vaccinated Persons

Preexposure vaccination should be offered to persons among high-risk groups, such as veterinarians, animal handlers, certain laboratory workers, and persons spending time (e.g., 1 month) in foreign countries where canine rabies is endemic. Other persons whose activities bring them into frequent contact with rabies virus or potentially rabid dogs, cats, skunks, raccoons, bats, or other species at risk of having rabies should also be considered for preexposure prophylaxis.

Preexposure prophylaxis is given for several reasons. First, it may provide protection to persons with inapparent exposures to rabies. Second, it may protect persons whose postexposure therapy might be delayed. Finally, although preexpo-

Table 8.19. Rabies Preexposure Prophylaxis Schedule, United States, 1991

Type of Vaccination	Route	Regimen
Primary	i.m.	HDCV or RVA, 1.0 ml (deltoid area), one each on
	i.d.	days 0, 7, and 21 or 28
		HDCV, 0.1 ml, one each on days 0, 7, and 21 or 28
Booster[a]	i.m.	HDCV or RVA, 1.0 ml (deltoid area), day 0 only
	i.d.	HDCV, 0.1 ml, day 0 only

[a] Administration of routine booster dose of vaccine depends on exposure risk category as noted in Table 8.18.

sure vaccination does not eliminate the need for additional therapy after a rabies exposure, it simplifies therapy by eliminating the need for HRIG and decreasing the number of doses of vaccine needed—a point of particular importance for persons at high risk of being exposed to rabies in areas where immunizing products may not be available or where they may carry a high risk of adverse reactions.

Primary Preexposure Vaccination

Intramuscular Primary Vaccination

Three 1.0-ml injections of HDCV or RVA should be given intramuscularly (deltoid area), one each on days 0, 7, and 21 or 28 (Table 8.19). In a study in the United States, >1000 persons received HDCV according to this regimen. Antibody was demonstrated in serum samples of all subjects when tested by the RFFIT. Other studies have produced comparable results (33, 56, 72, 73).

Intradermal Primary Vaccination

A regimen of three 0.1-ml doses of HDCV, one each on days 0, 7, and 21 or 28, (10, 33, 34, 36, 72, 73) is also used for preexposure vaccination (Table 8.19). The intradermal dose/route has been recommended previously by the ACIP as an alternative to the 1.0-ml intramuscular dose/route for rabies preexposure prophylaxis with HDCV (24, 74).

Pasteur-Merieux developed a syringe containing a single dose of lyophilized HDCV (Imovax™ Rabies I.D.) that reconstituted in the syringe just before administration. The syringe is designed to deliver 0.1 ml of HDCV reliably and was approved by the FDA in 1986 (24). The 0.1-ml intradermal doses, given in the area over the deltoid (lateral aspect of the upper arm) on days 0, 7, and 21 or 28, are used for primary preexposure vaccination. One 0.1-ml intradermal dose is used for booster vaccination (Table 8.18). The 1.0-ml vial is not approved for multidose intradermal use. *RVA should not be given by the intradermal dose/route* (26).

Chloroquine phosphate (administered for malaria chemoprophylaxis) interferes with the antibody response to HDCV (75). Accordingly, HDCV should not be administered by the intradermal dose/route to persons traveling to malaria-endemic countries while the person is receiving chloroquine (76). The intramuscular dose/route of preexposure prophylaxis provides a sufficient margin of safety in this situation (76). For persons who will be receiving both rabies preexposure prophylaxis and chloroquine in preparation for travel to a rabies-enzootic area, the intradermal dose/route should be initiated at least 1 month before travel to allow for completion of the full three-dose vaccine series before antimalarial prophylaxis begins. If this schedule is not possible, the intramuscular dose/route should be used. Although interference with the immune response to rabies vaccine by other antimalarials structurally related to chloroquine (e.g., mefloquine) has not been evaluated, it would seem prudent to follow similar precautions for persons receiving these drugs.

BOOSTER VACCINATION

Preexposure Booster Doses of Vaccine

Persons who work with live rabies virus in research laboratories or vaccine production facilities (continuous risk category; see Table 8.18) are at the highest risk of inapparent exposures. Such persons should have a serum sample tested for rabies antibody every 6 months (Table 8.19). Booster doses (intramuscular or intradermal) of vaccine should be given to maintain a serum titer corresponding to at least complete neutralization at a 1:5 serum dilution by the RFFIT. The frequent risk category includes other laboratory workers, such as those doing rabies diagnostic testing, spelunkers, veterinarians and staff, animal-control and wildlife officers in areas where animal rabies is epizootic, and international travelers living or visiting (for >30 days) in areas where canine rabies is endemic. Persons among this group should have a serum sample tested for rabies antibody every 2 years and, if the titer is less than complete neutralization at a 1:5 serum dilution by the RFFIT, should have a booster dose of vaccine. Alternatively, a booster can be administered in lieu of a titer determination. Veterinarians and animal-control and wildlife officers working in areas of low rabies enzooticity (infrequent exposure group) do not require routine preexposure booster doses of HDCV or RVA after completion of primary preexposure vaccination (Table 8.18).

Postexposure Therapy of Previously Vaccinated Persons

If exposed to rabies, persons previously vaccinated should receive two intramuscular doses (1.0 ml each) of vaccine, one immediately and one 3 days later. Previously vaccinated refers to persons who have received one of the recommended preexposure or postexposure regimens of HDCV or RVA, or those who received another vaccine and had a documented rabies antibody titer. HRIG is unnecessary and should not be given in these cases because an anamnestic antibody response will follow the administration of a booster regardless of the prebooster antibody titer (77).

PREEXPOSURE VACCINATION AND SEROLOGIC TESTING

Because the antibody response after these recommended preexposure prophylaxis vaccine regimens has been satisfactory, serologic testing is not necessary except for persons suspected of being immunosuppressed. Patients who are immunosuppressed by disease or medications should postpone preexposure vaccinations. Immunosuppressed persons who are at risk of rabies exposure should be vaccinated and their antibody titers checked.

Unintentional Inoculation with Modified Live Rabies Virus

Veterinary personnel may be inadvertently exposed to attenuated rabies virus while administering modified live rabies virus (MLV) vaccines to animals. Although there have been no reported rabies cases among humans resulting from exposure to needlesticks or sprays with licensed MLV vaccines, vaccine-induced rabies has occurred among animals given these vaccines. Absolute assurance of a lack of risk for humans, therefore, cannot be given. The best evidence for low risk is the absence of recognized cases of vaccine-associated disease among humans despite frequent inadvertent exposures.

MLV animal vaccines that are currently available are made with one attenuated strain of rabies virus: high egg passage (HEP) Flury strain. The HEP Flury strain has been used in animal vaccines for more than 25 years without evidence of associated disease among humans; therefore, postexposure treatment is not recommended following exposure to this type of vaccine by needlesticks or sprays.

Because the data are insufficient to assess the true risk associated with any of the MLV vaccines, preexposure vaccination and periodic boosters are recommended for all persons whose activities either bring them into contact with potentially rabid animals or who frequently handle attenuated animal rabies vaccine.

Adverse Reactions

HUMAN DIPLOID CELL RABIES VACCINE AND RABIES VACCINE, ADSORBED

Reactions after vaccination with HDCV and RVA are less serious and common than with previously available vaccines (78, 79). In studies using a three-dose postexposure regimen of HDCV, local reactions, such as pain, erythema, and swelling or itching at the injection site, have been reported among 30 to 74% of recipients. Systemic reactions, such as headache, nausea, abdominal pain, muscle aches, and dizziness have been reported among 5 to 40% of recipients. Three cases of neurologic illness resembling Guillain-Barré syndrome that resolved without sequelae in 12 weeks have been reported (18, 80, 81). In addition, a few other subacute central and peripheral nervous system disorders have been temporally associated with HDCV vaccine, but a causal relationship has not been established (82).

An immune complex-like reaction occurs among approximately 6% of persons receiving booster doses of HDCV (11, 12), 2 to 21 days after administration of the booster dose. These patients develop a generalized urticaria, sometimes accompanied by arthralgia, arthritis, angioedema, nausea, vomiting, fever, and malaise. In no cases have the illnesses been life-threatening. This reaction occurs much less frequently among persons receiving primary vaccination.

The reaction has been associated with the presence of β-propiolactone-altered human serum albumin in the HDCV and the development of IgE antibodies to this allergen (83, 84). Among persons who have received their primary vaccination series with HDCV, administration of boosters with a purified HDCV produced in Canada (Connaught Laboratories Ltd., Rabies Vaccine Inactivated (Diploid Cell Origin)-Dried) does not appear to be associated with this reaction. This vaccine is not yet licensed in the United States.

VACCINES AND IMMUNE GLOBULINS USED IN OTHER COUNTRIES

Many developing countries use inactivated nerve tissue vaccines made from the brains of adult animals or suckling mice. Nerve tissue vaccine (NTV) is reported to induce neuroparalytic reactions among approximately 1 per 200 to 1 per 2000 vaccinees; suckling mouse brain vaccine (SMBV) causes reactions in among approximately 1 per 8000 (17).

HUMAN RABIES IMMUNE GLOBULINS

Local pain and low-grade fever may follow receipt of HRIG. Although not reported specifically for HRIG, angioneurotic edema, nephrotic syndrome, and anaphylaxis have been reported after injection of IG. These reactions occur so rarely that a causal relationship between IG and these reactions is not clear.

There is no evidence that hepatitis B virus (HBV), human immunodeficiency virus (HIV, the causative agent of acquired immunodeficiency syndrome (AIDS)), or other viruses have ever been transmitted by commercially available HRIG in the United States.

MANAGEMENT OF ADVERSE REACTIONS

Once initiated, rabies prophylaxis should not be interrupted or discontinued because of local or mild systemic adverse reactions to rabies vaccine. Usually such reactions can be successfully managed with antiinflammatory and antipyretic agents (e.g., aspirin).

When a person with a history of serious hypersensitivity to rabies vaccine must be revaccinated, antihistamines may be given. Epinephrine should be readily available to counteract anaphylactic reactions, and the person should be observed carefully immediately after vaccination.

Although serious systemic, anaphylactic, or neuroparalytic reactions are rare during and after the administration of rabies vaccines, such reactions pose a serious dilemma for the attending physician (11). A patient's risk of acquiring rabies must be carefully considered before deciding to discontinue vaccination. Advice and assistance on the management of serious adverse reactions for persons receiving rabies vaccines may be sought from the state health department or CDC.

All serious systemic, neuroparalytic, or anaphylactic reactions to HDCV should be reported immediately to Connaught Laboratories, Inc., Swiftwater, PA 18370. Telephone: (800) VACCINE or (717) 839-7187. Serious reactions after the administration for RVA should be reported immediately to Coordinating Physicians, Bureau of Laboratories and Epidemiological Services, Michigan Department of Public Health, P.O. Box 30035, 3500 N. Logan, Lansing, MI 48909. Telephone: (517) 335-8050.

Precautions and Contraindications

IMMUNOSUPPRESSION

Corticosteroids, other immunosuppressive agents, antimalarials, and immunosuppressive illnesses can interfere with the development of active immunity after vaccination and may predispose the patient to rabies (75, 85). Preexposure prophylaxis should be administered to such persons with the awareness that the immune response may be inadequate (see Intradermal Primary Vaccination). Immunosuppressive agents should not be administered during postexposure therapy unless essential for the treatment of other conditions. When rabies postexposure prophylaxis is administered to persons receiving steroids or other immunosuppressive therapy, it is especially important that a serum sample be tested for rabies antibody to ensure that an acceptable antibody response has developed (see Vaccination and Serologic Testing).

PREGNANCY

Because of the potential consequences of inadequately treated rabies exposure, and because there is no indication that fetal abnormalities have been associated with rabies vaccination, pregnancy is not considered a contraindication to postexposure prophylaxis (86). If there is substantial risk of exposure to rabies, preexposure prophylaxis may also be indicated during pregnancy.

ALLERGIES

Persons who have a history of serious hypersensitivity to rabies vaccine should be revaccinated with caution (see Management of Adverse Reactions).

REFERENCES

1. Reid-Sanden FL, Dobbins JG, Smith JS, Fishbein DB. Rabies surveillance, United States during 1989. J Am Vet Med Assoc 1990;197:1571-1583.
2. Helmick CG. The epidemiology of human rabies postexposure prophylaxis, 1980-1981. JAMA 1983;250:1990-1996.
3. CDC. Human rabies diagnosed 2 months postmortem—Texas. MMWR 1985;34:700, 705-707.

4. CDC. Human rabies acquired outside the United States. MMWR 1985;34:235–236.
5. CDC. Human rabies—California, 1987. MMWR 1988;37:305–308.
6. CDC. Human rabies—Oregon, 1989. MMWR 1989;38:335–337.
7. CDC. Human rabies—Texas. MMWR 1984;33:469–470.
8. CDC. Imported human rabies. MMWR 1983;32:78–80, 85–86.
9. CDC. Human rabies acquired outside the United States from a dog bite. MMWR 1981;30:537–540.
10. Bernard KW, Smith PW, Kader FJ, Moran MJ. Neuroparalytic illness and human diploid cell rabies vaccine. JAMA 1982;248:3136–3138.
11. CDC. Systemic allergic reactions following immunization with human diploid cell rabies vaccine. MMWR 1984;33:185–187.
12. Dreesen DW, Bernard KW, Parker RA, Deutsch AJ, Brown J. Immune complex-like disease in 23 persons following a booster dose of rabies human diploid cell vaccine. Vaccine 1986;4:45–49.
13. Aoki FY, Tyrrell DA, Hill LE. Immunogenicity and acceptability of a human diploid-cell culture rabies vaccine in volunteers. Lancet 1975;1:660–662.
14. Cox JH, Schneider LC. Prophylactic immunization of humans against rabies by intradermal inoculation of human diploid cell culture vaccine. J Clin Microbiol 1976;3:96–101.
15. Anderson LJ, Sikes RK, Langkop CW, et al. Postexposure trial of a human diploid cell strain rabies vaccine. J Infect Dis 1980;142:133–138.
16. Bahmanyar M, Fayaz A, Nour-Salehi S, Mohammadi M, Koprowski H. Successful protection of humans exposed to rabies infection. Postexposure treatment with the new human diploid cell rabies vaccine and antirabies serum. JAMA 1976;236:2751–2754.
17. Hattwick MAW. Human rabies. Public Health Rev 1974;3:229–274.
18. Wiktor TJ, Plotkin SA, Koprowski H. Development and clinical trials of the new human rabies vaccine of tissue culture (human diploid cell) origin. Dev Biol Stand 1978;40:3–9.
19. World Health Organization. WHO expert committee on rabies. WHO Tech Rep Ser 1984;709:1–104.
20. Kuwert EK, Werner J, Marcus I, Cabasso VJ. Immunization against rabies with rabies immune globulin, human (RICH) and a human diploid cell strain (HDCS) rabies vaccine. J Biol Stand 1978;6:211–219.
21. Winkler WG, Schmidt RC, Sikes RK. Evaluation of human rabies immune globulin and homologous and heterologous antibody. J Immunol 1969;102:1314–1321.
22. Cabasso VJ, Loofbourow JC, Roby RE, Anuskiewicz W. Rabies immune globulin of human origin: preparation and dosage determination in non-exposed volunteer subjects. Bull WHO 1971;45:303–315.
23. Wiktor TJ, Sokol F, Kuwert E, Koprowski H. Immunogenicity of concentrated and purified rabies vaccine of tissue culture origin. Proc Soc Exp Biol Med 1969;131:799–805.
24. CDC. Rabies prevention: supplementary statement on the preexposure use of human diploid cell rabies vaccine by the intradermal route. MMWR 1986;35:767–768.
25. CDC. Rabies postexposure prophylaxis with human diploid cell rabies vaccine: lower neutralizing antibody titers with Wyeth vaccine. MMWR 1985;34:90–92.
26. CDC. Rabies vaccine, adsorbed: a new rabies vaccine for use in humans. MMWR 1988;37:217–218, 223.
27. Burgoyne GH, Kajiya KD, Brown DW, Mitchell JR. Rhesus diploid rabies vaccine (adsorbed): a new rabies vaccine using FrhL-2 cells. J Infect Dis 1985;152:204–210.
28. Levenbook IS, Elisberg BL, Driscoll BF. Rhesus diploid rabies vaccine (adsorbed): neurological safety in guinea pigs and Lewis rats. Vaccine 1986;4:225–227.
29. Berlin BS, Goswick C. Rapidity of booster response to rabies vaccine produced in cell culture [Letter]. J Infect Dis 1984;150:785.
30. Berlin BS, Mitchell JR, Burgoyne GH, Brown WE, Coswick C. Rhesus diploid rabies vaccine (adsorbed), a new rabies vaccine. II. Results of clinical studies simulating prophylactic therapy for rabies exposure. JAMA 1983;249:2663–2665.
31. Berlin BS, Mitchell JR, Burgoyne GH, et al. Rhesus diploid rabies vaccine (adsorbed), a new rabies vaccine. Results of initial clinical studies of preexposure vaccination. JAMA 1982;247:1726–1728.
32. Berlin BS. Rabies vaccine adsorbed: neutralizing antibody titers after three-dose preexposure vaccination. Am J Public Health 1990;80:476–477.
33. Nicholson KG, Turner GS, Aoki FY. Immunization with a human diploid cell strain of rabies virus vaccine: two-year results. J Infect Dis 1978;137:783–788.

34. Bernard KW, Roberts MA, Sumner J, et al. Human diploid cell rabies vaccine. Effectiveness of immunization with small intradermal or subcutaneous doses. JAMA 1982;247:1138–1142.
35. Bernard KW, Mallonee J, Wright JC, et al. Preexposure immunization with intradermal human diploid cell rabies vaccine. Risks and benefits of primary and booster vaccination. JAMA 1987;257:1059–1063.
36. Fishbein DB, Pacer RE, Holmes DF, Ley AB, Yager P, Tong TC. Rabies preexposure prophylaxis with human diploid cell rabies vaccine: a dose-response study. J Infect Dis 1987;156:50–55.
37. Afshar A. A review of non-bite transmission of rabies virus infection. Br Vet J 1979;135:142–148.
38. Winkler WC, Fashinell TR, Leffingwell L, Howard P, Conomy P. Airborne rabies transmission in a laboratory worker. JAMA 1973;226:1219–1221.
39. CDC. Rabies in a laboratory worker—New York. MMWR 1977;26:183–184.
40. CDC. Human-to-human transmission of rabies via corneal transplant—Thailand. MMWR 1981;30:473–474.
41. Gode GR, Bhide NK. Two rabies deaths after corneal grafts from one donor [Letter]. Lancet 1988;2:791.
42. CDC. Human-to-human transmission of rabies via a corneal transplant—France. MMWR 1980;29:25–26.
43. Houff SA, Burton RC, Wilson RW, et al. Human-to-human transmission of rabies virus by corneal transplant. N Engl J Med 1979;300:603–604.
44. Helmick CG, Tauxe RV, Vernon AA. Is there a risk to contacts of patients with rabies? Rev Infect Dis 1987;9:511–518.
45. Garner JS, Simmons BP. Guidelines for isolation precautions in hospitals. Infect Control 1983;4(suppl):245–325.
46. National Association of State Public Health Veterinarians. Compendium of animal rabies control. J Am Vet Med Assoc 1990;196:36–39.
47. Fishbein DB, Belotto AJ, Pacer RE, et al. Rabies in rodents and lagomorphs in the United States, 1971–1984: increased cases in the woodchuck (*Marmota monax*) in mid-Atlantic states. J Wildl Dis 1986;22:151–156.
48. CDC. Imported dog and cat rabies—New Hampshire, California. MMWR 1988;37:559–560.
49. Eng TR, Fishbein DB. Epidemiologic factors, clinical findings, and vaccination status of rabies in cats and dogs in the United States in 1988. J Am Vet Med Assoc 1990;197:201–209.
50. Dean DJ, Baer GM. Studies on the local treatment of rabies infected wounds. Bull WHO 1963;28:477–486.
51. Kaplan MM, Cohen D, Koprowski H, Dean D, Ferrigan L. Studies on the local treatment of wounds for the prevention of rabies. Bull WHO 1962;26:765–775.
52. Fishbein DB, Sawyer LA, Reid-Sanden FL, Weir EH. Administration of human diploid-cell rabies vaccine in the gluteal area [Letter]. N Engl J Med 1988;318:124–125.
53. Helmick CG, Johnstone C, Sumner J, Winkler WG, Fager S. A clinical study of Merieux human rabies immune globulin. J Biol Stand 1982;10:357–367.
54. Roumiantzeff M. The present status of rabies vaccine development and clinical experience with rabies vaccine. Southeast Asian J Trop Med Public Health 1988;19:549–561.
55. Kuwert EK, Marcus I, Werner J, et al. Post-exposure use of human diploid cell culture rabies vaccine. Dev Biol Stand 1976;37:273–286.
56. CDC. Recommendation of the Immunization Practices Advisory Committee (ACIP). Supplementary statement on pre-exposure rabies prophylaxis by the intradermal route. MMWR 1982;31:279–280, 285.
57. Fishbein DB, Dreesen DW, Holmes DF, et al. Human diploid cell rabies vaccine purified by zonal centrifugation: a controlled study of antibody response and side effects following primary and booster pre-exposure immunization. Vaccine 1990;7:437–442.
58. Richardson JH, Barkley WE, eds. Biosafety in Microbiological and Biomedical Laboratories. 2nd ed. Washington, DC: U.S. Government Printing Office, 1988. HHS Publication No. (NIH) 88-8395.
59. Nicholson KG. Rabies. Lancet 1990;335:1201–1205.
60. Warrell MJ, Nicholson KG, Warrell DA, et al. Economical multiple-site intradermal immunisation with human diploid-cell-strain vaccine is effective for post-exposure rabies prophylaxis. Lancet 1985;1:1059–1062.
61. Chutivongse S, Wilde H, Supich C, Baer GM, Fishbein DB. Postexposure prophylaxis for rabies with antiserum and intradermal vaccination. Lancet 1990;335:896–898.

62. Anderson LJ, Baer GM, Smith JS, Winkler WG, Holman RC. Rapid antibody response to human diploid rabies vaccine. Am J Epidemiol 1981;113:270–275.
63. Vodopija I, Sureau P, Lafon M, et al. An evaluation of second generation tissue culture rabies vaccines for use in man: a four-vaccine comparative immunogenicity study using a pre-exposure vaccination schedule and an abbreviated 2-1-1 postexposure schedule. Vaccine 1986;4:245–248.
64. Vodopija I, Sureau P, Smerdel S, et al. Comparative study of two human diploid rabies vaccines administered with antirabies globulin. Vaccine 1988;6:489–490.
65. Vodopija I, Sureau P, Smerdel S, et al. Interaction of rabies vaccine with human rabies immunoglobulin and reliability of a 2-1-1 schedule application for postexposure treatment. Vaccine 1988;6:283–286.
66. Wilde H, Chomchey P, Prakongsri S, Punyaratabandhu P. Safety of equine rabies immune globulin [Letter]. Lancet 1987;2:1275.
67. Wilde H, Chomchey P, Prakongsri S, Punyaratabandhu P, Chutivongse S. Adverse effects of equine rabies immune globulin. Vaccine 1989;7:10–11.
68. Wilde H, Chomchey P, Punyaratabandhu P. Purified equine rabies immune globulin; a safe and affordable alternative to human rabies immune globulin (experience with 3156 patients). Bull WHO 1989;67(6):731–736.
69. CDC. Human rabies despite treatment with rabies immune globulin and human diploid cell rabies vaccine—Thailand. MMWR 1987;36:759–760, 765.
70. Shill M, Baynes RD, Miller SD. Fatal rabies encephalitis despite appropriate post-exposure prophylaxis. A case report. N Engl J Med 1987;316:1257–1258.
71. Wilde H, Choomkasien P, Hemachudha T, Supich C, Chutivongse S. Failure of rabies postexposure treatment in Thailand. Vaccine 1989;7:49–52.
72. Turner GS, Nicholson KG, Tyrrell DA, Aoki FY. Evaluation of a human diploid cell strain rabies vaccine: final report of a three year study of pre-exposure immunization. J Hyg (Lond) 1982;89:101–110.
73. Cabasso VJ, Dobkin MB, Roby RE, Hammar AH. Antibody response to a human diploid cell rabies vaccine. Appl Microbiol 1974:27:553–561.
74. CDC. Rabies prevention—United States, 1984. MMWR 1984:33:393–402, 407–408.
75. Pappaioanou M, Fishbein DB, Dreesen DW, et al. Antibody response to preexposure human diploid-cell rabies vaccine given concurrently with chloroquine. N Engl J Med 1986;314:280–284.
76. Bernard KW, Fishbein DB, Miller KD, et al. Pre-exposure rabies immunization with human diploid cell vaccine: decreased antibody responses in persons immunized in developing countries. Am J Trop Med Hyg 1985;34:633–647.
77. Fishbein DB, Bernard KW, Miller KD, et al. The early kinetics of the neutralizing antibody response after booster immunizations with human diploid cell rabies vaccine. Am J Trop Med Hyg 1986;35:663–670.
78. Rubin RH, Hattwick MA, Jones S, Gregg MB, Schwartz VD. Adverse reactions to duck embryo rabies vaccine. Range and incidence. Ann Intern Med 1973;78:643–649.
79. Corey L, Hattwick MA, Baer GM, Smith JS. Serum neutralizing antibody after rabies postexposure prophylaxis. Ann Intern Med 1976;85:170–176.
80. Boe E, Nylan H. Guillain-Barré syndrome after vaccination with human diploid cell rabies vaccine. Scand J Infect Dis 1980;12:231–232.
81. Knittel T, Ramadori G, Mayet WJ, Lohr H, Meyer zum Buschenfelde KH. Guillain-Barré syndrome and human diploid cell rabies vaccine [Letter]. Lancet 1989;1:1334–1335.
82. Tornatore CS, Richert JR. CNS demyelination associated with diploid cell rabies vaccine [Letter]. Lancet 1990;335:1346–1347.
83. Anderson MC, Baer H, Frazier DJ, Quinnan GV. The role of specific IgE and beta-propiolactone in reactions resulting from booster doses of human diploid cell rabies vaccine. J Allergy Clin Immunol 1987;80:861–868.
84. Swanson MC, Rosanoff E, Gurwith M, Deitch M, Schnurrenberger P, Reed CE. IgE and IgG antibodies to beta-propiolactone and human serum albumin associated with urticarial reactions to rabies vaccine. J Infect Dis 1987;155:909–913.
85. Enright JB. The effects of corticosteroids on rabies in mice. Can J Microbiol 1974;16:667.
86. Varner MW, McGuinness GA, Galask RP. Rabies vaccination in pregnancy. Am J Obstet Gynecol 1982;143:717–718.

Smallpox Vaccine and Vaccinia Immune Globulin (VIG)[e, f]

SMALLPOX VACCINE

These revised ACIP recommendations on smallpox vaccine update the previous recommendations (MMWR 1980;29:417–420) to include current information on the changes in the International Health Regulations and the ending of distribution of smallpox vaccine to civilians. The basic recommendation is unchanged— smallpox vaccine is only indicated for civilians who are laboratory workers occupationally exposed to smallpox or other closely related orthopox viruses.

Smallpox vaccine (vaccinia virus) is a highly effective immunizing agent against smallpox. The judicious use of smallpox vaccine has eradicated smallpox. At the World Health Assembly in May 1980, the World Health Organization (WHO) declared the world free of smallpox (1–4).

Smallpox vaccination of civilians is now indicated *only* for laboratory workers directly involved with smallpox (variola virus) or closely related orthopox viruses (e.g., monkeypox, vaccinia, and others).

Surveillance of Suspected Cases of Smallpox

There is no evidence of smallpox transmission anywhere in the world. WHO has coordinated the investigation of 173 rumors of smallpox between 1979 and 1984 (5–7). All have been diseases other than smallpox, most commonly chickenpox or other rash illnesses. Even so, a suspected case of smallpox is a public health emergency and must be promptly investigated. Assistance in the clinical evaluation, collection of laboratory specimens, and preliminary laboratory diagnosis is available from state health departments and CDC (Telephone: (404) 329-3145 during the day and (404) 329-2888 outside usual working hours).

Misuse of Smallpox Vaccine

There is no evidence that smallpox vaccination has any value in the treatment or prevention of recurrent herpes simplex infection, warts, or any disease other than those caused by orthopox viruses (8). Misuse of smallpox vaccine to treat herpes infections has been associated with severe complications (9–11). Smallpox vaccine should never be used therapeutically.

Smallpox Vaccination Not Required for International Travel

Smallpox vaccination is no longer required for international travel. In January 1982, the International Health Regulations were changed deleting smallpox from

---

[e] Modified and abstracted from Center for Disease Control. immunobiologic agents and drugs available from the Centers for Disease Control—descriptions, recommendations, and adverse reactions. 2nd ed. Atlanta: Centers for Disease Control, 1979.
[f] From Advisory Committee on Immunization Practices. Recommendations of the Smallpox Vaccine Immunization Practices Advisory Committee. MMWR 34(23):341–342.

the Regulations (12). The International Certificates of Vaccination no longer include a smallpox vaccination certificate.

Smallpox Vaccine No Longer Available for Civilians

In May 1983, the only active, licensed producer of smallpox vaccine in the United States discontinued distribution of smallpox vaccine to civilians (13). As a result, smallpox vaccine is no longer available to civilians.

Smallpox Vaccine Available to Protect At-Risk Laboratory Workers

CDC provides smallpox vaccine to protect laboratory workers occupationally exposed to smallpox virus and other closely related orthopox viruses (14). Vaccine will be provided *only* for the protection of personnel of such laboratories. The vaccine should be administered to eligible employees under the supervision of a physician selected by the laboratory. Vaccine will be shipped to physicians responsible for vaccinating at-risk workers. Requests for vaccine should be sent to:

Drug Immunobiologic and Vaccine Service
Center for Infectious Diseases
Building 1, Room 1259
Centers for Disease Control and Prevention
Atlanta, GA 30333
(404) 329-3356

Smallpox Vaccination of Military Personnel

U.S. military personnel are routinely vaccinated against smallpox.

Consultation for Complications of Smallpox Vaccination

CDC can assist physicians in the diagnosis and management of patients with suspected complications of smallpox vaccination. Vaccinia immune globulin (VIG) is available when indicated. Physicians should call (404) 329-3145 during the day and (404) 329-2888 evenings and weekends.

The majority of persons with such complications are likely to be recently vaccinated military personnel or their contacts infected through person-to-person spread of vaccinia virus (15–17). Such person-to-person spread can be extremely serious if the person infected has eczema or is immunocompromised.

Health-care workers are requested to report complications of smallpox vaccination to CDC through state and local health departments.

REFERENCES

1. WHO. Smallpox eradication. Wkly Epidemiol Rec 1980;55:33–40.
2. WHO. Smallpox eradication. Wkly Epidemiol Rec 1980;55:121–128.
3. WHO. Declaration of global eradication of smallpox. Wkly Epidemiol Rec 1980;55:145–152.
4. WHO. Smallpox vaccination policy. Wkly Epidemiol Rec 1980;55:153–160.
5. CDC. Investigation of a smallpox rumor—Mexico. MMWR 1985;34:343–344.

6. WHO. Orthopox virus surveillance: post-smallpox eradication policy. Wkly Epidemiol Rec 1983;58:149–156.
7. WHO Smallpox Eradication Unit. Personal communication.
8. Kern AB, Schiff BL. Smallpox vaccinations in the management of recurrent herpes simplex: a controlled evaluation. J Invest Dermatol 1959;33:99–102.
9. CDC. Vaccinia necrosum after smallpox vaccination—Michigan. MMWR 1982;31:501–502.
10. U.S. Food and Drug Administration. Inappropriate use of smallpox vaccine. FDA Drug Bull 1982;12:12.
11. Freed ER, Duma RJ, Escobar MR. Vaccinia necrosum and its relationship to impaired immunologic responsiveness. Am J Med 1972;52:411–420.
12. WHO. Smallpox vaccination certificates. Wkly Epidemiol Rec 1981;39:305.
13. CDC. Smallpox vaccine no longer available for civilians—United States. MMWR 1983;32:387.
14. CDC. Smallpox vaccine available for protection of at-risk laboratory workers. MMWR 1983;32:543.
15. CDC. Contact spread of vaccinia from a recently vaccinated marine—Louisiana. MMWR 1984;33:37–38.
16. CDC. Contact spread of vaccinia from a National Guard vaccinee—Wisconsin. MMWR 1985;34:182–183.
17. Urdahl P, Rosland JH. Vaccinia genitalis. Tidsskr Nor Laegeforen 1982;102:1453–1454.

Varicella-Zoster Immune Globulin (VZIG) (1)

Chickenpox or varicella is usually a benign, highly contagious disease caused by varicella-zoster (VZ) virus. The disease occurs primarily among preschool and young, school-aged children. More than 90% of cases are reported among persons under 15 years of age. Epidemiologic and serologic studies confirm that susceptibility among adults is substantially lower than that among children. Varicella is highly communicable; secondary clinical attack rates of about 90% follow exposure of household contacts (1). The period of communicability of patients with varicella is estimated to range from 1 to 2 days before rash onset through the first 5 to 6 days after rash onset. Persons with progressive varicella may be communicable for longer periods, presumably because their immune response is to some degree depressed, allowing viral replication to persist.

Because of the large number of varicella cases among normal children, children account for the greatest number of complications from this disease. However, the risk of complications for normal children is small compared to that for immunocompromised children, whose varicella can frequently be life-threatening. (Immunocompromised persons include individuals with congenital or acquired immunodeficiency diseases and persons with suppressed immune responses, such as those that occur with leukemia, lymphoma, generalized malignancy, and therapy with immunosuppressive drugs, including steroids, alkylating drugs, antimetabolites, or radiation.) The risk of serious morbidity and mortality from varicella is directly related to host immunodeficiency.

Varicella can also be life-threatening to neonates who acquire infection transplacentally just before delivery. Term infants born to women who had onset of varicella rash within 4 days before delivery appear to have an increased mortality rate from varicella. Infants born to mothers with onsets of varicella rash 5 or more days before delivery usually have a benign course, presumably because of passive transfer of maternal antibody.

Although intrauterine infection acquired shortly before delivery increases the risk of neonatal complications, infection of mothers during the first 16 weeks of pregnancy only rarely leads to fetal damage (low birth weight, hypotrophic limbs, ocular abnormalities, brain damage, and mental retardation). This "syndrome" is so uncommon that two large studies of pregnancies complicated by varicella have not shown an increased incidence rate of congenital defects compared with that of controls (2, 3). However, review of available case records clearly supports its existence.

Although few adults are susceptible to varicella, those who develop the disease are more likely to experience complications. Persons 20 years of age or older account for a disproportionate amount of encephalitis and death. Although less than 2% of reported cases occur among individuals 20 years of age or older, almost a quarter of all the mortality is reported in this age group. Pneumonia also appears to be more common among adults with varicella.

Following chickenpox, VZ virus may persist in latent form without clinical manifestations. Upon reactivation, the latent virus can cause zoster or "shingles," a painful, vesicular, pustular eruption in the distribution of one or more sensory-nerve roots. Zoster is more common among the elderly and among immunocompromised patients, who are also more prone than the general population to develop disseminated zoster with generalized skin eruptions and central nervous system, pulmonary, hepatic, and pancreatic involvement.

Prevention of Varicella by Varicella-Zoster Immune Globulin

In 1969, zoster immune globulin (ZIG), prepared from patients convalescing from herpes zoster, was shown to prevent clinical varicella in susceptible, normal children if administered within 72 hours after exposure. Subsequent uncontrolled studies of immunocompromised patients who received ZIG after exposure to VZ virus showed that they also tended to have lower-than-expected clinical attack rates and higher-than-expected rates of subclinical infection when ZIG was administered no later than 96 hours after exposure. Patients who became ill tended to have modified illnesses with a low complication rate. The efficacy of ZIG in immunocompromised persons was further demonstrated by a study comparing the use of low-titer versus high-titer lots; patients who received the high-titer ZIG had significantly lower risks of complications.

In 1978, VZIG became available. Both serologic and clinical evaluations have demonstrated that the product is equivalent to ZIG in preventing or modifying clinical illness in susceptible, immunocompromised patients exposed to varicella. VZIG has been licensed by the FDA's Office of Biologics. VZIG is prepared from plasma found in routine screening of normal, volunteer blood donors to contain high antibody titers to VZ. VZIG (human) is a sterile, 10 to 18% solution of the globulin fraction of human plasma, primarily immunoglobulin G (IgG) in 0.3 M glycine as a stabilizer and 1:10,000 thimerosol as a preservative. It is prepared by Cohn cold ethanol precipitation.

ZIG was in short supply because of the continuous need to find new donors convalescing from herpes zoster. Because of the method of routinely screening plasma from regular blood donors for high titers of VZ antibody and using those units to prepare VZIG, supplies became substantially greater.

Indications for Use

When deciding whether to administer VZIG, the clinician must determine whether the patient is likely to be susceptible, whether the exposure is likely to result in infection, and whether the patient is at greater risk of complications from varicella than is the general population. Whereas risks of VZIG administration appear to be negligible, costs of administration can be substantial (approximately $95 per 125 units, or $475 for persons over 40 kg (88 lbs) body weight, i.e., for the maximum recommended dose). (VZIG is, however, distributed free of charge to Massachusetts residents.) In addition, it is not known whether modified infection will lead to lifelong immunity or whether modified infections will increase or decrease the risk of later developing zoster. The following recommendations are made taking these factors into account. In some instances, VZIG is routinely recommended; in others, administration should be evaluated on an individual basis.

DETERMINATION OF SUSCEPTIBILITY

Both normal and immunocompromised adults and children, who are believed to have had varicella based on a carefully obtained history by an experienced interviewer, can be considered immune (except bone marrow recipients) (Table 8.20). Reports of second attacks of clinical varicella are rare.

Since subclinical primary infections appear rare (less than 5% of infections among normal children), children (under 15 years old) without histories of clinical varicella should be considered susceptible unless proven otherwise (see below). On the other hand, most normal adults with negative or unknown histories of varicella are probably immune since attack rates of varicella in such adults after household or hospital exposure have ranged from only 5 to 15%. (Susceptibility rates of adults who were raised in some tropical areas, such as Puerto Rico, and particularly remote areas may be somewhat higher.)

Antibody Assays

Laboratory determination of susceptibility to varicella is often impractical. The most commonly available serologic assay for varicella antibodies, the complement-fixation (CF) test, is insensitive and may not be specific, particularly at low titers. One year after clinical varicella, approximately two of three patients will lack detectable CF antibody to varicella.

Other antibody assays are more sensitive and specific indicators of varicella immunity in normal hosts but are not generally available. These tests include fluorescent antibody against membrane antigen (FAMA), immune adherence

Table 8.20. Determination of Susceptibility to Varicella in Some Selected Situations[a]

Group	Immune Status	Carefully Obtained Prior History of Varicella	Detectable Varicella Antibody by a Reliable Test[b]	Susceptibility Status
Children (<15 years)	Immunocompromised	Yes	Unnecessary to perform	Immune
		No or unknown	—[c]	Susceptible
Adolescents and adults (≥15 years)	Normal	Yes	Unnecessary to perform	Immune
		No or unknown	Not performed	Generally consider immune[d]
			Yes	Immune
			No	Susceptible
	Immunocompromised	Yes	Unnessary to perform	Immune
		No or unknown	—[c]	Consider susceptible[d]

[a] This table provides general guidelines for determining susceptibility in frequently encountered situations. Not all potential scenarios are considered. In all situations, individual judgment should also be used. See text for details.
[b] Reliable tests are discussed in the text.
[c] Some immunocompromised persons with detectable antibody before VZIG administration, presumably passively transferred by recent transfusions, have developed clinical varicella. Until further evaluation of serologic tests in the immunocompromised has been completed, one may need to rely on a carefully obtained clinical history by an experienced interviewer to determine susceptibility (i.e., the absence of a history of clinical varicella).
[d] More than 85% and probably more than 95% of such persons are immune.

hemagglutination (IAHA), enzyme-linked immunosorbent assay (ELISA), and neutralizing antibody. Commercial kits are available that utilize these sensitive antibody detection methods, although they have not been fully evaluated, particularly in immunocompromised populations. (Some research laboratories have used experimental varicella skin-test antigens on a limited basis in selected populations, but their utility in routine screening programs has not been established.) When sensitive tests are available, they can be used when a determination of susceptibility is necessary.

In some instances there have been difficulties in interpreting results of some current sensitive antibody assays in immunocompromised persons. Low levels of such antibodies have been detected in the sera of some immunocompromised persons lacking histories of chickenpox who subsequently developed clinical varicella. While present, these antibodies did not prevent illness. Presumably, most if not all these persons had passively acquired antibodies as a result of recent transfusions of blood, blood derivatives, or blood products containing antibody. Investigation of other immunocompromised persons has demonstrated that serum antibodies are frequently present following transfusions. In addition, some of these sensitive antibody assays may be measuring nonspecific activity rather than antibody. Little is known about the cellular immune status of immunocompromised individuals. Therefore, until data are collected that allow further evaluation of serologic tests in the immunocompromised, in routine circumstances, one may need to rely primarily on a carefully obtained history of prior clinical chickenpox to define susceptibility. The history should be taken by an experienced interviewer. Additional studies to evaluate serologic tests of immunocompromised patients are in progress.

In addition, sensitive antibody assays may not be useful in assessing the likelihood that neonates and young infants exposed to varicella will develop clinical disease. Some infants have developed varicella after exposure, despite the presence of detectable antibody, although in most circumstances, such illnesses have been of modified severity.

Bone Marrow Recipients

Because data correlating a prior history of varicella in the bone marrow donor or recipient with actual immunity to chickenpox in the recipient are lacking, children or adults who have received bone marrow transplants should be considered susceptible, regardless of prior histories of clinical chickenpox either in themselves or in the transplant donor. However, bone marrow recipients who develop varicella or zoster following transplantation can subsequently be considered immune.

Types of Exposure

Several types of exposure are likely to place a susceptible person at risk for varicella (Table 8.21); persons continuously exposed in the household to patients with varicella are at greatest risk. Approximately 90% of such exposed, suscepti-

Table 8.21. Exposure Criteria for Which Varicella-Zoster Immune Globulin (VZIG) Is Indicated[a]

1. One of the following types of exposure to persons with chickenpox or zoster:
   a. Continuous household contact.
   b. Playmate contact (generally >1 hr of play indoors).
   c. Hospital contact (in same two- or four-bed room or adjacent beds in a large ward or prolonged face-to-face contact with an infectious staff member or patient)
   d. Newborn contact (newborn of mother who had onset of chickenpox 5 days or less before delivery or within 48 hours after delivery).
      AND
2. Time elapse after exposure is such that VZIG can be administered within 96 hr but preferably sooner.

[a] Patients should meet both criteria.

ble patients contract varicella after a single exposure. Data are not available from immunocompromised susceptible populations to directly compare the risk of varicella after playmate or hospital exposure with the risk of household exposure. However, clinical attack rates among immunocompromised patients treated with VZIG allow some comparison; approximately one-third to one-half of VZIG-treated immunocompromised children with negative histories of prior varicella become ill after household exposure. The risks of disease following playmate and hospital exposure are approximately one-fifth the risk after household exposure. Significant playmate contact generally consists of longer than 1 hour of play indoors. Significant exposure for hospital contacts consists either of sharing the same two- to four-bed hospital room with an infectious patient or of prolonged, direct face-to-face contact with an infectious person (e.g., nurses or doctors who care for the patient). Transient contacts (e.g., x-ray technicians and maintenance personnel) are less likely to result in transmission than are more prolonged contacts.

The clinical attack rate in VZIG-treated, normal infants who have been exposed in utero shortly before delivery is as high as 30 to 40%, which is not substantially different from reported rates without VZIG. However, complications are much lower in VZIG-treated infants.

Recommendations for Use of VZIG

INFANTS AND CHILDREN

Immunocompromised Children

The most important use of VZIG is for passive immunization of susceptible, immunocompromised children after significant exposure to chickenpox or zoster (Table 8.22). This includes children with primary immune deficiency disorders and neoplastic diseases and children currently receiving immunosuppressive treatment.

Table 8.22. Candidates for Whom Varicella-Zoster Immune Globulin (VZIG) Is Indicated[a]

1. Susceptible to varicella-zoster (see text and Table 8.20)
2. Significant exposure (see Table 8.21)
3. Age of <15 years, with administration to immunocompromised adolescents and adults and to other older patients on an individual basis (see text)
4. One of the following underlying illnesses or conditions:
   a. Leukemia or lymphoma
   b. Congenital or acquired immunodeficiency
   c. Immunosuppressive treatment
   d. Newborn of mother who had onset of chickenpox within 5 days before delivery or within 48 hr after delivery
   e. Premature infant (≥28 weeks' gestation) whose mother lacks a prior history of chickenpox
   f. Premature infants (<28 weeks' gestation of ≤1000 gm) regardless of maternal history

[a] Patients should meet the four criteria for VZIG candidates.

Newborns of Mothers with Varicella Shortly Before Delivery

VZIG is indicated for newborns of mothers who develop chickenpox within 5 days before and 48 hours after delivery. VZIG is probably not necessary for newborns whose mothers develop varicella more than 5 days before delivery, since those infants should be protected from complications of varicella by transplacentally acquired maternal antibody. There is no evidence to suggest that infants born to mothers who develop varicella more than 48 hours after delivery are at increased risk of complications of disease.

Postnatal Exposure of Newborn Infants

Premature infants who have significant postnatal exposure should be evaluated on an individual basis. Most premature infants of 28 weeks' gestation or more will have transplacentally acquired maternal antibodies and are protected from complications of disease if the mother is immune. The risk of complications of postnatally acquired varicella in the premature infant is unknown. However, since their immune systems may be compromised, it seems prudent to administer VZIG to exposed premature infants whose mothers have negative or uncertain histories of varicella. Such infants should be considered at risk as long as they require continued hospital care. Exposed infants of less than 28 weeks' gestation, or birth weight of 1000 gm or less, probably should receive VZIG regardless of maternal history, because they may not yet have acquired transplacental maternal antibody.

Normal-term infants who develop varicella following postnatal exposure are not known to be at any greater risk from complications of chickenpox than are older children. VZIG is not recommended for normal-term infants exposed postnatally even if their mothers do not have prior history of varicella.

ADULTS

Immunocompromised Adults

The complication rate of immunocompromised adults who contract varicella is likely to be substantially greater than that for normal adults. Most (85 to 95%) immunocompromised adults with negative or unknown histories of prior varicella are likely to be immune. After careful evaluation, adults who are believed susceptible and who have had significant exposures should receive VZIG to prevent complications.

Normal Adults

Chickenpox can be severe in normal adults. Based on available epidemiologic and clinical data, normal adults who develop varicella have a 9- to 25-fold greater risk of complications, including death, than do normal children. The estimated risk of death following varicella in normal adults is 50/100,000, compared with an estimated 2/100,000 among normal children. The decision to administer VZIG to an adult should be evaluated on an individual basis. Approximately 85 to 95% of adults with negative or uncertain histories of varicella will be immune. The objective is to modify rather than prevent illness in hopes of inducing lifelong immunity. The clinician should consider the patient's health status, type of exposure, and likelihood of previous infection when deciding whether to administer VZIG. Adults who are older siblings of large families and adults whose children have had varicella are probably immune. If sensitive laboratory screening tests for varicella are available, they might be used to determine susceptibility, if time permits. If, after careful evaluation, a normal adult with significant exposure to varicella is believed susceptible, VZIG may be administered. However, it should be noted that VZIG supplies are still limited and that the cost of VZIG is substantial (an adult dose costs $475).

Indiscriminate use of VZIG in normal adults would quickly exhaust supplies and prevent prophylaxis of known high-risk individuals, such as immunocompromised children and high-risk neonates. Persons in the latter two groups who develop varicella have estimated death-to-case ratios of at least 7,000/100,000 and 31,000/100,000, respectively, compared with 50/100,000 for normal adults.

Pregnant Women

Pregnant women should be evaluated the same way as other adults. Some experts have recommended VZIG administration for pregnant women with negative or uncertain prior histories of varicella who are exposed in the first or second trimester to prevent congenital varicella syndrome or in the third trimester to prevent neonatal varicella. However, there is no evidence that administration of VZIG to a susceptible, pregnant woman will prevent viremia, fetal infection, or congenital varicella syndrome. Because most immunosuppressed persons who receive VZIG after a significant exposure develop modified clinical disease or subclinical infection, it is theoretically possible that VZIG may prevent or suppress clinical disease in the normal mother without preventing fetal infection and disease. In the absence of evidence that VZIG can prevent congenital varicella syndrome or neonatal varicella, the primary indication for VZIG in pregnant women is to prevent complications of varicella in a susceptible adult patient rather than to prevent intrauterine infection. Neonates born to mothers who develop varicella within the 5 days preceding or 48 hours after delivery should receive VZIG regardless of whether the mother received VZIG.

HOSPITAL SETTINGS

Personnel

After exposure, hospital personnel with negative or uncertain prior histories of chickenpox should be evaluated in the same manner as other adults. When deciding whether to give VZIG to exposed hospital personnel, types of exposure and histories of prior exposure to patients with varicella should be taken into account. If available, sensitive laboratory tests for determining susceptibility can be used to assess candidacy for VZIG and whether work restrictions are necessary during the incubation period.

Hospital Management of Varicella

Ideally, health-care personnel caring for patients with chickenpox or zoster should be immune to varicella. Proper control measures to prevent or control varicella outbreaks in hospitals should include strict isolation precautions (whenever possible, patients should be in a negative-pressure room), cohorting of exposed patients (exposed persons can share a room), early discharge when possible, and the use of immune staff. (Most studies indicate that almost all adults with prior histories of varicella are immune. Thus, staff with positive histories should be considered immune. Serologic screening may be useful in defining immunity of staff with negative or uncertain histories.) Potentially susceptible hospital personnel (Table 8.20) with significant exposure should not have direct patient contact from the 10th through the 21st day after exposure, if they do not develop varicella. This is the period during which chickenpox may occur. If they develop varicella, they should not have direct patient contact until all lesions have dried and crusted, generally 6 days after rash onset. It should be remembered that staff with varicella may be contagious 1 to 2 days before onset of rash.

In general, the same control measures should apply regardless of whether potentially susceptible personnel or patients receive VZIG. Data on clinical attack rates and incubation periods of varicella following VZIG administration to normal adults are lacking. Studies of immunocompromised children with negative histories of previous varicella treated with VZIG, who have had intense exposures, such as in the household setting, demonstrate that approximately one-third to one-half will develop clinical varicella and could be infectious. Many of the remaining susceptible population develop subclinical infections that theoretically may be infectious. In addition, VZIG may prolong the average incubation period of immunocompromised patients from 14 to 18 days. The vast majority of cases occur within 28 days of exposure in immunocompromised, VZIG-treated patients. Because of the potential of a prolonged incubation period, personnel who receive VZIG should probably not work in patient areas for 10 to 28 days following exposure if no illness occurs.

Use

ADMINISTRATION

VZIG is of maximum benefit when administered as soon as possible after the presumed exposure, but may be effective given as late as 96 hours after exposure. VZIG has not been evaluated more than 96 hours after initial exposure.

VZIG is not known to be useful in treating clinical varicella or zoster or in preventing disseminated zoster, and it is not recommended for such use. The duration of protection after VZIG administration is unknown, but it seems reasonable that protection should last for at least one half-life of immune globulin—approximately 3 weeks (in the absence of increased loss or turnover of immunoglobulin, e.g., nephrotic syndrome or Wiskott-Aldrich syndrome). To be safe, high-risk susceptible persons who are again exposed more than 3 weeks after a prior dose of VZIG should receive another full dose.

Dosage

VZIG is supplied in vials containing 125 U per vial (volume is approximately 1.25 ml). The recommended dose is 125 U/10 kg (22 lbs) body weight, up to a maximum of 625 U (i.e., 5 vials). The minimum dose is 125 U. Fractional doses are not recommended. Some experts recommend 125 U/10 kg body weight without limiting the total dose to 625 U. VZIG has not been evaluated as a prophylactic measure for prevention or attenuation of varicella in normal or immunocompromised adults. Therefore, data do not exist with which to calculate the appropriate dose in adults. However, it seems likely that 625 U should be sufficient to prevent or modify infection in normal adults. Higher doses may be needed in immunocompromised adults.

Route

VZIG should be administered intramuscularly as directed by the manufacturer. *It should never be administered intravenously.*

Supply

VZIG is produced by the Massachusetts Public Health Biologic Laboratories. Outside Massachusetts, distribution is arranged by the American Red Cross Blood Services-Northeast Region, through other centers. VZIG is distributed within Massachusetts by the Massachusetts Public Health Biologic Laboratories.

Adverse Reactions and Precautions

The most frequent adverse event following VZIG is local discomfort at the injection site. Pain, redness, or swelling occurs at the injection site in about 1% of patients. Less frequent adverse reactions are gastrointestinal symptoms, malaise, headache, rash, and respiratory symptoms that occur in approximately 0.2% of recipients. Severe reactions, such as angioneurotic edema and anaphylactic shock, are rare (less than 0.1%).

When VZIG is indicated for patients with severe thrombocytopenia or any other coagulation disorder that would ordinarily contraindicate intramuscular injections, the expected benefits should outweigh the risks.

REFERENCES

1. Modified from ACIP. Recommendations of the Immunization Practices Advisory Committee (ACIP): varicella-zoster immune globulin for the prevention of chickenpox. MMWR 1984;33:84, 95, 100.
2. Ross AH. Modification of chickenpox in family contacts by administration of gamma globulin. N Engl J Med 1962;267:369.
3. Siegel M. Congenital malformations following chickenpox, measles, mumps and hepatitis. Results of a cohort study. JAMA 1973;226:1521.
4. Manson MM, Logan WPD, Loy RM. Rubella and other virus infections in pregnancy. Report on Public Health and Medical Subject, 1960; No. 101. London, England: Ministry of Health.

SUGGESTED READINGS

Brunell PA, Ross A, Miller LH, et al. Prevention of varicella by zoster immunoglobulin. N Engl J Med 1969;280:1191–1194.
Brunnell PA. Fetal and neonatal varicella-zoster infections. Semin Perinatol 1983;7:47– 56.
Feldman S, Hughes WT, Daniel CB. Varicella in children with cancer: seventy-seven cases. Pediatrics 1975;56:388–397.
Gershon AA et al. Antibody to varicella-zoster virus in parturient women and their offspring during the first year of life. Pediatrics 1976;58:692–696.
Gershon AA, Steinberg S, Brunell PA. Zoster immune globulin. A further assessment. N Engl J Med 1974;290:243.
Gustafson TL, Shehab Z, Brunell PA. Outbreak of varicella in a newborn intensive care nursery. Am J Dis Child 1984;158(6):548–550.
Meyers JD. Congenital varicella in term infants: risk reconsidered. J Infect Dis 1974;129:215.
Meyers JD, Witte JJ. Zoster-immune globulin in high-risk children. J Infect Dis 1974;129:616.
Orenstein WA et al. Prophylaxis of varicella in high-risk children. Dose-response effect of zoster immune globulin. J Pediatr 1981;98:368.
Preblud SR. Age-specific risks of varicella complications. Pediatrics 1981;68:14.
Preblud SR, D'Angleo LJ. Chickenpox in the United States, 1972–1977. J Infect Dis 1979;140:257.
Raker RK, Steinberg S, Drusin, LM, Gershon A. Antibody to varicella zoster virus in low-birth-weight newborn infants. J Pediatr 1978;93:505.
Straus SE et al. Varicella-zoster virus infections. Ann Intern Med 1988;108(2):221.
Wang EEL, Prober CG, Arvin AN. Varicella-zoster virus antibody titers before and after administration of zoster immune globulin to neonates in an intensive care nursery. J Pediatr 1983;103:113.
Zaia JA et al. Evaluation of varicella-zoster immune globulin: protection of immunosuppressed children after household exposure to varicella. J Infect Dis 1983;147:737.
Zaia JA, Levin MJ, Preblud SR. The status of passive immunization for Herpesvirus infections. In: Alving BM, Finlayson JS, eds. Immunoglobulins: characteristics and use of intravenous preparations. Bethesda, MD: Department of Health and Human Services, 1980 (DHHS publication no. (FDA) 809005).

Zaia JA, Levin MJ, Wright GG, Grady GF. A practical method for preparation of varicella-zoster immune globulin. J Infect Dis 978;137:601.

Hepatitis B Immunization

Table 8.23. Preexposure Hepatitis B Immunization

All infants
Preadolescents (starting at 10 years), adolescents, young adults
    Striving to protect as many persons as possible, immunizing these young people will protect them before they become sexually active or adopt other lifestyles exposing them to risk
Persons with occupational risk
    Now defined by the Occupational Safety and Health Administration, this includes health-care workers and many public service workers. For persons in health-care fields, vaccination should be completed during training before students encounter blood
Persons with lifestyle risk
    Heterosexual persons with multiple partners (more than one partner in the preceding 6 months) or any sexually transmitted disease, homosexual and bisexual men, injecting drug users
Special patient groups
    Hemophiliac persons
    Hemodialysis patients
Environmental risk factors
    Household and sexual contacts of hepatitis B virus (HBV) carriers, clients and staff of institutions for the developmentally disabled, prison inmates, immigrants and refugees from areas where HBV is highly endemic, international travelers to HBV endemic areas who are health-care workers, who will reside there more than 6 months or anticipate sexual contact with local persons

Reprinted with permission from ACP Task Force on Adult Immunization and Infectious Diseases Society of America, Guide for Adult Immunization. 3rd ed. Philadelphia: American College of Physicians, United States of America, 1994:78–80.

Table 8.24. Postexposure Prophylaxis for Hepatitis B

Exposure	Hepatitis B Immune Globulin	Hepatitis B Vaccine
Perinatal	0.5 ml i.m. within 12 hr of birth	0.5 ml[a] i.m. within 12 hours of birth (no later than 7 days), and at 1 and 6 months[b]; test for HB$_s$Ag and anti-HB$_s$ at 12–15 months[c]
Sexual	0.06 ml kg i.m. within 14 days of sexual contact; a second dose should be given if the index patient remains HBAg-positive after 3 months and hepatitis B vaccine was not given initially	1.0 ml i.m. at 0, 1, and 6 months for homosexual and bisexual men and regular sexual contacts of persons with acute and chronic hepatitis B
Percutaneous: exposed person unvaccinated Source known HB$_s$Ag-positive	0.06 ml/kg i.m. within 24 hr	1.0 ml i.m. within 7 days, and at 1 and 6 months[d]
Source known, HB$_s$Ag status not known	Test source for HB$_s$Ag; if source is positive, give exposed person 0.06 ml/kg i.m. once within 7 days	1.0 ml i.m. within 7 days, and at 1 and 6 months[d]
Source not tested or unknown	Nothing required	1.0 ml i.m. within 7 days, and at 1 and 6 months
Percutaneous: exposed person vaccinated Source known HB$_s$Ag-positive	Test exposed person for anti-HB$_s$,[e] if titer is protective, nothing is required; if titer is not protective, give 0.06 ml/kg within 24 hr	Review vaccination status[f]

Table 8.24—continued

Exposure	Hepatitis B Immune Globulin	Hepatitis B Vaccine[f]
Source known, HB$_s$Ag status not known	Test source for anti-HB$_s$. If source is HB$_s$Ag-negative, or if source is HB$_s$Ag-positive but anti-HB$_s$ titer is protective, nothing is required. If source is HB$_s$Ag-positive and anti-HB$_s$ titer is not protective or if exposed person is a known nonresponder, give 0.06 ml/kg i.m. within 24 hr. A second dose of hepatitis B immune globulin can be given 1 month later if a booster dose of hepatitis B vaccine is not given.	Review vaccination status[f]
Source not tested or unknown	Test exposed person for anti-HB$_s$. If anti-HB$_s$ titer is protective, nothing is required. If anti-HB$_s$ titer is not protective, 0.06 ml/kg may be given along with a booster dose of hepatitis B vaccine	Review vaccination status[f]

Reprinted with permission from ACP Task Force on Adult Immunization and Infectious Diseases Society of America, Guide for Adult Immunization. 3rd ed. Philadelphia: American College of Physicians, United States of America, 1994:78–80.

[a] Each 0.5-ml dose of recombinant hepatitis B vaccine contains 5 μg (Merck, Sharp & Dohme) or 10 μg (SmithKline Beecham) of HB$_s$Ag.

[b] If hepatitis B immune globulin and hepatitis B vaccine are given simultaneously, they should be given at separate sites.

[c] HB$_s$Ag, hepatitis B surface antigen; anti-HB$_s$, antibody to hepatitis B surface antigen.

[d] If hepatitis B vaccine is not given, a second dose of hepatitis B immune globulin should be given 1 month later.

[e] Anti-HB, titers less than 10 standard ratio units (SRU) by radioimmunoassay or negative by enzyme immunoassay indicate lack of protection. Testing the exposed person for anti-HB$_s$ is not necessary if a protective level of antibody has been shown within the previous 24 months.

[f] If the exposed person has not completed a three-dose series of hepatitis B vaccine, the series should be completed. Test the exposed person for anti-HB$_s$. If the antibody level is protective, nothing is required. If an adequate antibody response in the past is shown on retesting to have declined to an inadequate level, a booster dose (1.0 ml) of hepatitis B vaccine should be given. If the exposed person has inadequate antibody or is a known nonresponder to vaccination, a booster dose can be given along with one dose of hepatitis B immune globulin.

Table 8.25. Recommended Doses of Currently Licensed Hepatitis B Vaccines

Group	Recombivax HB Dose[a, b]		Engerix-B Dose[b]	
	μg	ml	μg	ml
Infants of HB$_s$Ag-negative mothers and children <11 years old	2.5	0.5	10	0.5
Infants of HB$_s$Ag-positive mothers; prevention of perinatal infection	5	0.5	10	0.5
Children and adolescents 11 to 19 years old	5	0.5	20	1.0
Adults ≥20 years old	10	1.0	20	1.0
Dialysis patients and other immunocompromised persons	40	1.0[c]	40	2.0[d]

Reprinted with permission from ACP Task Force on Adult Immunization and Infectious Diseases Society of America, Guide for Adult Immunization. 3rd ed. Philadelphia: American College of Physicians, United States of America, 1994:78–80.
[a] HB, hepatitis B, HB$_s$Ag, hepatitis B surface antigen.
[b] Both vaccines are routinely administered in a three-dose series. Engerix-B has also been licensed for a four-dose series administered at 0, 1, 2, and 12 months.
[c] Special formulation.
[d] Two 1-ml doses administered at one site, in a four-dose schedule at 0, 1, 2, and 6 months.

SECTION 9
Drugs for Parasitic Infections

Parasitic infections are found throughout the world. With increasing travel, use of immunosuppressive drugs, and the spread of AIDS, physicians anywhere may see infections caused by previously unfamiliar parasites. Table 9.1 lists first-choice and alternative drugs for most parasitic infections. In every case, the need for treatment must be weighed against the toxicity of the drug. A decision to withhold therapy may often be correct, particularly when the drugs can cause severe adverse effects. When the first-choice drug is initially ineffective and the alternative is more hazardous, it may be prudent to try a second course of treatment with the first drug before using the alternative. Adverse effects of some antiparasitic drugs are also listed in this section.

Partial List of Antiparasitic Drugs

*albendazole—Zente (SmithKline Beecham)
**benznidazole—Pochagan (Roche, Brazil)
†bithionol—Bitin (Tanabe, Japan)
chloroquine—Aralen (Sanofi Winthrop), others
crotamiton—Eurax (Westwood-Squibb)
†dehydroemetine (paromomycin)—Humatin (Parke-Davis)
*diethylcarbamazine—Hetrazan (Lederle), others
†diloxanide furoate—Furamide (Boots, England)
*eflornithine (difluoromethylornithine, DFMO)—Ornidyl (Merrell Dow)
**flubendazole—(Janssen)
furazolidone—Furoxone (Roberts)
**halofantrine—Halfan (SmithKline Beecham)
hydroxychloroquine—Plaquenil (Sanofi Winthrop)
iodoquinol (diiodohydroxyquin)—Yodoxin (Glenwood), others
†ivermectin—Mectizan (Merck)
lindane (γ-benzene hexachloride)—Kwell (Reed & Carnick), others
malathion—Ovide (GenDerm)

---

* Available in the United States only from the manufacturer.
** Not available in the United States.
† Available from the CDC Drug Service, Centers for Disease Control and Prevention, Atlanta, GA 30333; Telephone: (404) 639-3670 (evenings, weekends, or holidays: (404) 639-2888).
‡ Available from the National Institute of Allergy and Infectious Diseases; Telephone: 800-537-9978.

mebendazole—Vermox (Janssen)
mefloquine—Lariam (Roche)
**meglumine antimoniate—Glucantime (Rhone-Poulenc Rorer, France)
†**melarsoprol**—Arsobal (Rhone Poulenc Rorer, France)
metronidazole—Flagyl (Searle), others
niclosamide—Niclocide (Miles)
‡**nifurtimox**— Lampit (Bayer, Germany)
**ornidazole—Tiberal (Hoffman-LaRoche, Switzerland)
oxamniquine—Vansil (Pfizer)
paromomycin—Humatin (Parke-Davis)
permethrin—Nix (Burroughs Wellcome), Elimite (Herbert)
pentamidine isethionate—Pentam 300 (Fujisawa), NebuPent (Fujisawa)
praziquantel—Biltncide (Miles)
primaquine phosphate—(Sanofi Winthrop)
**proguanil—Paludnne (Ayerst, Canada; ICI, England)
pyrantel pamoate—Antiminth (Pfizer)
pyrethrins and **piperonyl butoxide**—RID (Pfizer), others
pyrimethamine—Daraprim (Burroughs Wellcome)
pyrimethamine-sulfadoxine—Fansidar (Roche)
quinacrine—Atabrine (Sanofi Winthrop)
quinidine gluconate—many manufacturers
**quinine dihydrochloride
quinine sulfate—many manufacturers
*spiramycin—Flovamycine (Rhone-Poulenc Rorer)
†**stibogluconate sodium** (antimony sodium gluconate)—Pentostam (Burroughs Wellcome, England)
†**suramin**—Germanin (Bayer, Germany)
thiabendazole—Mintezol (Merck)
**tinidazole—Fasigyn (Pfizer)
**triclabendazole (Ciba-Geigy, France)
‡**trimetrexate**—Neutrexin (US Bioscience)
**tryparsamide

Table 9.1. Drugs for Treatment of Parasitic Infections

Infection	Drug	Adult Dosage	Pediatric Dosage
AMEBIASIS (*Entamoeba histolytica*)			
Asymptomatic	Drug of choice: iodoquinol[1] or paromomycin	650 mg t.i.d. × 20 d 25–30 mg/kg/d in 3 doses × 7 d	30–40 mg/kg/d in 3 doses × 20 d 25–30 mg/kg/d in 3 doses × 7 d
	Alternative: diloxanide furoate[2]	500 mg t.i.d. × 10 d	20 mg/kg/d in 3 doses × 10 d
Mild-to-moderate intestinal disease	Drugs of choice: metronidazole[3] or tinidazole[4] followed by	750 mg t.i.d. × 10 d 2 gm/d × 3 d	35–50 mg/kg/d in 3 doses × 10 d 50 mg/kg (max. 2 g) qd × 3 d
	iodoquinol[1] or paromomycin	650 mg tid × 20 d 25–30 mg/kg/d in 3 doses × 7 d	30–40 mg/kg/d in 3 doses × 20 d 25–30 mg/kg/d in 3 doses × 7 d
Severe intestinal disease	Drugs of choice: metronidazole[3] or tinidazole[4] followed by iodoquinol[1] or paromomycin	750 mg t.i.d. × 10 d 600 mg b.i.d. × 5 d 650 mg t.i.d. × 20 d 25–30 mg/kg/d in 3 doses × 7 d	35–50 mg/kg/d in 3 doses × 10 d 50 mg/kg (max. 2 g) qd × 3 d 30–40 mg/kg/d in 3 doses × 20 d 25–30 mg/kg/d in 3 doses × 7 d
	Alternatives: dehydroemetine[2,5] followed by iodoquinol[1]	1–1.5 mg/kg/d (max. 90 mg/d) i.m. for up to 5 d 650 mg t.i.d. × 20 d	1–1.5 mg/kg/d (max. 90 mg/d) i.m. in 2 doses for up to 5 d 30–40 mg/kg/d in 3 doses × 20 d
Hepatic abscess	Drugs of choice: metronidazole[3] or tinidazole[4] followed by iodoquinol[1]	750 mg t.i.d. × 10 d 800 mg t.i.d. × 5 d 650 mg t.i.d. × 20 d	35–50 mg/kg/d in 3 doses × 10 d 60 mg/kg (max. 2 gm) qd × 3 d 30–40 mg/kg/d in 3 doses × 20 d
	Alternatives: dehydroemetine[2,5] followed by chloroquine phosphate plus iodoquinol[1]	1–1.5 mg/kg/d (max. 90 mg/d) i.m. for up to 5 d 600 mg base (1 gm)/d × 2 d, then 300 mg base (500 mg)/d × 2–3 wk 650 mg t.i.d. × 20 d	1 to 1.5 mg/kg/d (max. 90 mg/d) i.m. in 2 doses for up to 5 d 10 mg base/kg (max. 300 mg base)/d × 2–3 wks 30–40 mg/kg/d in 3 doses × 20 d
AMEBIC MENINGOENCEPHALITIS, PRIMARY			
Naegleria	Drug of choice: amphotericin B[6,7]	1 mg/kg/d i.v., uncertain duration	1 mg/kg/d i.v., uncertain duration
Acanthamoeba	Drug of choice: See Footnote 8		

Ancylostoma duodenale (see Hookworm)

ANGIOSTRONGYLIASIS

		Adult	Pediatric
Angiostrongylus cantonensis	Drug of choice: mebendazole[7,9,10]	100 mg b.i.d. x 5 d	100 mg b.i.d. x 5 d
Angiostrongylus costaricensis	Drug of choice: thiabendazole[7,9]	75 mg/kg/d in 3 doses x 3 d[11] (max. 3 gm/d)	75 mg/kg/d in 3 doses x 3 d[11] (max. 3 gm/d)

ANISAKIASIS (*Anisakis*)   Treatment of choice: surgical or endoscopic removal

ASCARIASIS (*Ascaris lumbricoides*, roundworm)

		Adult	Pediatric
	Drug of choice: mebendazole	100 mg b.i.d. x 3 d	100 mg b.i.d. x 3 d
	or pyrantel pamoate	11 mg/kg once (max. 1 gm)	11 mg/kg once (max. 1 gm)
	or albendazole	400 mg once	400 mg once

BABESIOSIS (*Babesia*)

		Adult	Pediatric
	Drugs of choice:[12] clindamycin[7]	1.2 gm b.i.d. parenteral or 600 mg t.i.d. oral x 7 d	20–40 mg/kg/d in 3 doses x 7 d
	plus quinine	650 mg t.i.d. oral x 7 d	25 mg/kg/d in 3 doses x 7 d

BALANTIDIASIS (*Balantidium coli*)

		Adult	Pediatric
	Drug of choice: tetracycline[7]	500 mg q.i.d. x 10 d	40 mg/kg/d in 4 doses x 10 d (max. 2 gm/d)[13]
	Alternatives: iodoquinol[1,7] or	650 mg t.i.d. x 20 d	40 mg/kg/d in 3 doses x 20 d
	metronidazole[3,7]	750 mg t.i.d. x 5 d	35–50 mg/kg/d in 3 doses x 5 d

BAYLISASCARIASIS (*Baylisascaris procyonis*)   Drug of choice: see Footnote 14

BLASTOCYSTIS *hominis* infection   Drug of choice: see Foonote 15

CAPILLARIASIS (*Capillaria philippinensis*)

		Adult	Pediatric
	Drug of choice: mebendazole[7]	200 mg b.i.d. x 20 d	200 mg b.i.d. x 20 d
	Alternatives: albendazole	200 mg b.i.d. x 10 d	200 mg b.i.d. x 10 d
	Thiabendazole[7]	25 mg/kg/d in 2 doses x 30 d	25 mg/kg/d in 2 doses x 30 d

Chagas' disease, see TRYPANOSOMIASIS

Clonorchis sinensis, see FLUKE infection

Table 9.1—continued

Infection	Drug	Adult Dosage	Pediatric Dosage
CRYPTOSPORIDIOSIS (Cryptosporidium)	Drug of choice: see Footnote 16		
CUTANEOUS LARVA MIGRANS (creeping eruption)	Drug of choice:[17] thiabendazole	Topically and/or 50 mg/kg/d in 2 doses (max. 3 gm/d) × 2–5 d	Topically and/or 50 mg/kg/d in 2 doses (max. 3 gm/d) × 2–5 d[11]
Cysticercosis, see TAPEWORM infection			
DIENTAMOEBA *fragilis* infection	Drug of choice: iodoquinol[1]	650 mg t.i.d. × 20 d	40 mg/kg/d in 3 doses × 20 d
	or paromomycin	25–30 mg/kg/d in 3 doses × 7 d	25–30 mg/kg/d in 3 doses × 7 d
	or tetracycline[7]	500 mg q.i.d. × 10 d	40 mg/kg/d in 4 doses × 10 d (max. 2 gm/d)[13]
***Diphyllobothrium latum*, see TAPEWORM infection**			
DRACUNCULUS *medinensis* (guinea worm) infection	Drug of choice: metronidazole[3,7,18]	250 mg t.i.d. × 10 d	25 mg/kg/d (max. 750 mg/d) in 3 doses × 10 d
	Alternative: thiabendazole[7,18]	50–75 mg/kg/d in 2 doses × 3 d[11]	50–75 mg/kg/d in 2 doses × 3 d[11]
Echinococcus, see TAPEWORM infection			
***Entamoeba histolytica*, see AMEBIASIS**			
ENTAMOEBA *polecki* infection	Drug of choice: metronidazole[3,7]	750 mg t.i.d. × 10 d	35–50 kg/d in 3 doses × 10 d
ENTEROBIUS *vermicularis* (pinworm) infection	Drug of choice: pyrantel pamoate	11 mg/kg once (max. 1 gm); repeat after 2 wk	11 mg/kg once (max. 1 gm) repeat after 2 wk
	or mebendazole	A single dose of 100 mg; repeat after 2 wk	A single dose of 100 mg; repeat after 2 wk
	or albendazole	400 mg once, repeat in 2 wk	400 mg once, repeat in 2 wk

Fasciola hepatica, see FLUKE infection

FILARIASIS

Infection	Drug	Adult Dosage	Pediatric Dosage
Wuchereria bancrofti, Brugia malayi	Drug of choice:[19] diethylcarbamazine[20]	Day 1: 50 mg, oral, p.c. Day 2: 50 mg t.i.d. Day 3: 100 mg t.i.d. Days 4 through 21: 6 mg/kg/d in 3 doses[11]	Day 1: 1 mg/kg, oral, p.c. Day 2: 1 mg/kg t.i.d. Day 3: 1–2 mg/kg t.i.d. Days 4 through 21 6 mg/kg/d in 3 doses[21]
Loa loa	Drug of choice: diethylcarbamazine[20]	Day 1: 50 mg, oral, p.c. Day 2: 50 mg t.i.d. Day 3: 100 mg t.i.d. Days 4 through 21 9 mg/kg/d in 3 doses[21]	Day 1: 1 mg/kg, oral, p.c. Day 2: 1 mg/kg t.i.d. Day 3: 1–2 mg/kg t.i.d. Days 4 through 21 9 mg/kg/d in 3 doses[21]
Mansonella ozzardi	Drug of choice: see Footnote 19		
Mansonella perstans	Drug of choice:[22] mebendazole[7]	100 mg b.i.d. × 30 d	
Tropical pulmonary eosinophilia (TPE)	Drug of choice: diethylcarbamazine	6 mg/kg/d in 3 doses × 21 d	6 mg/kg/d in 3 doses × 21 d
Onchocerca volvulus	Drug of choice: ivermectin[2]	150 µg/kg oral once, repeated every 6–12 months	150 µg/kg oral once, repeated every 6–12 months

FLUKE, hermaphroditic, infection

Infection	Drug	Adult Dosage	Pediatric Dosage
Clonorchis sinensis (Chinese liver fluke)	Drug of choice: praziquantel	75 mg/kg/d in 3 doses	75 mg/kg/d in 3 doses
Fasciola hepatica (sheep liver fluke)	Drug of choice:[23] bithionol[2]	30–50 mg/kg on alternate days × 10–15 doses	30–50 mg/kg on alternate days × 10–15 doses
Fasciolopsis buski (intestinal fluke)	Drug of choice:[23]praziquantel[7] or niclosamide[7]	75 mg/kg/d in 3 doses × 1 d A single dose of 4 tablets (2 gm), chewed thoroughly	75 mg/kg/d in 3 doses × 1 d 11–34 kg, 2 tablets (1 gm) >34 kg, 3 tablets (1.5 gm)
Heterophyes heterophyes (intestinal fluke)	Drug of choice: praziquantel[7]	75 mg/kg/d in 3 doses × 1 d	75 mg/kg/d in 3 doses × 1 d
Metagonimus yokogawai (intestinal fluke)	Drug of choice: praziquantel[7]	75 mg/kg/d in 3 doses × 1 d	75 mg/kg/d in 3 doses × 1 d
Nanophyetus salmincola	Drug of choice: praziquantel[7]	60 mg/kg/d in 3 doses × 1 d	60 mg/kg/d in 3 doses × 1 d

Table 9.1—continued

Infection	Drug	Adult Dosage	Pediatric Dosage
Opisthorchis viverrini (liver fluke)	Drug of choice: praziquantel	75 mg/kg/d in 3 doses × 1 d	75 mg/kg/d in 3 doses × 1 d
Paragonimus westermani (lung fluke)	Drug of choice: praziquantel[7] Alternative: bithionol[2]	75 mg/kg/d in 3 doses × 2 d 30–50 mg/kg on alternate days × 10–15 doses	75 mg/kg/d in 3 doses × 2 d 30–50 mg/kg on alternate days × 10–15 doses
GIARDIASIS (*Giardia intestinalis,* formerly *G. lamblia*)	Drug of choice: Quinacrine HCl	100 mg t.i.d. p.c. × 5 d	6 mg/kg/d in 3 doses p.c. × 5 d (max. 300 mg/d)
	Alternatives: metronidazole,[3,7] tinidazole,[4] furazolidone, and paromomycin[24]	250 mg t.i.d. × 5 d 2 gm once 100 mg q.i.d. × 7–10 d 25–30 mg/kg/d in 3 doses × 7 d	15 mg/kg/d in 3 doses × 5 d 50 mg/kg once (max. 2 gm) 6 mg/kg/d in 4 doses × 7–10 d
GNATHOSTOMIASIS (*Gnathostoma spinigerum*)	Treatment of choice: surgical removal or mebendazole[7]		
HOOKWORM infection (*Ancylostoma duodenale, Necator americanus*)	Drug of choice: mebendazole or pyrantel pamoate[7] or albendazole	100 mg b.i.d. × 3 d 11 mg/kg (max. 1 gm) × 3 d 400 mg once	100 mg b.i.d. × 3 d 11 mg/kg (max. 1 gm\ × 3 d 400 mg once
Hydatid cyst, see TAPEWORM infection			
Hymenolepis nana, see TAPEWORM infection			
ISOSPORIASIS (*Isospora belli*)	Drug of choice: trimethoprim-sulfamethoxazole[7,25]	160 mg TMP, 800 mg SMX q.i.d. × 10 d, then bid × 3 wk	
LEISHMANIASIS (*L. mexicana, L. tropica, L. major, L. brazilliensis, L. donovani* [Kala-azar])	Drug of choice:[26] stibogluconate sodium[2] or meglumine antimoniate	20 mg Sb/kg/d i.v. or i.m. × 20–28 d[27] 20 mg Sb/kg/d × 20–28 d[27]	20 mg Sb/kg/d i.v. or i.m. × 20–28 d[27] 20 mg Sb/kg/d i.v. or i.m. × 20–28 d[27]
	Alternatives:[28] amphotericin B[7]	0.25–1 mg/kg by infusion over 1–4° daily or every 2 d for up to 8 wk	0.25–1 mg/kg by infusion over 1–4° daily or every 2 d for up to 8 wk

	Adult dose	Pediatric dose
Pentamidine isethionate[7]	2–4 mg/kg/d i.m. for up to 15 doses[27]	2–4 mg/kg/d i.m. for up to 15 doses[27]

LICE infestation (*Pediculus humanus, capitis; Phthirus pubis*)[30]
topical treatment[29]

	Adult dose	Pediatric dose
Drug of choice: 1% permethrin[31]	Topically	Topically
or 0.5% malathion	Topically	Topically
Alternatives: pyrethrins with piperonyl butoxide	Topically[32]	Topically[32]
Lindane	Topically[32]	Topically[32]

***Loa loa*, see FILARIASIS**

MALARIA, Treatment of (*Plasmodium falciparum, P. ovale, P. vivax, and P. malariae*)
All *Plasmodium*, except Chloroquine-resistant *P. falciparum*

		Adult dose	Pediatric dose
Oral	Drug of choice: chloroquine phosphate	600 mg base (1 gm), then 300 mg base (500 mg salt) 6 hr later, then 300 mg base (500 mg salt) at 24 and 48 hr	10 mg base/kg (max 600 mg base), then 5 mg base/kg 6 hr later, then 5 mg base/kg at 24 and 48 hr
Parenteral	Drug of choice:[35] quinidine gluconate[7,36]	10 mg/kg loading dose (max. 600 mg) in normal saline slowly over 1 hr, followed by continuous infusion of 0.02 mg/kg/min for 3 d max.	Same as adult dose
	or quinine dihydrochloride[37]	20 mg salt/kg loading dose in 10 ml/kg 5% dextrose over 4 hr, followed by 10 mg salt/kg over 2–4 hr q8h (max. 1800 mg/d) until oral therapy can be started	Same as adult dose

Table 9.1—continued

Infection	Drug	Adult Dosage	Pediatric Dosage
Chloroquine-resistant *P. falciparum*[38]			
Oral	Drugs of choice:[39] quinine sulfate[40,41]	650 mg t.i.d. × 3 d	25 mg/kg/d in 3 doses × 3 d
	plus pyrimethamine-sulfadoxine[42]	3 tablets at once on last day of quinine	<1 yr 1/4 tablet 1–3 yr 1/2 tablet 4–8 yr: 1 tablet 9–14 yr: 2 tablets
	or **plus** tetracycline[7,13]	250 mg q.i.d. × 7 d	20 mg/kg/d in 4 doses × 7 d[13]
	or **plus** clindamycin[7]	900 mg t.i.d. × 3 d	20–40 mg/kg/d in 3 doses × 3 d
	Alternatives: mefloquine[43,44]	1250 mg once[45]	25 mg/kg once[46] (<45 kg)
	halofantrine[47]	500 mg q6h × 3 doses	8 mg/kg q6h × 3 doses (<40 kg)
Parenteral	Drug of choice: quinidine gluconate[7,36]	Same as above	Same as above
	or quinine dihydrochloride[37]		
Prevention of relapses: *P. vivax* and *P. ovale* only	Drug of choice: primaquine phosphate[48]	15 mg base (26.3 mg)/d × 14 d or 45 mg base (79 mg)/wk × 8 wk	0.3-mg base/kg/d × 14 d
MALARIA, Prevention of[49]			
Chloroquine-sensitive areas	Drug of choice: chloroquine phosphate[50]	300 mg base (500 mg salt) orally, once/week, beginning 1 wk before and continuing for 4 wk after last exposure	5-mg/kg base (8.3 mg/kg salt) once/week, up to adult dose of 300-mg base
Chloroquine-resistant areas[38]	Drug of choice:[51] mefloquine[44,50,52]	250 mg oral once/wk[53]	15–19 kg: 1/4 tablet 20–30 kg 1/2 tablet 31–45 kg: 3/4 tablet > 45 kg: 1 tablet
	or doxycycline[7,50,54]	100 mg daily	> 8 years of age: 2 mg/kg/d orally, up to 100 mg/d
	or chloroquine phosphate[50]	As above	As above

	Adult dose	Pediatric dose
plus pyrimethamine-sulfadoxine[47] for presumptive treatment[55]	Carry a single dose (3 tablets) for self-treatment of febrile illness when medical care is not immediately available	<1 yr: 1/4 tablet 1–3 yr: 1/2 tablet 4–8 yr: 1 tablet 9–14 yr: 2 tablets
or **plus** proguanil[56] (in Africa south of the Sahara)	200 mg daily during exposure and for 4 wk afterwards	<2 yr: 50 mg daily 2–6 yr: 100 mg daily 7–10 yr: 150 mg daily

MICROSPORIDIOSIS
Enterocytozoon bieneusi Drug of choice: none[57]
Encephalitozoon hellem Drug of choice: none[58]

Mites, see SCABIES

***MONILIFORMIS moniliformis* infection**

Drug of choice: pyrantel pamoate[7]	11 mg/kg once, repeat twice, 2 wk apart	11 mg/kg once, repeat twice, 2 wk apart

***Naegleria* species (see AMEBIC MENINGOENCEPHALITIS, PRIMARY)**

***Necator americanus* (see HOOKWORM infection)**

***Onchocerca volvulus* (see FILARIASIS)**

***Opisthorchis viverrini* (see FLUKE infection)**

***Paragonimus westermani* (see FLUKE infection)**

***Pediculus capitis, humanus, Phthirus pubis* (see LICE)**

Pinworm (see ENTEROBIUS)

***PNEUMOCYSTIS carinii* pneumonia[59]**

Drug of choice: trimethoprim-sulfamethoxazole	TMP 15–20 mg/kg/d, SMX 75–100 mg/kg/d, oral or i.v. in 3 or 4 doses × 14–21 d	Same as adult dose

Table 9.1—continued

Infection	Drug	Adult Dosage	Pediatric Dosage
	or pentamidine	3–4 mg/kg i.v. qd × 14–21 days	Same as adult dose
	Alternatives: trimethoprim[7,60]	5 mg/kg p.o. q6h × 21 days	
	plus dapsone[7,48]	100 mg p.o. qd × 21 days	
	primaquine[7,48]	15 mg base p.o. qd × 21 days	
	plus clindamycin[7]	600 mg i.v. q6h × 21 days or 300–450 mg p.o. q6h × 21 days	
	trimetrexate	45 mg/m² i.v. qd × 21 days	
	plus folinic acid	20 mg/m² p.o. or i.v. q6h × 21 days	
Primary and secondary prophylaxis	Drug of choice: trimethoprim-sulfamethoxazole	1 DS[61] tablets p.o. qd, b.i.d. or 3 ×/week	
	Alternatives: dapsone[7,60]	25–50 mg p.o. qd, or 100 mg p.o. 2 ×/wk	
	Aerosol pentamidine	300 mg inhaled monthly via Respirgard II nebulizer	
Roundworm, see ASCARIASIS			
SCABIES (Sarcoptes scabiei)	Drug of choice: 5% permethrin	Topically	Topically
	Alternatives: lindane[32]	Topically	Topically
	10% crotamiton	Topically	Topically
SCHISTOSOMIASIS (Bilharziasis)			
S. haematobium	Drug of choice: praziquantel	40 mg/kg/d in 2 doses × 1 d	40 mg/kg/d in 2 doses × 1 d
S. japonicum	Drug of choice: praziquantel	60 mg/kg/d in 3 doses × 1 d	60 mg/kg/d in 3 doses × 1 d
S. mansoni	Drug of choice: praziquantel	40 mg/kg/d in 2 doses × 1 d	40 mg/kg/d in 2 doses × 1 d[63]
	Alternative: oxamniquine[62]	15 mg/kg once[63]	20 mg/kg/d in 2 doses × 1 d[63]
S. mekongi	Drug of choice: praziquantel	60 mg/kg/d in 3 doses × 1 d	60 mg/kg/d in 3 doses × 1 d
Sleeping sickness, see TRYPANOSOMIASIS			

STRONGYLOIDIASIS (*Strongyloides stercoralis*)

Drug of choice:[64] thiabendazole	50 mg/kg/d in 2 doses (max. 3 gm/d) × 2 d[11,65]	50 mg/kg/d in 2 doses (max. 3 gm/d× 2 d[11,65]
or ivermectin[2]	200 µg/kg/d × 1–2 d	
or albendazole	400 mg qd × 3 d	400 mg qd × 3 d

TAPEWORM infection-Adult (intestinal stage)
Diphyllobothrium latum (fish), *Taenia saginata* (beef), *Taenia solium* (pork), *Dipylidium caninum* (dog)

Drug of choice: praziquantel[7]	10–20 mg/kg once	10–20 mg/kg once
or Niclosamide	A single dose of 4 tablets (2 gm), chewed thoroughly	11–34 kg: a single dose of 2 tablets (1 gm); >34 kg: a single dose of 3 tablets (1.5 gm)

Hymenolepis nana (dwarf tapeworm)

Drug of choice: praziquantel[7]	25 mg/kg once	25 mg/kg once
Alternative: niclosamide	A single daily dose of 4 tablets (2 g), chewed thoroughly, then 2 tablets daily × 6 d	11–34 kg: a single dose of 2 tablets (1 g) × 1 d, then 1 tablet (0.5 gm)/d × 6 d; >34 kg: a single dose of 3 tablets (1.5 g) × 1 d, then 2 tablets (1 gm)/d × 6 d

Larval (tissue stage)
Echinococcus granulosus (hydatid cyst)
Echinococcus multilocularis

Drug of choice: albendazole[66]	400 mg b.i.d. × 28 d, repeated as necessary	15 mg/kg/d × 28 d, repeated as necessary
Treatment of choice: see footnote 67		

Cysticercus cellulosae (cysticercosis)

Drug of choice:[68] praziquantel[7]	50 mg/kg/d in 3 doses × 15 d	50 mg/kg/d in 3 doses × 15 d
or albendazole	15 mg/kg/d in 3 doses × 8 d, repeated as necessary	15 mg/kg/d in 3 doses × 8 d, repeated as necessary
Alternative: surgery		

Toxocariasis, see VISCERAL LARVA MIGRANS

TOXOPLASMOSIS (*Toxoplasma gondii*)[69]

Drugs of choice: pyrimethamine[70]	25–100 mg/d × 3–4 wk	2 mg/kg/d × 3 d, then 1 mg/kg/d (max. 25 mg/d) × 4 wk[71]
plus sulfadiazine	1–2 gm q.i.d. × 3–4 wk	100–200 mg/kg/d × 3–4 wk
Alternative: spiramycin	3–4 gm/d[72]	50–100 mg/kg/d × 3–4 wk

Table 9.1—continued

Infection	Drug	Adult Dosage	Pediatric Dosage
TRICHINOSIS (Trichinella spiralis)	Drugs of choice: steroids for severe symptoms plus mebendazole[7,73]	200–400 mg t.i.d. × 3 d, then 400–500 mg t.i.d. × 10 d	
TRICHOMONIASIS (Trichomonas vaginalis)	Drug of choice:[74] metronidazole[3]	2 gm once or 250 mg t.i.d. orally × 7 d	15 mg/kg/d orally in 3 doses × 7 d
	or tinidazole[4]	2 gm once	50 mg/kg once (max. 2 gm)
Trichostrongylus infection	Drug of choice: pyrantel pamoate[7]	11 mg/kg once (max. 1 gm)	11 mg/kg once (max. 1 gm)
	Alternative: mebendazole[7] or albendazole	100 mg b.i.d. × 3 d 400 mg once	100 mg b.i.d. × 3 d 400 mg once
Trichuriasis (Trichuris trichiura, whipworm)	Drug of choice: mebendazole or albendazole	100 mg b.i.d. × 3 d 400 mg once[75]	100 mg b.i.d. × 3 d 400 mg once[75]
TRYPANOSOMIASIS ***T. cruzi* (South American trypanosomiasis, Chagas' disease)**	Drug of choice: nifurtimox[2,76]	8–10 mg/kg/d orally in 4 doses × 120 d	1–10 yr: 15–20 mg/kg/d in 4 doses × 90 d; 11–16 yr: 12.5–15 mg/kg/d in 4 doses × 90 d
	Alternative: benznidazole[77]	5–7 mg/kg/d × 30–120 d	
***T. brucei gambiense; T.b. rhodesiense* (African trypanosomiasis, sleeping sickness)** Hemolymphatic stage	Drug of choice: suramin[2]	100–200 mg (test dose) i.v., then 1 gm i.v. on days 1, 3, 7, 14, and 21	20 mg/kg on days 1, 3, 7, 14, and 21
	or Eflornithine	See Footnote 78	
	Alternative: pentamidine isethionate[7]	4 mg/kg/d i.m. × 10 d	

Infection	Drug	Adult Dosage	Pediatric Dosage
Late disease with CNS involvement	Drug of choice: Melarsoprol[2,79]	2-3.6 mg/kg/d i.v. × 3 doses; after 1 week 3.6 mg/kg/d i.v. × 3 doses; repeat again after 10-21 d	18-25 mg/kg total over 1 month; initial dose of 0.36 mg/kg/d i.v., increasing gradually to max. 3.6 mg/kg at intervals of 1-5 d for total of 9-10 doses.
	or eflornithine	See Footnote 78	
	Alternative: tryparsamide	One injection of 30 mg/kg (max. 2 gm) i.v. every 5 d to total of 12 injections; may be repeated after 1 month	
	plus suramin[2]	One injection of 10 mg/kg i.v. every 5 to total of 12 injections; may be repeated after 1 month	
VISCERAL LARVA MIGRANS[80]	Drug of choice:[81] diethylcarbamazine[7]	6 mg/kg/d in 3 doses × 7-10 d	6 mg/kg/d in 3 doses × 7-10 d
	Alternatives: thiabendazole	50 mg/kg/d in 2 doses × 5 d (max. 3 gm/d)[11]	50 mg/kg/d in 2 doses × 5 d (max. 3 gm/d)[11]
	or mebendazole[7]	100-200 mg b.i.d. × 5 d[82]	
Whipworm (see Trichuriasis)			
Wuchereria bancrofti (see Filariasis)			

[1] Dosage and duration of administration should not be exceeded because of possibility of causing optic neuritis; maximum dosage is 2 gm/day.

[2] In the United States, this drug is available from the CDC Drug Service, Centers for Disease Control, Atlanta, GA 30333; Telephone: (404) 639-3670 (evenings, weekends, and holidays: (404) 639-2888).

[3] Metronidazole is carcinogenic in rodents and mutagenic in bacteria; it should generally not be given to pregnant women, particularly in the first trimester.

[4] A nitroimidazole similar to metronidazole but not marketed in the United States, tinidazole appears to be at least as effective as metronidazole and better tolerated. Ornidazole, a similar drug, is also used outside the United States.

[5] Contraindicated in pregnancy.

[6] One patient with a Naegleria infection was successfully treated with amphotericin B, miconazole, and rifampin (Seidel JS, et al. N Engl J Med 1982; 306:346).

[7] An approved drug but considered investigational for this condition by the U.S. Food and Drug Administration.

[8] Strains of Acanthamoeba isolated from fatal granulomatous amebic encephalitis are usually sensitive in vitro to pentamidine, ketoconazole (Nizoral), 5-fluorocytosine, and (less so) to amphotericin B (Duma RJ et al. Antimicrob Agents Chemother 1976;10:370). For treatment of keratitis caused by Acanthamoeba, concurrent topical use of 0.1% propamidine isethionate (Broline, Rhone-Poulenc Rorer, Canada) plus neosporin, or oral itraconazole (Sporanox (Janssen)) plus topical miconazole, has been successful (Moore MB, McCulley JP. Br J Ophthalmol 1989;73:271; Ishibashi Y, et al. Am J Ophthalmol 1990; 109:121).

[9] Effectiveness documented only in animals.

Table 9.1—continued

[10] Most patients recover spontaneously without antiparasitic drug therapy. Analgesics and corticosteroids, and careful removal of CSF at frequent intervals can relieve symptoms (Koo J, et al. Rev Infect Dis 1988;10:1155). Albendazole, levamisole (Ergamisol), or ivermectin have also been used successfully in animals.

[11] This dose is likely to be toxic and may have to be decreased.

[12] Azithromycin (Zithromax) 150 mg/kg plus quinine has been effective in experimental animals. Concurrent use of pentamidine and trimethoprim-sulfamethoxazole has been reported to cure an infection with B. divergens (Raoult D, et al. Ann Intern Med 1987;107:944).

[13] Not recommended for children less than 8 years old.

[14] Drugs that could be tried include diethylcarbamazine, levamisole, fenbendazole (Kazacos KR. J Am Vet Med Assoc 1989;195:894), and ivermectin. Steroid therapy may be helpful, especially in eye or CNS infection. Ocular baylisascariasis has been treated successfully, using laser therapy to destroy intraretinal larvae.

[15] Clinical significance of these organisms is controversial, but metronidazole 750 mg three times a day x 10 days or iodoquinol 650 mg three times a day x 20 days anecdotally have been reported to be effective (Miller RA, Minshew BH. Rev Infect Dis 1988;10:930; Doyle PW, et al. J Clin Microbiol 1990; 28:116).

[16] Infection is self-limited in immunocompetent patients. In AIDS patients with large-volume intractable diarrhea, octreotide (Sandostatin) 300–500 mg three times a day subcutaneously may control the diarrhea but not the infection (Cook DJ, et al. Ann Intern Med 1978;108:708). Paromomycin may be helpful in some patients (Clezy K, et al. AIDS 1991;5:1146; Gathe J Jr, et al. Int Conference on AIDS 1990;6:384.

[17] Albendazole 200 mg twice a day x 3 days has also been reported to be effective (Jones SK, et al. Br J Dermatol 1990;122:9.

[18] Not curative but decreases inflammation and facilitates removing the worm. Mebendazole 400–800 mg/day for 6 days has been reported to kill the worm directly.

[19] A single dose of ivermectin 25–200 µg/kg has been reported to be effective for treatment of microfilaremia due to W. bancrofti and M. ozzardi (Ottesen EA, et al. N Engl J Med 1990;322:1113; Sabry M, et al. Trans R Soc Trop Med Hyg 1991;85:640; Nutman TB, et al. J Infect Dis 1987;156:662).

[20] Antihistamines or corticosteroids may be required to decrease allergic reactions due to disintegration of microfilariae in treatment of filarial infections, especially those caused by Loa loa. Diethylcarbamazine should be adminstered with special caution in heavy infections with Loa loa, because it can provoke an encephalopathy (Carme B, et al. Am J Trop Med Hyg 1991;44:684). Apheresis has been reported to be effective in lowering microfilarial counts in patients heavily infected with loiasis. Diethylcarbamazine 300 mg once weekly has been recommended for prevention of loiasis (Nutman TB, et al. N Engl J Med 1988;319:752.

[21] For patients with no microfilaremia in the blood or skin, full doses can be given from day 1.

[22] Ivermectin may also be effective.

[23] Unlike infections with other flukes, hepatica infections may not respond to praziquantel. Limited data, however, indicate that triclabendazole (Fasinex), a veterinary fasciolide, is safe and effective in a single oral dose of 10 mg/kg (Loutan L, et al. Lancet 1989;2:383).

[24] Not absorbed; may be useful for treatment of giardiasis in pregnant women.

[25] In sulfonamide-sensitive patients, such as some patients with AIDS, pyrimethamine 50–75 mg daily has been effective (Weiss LM, et al. Ann Intern Med 1988;109:474). In immunocompromised patients, it may be necessary to continue therapy indefinitely.

[26] Limited data indicate that ketoconazole 400 to 600 mg daily for 4–8 weeks may be effective for treatment of cutaneous and mucosal leishmaniasis (Saenz RE, et al. Am J Med 1990;89:147).

[27] May be repeated or continued. A longer duration may be needed for some forms of visceral leishmaniasis.

[28] Recent studies indicate that stibogluconate (pentavalent antimony)-resistant L. donovani may respond to recombinant human γ-interferon in addition to antimony (Badaro R, et al. N Engl J Med 1990;322:16); pentamidine followed by a course of antimony (Thakur CP, et al. Am J Trop Med Hyg 1991;45:435) or ketoconazole (Wali JP, et al. Lancet 1990;336:810). Recently, liposomal-encapsulated amphotericin b (AmBisome (Vestar, San Dimas, CA) was used successfully to treat multiple drug-resistant visceral leishmaniasis (Davidson RN, et al. Lancet 1991;337:1061).

[29] Application of heat 39–42 °C directly to the lesion for 20 to 32 hours over a period of 10–12 days has been reported to be effective in cutaneous L. tropica (Neva FA, et al. Am J Trop Med Hyg 1984;33:800).

[30] For infestation of eyelashes with crab lice, use petrolatum.

[31] FDA-approved only for head lice.

[32] Some consultants recommend a second application 1 week later to kill hatching progeny. Seizures have been reported in association with the use of lindane. Do not use higher-than-recommended doses and avoid warm baths before application (Tenenbein IM. J Am Geriatr Soc 1991;39:394. Prolonged use of lindane has been associated with aplastic anemia (Rauch AE, et al. Arch Intern Med 1990;150:2393).

[33] If chloroquine phosphate is not available, hydroxychloroquine sulfate is as effective; 400 mg of hydroxychloroquine sulfate is equivalent to 500 mg of chloroquine phosphate.

[34] In P. falciparum malaria, if the patient has not shown a response to conventional doses of chloroquine in 48 to 72 hours, parasitic resistance to this drug should be considered. P. vivax with decreased susceptibility to chloroquine has been reported from Papua, New Guinea (Rieckmann KH, et al. Lancet 1989;2:1183); and from Indonesia (Schwartz IK, et al. N Engl J Med 1991;324:927). Intramuscular injection of chloroquine can be painful and has been reported to cause abscesses.

[35] A recent study found artemether, a Chinese drug, effective for parenteral treatment of severe malaria in children (White NJ, et al. Lancet 1992;339:317).

[36] Some experts consider quinidine more effective than quinine. ECG monitoring is necessary to detect arrhythmias. Oral drugs should be substituted as soon as possible.

[37] Not available in the United States. P. falciparum infections with a high parasitemia may require a loading dose of 20 mg/kg (White NJ, et al. Am J Trop Med Hyg 1983;32:1). Intravenous administration of quinine dihydrochloride can be hazardous: constant monitoring of the pulse and blood pressure is necessary to detect arrhythmia or hypotension. Use of parenteral quinine may also lead to severe hypoglycemia; blood glucose should be monitored. Oral drugs should be substituted as soon as possible.

[38] Chloroquine-resistant P. falciparum infections have been reported in all areas that have malaria, except Central America north of Panama, Mexico, Haiti, the Dominican Republic, and the Middle East (including Egypt). In pregnancy, chloroquine prophylaxis has been used extensively and safely, but the safety of other prophylactic antimalarial agents in pregnancy is unclear. Therefore, travel during pregnancy to chloroquine-resistant areas should be discouraged. For chloroquine-resistant parasitemia >10%, exchange transfusion has been used (Miller KD, et al. N Engl J Med 1989;321:65; Saddler, et al. Vachon F, et al. Miller KD, et al. N Engl J Med 1990;322:56.

[39] Chloroquine-resistant falciparum malaria acquired outside of Southeast Asia, East Africa, Bangladesh, Oceania, and the Amazon basin is likely to respond to quinine (or quinidine) plus pyrimethamine sulfadoxine. In pregnancy, quinine (or quinidine) plus clindamycin is a reasonable alternative.

[40] Although quinine will usually control an attack of resistant falciparum malaria, in a substantial number of infections from Southeast Asia, Bangladesh, Oceania, East Africa, and the Amazon region it fails to prevent recurrence. In these regions, there may be pyrimethamine-sulfadoxine resistance, and addition of tetracycline or clindamycin may decrease the rate of occurrence.

[41] In Southeast Asia, there is a relative increase in resistance to quinine, and the usual treatment dose should be extended to 7 days.

[42] Fansidar tablets contain 25 mg of pyrimethamine and 500 mg of sulfadoxine.

[43] At this dosage, adverse effects including nausea, vomiting, diarrhea, dizziness, disturbed sense of balance, toxic psychosis, and seizures can occur. Mefloquine is teratogenic in animals. It should not be given together with quinine or quinidine, and caution is required in using quinine or quinidine to treat patients with malaria who have taken mefloquine for prophylaxis. The pediatric dosage has not been approved by the FDA.

[44] In the United States a 250-mg tablet of mefloquine contains 228 mg of mefloquine base. Outside the United States, each 274-mg tablet contains 250-mg base.

[45] Outside the United States, the manufacturer recommends dividing the 1250-mg dose into 750 mg, followed 6 to 8 hours later by 500 mg (Kingston D. Med J Aust 1990;153:235).

[46] White NJ. Eur J Clin Pharmacol 1988;34:1.

[47] May be effective in multiple-drug-resistant falciparum malaria (Editorial. Lancet 1989;2:537). Failures in treatment of multiple-drug-resistant malaria have, however, been reported (Shanks GD, et al. Am J Trop Med Hyg 1991;45:488). For patients with minimal previous exposure to malaria, a second course of therapy is recommended 1 week after the first course.

Table 9.1—continued

[48]Primaquine phosphate can cause hemolytic anemia, especially in patients whose red cells are deficient in glucose-6-phosphate dehydrogenase (G-6-PD). This deficiency is most common in blacks, Asians, and Mediterranean peoples. Patients should be screened for G-6-PD deficiency before treatment. Primaquine should not be used during pregnancy.

[49]At present no drug regimen guarantees protection against malaria. If fever develops within a year (particularly within the first 2 months) after travel to malarious areas, travelers should be advised to seek medical attention. Insect repellents, insecticide-impregnated bed nets, and proper clothing are important adjuncts for malaria prophylaxis.

[50]For prevention of attack after departure from areas where P. vivax and P. ovale are endemic, which includes almost all areas where malaria is found (except Haiti), some experts in addition prescribe primaquine phosphate 15-mg base (26.3 mg)/day or, for children, 0.3 mg base/kg/day during the last 2 weeks of prophylaxis. Others prefer to avoid the toxicity of primaquine and rely on surveillance to detect cases when they occur, particularly when exposure was limited or doubtful. See also Footnote 48.

[51]For prophylaxis where both chloroquine and pyrimethamine/sulfadoxine resistance coexist, mefloquine is the usual drug of choice. In mefloquine-resistant areas such as Thailand, doxycycline is recommended.

[52]The pediatric dosage has not been approved by the FDA, and the drug has not been approved for use during pregnancy. Women should take contraceptive precautions while taking mefloquine and for 2 months after the last dose. Mefloquine is not recommended for children weighing less than 15 kg or for patients taking β-blockers, calcium-channel blockers, or other drugs that may prolong or otherwise alter cardiac conduction. Patients with a history of seizures or psychiatric disorders and those whose occupation requires fine coordination or spatial discrimination should probably avoid mefloquine (Med Lett 1990;32:13).

[53]Beginning 1 week before travel and continuing weekly for the duration of stay and for 4 weeks after leaving.

[54]Beginning 1 day before travel and continuing for the duration of stay and for 4 weeks after leaving. The FDA considers use of tetracyclines as antimalarials to be investigational. Use of tetracyclines is contraindicated in pregnancy and in children less than 8 years old. Physicians who prescribe doxycycline as malaria chemoprophylaxis should advise patients to use an appropriate sunscreen (Med Lett 1989;31:59) to minimize the possibility of a photosensitivity reaction and should warn women that Candida vaginitis is a frequent adverse effect.

[55]Resistance to fansidar should be anticipated in Southeast Asia, Bangladesh, Oceania, the Amazon basin, and East Africa. Use of Fansidar is contraindicated in patients with a history of sulfonamide or pyrimethamine intolerance. In pregnancy at term and in infants less than 2 months old, pyrimethamine sulfadoxine may cause hyperbilirubinemia.

[56]Proguanil (Paludrine (Ayerst, Canada; ICI, England)), which is not available in the United States but is widely available overseas, is recommended mainly for use in Africa south of the Sahara. Failures in prophylaxis with chloroquine and proguanil have, however, been reported in travelers to Kenya (Rarnes AJ. Lancet 1991;338:1338).

[57]In a limited number of patients with severe diarrhea, albendazole 400 mg 2 times a day for 4 to 6 weeks was reported to produce remission (Bianshard C, et al. Int Conference on AIDS 1991;7:248). Octreotide (Sandostatin, Sandoz) has provided symptomatic relief (JP Ceilo, et al. Ann Intern Med 1991;115:705).

[58]A keratopathy in an AIDS patient was treated successfully with surgical debridement, topical antibiotics, and itraconazole (Sporanox, Janssen) (Yee RW, et al. Ophthalmology 1991;98:196).

[59]AIDS patients should be treated for 21 days. In moderate or severe PCP with room air PO_2 <70 mm Hg or Aa gradient ≥35 mm Hg, prednisone should also be used (Med Lett 1991;33:101).

[60]Assay for G-6-PD deficiency recommended at start of therapy.

[61]Each double-strength tablet contains 160 mg TMP and 800 mg SMX.

[62]Contraindicated in pregnancy. Neuropsychiatric disturbances and seizures have been reported in some patients (Stokvis H, et al. Am J Trop Med Hyg 1986;35:330).

[63]In East Africa, the dose should be increased to 30 mg/kg, and in Egypt and South Africa, 30 mg/kg/day × 2 days. Some experts recommend 40 to 60 mg/kg over 2 to 3 days in all of Africa (Shekhar KC. Drugs 1991;42:379).

[64]In immunocompromised patients it may be necessary to continue therapy or use other agents.

[65] In disseminated strongyloidiasis, thiabendazole therapy should be continued for at least 5 days.

[66] With a fatty meal to enhance absorption. Some patients may benefit from or require surgical resection of cysts (Tompkins RK. Mayo Clin Proc 1991;66:1281). Praziquantel may also be useful preoperatively or in case of spill during surgery.

[67] Surgical excision is the only reliable means of treatment, although some reports have suggested use of albendazole or mebendazole (Wilson JF, et al. Am J Trop Med Hyg 1987;37:162; Davis A., et al. WHO 1986;64:383).

[68] Corticosteroids should be given for 2 to 3 days before and during drug therapy. Any cysticercocidal drug may cause irreparable damage when used to treat ocular or spinal cysts, even when corticosteroids are used.

[69] In ocular toxoplasmosis, corticosteroids should also be used for anti-inflammatory effect on the eyes.

[70] Pyrimethamine is teratogenic in animals. To prevent hematological toxicity from pyrimethamine, it is advisable to give leucovorin (folinic acid), about 10 mg/day, either by injection or orally. Some clinicians use pyrimethamine (50 to 100 mg daily) after a loading dose of 200 mg with a sulfonamide to treat CNS toxoplasmosis in patients with AIDS and, when sulfonamide sensitivity developed, have given clindamycin 1.8 to 2.4 gm/day in divided doses instead of the sulfonamide. In AIDS patients, chronic suppressive treatment with lower dosage should continue indefinitely (Med Lett 1991;34:95; Daneman B, et al. Ann Intern Med 1992;116:33).

[71] Congenitally infected newborns should be treated with pyrimethamine every 2 or 3 days and a sulfonamide daily for about 1 year (Remington JS, Desmonts G. In Remington JS, Klein JO, eds. Infectious disease of the fetus and newborn infant. 3rd ed. Philadelphia: WB Saunders, 1990:89).

[72] For treatment during pregnancy, continue the drug until delivery.

[73] Albendazole or flubendazole (not available in the United States) may also be effective for this indication.

[74] Sexual partners should be treated simultaneously. Outside the United States, ornidazole has also been used for this condition. Metronidazole-resistant strains have been reported; higher doses of metronidazole for longer periods are sometimes effective against these strains (Lossick J. Rev Infect Dis 1990;12:S665).

[75] In heavy infection it may be necessary to extend therapy for 3 days.

[76] The addition of γ-interferon to nifurtimox for 20 days in a limited number of patients and in experimental animals appears to have shortened the acute phase of Chagas' disease (McCabe RE, et al. J Infect Dis 1991;163:912).

[77] Limited data.

[78] In *Trypanosoma brucei gambiense* infections, eflornithine is highly effective in both the hemolymphatic and CNS stages. Its effectiveness in *Trypanosoma brucei rhodesiense* infections has been variable. Some clinicians have given 400 mg/kg/d intravenously in 4 divided doses for 14 days, followed by oral treatment with 300 mg/kg/day for 3 to 4 weeks. (Doua F, et al. Am J Trop Med Hyg 1987;37:525).

[79] In frail patients, begin with as little as 18 mg and increase the dose progressively. Pretreatment with suramin has been advocated for debilitated patients.

[80] For severe symptoms or eye involvement, corticosteroids can be used in addition.

[81] Ivermectin or albendazole may also be effective. (Sturchler D, et al. Ann Trop Med Parasitol 1989;83:473).

[82] One report of a cure using 1 gm three times a day for 21 days has been published. (Bekhti A. Ann Intern Med 1984;100:463).

Adverse Effects of Some Antiparasitic Drugs[a]

ALBENDAZOLE (Zentel)
Occasional: diarrhea; abdominal pain; migration of ascaris through mouth and nose **Rare:** leukopenia; alopecia; increased serum transaminase activity

BENZNIDAZOLE (Rochagan)
Frequent: allergic rash; dose-dependent polyneuropathy; gastrointestinal disturbances; psychic disturbances

BITHIONOL (Bitin)
Frequent: photosensitivity reactions; vomiting; diarrhea; abdominal pain; urticaria
Rare: leukopenia toxic hepatitis

CHLOROQUINE HCl and CHLOROQUINE PHOSPHATE (Aralen and others)
Occasional: pruritus; vomiting; headache; confusion; depigmentation of hair; skin eruptions; corneal opacity; weight loss; partial alopecia; extraocular muscle palsies; exacerbation of psoriasis, eczema, and other exfoliative dermatoses; myalgias; photophobia
Rare: irreversible retinal injury (especially when total dosage exceeds 100 gm); discoloration of nails and mucus membranes; nerve-type deafness; peripheral neuropathy and myopathy; heart block; blood dyscrasias; hematemesis

CROTAMITON (Eurax)
Occasional: rash; conjunctivitis

DEHYDROEMETINE
Frequent: cardiac arrhythmias; precordial pain; muscle weakness; cellulitis at site of injection
Occasional: diarrhea; vomiting; peripheral neuropathy; heart failure; headache; dyspnea

DIETHYLCARBAMAZINE CITRATE USP (Hetrazan)
Frequent: severe allergic or febrile reactions in patients with microfilaria in the blood or the skin; GI disturbances
Rare: encephalopathy

DILOXANIDE FUROATE (Furamide)
Frequent: flatulence
Occasional: nausea; vomiting; diarrhea
Rare: diplopia; dizziness; urticaria; pruritus

EFLORNITHINE (Difluoromethylornithine, DFMO, Ornidyl)
Frequent: anemia; leukopenia
Occasional: diarrhea; thrombocytopenia; seizures
Rare: hearing loss

FLUBENDAZOLE—Similar to mebendazole

[a]Modified and reprinted from The Medical Letter, Inc. 34 (Issue 865);March 6, 1992.

FURAZOLIDONE (Furoxone)
Frequent: nausea; vomiting
Occasional: allergic reactions, including pulmonary infiltration, hypotension, urticaria, fever, vesicular rash; hypoglycemia; headache
Rare: hemolytic anemia in G-6-PD deficiency and neonates; disulfiram-like reaction with alcohol; MAO-inhibitor interactions; polyneuritis

HALOFANTRINE (Halfan)
Occasional: diarrhea; abdominal pain; pruritus

IODOQUINOL (Yodoxin)
Occasional: rash; acne; slight enlargement of the thyroid gland nausea; diarrhea; cramps; anal pruritus
Rare: optic atrophy, loss of vision, peripheral neuropathy after prolonged use in high dosage (for months); iodine sensitivity

IVERMECTIN (Mectizan)
Occasional: Mazzotti-type reaction seen in onchocerciasis, including fever, pruritus, tender lymph nodes, headache, and joint and bone pain
Rare: hypotension

LINDANE (Kwell and others)
Occasional: eczematous rash; conjunctivitis
Rare: convulsions; aplastic anemia

MALATHION (Ovide)
Occasional: local irritation

MEBENDAZOLE (Vermox)
Occasional: diarrhea; abdominal pain; migration of ascaris through mouth and nose
Rare: leukopenia; agranulocytosis; hypospermia

MEFLOQUINE (Lariam)
Frequent: vertigo; lightheadedness: nausea; other gastrointestinal disturbances; nightmares; visual disturbances; headache
Occasional: confusion
Rare: psychosis; hypotension; convulsions; coma

MEGLUMINE ANTIMONIATE (Glucantime)—Similar to stibogluconate sodium

MELARSOPROL (Arsobal)
Frequent: myocardial damage; albuminuria; hypertension; colic; Herxheimer-type reaction; encephalopathy; vomiting; peripheral neuropathy
Rare: shock

METRONIDAZOLE (Flagyl and others)
Frequent: nausea; headache; dry mouth; metallic taste
Occasional: vomiting; diarrhea; insomnia; weakness; stomatitis; vertigo; paresthesias; rash; dark urine; urethral burning; disulfiram-like reaction with alcohol
Rare: seizures; encephalopathy; pseudomembranous colitis; ataxia; leukopenia; peripheral neuropathy; pancreatitis

NICLOSAMIDE (Niclocide)
Occasional: nausea; abdominal pain

NIFURTIMOX (Lampit)
Frequent: anorexia; vomiting; weight loss; loss of memory; sleep disorders; tremor; paresthesias; weakness; polyneuritis
Rare: convulsions; fever; pulmonary infiltrates and pleural effusion

ORNIDAZOLE (Tiberal)
Occasional: dizziness; headache; gastrointestinal disturbances
Rare: reversible peripheral neuropathy

OXAMNIQUINE (Vansil)
Occasional: headache; fever; dizziness; somnolence; nausea; diarrhea; rash; insomnia; hepatic enzyme changes; ECG changes; EEG changes; orange-red discoloration of urine
Rare: seizures; neuropsychiatric disturbances

PAROMOMYCIN (Humatin)
Frequent: GI disturbances
Rare: eighth-nerve damage (mainly auditory); renal damage

PENTAMIDINE ISETHIONATE (Pentam 300, NebuPent)
Frequent: hypotension; hypoglycemia often followed by diabetes mellitus; vomiting; blood dyscrasias; renal damage; pain at injection site; GI disturbances
Occasional: May aggravate diabetes; shock; hypocalcemia; liver damage; cardiotoxicity; delirium; rash
Rare: Herxheimer-type reaction; anaphylaxis; acute pancreatitis; hyperkalemia

PERMETHRIN (Nix, Elimite)
Occasional: burning; stinging; numbness; increased pruritus; pain; edema; erythema; rash

PRAZIQUANTEL (Biltricide)
Frequent: malaise; headache; dizziness
Occasional: sedation; abdominal discomfort; fever; sweating; nausea; eosinophilia; fatigue
Rare: pruritus; rash

PRIMAQUINE PHOSPHATE USP
Frequent: hemolytic anemia in G-6-PD deficiency
Occasional: neutropenia; GI disturbances; methemoglobinemia in G-6-PD deficiency
Rare: CNS symptoms; hypertension; arrhythmias

PROGUANIL (Paludrine)
Occasional: oral ulceration; hair loss; scaling of palms and soles
Rare: hematuria (with large doses); vomiting; abdominal pain; diarrhea (with large doses)

PYRANTEL PAMOATE (Antiminth)
Occasional: GI disturbances; headache; dizziness; rash; fever

PYRETHRINS and PIPERONYL BUTOXIDE (RID and others)
Occasional: allergic reactions
PYRIMETHAMINE USP (Daraprim)
Occasional: blood dyscrasias; folic acid deficiency
Rare: rash; vomiting; convulsions; shock; possibly pulmonary eosinophilia
QUINACRINE HCl USP (Atabrine)
Frequent: dizziness; headache; vomiting; diarrhea
Occasional: yellow staining of skin; toxic psychosis; insomnia; bizarre dreams; blood dyscrasias; urticaria; blue and black nail pigmentation; psoriasis-like rash
Rare: acute hepatic necrosis; convulsions; severe exfoliative dermatitis; ocular effects similar to those caused by chloroquine
QUININE DIHYDROCHLORIDE and SULFATE
Frequent: cinchonism (tinnitus, headache, nausea, abdominal pain, visual disturbance)
Occasional: deafness; hemolytic anemia; other blood dyscrasias; photosensitivity reactions; hypoglycemia; arrhythmias; hypotension; drug fever
Rare: blindness; sudden death if injected too rapidly
SPIRAMYCIN (Rovamycine)
Occasional: GI disturbances
Rare: allergic reactions
STIBOGLUCONATE SODIUM (Pentostam)
Frequent: muscle pain and joint stiffness; nausea; transaminase elevations; T-wave flattening or inversion
Occasional: weakness; colic; liver damage; bradycardia; leukopenia
Rare: diarrhea; rash; pruritus; myocardial damage; hemolytic anemia; renal damage; shock; sudden death
SURAMIN SODIUM (Germanin)
Frequent: vomiting; pruritus; urticaria; paresthesias; hyperesthesia of hands and feet; photophobia; peripheral neuropathy
Occasional: kidney damage; blood dyscrasias; shock; optic atrophy
THIABENDAZOLE (mintezol)
Frequent: nausea; vomiting; vertigo
Occasional: leukopenia; crystalluria; rash; hallucinations; olfactory disturbance; erythema multiforme; Stevens-Johnson syndrome
Rare: shock; tinnitus; intrahepatic cholestasis; convulsions; angioneurotic edema
TINIDAZOLE (Fassyn)
Occasional: metallic taste; nausea; vomiting; rash
TRIMETREXATE (with ''leucovorin rescue'')
Occasional: rash; peripheral neuropathy; bone marrow depression; increased serum aminotransferase concentrations
TRYPARSAMIDE
Frequent: nausea; vomiting
Occasional: impaired vision; optic atrophy; fever; exfoliative dermatitis; allergic reactions; tinnitus

Table 9.2. Classification of the Major Helminths and Drugs Used to Treat Helminthiasis

Disease Name(s)	Parasite	Geographical Distribution	Usual Source and Route of Infection	Vector or Intermediate Host	Stage(s) in Humans	Site(s) of Involvement	Drug(s) of Choice	Alternative Drugs
CESTODES (Tapeworms)								
Intestinal Infections								
Diphyllobothriasis	*Diphyllobothrium latum* Fish tapeworm	Cosmopolitan (more common in temperate areas)	Freshwater Crustacea to fish to humans	Freshwater Crustacea to fish to humans	Adults	Ileum	Niclosamide or praziquantel	None
Dipylidiasis	*Dipylidium caninum* Dog tapeworm	Cosmopolitan	Dog or cat fleas to mouth	Dog or cat flea	Adults	Small intestine	Niclosamide or praziquantel	None
Hymenolepiasis	*Hymenolepis nana* Dwarf tapeworm	Cosmopolitan	Human feces to soil to food. Fecal contamination	None	Larvae and adults	Small intestine	Praziquantel	Niclosamide
Taeniasis	*Taenia saginata* Beef tapeworm	Cosmopolitan (mainly Middle East, Kenya, Ethiopia, South America, Mexico, Russia)	Beef as food	Cattle	Adults	Small intestine	Niclosamide or praziquantel	Albendazole*
Taeniasis	*Taenia solium* Pork tapeworm	Cosmopolitan (common in Mexico, Central and South America, India, China, South Africa)	Pork as food	Swine	Adults	Small intestine	Niclosamide or praziquantel	Albendazole*
Tissue Infections								
Cysticercosis (neurocysticercosis)	*Cysticercus cellulosae* Cysticercoid stage of *Taenia solium*	Cosmopolitan (common in Mexico, Central and South America, India, China)	*T. solium* eggs in fecal-contaminated food or soil, carrier self-contamination, or reverse peristalsis	Swine	Larvae	Any tissue, especially skeletal muscle, central nervous system, and eye	Albendazole*	Praziquantel

Disease	Organism	Distribution	Transmission	Reservoir hosts	Stage	Location	Drug of choice	Alternative drugs
Echinococcosis Alveolar hydatid disease	Echinococcus multilocularis	Cosmopolitan (domestic cycle involving dogs and domestic herbivores; sylvatic cycle involving foxes and rodents (primarily in Northern Hemisphere)	Canine fecal contamination	Wild rodents (lemmings, mice, shrews, voles) Humans (abnormal host)	Larvae	Liver, with contiguous structural invasion and metastasis to distant sites (brain, lung, mediastinum)	Surgery plus adjunctive use of albendazole[a] or mebendazole	Albendazole[a] or mebendazole for inoperable cases
Cystic hydatid Disease	Echinococcus granulosus	Cosmopolitan (primarily involving domestic dogs and herbivores; northern sylvatic cycle also exists)	Canine fecal contamination	Herbivores (camels, goats, horses, pigs, sheep, yaks) Humans	Larvae	Primarily liver, lung; other sites, including muscle, bone, kidney, spleen, brain; noninvasive encapsulated cysts	Surgery plus adjunctive use of albendazole[a] or mebendazole	Albendazole[a] or mebendazole for inoperable cases

NEMATODES (Roundworms)
Intestinal Infections

Disease	Organism	Distribution	Transmission	Reservoir hosts	Stage	Location	Drug of choice	Alternative drugs
Ascariasis	Ascaris lumbricoides Roundworm	Cosmopolitan (more common in tropics)	Human feces to soil to food	None	Larvae and adults	Small intestine	Pyrantel pamoate or mebendazole	Albendazole[a] Piperazine citrate
Enterobiasis	Enterobius vermicularis Pinworm, seatworm	Cosmopolitan (less common in tropics)	Anal contact Fecal or soil contamination to food	None	Larvae and adults	Cecum, ascending colon, ileum	Pyrantel pamoate or mebendazole	Albendazole[a] Piperazine citrate
Strongyloidiasis (Cochin-China diarrhea)	Strongyloides stercoralis Threadworm	Tropics and subtropics (more common in tropics)	Human feces to soil to skin	None	Larvae and adults	Small intestine, lung	Thiabendazole[b]	Albendazole[a] Mebendazole Ivermectin
Trichuriasis	Trichuris trichiura Whipworm	Cosmopolitan (more common in tropics)	Human feces to soil to food	None	Larvae and adults	Cecum, upper colon, rectum, appendix	Mebendazole[b]	Albendazole[a]
Uncinariasis (ancylostomiasis, Miner's anemia)	Ancylostoma duodenale Old World, European, or Common hookworm	Tropics and subtropics (Europe, North Africa, Middle and Far East, South America)	Human feces to soil to skin or food	None	Larvae and adults	Small intestine	Pyrantel pamoate or mebendazole	Albendazole[a]

Table 9.2—continued

Disease Name(s)	Parasite	Geographical Distribution	Usual Source and Route of Infection	Vector or Intermediate Host	Stage(s) in Humans	Site(s) of Involvement	Drug(s) of Choice	Alternative Drugs
Uncinariasis (Necatoriasis)	Necator americanus New World or American hookworm	Tropics and subtropics (Americas, Italy, tropical Africa, Asia)	Human feces to soil to skin	None	Larvae and adults	Small intestine	Pyrantel pamoate or mebendazole	Albendazole[a]
Tissue Infections Cutaneous larva migrans (creeping eruption)	Ancylostoma braziliense	Tropics and subtropics (Asia, Africa, Americas, Pacific)	Cat and dog feces to soil to skin	Cats, dogs	Larvae only (in epidermis)	Skin	Thiabendazole (oral and topical)	Albendazole (oral)
Dracunculiasis (dracontiasis, dirofilariasis, Guinea worm infection)	ciDracunculus medinensis Guinea worm	Subsaharan Africa, India, Pakistan	Ingesting infected water fleas	Cyclops Water flea	Cyclops Water flea	Larvae and adults	Loose connective tissue and skin	Anthelmintic therapy not indicated.[c] Topical antibiotics and tetanus toxoid may be useful.
Filariasis Brugiasis	Brugia (species unknown)	North American (Eastern United States)	Insect bite	Unknown	Adults (macrofilariae)	Lymph nodes	Drug therapy not indicated: surgery when necessary	None
Brugiasis (lymphatic, Malayan, or Brug's filariasis)	Brugia malayi, B. timori	Southeast Asia (Malaya, Borneo, India, Ceylon, tropical China)	Insect bite	Mansonoides mosquito	Larvae (microfilariae in blood) and adults (macrofilariae)	Lymphatics, blood	Diethylcarbamazine citrate	None
Loiasis (eyeworm disease of Africa, Calabar swelling disease)	Loa loa	West and Central Africa (rain forest)	Insect bite	Chrysops fly	Larvae (microfilariae in blood) and adults (macrofilariae)	Lymphatics, blood, subcutaneous tissue, skin	Diethylcarbamazine citrate	Mebenedazole
Lymphatic filariasis (Bancroftian or Wuchereriasis)	Wuchereria bancrofti	Asia, Africa, Pacific, South America	Insect bite	Culex, Aedes, and Anopheles mosquitoes	Larvae (microfilariae in blood) and adults (macrofilariae)	Lymphatics, blood	Diethylcarbamazine citrate	Ivermectin[a]

Disease	Organism	Transmission	Geographic distribution	Vector/reservoir	Stage	Location in body	Drug of choice	Alternative drug
Mansonellosis (dipetalonemiasis)	Mansonella perstans	Insect bite	West and Central Africa, South America	Culicoides midge	Larvae (microfilariae in blood) and adults (macrofilariae)	Lymphatics, blood, serous cavities	Diethylcarbamazine citrate	Mebendazole
Onchocerciasis (river blindness)	Onchocerca volvulus	Insect bite	Africa, Yemen, Central and South America	Simulium (black fly)	Larvae (microfilariae) migrate and adults (macrofilariae) in skin	Lymphatics, blood, skin, subcutaneous tissue, eye	Ivermectin*	Diethylcarbamazine citrate followed by suramin*
Ozzardi filariasis	Mansonella ozzardi	Insect bite	South America, West Indies	Culicoides and Simulium	Larvae (microfilariae in blood) and adults (macrofilariae)	Lymphatics, blood, visceral adipose tissue	Ivermectin*	None
Pulmonary dirofilariasis	Dirofilaria immitis	Insect bite	Cosmopolitan	Mosquito	Adults only	Lung	Drug therapy not indicated; surgery when necessary	
Toxocariasis (visceral larva migrans)	Toxocara canis, T. cati	Cat and dog feces to soil to skin	Cosmopolitan (common in North America and Europe)	Dogs, cats	Larvae only	Liver, lungs; occasionally kidney, brain, eye	Mebendazole or thiabendazole plus corticosteroids* if symptoms are severe, especially if there is ocular involvement	Albendazole* Diethylcarbamazine citrate
Trichinosis (trichinelliasis)	Trichinella spiralis Pork roundworm	Meat as food (usually pork)	Cosmopolitan (more common in Northern Hemisphere than in tropics)	Swine (mainly)	Larvae and adults	Small intestine	Thiabendazole plus corticosteroids*	Mebendazole* Pyrantel pamoate (kills only adult worms) Albendazole*
TREMATODES (Flukes) Clonorchiasis	Clonorchis sinensis Chinese liver fluke	Human and animal feces to water to soil to fish as food	Far East, mainly Japan, Korea, China, Vietnam	Snail, fish (other definitive hosts are cats, dogs, rats)	Larvae and adults	Biliary tract	Praziquantel	None
Fascioliasis	Fasciola hepatica Sheep liver fluke	Sheep feces to water to snail to wild watercress and other pasture food plants	Cosmopolitan (more common in Europe, Cuba, and Chile)	Snail (sheep and cattle are definitive hosts)	Larvae and adult	Biliary tract	Praziquantel	Bithionol*

Table 9.2—continued

Disease Name(s)	Parasite	Geographical Distribution	Usual Source and Route of Infection	Vector or Intermediate Host	Stage(s) in Humans	Site(s) of Involvement	Drug(s) of Choice	Alternative Drugs
Fasciolopsiasis	*Fasciolopsis buski* Giant intestinal fluke	China, India, Indonesia, Thailand, Malaya, Taiwan	Swine feces to soil to snail to water plants (e.g., water chestnuts)	Snail, freshwater plants	Adults	Small intestine	Praziquantel	Niclosamide
Opisthorchiasis	*Opisthorchis viverrini* liver fluke	Far East, mainly Japan, Korea, China, Vietnam	Human and animal feces to water to snail to soil to fish as food	Snail, fish (other definitive hosts are cats, dogs, rats)	Larvae and adults	Biliary tract	Praziquantel	None
Paragonimiasis	*Paragonimus westermani* Lung fluke	Far East, Central and South America	Human sputum and feces to soil to snail to freshwater crabs used as food	Snail, freshwater crabs	Larvae and adults	Lung; occasionally central nervous and gastrointestinal systems	Praziquantel	Bithionol*
Schistosomiasis (African)	*Schistosoma intercalatum* African blood fluke	Africa	Skin penetration from contaminated water	Freshwater snail	Larvae (penetrate the skin) and adults	Veins of small and large intestine, other tissues	Praziquantel	None
Schistosomiasis (Chinese or Oriental)	*Schistosoma japonicum, S. mekongi* Oriental blood fluke	Japan, China, Philippines, Celebes	Skin penetration from contaminated water	Freshwater snail	Larvae (penetrate the skin) and adults	Veins of small and large intestine, other tissues	Praziquantel	None
Schistosomiasis (intestinal)	*Schistosoma mansoni* Blood fluke	Africa, West Indies, South America, Middle East	Skin penetration from contaminated water	Freshwater snail	Larvae (penetrate the skin) and adults	Veins of small and large intestines, other tissues	Praziquantel	Oxaminiquine
Schistosomiasis (urinary)	*Schistosoma haematobium* Blood fluke	Iraq, Africa, Near East, Madagascar	Skin penetration from contaminated water	Freshwater snail	Larvae (penetrate the skin) and adults	Veins of urinary bladder, other tissues	Praziquantel	Metrifonate*

Reprinted with permission from The American Medical Association Drug Evaluations Annual, 1994.

[a] Investigational drug in the United States.

[b] Follow-up threapy with pyrantel pamoate may be indicated if multiple infection with *Ascaris* roundworms and pinworms also present.

[c] Although nitroimidazoles (e.g., metronidazole, niridazole) are used in this disease, their beneficial effect appears to be unrelated to any antiparasitic action; they probably minimize the high risk of secondary skin infection and inflammation that accompany the primary lesion.

[d] Thiabendazole is nematocidal in conventional doses during early larval migration; corticosteroids reduce the marked inflammation that usually occurs during the migration.

[e] Mebendazole, used in a larger dose and for a longer duration than for intestinal worms, kills encysted larvae (Levin ML. Treatment of trichinosis with mebendazole. Am J Trop Med Hyg 1983;32(5):980–983.

SECTION 10

Tuberculosis

Preventing Transmission of Tuberculosis in Health-Care Facilities[a]

I. Introduction

A. OVERVIEW

This summary emphasizes the importance of (1) the hierarchy of control measures including administrative and engineering controls and personal respiratory protection, (2) health-care facility risk assessment and development of a written tuberculosis (TB) control plan, (3) early diagnosis and management of persons with TB, (4) purified protein derivative (PPD) skin testing programs, and (5) health-care worker (HCW) education (1).

Transmission of TB is a recognized risk in health-care facilities. Transmission is most likely to occur from patients with unrecognized pulmonary or laryngeal TB who are not receiving effective antituberculosis therapy and have not been placed in TB isolation. Several recent TB outbreaks in health-care facilities, including outbreaks of multidrug-resistant TB (MDR-TB), have heightened concern about nosocomial transmission. Increases in TB in many areas are related to the high risk of TB among immunosuppressed persons, particularly those infected with the human immunodeficiency virus (HIV). Transmission of *Mycobacterium tuberculosis* infection to persons with HIV infection is of particular concern because they are at high risk of developing active TB if infected. Thus, health-care facilities should be particularly alert to the need for preventing TB transmission in settings in which persons with HIV infection work or receive care.

An effective TB infection control program requires early diagnosis, isolation, and treatment of persons with active TB. The primary emphasis of the TB infection control plan should be achieving these three goals by the application of a hierarchy of control measures, including (1) the use of administrative measures to reduce the risk of exposure to persons with infectious TB, (2) the use of engineering controls to prevent the spread and reduce the concentration of infectious droplet nuclei, and (3) the use of personal respiratory protective equipment in areas where there is still a risk of exposure to *M. tuberculosis*, such as

---

[a]Modified and reprinted from Centers for Disease Control and Prevention draft guidelines for preventing the transmission of tuberculosis in health-care facilities. Federal Register, October 12, 1993. Atlanta: Department of Health and Human Services. 1993;Part II:52810-54.

332

TB isolation rooms. Implementation of an optimum TB control program requires risk assessment; early identification and isolation of infectious TB patients; effective engineering controls; an appropriate respiratory protection program; and HCW TB education, counseling, screening, and evaluation.

B. EPIDEMIOLOGY, TRANSMISSION, AND PATHOGENESIS

TB is not evenly distributed throughout all segments of the U.S. population. Some subgroups or individuals have a higher risk of TB either because they are more likely than the general population to have been exposed to and infected by *M. tuberculosis* or because they are more likely to progress to active TB once infected (3). In some cases, both of these factors may be present. Groups known to have a higher prevalence of TB infection include medically underserved populations (including some African-Americans, Hispanics, Asians and Pacific Islanders, American Indians, and Alaskan Natives), homeless persons, current or past prison inmates, alcoholics, injecting drug users, the elderly, foreign-born persons from areas of the world with a high prevalence of TB (e.g., Asia, Africa, the Caribbean, and Latin America), and contacts to persons with active TB. Groups with a higher risk of progression from latent TB infection to active disease include persons with certain medical conditions, including HIV infection, silicosis, status post gastrectomy, jejunoileal bypass surgery, being ≥10% below ideal body weight, chronic renal failure, diabetes mellitus, immunosuppression due to receipt of high-dose corticosteroid or other immunosuppressive therapy, and some malignancies; persons who have been recently infected (within the past 2 years); young children (≤5 years old); and persons with fibrotic lesions on chest radiograph (3).

   M. tuberculosis is carried in airborne particles, known as droplet nuclei, that can be generated when persons with pulmonary or laryngeal TB sneeze, cough, speak, or sing (4). The particles are estimated to be approximately 1 to 5 μm in size, and normal air currents keep them airborne and can spread them throughout a room or building (5). Infection occurs when a susceptible person inhales droplet nuclei containing *M. tuberculosis*, and bacilli are able to traverse the mouth or nasal passages, upper respiratory tract, and bronchi to reach the alveoli of the lungs. Once in the alveoli, the organisms are taken up by alveolar macrophages and spread throughout the body. Usually within 2 to 10 weeks after initial infection with *M. tuberculosis*, the immune response limits further multiplication and spread of the tubercle bacilli; however, some of the bacilli remain dormant and viable for many years. This is known as latent TB infection. Persons with latent TB infection usually have a positive PPD skin test, but they have no symptoms of active TB, and they are not infectious. In general, persons with latent TB infection have approximately a 10% risk during their lifetime for the development of active TB. The risk is greatest in the first 2 years after infection, but some risk persists for decades.

   Persons with immunocompromising conditions have a greater risk for the progression of latent TB infection to active disease. HIV infection is the strongest known risk factor yet identified for the progression from latent TB infection to active TB disease. Persons with latent TB infection who become infected with HIV have approximately an 8 to 10% risk per year for the development of active TB (6). Persons who are infected with HIV and become newly infected with TB have an even greater risk for the development of active TB (7–10).

The probability that a susceptible person will become infected with *M. tuberculosis* depends primarily upon the concentration of infectious droplet nuclei in the air and the duration of exposure. Characteristics of the TB patient that enhance transmission include (1) disease in the lungs, airways, or larynx; (2) presence of cough or other forceful expiratory measures; (3) presence of acid-fast bacilli (AFB) in the sputum; (4) failure of the patient to cover the mouth and nose when coughing; (5) presence of cavitation on chest radiograph; (6) short duration of adequate chemotherapy; and (7) administration of procedures that can induce coughing or cause aerosolization of *M. tuberculosis* (e.g., sputum induction). Environmental factors that enhance the likelihood of transmission include (1) exposure of susceptible persons to an infectious person in relatively small, enclosed spaces; (2) inadequate local or general ventilation that results in insufficient dilution and/or removal of infectious droplet nuclei; and (3) recirculation of air containing infectious droplet nuclei.

C. RISK OF NOSOCOMIAL TB TRANSMISSION

TB transmission is a recognized risk in health-care facilities (11–19). The magnitude of the risk varies considerably by type of health-care facility; prevalence of TB in the community, patient population served, job category, area of the health-care facility in which a person works; and the effectiveness of TB infection control interventions. The risk may be higher in areas where patients with TB are provided care before diagnosis and initiation of TB isolation precautions (e.g., clinic waiting areas and emergency rooms) or where diagnostic or treatment procedures that stimulate coughing are performed. Nosocomial transmission of TB has been associated with close contact with infectious patients or HCWs, and during procedures such as bronchoscopy (14), endotracheal intubation and suctioning (15), open abscess irrigation (17), and autopsy (18, 19). Sputum induction and aerosol treatments that induce cough may also increase the potential for TB transmission (20, 21). Health-care facility personnel should be particularly alert to the need for preventing TB transmission in health-care facilities in which immunocompromised persons, such as persons with HIV infection, work and/or receive care, especially if cough-inducing procedures, such as sputum induction and aerosolized pentamidine treatments, are being performed.

Several TB outbreaks in health-care facilities have been reported during the past several years (9, 21–26). Many of these outbreaks involved transmission of MDR strains of *M. tuberculosis* to both patients and HCWs. Most of the patients and some of the HCWs were HIV-infected persons in whom new infection progressed rapidly to active disease. Mortality associated with those outbreaks was very high (range 43 to 93%). Furthermore, the time between diagnosis and death was very short, with the median interval ranging from 4 to 16 weeks. Factors contributing to these outbreaks included delayed diagnosis of patients with TB, delayed recognition of drug resistance, delayed initiation of effective therapy resulting in prolonged infectiousness, delayed initiation and inadequate duration of TB isolation, inadequate ventilation in TB isolation rooms, lapses in TB isolation practices, and inadequate precautions for cough-inducing procedures. There is evidence from three of the facilities that MDR-TB transmission decreased significantly or ceased in areas where measures similar to those in the previously published CDC guidelines were implemented (2, 27–30). Since several interventions were implemented simultaneously, it cannot be determined which played the most important role in reducing transmission.

D. FUNDAMENTALS OF TB INFECTION CONTROL

An effective TB control program requires early identification, isolation, and treatment of persons with active TB. The primary emphasis of the TB infection control plan should be achieving these three goals. In all health-care facilities, particularly those in which persons who are at high risk for TB work or receive care, policies and procedures for TB control should be developed, periodically reviewed, and evaluated for effectiveness to determine the actions necessary to minimize the risk of TB transmission.

The TB control program should be based on a hierarchy of control measures. The first and most important level of the hierarchy is the use of administrative measures to reduce the risk of exposure to persons with infectious TB. This includes developing and implementing effective written policies and protocols to ensure the rapid identification, isolation, diagnostic evaluation, and treatment of persons likely to have TB, as well as implementing effective work practices by persons working in the health-care facility.

The second level of the hierarchy is the use of engineering controls to prevent the spread and reduce the concentration of infectious droplet nuclei. This includes (1) direct source control using local exhaust ventilation, (2) controlling direction of air flow to prevent contamination of air in areas adjacent to the infectious source, (3) dilution and removal of contaminated air via general ventilation, and (4) air cleaning via air filtration or ultraviolet germicidal irradiation (UVGI).

The first two approaches minimize the number of areas in the health-care facility where exposure to infectious TB may occur and reduce, but do not eliminate, the risk in those few areas (e.g., TB isolation rooms and treatment rooms where cough-inducing procedures are performed) where exposure may still occur. Because persons entering isolation and treatment rooms may be exposed to *M. tuberculosis*, the third level of the hierarchy is the use of personal respiratory protective equipment in these and a few other situations of probable relatively higher risk.

Specific measures to reduce the risk of TB transmission include the following:

Assigning supervisory responsibility for the design, implementation, and maintenance of the TB infection control program to specific persons in the health-care facility (Part II.A);

Conducting a risk assessment to evaluate the risk of TB transmission in all parts of the health-care facility, developing a written TB control program based on the risk assessment, and periodically repeating the risk assessment to evaluate the effectiveness of the TB infection control program (Part II.B);

Developing, implementing, and enforcing policies and protocols to ensure early identification of patients who may have infectious TB (Parts II.C and III.A);

Providing prompt triage and appropriate management of patients who may have infectious TB in the outpatient setting (Part II.D);

Promptly initiating and maintaining TB isolation, diagnostic evaluation, and treatment for persons who may have infectious TB and who are admitted to the inpatient setting (Part II.E); Developing, installing, maintaining, and evaluating ventilation and other engineering controls to reduce the potential for airborne exposure to *M. tuberculosis* (Part II.F) (1);

Developing, implementing, maintaining, and evaluating a respiratory protection program (Parts II.G and III.C);

Using appropriate precautions for cough-inducing procedures (Part II.H) (1);

Educating and training HCWs about TB, effective methods for prevention of TB transmission, and the benefits of medical screening programs (Part II.I);

Developing and implementing a program for routine periodic screening of HCWs for active TB and TB infection (Parts II.J and III.B);

Promptly evaluating possible episodes of transmission of TB in health-care facilities, including HCW PPD skin test conversions, clusters of cases in HCWs or patients, and contacts of TB patients who were not promptly identified and isolated (Part II.K);

Coordinating activities with the local public health department, emphasizing reporting, adequate discharge follow-up, and ensuring continuation and completion of therapy (Part II.L).

II. Recommendations

A. ASSIGNMENT OF RESPONSIBILITY

Supervisory responsibility for the TB control program should be assigned to designated persons with expertise in infection control, occupational health, and engineering.

B. RISK ASSESSMENT, DEVELOPMENT OF THE TB CONTROL PLAN, AND PERIODIC REASSESSMENT

1. Risk Assessment
a. General.   TB control measures for each health-care facility should be based on a careful assessment of the risk of TB transmission in that setting. Therefore, the first step in developing the TB control program should be conducting an initial risk assessment (Fig. 10.1). The purpose of this assessment is to evaluate the risk of TB transmission in each area and occupational group in the

Analyze purified protein derivative (PPD) test conversion data, number of TB cases, and other risk factors by area and occupation group

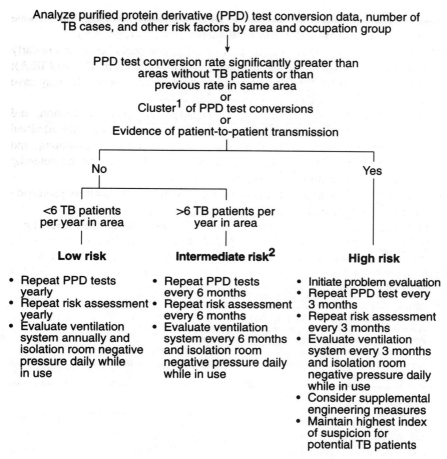

Figure 10.1. Risk assessment. *1*, Cluster refers to two or more PPD conversions in one area or in a single occupational group that works in multiple areas over a 3-month period. *2*, Occurrence of a drug-resistant TB in the facility or the community, or high prevalence of HIV infection among patients or workers in the facility may warrant a higher risk.

facility so that appropriate infection control interventions can be developed based on actual risk.[b]

The risk assessment should be conducted by a group of qualified personnel, which may include hospital epidemiologists, infectious disease specialists, pulmonary disease specialists, infection control practitioners, health-care administrators, occupational health personnel, engineers, HCWs, and local public health authorities.

---

[b]Regardless of risk level, the management of patients with known or suspected infectious TB will not vary. However, the index of suspicion for infectious TB among patients, the frequency of HCW PPD skin testing, the number of TB isolation rooms, and other factors will vary by whether the risk of TB transmission in the facility, area, or occupational group is high, intermediate, or low.

Table 10.1. Elements of the Risk Assessment

1. Review the number of TB patients seen by area (inpatient and outpatient). (This information can be obtained by laboratory surveillance or medical record review).
2. Review the drug susceptibility patterns of TB patients seen at the facility.
3. Analyze HCW PPD test data by area (or by occupational group for persons not assigned to a specific area such as respiratory therapists).

Review medical records of a sample of consecutive TB patients seen at the facility to evaluate infection control parameters.
Calculate intervals from:
   Admission until TB suspected
   Admission until TB evaluation performed
   Admission under AFB specimens ordered
   AFB specimens ordered until AFB specimens collected
   AFB specimens collected until AFB smears done and reported
   AFB specimens collected until cultures done and reported
   AFB specimens collected until species identification done and reported
   AFB specimens collected until drug susceptibility tests done and reported
   Admission until TB isolation initiated
   Admission until TB treatment initiated
   Duration of TB isolation
Additional information:
   Were appropriate criteria used for discontinuing isolation?
   History of prior admission to facility
   Adequacy of TB treatment regimen
   Were follow-up sputum specimens collected appropriately?
   Was appropriate discharge planning conducted?
   Perform an observational review of TB infection control practices.
   Perform a review of the most recent environmental evaluation and maintenance procedures.

The risk assessment should be done for the facility as a whole and for individual areas of the institution (e.g., medical, TB, pulmonary, or HIV wards; HIV, infectious disease, or pulmonary clinics; emergency departments or areas where TB patients may receive care or where cough-inducing procedures are performed, etc.). In addition, risk assessments should be done for individual groups of HCWs that work throughout the institution (e.g., respiratory therapists, bronchoscopists, environmental services, dietary, maintenance, housestaff by specialty, etc.).

The elements of a risk assessment are summarized in Table 10.1. Classification of risk as high, intermediate, or low in a specific area and for a specific occupational category should be based on (1) the number of infectious TB patients admitted to the area or ward or the estimated number of infectious TB patients to whom HCWs in an occupational category may be exposed and (2) the results of analysis of HCW PPD test conversions and possible patient-to-patient TB transmission (Fig. 10.1).

All TB infection control programs should include periodic PPD testing and reassessment of risk. The frequency of repeat skin testing and risk assessment should be selected on the basis of the most recent risk assessment (Fig. 10.1):

"Low-risk" areas or groups are those in which (1) the PPD test conversion rate is not greater than in areas or groups without occupational exposure to TB patients or than previous rates in the same area or group, (2) there are no clusters of PPD test conversions, (3) there is no evidence of patient-to patient transmission, and (4) (in the case of an area) there are <6 TB patients hospitalized per year.

"Intermediate-risk" areas or groups are those in which (1) the PPD test conversion rate is not greater than in areas without occupational exposure to TB patients or than previous rates in the same area or group, (2) there are no clusters of PPD conversions, (3) there is no evidence of patient-to-patient transmission, and (4) there are ≥6 TB patients hospitalized per year. (NOTE: Even if there is no evidence of *M. tuberculosis* transmission, areas or groups encountering ≥6 TB patients per year still have a potential for transmission and should be classified as intermediate risk.)

"High-risk" areas or groups are those in which (1) the PPD test conversion rate is significantly greater than that in areas without occupational exposure to TB patients or than previous rates in the same area or group, or (2) there is a cluster of PPD test conversions, or (3) there is other evidence of patient-to-patient or patient-to-HCW transmission of *M. tuberculosis*. If no data or insufficient data for determination of risk have been collected on PPD test conversions among HCWs, the number of TB patients who have received care in that area, or from an occupational group, these data should be compiled, analyzed, and reviewed expeditiously. Until such data are analyzed and found to warrant a lesser risk rating, all acute care areas and occupational groups likely to encounter TB patients or be exposed to *M. tuberculosis* should be considered high risk.

b. Case Surveillance.   Data on the number of active TB cases among patients and HCWs in the facility should be systematically collected, reviewed, and used to estimate the number of isolation rooms needed, recognize clusters of nosocomial transmission, and assess the level of potential occupational risk. Information regarding the number of TB patients by specific area can be obtained by review of laboratory surveillance data on specimens positive for AFB smears and/or *M. tuberculosis* cultures.

Drug-susceptibility characteristics of *M. tuberculosis* isolates (i.e., the antituberculous agents to which each isolate is susceptible and those to which it is resistant) from TB patients seen in the facility should be reviewed to identify the frequency and patterns of drug resistance. This information may indicate a need to modify the initial treatment regimen or may suggest evidence of nosocomial transmission or increased occupational risk.

c. Analysis of HCW PPD Test Screening Data.   In addition to being recorded in individual HCWs employee health records, results of PPD testing should also be recorded in a retrievable aggregate data base of all HCW PPD test results. Identifying information should be handled confidentially. PPD test conversion rates should be calculated at appropriate intervals to estimate the risk of PPD test conversion for each area in the facility and for each specific occupational group not assigned to a specific area. In order to calculate PPD test conversion rates, it is necessary to know the total number of PPD-negative persons working in each area or group (denominator) and the number of PPD test conversions among HCWs in each area or group (numerator).

PPD test conversion rates for each area should be compared to rates in areas without occupational exposure to *M. tuberculosis* and to previous rates in the same area to identify areas where the risk of occupational PPD test conversion may be increased. When comparing conversion rates by area, a low number of HCWs in a specific area may result in a greatly increased rate of conversion for that area although the risk may not actually be meaningfully higher than for other areas. Testing for statistical significance (e.g., Fisher's exact test or chi square) may assist interpretation. However, lack of statistical significance may not rule out a problem because, if the number of HCWs tested is low, there may not be adequate statistical power to detect a significant difference. Thus, some interpretation of individual situations is indicated.

Any time a cluster of PPD test conversions is noted, further evaluation is indicated (Part II.K.1). A cluster is defined as PPD test conversions in ≥ 2 persons in one area, or in a single occupational group that works in multiple areas (e.g., respiratory therapy, dietary, etc.), over a 3-month time period.

The frequency and comprehensiveness of the HCW PPD testing program should be evaluated periodically to assure that all HCWs are being included in the program and tested at appropriate intervals. For surveillance purposes, it may be advantageous to stagger the testing of HCWs in a given area or occupational group, since this may lead to earlier detection of transmission (Part II.J.3).

d. Review of TB Patient Medical Records.   The medical records of a sample of consecutive TB patients admitted to the facility should be reviewed periodically to evaluate infection control parameters (Table 10.1). Parameters to examine include the intervals from date of admission until TB was suspected, specimens for AFB smears were ordered and collected, tests performed, and results reported. Adequacy of TB treatment regimens should also be evaluated.

Medical record reviews should also note previous admissions before onset of TB. Patient-to-patient transmission may be suspected if active TB occurs in a patient with a prior hospitalization during which exposure to another TB patient occurred or if ≥ 2 patients with a characteristic drug susceptibility or DNA fingerprint pattern are detected.

Data from the case review should be used to determine if there is a need to modify (1) protocols for identifying and isolating patients who may have infectious TB, (2) laboratory procedures, (3) administrative policies and practices, or (4) protocols for patient management.

e. Observation of Infection Control Practices.   Assessment of adherence to the policies of the TB control program should be part of the evaluation process. This assessment should be performed on a regular basis and whenever there is an increase in HCW PPD test conversions or number of TB patients. Areas at high risk for TB transmission should be monitored more frequently. The review of patient records discussed above provides information on HCW adherence to a portion of the policies. In addition, observation of work practices related to

TB isolation should be done to determine if employers are enforcing and HCWs are adhering to the policies and enforcing patient adherence. Whenever poor adherence to policies is recognized, the situation should be evaluated to determine if problems exist that interfere with adherence to procedures, and appropriate education and other corrective action should be implemented.

   f. Engineering Evaluation.   Engineering measures should be evaluated and monitored according to the appropriate TB control protocol schedule (Part II.B.2) (1). Data from the most recent evaluation and from review of maintenance procedures and logs should be carefully reviewed as a part of the risk assessment.

2. Development of the TB Infection Control Plan

   Based on the risk assessment, a written TB infection control plan should be developed and implemented for each area of the facility (or occupational group for those HCWs not assigned to a specific area of the facility). There are optimum measures that all health-care facilities should implement to ensure that a program suitable to the needs of HCWs and patients is in place (Table 10.2). Additional measures may be necessary in facilities with a greater potential for TB transmission.

   In low-risk areas, PPD testing of HCWs should be done annually, a repeat risk assessment should be done annually, the ventilation system should be evaluated annually, and TB isolation room negative pressure should be checked daily when in use.

   In intermediate-risk areas, PPD testing of HCWs should be done every 6 months, a repeat risk assessment should be done every 6 months, the ventilation system should be evaluated every 6 months, and TB isolation room negative pressure should be checked daily when in use.

   In high-risk areas, problem evaluation should be immediately conducted (Part II.K), PPD testing should be done every 3 months, a repeat risk assessment should be done every 3 months, the ventilation system should be evaluated every 3 months, and TB isolation room negative pressure should be checked daily when in use.

   Areas in which cough-inducing procedures are performed on patients who may have TB should, at the minimum, implement the intermediate protocol.

   The occurrence of drug-resistant TB in the facility or the community or a high prevalence of HIV infection among patients or HCWs in the facility may increase the concern about transmission of TB and may influence the decision regarding the protocol to follow in favor of a higher risk classification.

   Health-care facilities are likely to have a combination of low-, intermediate-, and high-risk areas or groups in the same time period and may not follow the same protocol in all areas. The appropriate protocol should be implemented for each area or occupational group.

   The number of rooms available for TB isolation should be determined by the number of TB patients seen in the area or by the occupational groups (Part II.E.5).

Table 10.2. Optimum TB Control Program for All Health-Care Facilities

I. Initial and periodic risk assessment
  A. Evaluate HCW PPD test conversion data
  B. Determine TB prevalence among patients
  C. Reassess risk each PPD testing period
II. Written TB infection control program
  A. Document all aspects of TB control
  B. Identify individual(s) responsible for TB control program
  C. Explain and emphasize hierarchy of controls
III. Implementation
  A. Assignment of responsibility
    1. Assign responsibility for TB control program to individual(s)
    2. Ensure that persons with expertise in infection control, occupational health, and engineering are identified and included
  B. Risk assessment and periodic reassessment of the program
    1. Select initial risk protocols
    2. Observe HCW infection control practices
    3. Repeat risk assessment at appropriate intervals
  C. Early detection of patients with TB
    1. Symptom screen for each patient
      a. On initial encounter in ER or ambulatory care setting
      b. Before or at admission
    2. Radiologic and bacteriologic screening for patients with symptoms of TB
  D. Management of outpatients with possible infectious TB
    1. Promptly initiate TB precautions
    2. Place patients in separate waiting areas or TB isolation rooms
    3. Give patients mask, box of tissues, instructions
  E. Isolation for infectious TB patients
    1. Prompt isolation and initiation of treatment for patients with suspected or known infectious TB
    2. Monitoring of response to treatment
    3. Appropriate criteria for discontinuation of isolation
  F. Engineering recommendations
    1. Local exhaust and general ventilation should be designed in collaboration with persons with expertise in ventilation engineering
    2. In areas where infectious TB patients receive care, use single-pass system or recirculation after HEPA filtration
    3. Use additional measures if needed in areas where TB patients may receive care
    4. Health-care facilities should be designed to achieve the best possible ventilation air flows
    5. Regularly monitor and maintain engineering controls
    6. Monitor and maintain TB isolation room negative pressure daily while in use relative to hallway and all surrounding areas
    7. Exhaust TB isolation room air to outside or, if unavoidable, recirculate after HEPA filtration
  G. Respiratory protection
    1. Respiratory protective devices should meet recommended performance criteria
    2. Should be worn by persons in settings where administrative and engineering controls are not likely to provide adequate protection (e.g., TB isolation rooms, treatment rooms, and other high-risk areas)
    3. A respiratory protection program is required where respiratory protection is used
  H. Cough-inducing procedures
    1. Should not be performed on TB patients unless absolutely necessary
    2. Should be performed using local exhaust or in individual TB isolation room

Table 10.2—*continued*

---

    3. After completion, TB patients should remain in booth or enclosure until cough subsides
  I. HCW TB education
    1. All HCWs should receive periodic education appropriate to their job
    2. Should include epidemiology of TB in the facility
    3. Should emphasize concepts of pathogenesis and occupational risk
    4. Should describe practices that reduce TB transmission
  J. HCW counseling and screening
    1. Counsel all HCWs regarding TB and TB infection
    2. Counsel all HCWs about increased risk if immunocompromised
    3. PPD test all HCWs on employment and repeat at periodic intervals
    4. Screen symptomatic HCWs for active TB
  K. Evaluate HCW PPD test conversions and possible nosocomial TB transmission
  L. Coordinate Efforts with Public Health Department

Protocols for detection of patients who may have active TB should be based on the number and characteristics of TB patients seen in the area or by the occupational group (Part II.C).

3. Periodic Reassessment

Follow-up risk assessment should be performed at the interval indicated by the most recent risk assessment (Fig. 10.1). Based on the follow-up assessment, problem evaluation may need to be conducted or the protocol modified to a higher or lower risk level.

Following each risk assessment, the staff responsible for TB control, in conjunction with other appropriate HCWs, should review all TB control policies to assure that they are effective and meet current needs.

4. Examples of Risk Assessment and Selection of TB Control Protocol

Below are described four hypothetical situations, and how surveillance data are used to select a TB control protocol.

Hospital A.   The health-care facility overall HCW PPD test conversion rate is 1.6%. No areas or occupational groups have a significantly greater PPD test conversion rate than areas without occupational exposure to TB patients (and than previous rates in the same area or group). There is no clustering of PPD test conversions. There is no evidence of patient-to-patient transmission. No area admits ≥6 TB patients per year. They will follow the low-risk protocol in all areas.

Hospital B.   Hospital B has an overall HCW PPD conversion rate of 1.8%. The medical intensive care unit (MICU) rate is significantly higher. No other area has a rate that high. They institute problem identification (Part II.K). No patient is found that was not isolated appropriately. Other potential problems are then evaluated and no cause is found. The high-risk protocol is followed in the MICU until the PPD conversion rate is documented to be similar to areas of the facility without occupational exposure to TB patients for two consecutive 3-month periods. If the rate remains significantly higher, further evaluation, including environmental and procedural studies (Table 10.2), will be performed to identify possible reasons for the high conversion rate.

Hospital C. The overall HCW PPD conversion rate is 2.4%. Rates range from 0 to 2.6% in individual areas and departments. None of these rates is significantly higher than rates in areas without occupational exposure to infectious TB patients. No particular HCW group has higher conversion rates than others. No clusters of HCW PPD conversions have occurred. Two units cared for >6 TB patients last year. These units will follow the intermediate protocol, and the remainder of the hospital will follow the low-risk protocol. This hospital is in the southeastern United States and these conversion rates may reflect cross-reactivity with nontuberculous mycobacteria.

Hospital D. The overall HCW PPD conversion rate is 1.2%. No area cared for >6 TB patients last year. Respiratory therapy HCWs had a PPD conversion rate of 15% (3/20 therapists). It was determined that HCWs who had PPD conversions spent all or part of their time in the pulmonary function laboratory where induced sputum specimens were obtained. Low-risk protocol is maintained for all areas of the facility except in the pulmonary function laboratory, where problem evaluation is conducted (Part II.K), and it is determined that the ventilation in the area is not adequate. The high-risk protocol is implemented and booths are installed for sputum induction. Once the booths are installed, after there are two consecutive 3-month periods with a PPD test conversion rate similar to areas of the facility without occupational exposure to *M. tuberculosis*, respiratory therapy HCWs will return to the low-risk protocol.

C. DETECTION OF PATIENTS WHO MAY HAVE ACTIVE TB

The most important steps in preventing TB transmission are early identification of patients who may have infectious TB, prompt application of TB isolation precautions for such patients, and prompt initiation of effective treatment in those in whom the diagnosis of TB is likely.

Health-care personnel assigned responsibility for TB infection control in ambulatory care and inpatient settings should develop, implement, and enforce protocols for early identification of patients who may have infectious TB.

The criteria used in these protocols should be based on the prevalence and characteristics of TB in the population served by the specific facility. Review of medical records of patients seen in the facility who were found to have TB may serve as a guide for developing or revising these protocols.

A diagnosis of TB should be considered in any patient with persistent cough (>2 weeks duration) or other sign or symptoms compatible with TB such as complaints of bloody sputum, night sweats, weight loss, anorexia, or fever. The index of suspicion for TB should be very high in areas or among groups of patients in which the prevalence of TB is high (Part I.B).

Diagnostic measures for identifying TB should be instituted among such patients. These measures include history, physical examination, PPD test, chest radiograph, and microscopic examination and culture of sputum or other appropriate specimens (4, 31, 32). Other diagnostic methods, such as bronchoscopy or biopsy, may be indicated for some patients (Part III.B) (33, 34).

Laboratories should use the most rapid methods available (e.g., fluorescent microscopy for AFB smears; radiometric culture methods for isolation of mycobacteria; p-nitro-α-acetylamino-β-hydroxy-proprophenone (NAP) test, nucleic acid probes, or high-pressure liquid chromatography (HPLC) for species identification; radiometric methods for drug susceptibility testing). As other more rapid or sensitive tests become available, practical, and affordable, such tests should be promptly incorporated into the mycobacteriology laboratory.

Results of AFB smears of sputum should be available in ≤ 24 hours of specimen collection. In some cases, availability of "stat" AFB smears may facilitate screening for TB.

The probability of TB is higher among patients with a positive PPD test or history of a positive PPD test, previous TB, exposure to TB, and among patients who belong to a group at high risk for TB (Part I.B). Active TB is strongly suggested if the diagnostic evaluation reveals AFB in sputum, a chest radiography is suggestive of TB, or symptoms are highly suggestive of TB. TB may occur simultaneously in immunosuppressed persons with pulmonary infections due to other organisms, such as *Pneumocystis carinii* or *Mycobacterium avium* complex, and should be sought in the diagnostic evaluation of all patients with symptoms compatible with TB (Parts III.A and B).

In addition to other measures for detecting patients with TB, immunosuppressed patients with pulmonary signs or symptoms that are initially ascribed to other etiologies should be evaluated for coexisting TB initially, and the evaluation should be repeated if the patient does not respond to appropriate therapy for the presumed etiology of the pulmonary abnormalities (Parts III.A and B).

TB may be more difficult to diagnose among persons with HIV infection or other conditions associated with severe suppression of cell-mediated immunity; the diagnosis may be overlooked because of an unusual or atypical clinical or radiographic presentation and/or the simultaneous occurrence of other pulmonary infections (e.g., *P. carinii* pneumonia). Among persons with HIV infection, the difficulty in making a diagnosis may be further compounded by impaired responses to PPD tests (35, 36), possibly lower sensitivity of sputum smears of detecting AFB (37), or overgrowth of cultures with M. avium complex among patients with both *M. avium* complex and *M. tuberculosis* (38).

Patients with suspected or confirmed TB should be reported to the appropriate health department immediately so that standard procedures for identifying and evaluating TB contacts can be initiated.

D. MANAGEMENT OF PATIENTS IN AMBULATORY CARE SETTINGS AND EMERGENCY ROOMS

Triage of patients should include vigorous efforts to promptly identify patients with active TB. HCWs who are the first points of contact in facilities serving patients at risk for TB should be trained to ask appropriate questions that will help recognize and detect patients with signs and symptoms suggestive of TB.

Patients with signs or symptoms suggestive of TB should be evaluated promptly to minimize the time spent in ambulatory care areas. Such patients should also have TB precautions applied while the diagnostic evaluation is being conducted. TB precautions in the ambulatory care setting consist of (1) placing the patient in a separate waiting area apart from other patients and not in open waiting areas, ideally, in a room meeting TB isolation requirements, and (2) giving the patient a surgical mask and instruction to keep it on. Patients should also be given tissues and instructed to cover their mouths and noses when coughing or sneezing, if they must remove their mask to facilitate respiratory clearance.

Patients who are known to have active TB and who have not completed therapy should have TB precautions applied until they are documented to be noninfectious (Part III.A).

Patients with active TB who need to be seen in a clinic should have appointments scheduled to avoid exposing HIV-infected or otherwise severely immunocompromised persons. This could be accomplished by setting aside certain times of the day for appointments for these patients or having them seen in areas where immunocompromised persons are not treated.

Ventilation in ambulatory care areas serving patients at high risk for TB should be designed and maintained to reduce the risk of TB transmission. General-use (e.g., waiting rooms) and special areas (e.g., treatment or TB isolation rooms in ambulatory areas) should be ventilated in the same manner as described for similar inpatient areas (Parts II.E.4 and F). Enhanced general ventilation or the use of air disinfection techniques, such as in-room recirculation of air through high-efficiency particulate air (HEPA) filters or UVGI may be useful in facilities where many infectious TB patients receive care in general-use areas for reducing the risk of transmission in these areas (see Part II.F for specific details and limitations of these disinfection techniques).

Ambulatory care settings in which patients with TB are frequently seen should have TB isolation room(s) available. In ambulatory care settings where cough-inducing procedures are performed, the additional guidelines in Part II.H should be followed.

E. MANAGEMENT OF HOSPITALIZED PATIENTS WITH TB

1. Evaluation for TB

Vigorous efforts should be made to detect patients with TB and initiate appropriate therapy promptly. Pulmonary TB should always be included in the differential diagnosis of persons with signs and symptoms suggestive of TB, and appropriate diagnostic measures should be used.

2. Initiation of Treatment

Patients who have confirmed active TB or are considered highly likely to have active TB should be started on appropriate treatment promptly, according to current guidelines (Part III.B) (39). In areas or facilities in which there is a high prevalence of MDR-TB, the initial regimen used (while results of drug-susceptibility tests are pending) may need to be enhanced. The decision should be based on analysis of surveillance data.

While the patient is in the health-care facility, antituberculosis drugs should be administered by directly observed therapy (DOT), in which a HCW observes the patient ingesting the medications. Strong consideration should be given to continuing DOT when the patient is discharged. This decision and arrangements for providing outpatient DOT should be made in collaboration with the health department.

3. Initiation of TB Isolation

In hospitals and other inpatient facilities, any patient suspected or known to have infectious TB should be placed in TB isolation in a private room with appropriate ventilation (Part II.E.5). There should be written policies for initiating TB isolation that specify (1) the indications for isolation, (2) who is authorized to initiate and discontinue isolation, (3) isolation practices, (4) monitoring of isolation, (5) management of patients who will not comply with isolation practices, and (6) criteria for discontinuing isolation.

Pediatric patients with suspected or confirmed TB should be evaluated for potential infectiousness as are adults, on the basis of symptoms, sputum AFB smears, radiologic findings, and other criteria. Those with pulmonary or laryngeal TB should be placed in TB isolation until they are determined to be noninfectious.

Intensive care unit patients, like patients in noncritical care settings, should be placed in TB isolation and have respiratory secretions submitted for AFB smear and culture if they have undiagnosed pulmonary symptoms suggestive of TB.

When patients with previously diagnosed TB are readmitted to an inpatient facility before confirmation of complete cure, they should be placed in TB isolation until infectiousness has been ruled out.

4. TB Isolation Practice

Patients who are placed in TB isolation should be educated about the transmission of TB and the reasons for TB isolation. They should be taught to cover their mouths and noses with a tissue when coughing or sneezing, even while in the TB isolation room, thus containing most liquid drops and droplets before they are expelled into the air (40).

Patients in TB isolation should remain in the isolation room with the door closed. Diagnostic and treatment procedures should be performed in the isolation room whenever possible to avoid transportation of the patient throughout the institution. If a patient who may have infectious TB must be transported outside the TB isolation room for a medically essential procedure that cannot be done in the room, he or she should wear a surgical mask covering the nose and mouth when transported outside the TB isolation room. The person transporting the patient does not need to wear respiratory protection outside of the isolation room. Efforts should be made to schedule the procedure at a time when it can be performed rapidly and when waiting areas are less crowded.

Treatment and procedure rooms where patients who have infectious TB or undiagnosed pulmonary disease and are at high risk for active TB receive care should meet the ventilation recommendations for TB isolation rooms (Part II.E.5, see below). Ideally, an area in the radiology department should be separately ventilated for TB patients. If this is not possible, the patient should be masked and spend the minimum amount of time possible in the radiology suite and returned promptly to the isolation room.

Efforts should be made to facilitate patient adherence to TB isolation measures, such as staying in the room. Such efforts might include the use of incentives, such as providing telephones, televisions, or radios in the room, or allowing special dietary requests. Efforts should also be made to address other problems that may interfere with adherence to isolation. Withdrawal from addictive substances (including tobacco) should be appropriately managed.

The number of persons entering the TB isolation room should be kept to a minimum. All persons who enter a TB isolation room or other room where known or suspected TB patients are receiving care should wear respiratory protection (Parts II.G and III.C).

5. TB Isolation Room

The TB isolation rooms should be single-patient rooms with special ventilation characteristics appropriate for the purposes of TB isolation (see below). The primary purposes of the isolation room are to (1) isolate patients who are likely to have infectious TB from other people; (2) prevent escape of droplet nuclei from the room, thus preventing entry of *M. tuberculosis* into the corridor and other areas of the facility; and (3) provide an environment that will allow reduction of the concentration of droplet nuclei through various engineering controls.

The isolation room should be maintained under negative pressure. TB isolation room doors should be kept closed, except when patients or personnel must enter or exit the room, in order to maintain negative pressure. Negative pressure should be monitored daily while the room is being used for TB isolation.

The American Society of Heating, Refrigerating and Air Conditioning Engineers (ASHRAE) (41), the American Institute of Architects (AIA) (42), and the federal Health Resources and Services Administration (43) recommend a minimum of 6 air changes/hr (ACH) for isolation and treatment rooms based on comfort and odor control considerations. The efficiency of this or any other level of air flow in reducing transmission of airborne pathogens has not been evaluated. Some reports suggest that ventilation rates substantially higher than 6 ACH produce a greater reduction in the concentration of bacteria in a room (44–46). However, accurate quantitation of decreases in risk that would result from specific increases in general ventilation levels from 6 ACH to substantially higher values is not possible. Under some experimental conditions, increasing ACH to 37 yielded substantial reductions in concentration of nonmycobacterial test organisms; further increases up to 60 ACH continued to be associated with reductions in concentrations of test organisms, but these reductions were more modest (44–46). It is unclear if these data can be extrapolated to TB control. However, ventilation air flows substantially >6 ACH would be expected to result in greater dilution of droplet nuclei. Therefore, it is recommended that health-care facilities be designed to achieve the best possible ventilation air flows.

Air from isolation rooms should be exhausted to the outside in accordance with applicable federal, state, and local regulations. The air should not be recirculated into the general ventilation. However, if recirculation of air into the general ventilation system from rooms or areas used to treat patients with known or suspected infectious TB is unavoidable (e.g., the ventilation system or facility configuration is such that it is impossible to vent the exhaust to the outside), HEPA filters should be used in the exhaust duct to the general ventilation system to remove infectious organisms and particulates the size of droplet nuclei from the air before the air is returned to the general ventilation system (Part II.F).

Although not required, an anteroom may increase the effectiveness of the isolation room by serving as an airlock to minimize the potential for droplet nuclei to escape into the corridor when the door is opened. To work effectively, the anteroom should have positive air pressure in relation to the TB isolation room. The pressure relationship between the anteroom and the corridor may vary according to ventilation design.

Upper air UVGI or in-room recirculation of air through UVGI devices may be used as adjuncts to general ventilation in the TB isolation room.

There should be enough TB isolation rooms to appropriately isolate all patients with suspected or confirmed active TB. This number should be derived through the risk assessment of the health-care facility. All acute care inpatient health-care facilities should have at least one TB isolation room.

Grouping TB isolation rooms together in one area of the facility may facilitate care of TB patients and installation and maintenance of optimal engineering (particularly ventilation) strategies, and reduce the possibility or transmission of TB to other patients.

6. Discontinuation of TB Isolation

The length of time required for a patient to become noninfectious after starting antituberculous therapy varies considerably (Part III.A). TB isolation should be discontinued only when the patient is on effective therapy and is improving clinically and the sputum smear is negative for AFB on 3 consecutive days.

Patients with active TB should be monitored for relapse with sputum smears on a regular basis (e.g., every 2 weeks). Failure to take medications as prescribed and the presence of drug-resistant TB are the two most common reasons for a patient remaining infectious. Thus, nonadherence to therapy or drug resistance should be considered in any patient who does not clinically respond to therapy within 2 to 3 weeks.

Consideration should be given to continuing isolation for patients with multidrug-resistant TB throughout their hospitalization because of the tendency to treatment failure or relapse (i.e., difficulty in maintaining noninfectiousness) that has been observed in such patients.

7. Discharge Planning

Before a TB patient is discharged from the health-care facility, the facility's staff and public health authorities should collaborate to ensure continuation of therapy. Discharge planning in the health-care facility should include, at a minimum, (1) a confirmed appointment with the provider who will follow the patient until cure; (2) sufficient medication to take until the outpatient appointment; and (3) placement into case management, such as directly observed therapy, or outreach programs of the local health department. It is essential that these plans be initiated and in place well before the patient's discharge.

Patients who may be infectious at the time of discharge should be discharged only to facilities with TB isolation capability or to home. However, they should not be discharged to home if there are persons in the household who are at a high risk of active TB if infected (e.g., HIV-infected or otherwise severely immunocompromised persons or children ≤5 years old).

F. ENGINEERING CONTROL RECOMMENDATIONS

1. General Ventilation

This part deals only with engineering controls for general-use areas of the health-care facility (e.g., waiting areas or emergency departments). Recommendations for engineering controls for specific areas of the facility (e.g., TB isolation rooms) are contained in the parts dealing with those areas.

Staff of health-care facilities should either include an engineer or other professional with expertise in ventilation or the facility should have this expertise available from a consultant who is an expert in ventilation engineering and who also has hospital experience. These persons should work closely with infection control staff to assist in the control of airborne infections.

Health-care facility ventilation system design should meet federal (e.g., Environmental Protection Agency), state, and local requirements.

The direction of air flow in health-care facilities should be set up and maintained so that air flows from clean areas to less-clean areas. In areas of a facility in which TB transmission is a potential problem, direction of air flow should be monitored with smoke tubes at intervals defined by the TB control plan.

Health-care facilities serving populations with a high prevalence of TB may need to supplement general ventilation or use additional engineering approaches (UVGI, HEPA filtration) in general-use areas of the health-care facilities where patients with TB are likely to be found (e.g., waiting areas, emergency rooms, or radiology suites). A single-pass, nonrecirculating system with air exhausted to the outside or a recirculation system with the air passed through HEPA filters before recirculation to the general ventilation system may be used in general-use areas where infectious TB patients are likely to be found.

2. Additional Engineering Control Approaches

a. HEPA Filtration.   HEPA filters may be used in a number of ways to reduce or eliminate infectious droplet nuclei from room air or exhaust. These methods include placement of HEPA filters (1) in exhaust ducts to remove droplet nuclei from air being discharged to the outside, either directly or through ventilation equipment; (2) in exhaust ducts discharging air from booths or enclosures into the surrounding room; (3) in ducts discharging room air into the general ventilation system; and (4) in ducts for individual room air recirculation. It should be noted that, although portable HEPA filtration units are available, the effectiveness of such units has not been adequately evaluated, and there is likely to be considerable variation in the effectiveness of these devices. In any application, HEPA filters need to be carefully installed and meticulously maintained to ensure adequate function.

b. Ultraviolet Germicidal Irradiation. For settings in which the risk of TB transmission is high, UV lamps may be used as a supplemental method of reducing the concentration of infectious droplet nuclei. However, the effectiveness of such units has not been adequately evaluated to permit their being substituted for other controls. UV units can be installed in a room or corridor to irradiate the air in the upper portion of the room (upper air irradiation) or they can be installed in ducts to irradiate air passing through the ducts. UV units installed in ducts should not be used as a substitute for HEPA filters prior to recirculation of air from a TB isolation room back into the general ventilation system. However, they may be used in ducts recirculating air back into the same room.

To function properly and decrease hazards to HCWs and others in the health-care facility, UV lamps should be properly installed and adequately maintained (with radiation levels monitored). UV tubes should be changed according to manufacturer's instructions or when meter readings indicate tube failure. A trained individual should be responsible for these measures and for keeping maintenance records. Applicable safety guidelines should be followed. Care should be taken to protect HCWs, patients, visitors, and others from excessive exposure to UV radiation.

G. RESPIRATORY PROTECTION

Respiratory protective devices used for *M. tuberculosis* should meet the following criteria:

1. The ability to filter particles 1 μm in size in the unloaded state with a filter efficiency of $\geq 95\%$ (i.e., filter leakage of $\leq 5\%$), given flow rates of up to 50 liters/min. Available evidence suggests that infectious droplet nuclei are in the 1- to 5-μm size range; therefore respirators used in health-care settings should be able to filter the smallest particles in this range efficiently. Fifty liters per minute is a reasonable estimate of the highest flow rate a HCW is likely to achieve during breathing even with strenuous work activities.
2. The ability to be qualitatively or quantitatively fit tested in a reliable way (47) to obtain a face-seal leakage of no more than 10% for most workers.
3. The ability to fit HCWs with different facial sizes and characteristics, which can usually be met by the availability of at least three sizes of respirators.

4. To ensure proper protection, the facepiece fit should be checked by the wearer each time he or she puts on the respirator, in accordance with OSHA's standard and good industrial hygiene practice.

The OSHA respiratory protection standard requires that all respiratory protective devices be certified by the National Institute of Occupational Safety and Health (NIOSH) (48). Respirators with HEPA filters are the only currently available certified respirators that meet or exceed the performance criteria stated above. Although dust-mist (DM) and dust-fume-mist (DFM) filters are certified, these criteria are not evaluated. Current NIOSH certification procedures require that DM and DFM filters filter 99% of silica dust, but the certification process does not include adequate tests for filter efficacy against low-concentration aerosols in the size range of droplet nuclei. There is evidence that some respirators with DM and DFM filters do meet these criteria. However, at the present time, the certification process does not determine which NIOSH-certified DM and DFM filters meet these performance criteria.

Appropriate respiratory protection should be worn by persons potentially exposed to *M. tuberculosis* in settings where administrative and engineering controls may not provide adequate protection (Part III.C). Such settings include TB isolation rooms and rooms or enclosures in which patients who may have infectious TB are undergoing cough-inducing or aerosol-generating procedures. Other such settings may include transport of patients who may have infectious TB in emergency transport vehicles or when urgent surgical or dental care must be provided to a patient who may have infectious TB before the patient can be treated with anti-TB medications and rendered noninfectious.

In some settings, the risk of TB transmission may be estimated in the risk assessment or the best judgment of infection control staff to be so high that respiratory protection exceeding these criteria may be considered appropriate. In such settings, consideration may be given to the use of higher levels of protection (Table 10.3). Characteristics of a variety of currently available respiratory protection devices are summarized in Table 10.3.

Health-care facilities in which respiratory protection is used for protection against inhalation of *M. tuberculosis* are required to develop, implement, and maintain a respiratory protection program (Part III.C). All HCWs who need to use respiratory protection should be included in this program.

H. COUGH-INDUCING PROCEDURES

1. General Guidelines

Procedures that involve instrumentation of the lower respiratory tract or induce cough may increase the probability of droplet nuclei being expelled into the air. These cough-inducing procedures include endotracheal intubation and suctioning, diagnostic sputum induction, aerosol treatments (including pentamidine therapy), and bronchoscopy. Other procedures that may generate aerosols (e.g., irrigation of tuberculosis abscesses, homogenizing or lyophilizing tissue) are also included in these recommendations.

Table 10.3. Summary of Features of Respiratory Protective Devices

	Surgical Masks	Disposable, Negative-Pressure Particulate Respirators	Reusable, Negative-Pressure Particulate Respirators	Tight-Fitting, Positive-Pressure Particulate Respirators
Fit test	Fit tests cannot be performed.	DM & DFM: Qualitative HEPA: Qualitative and quantitative	Both qualitative and quantitative fit tests can be performed reliably	Both qualitative and quantitative fit tests can be performed reliably
Fit check	Fit checks cannot be performed	Some currently available cannot be fit checked with current technology	Fit checks can be performed reliably	Fit checks can be performed reliably
Face-seal leakage[a]	10–20%	DM or DFM: 10–20%[b] HEPA: ≤10%	Half-masks: ≤10% Full-mask: <2%	<2%
Filter leakage	25–85%[c]	DM or DFM: 0–40%[c] HEPA: <0.03%[d]	DM or DFM: 0–40%[c] HEPA: <0.03%[d]	HEPA: <0.03%[d]
Facepiece sizes	One[e]	Up to 3	Up to 3	Up to 3

[a] For respirable aerosols (i.e., less than 10 µm).
[b] Less than 10% face-seal leakage should be achievable if more sizes become available and if fit testing and fit checking is performed.
[c] At 30 L/min over a particle size range of 1–5 µm.
[d] For aerosols 0.3 µm.
[e] Currently, only one facepiece size is generally available, tending to produce higher face-seal leakages on small facial sizes.

Cough-inducing procedures should not be performed on patients who may have infectious TB unless absolutely necessary. All cough-inducing procedures performed on patients who may have infectious TB should be performed using local exhaust ventilation devices (e.g., booths or special enclosures) or, if that is not feasible, in a room that meets the ventilation requirements for TB isolation.

HCWs should wear respiratory protection when present in rooms or enclosures where cough-inducing procedures are being performed on patients who have, or are at high risk of having, infectious TB. After completion of cough-inducing procedures, patients with known or suspected TB should remain in the isolation room or enclosure and not return to common waiting areas until coughing subsides. They should be given tissues and instructed to cover their mouth and nose when coughing. If they must recover from sedatives or anesthesia following procedures such as bronchoscopy, they should be monitored in a separate TB isolation room and not in recovery rooms with other patients.

Before the booth, enclosure, or room is used for another patient, adequate time should be allowed to pass so that any droplet nuclei that have been expelled into the air are removed. This time will vary according to the efficiency of the ventilation or filtration used.

2. Additional Considerations for Bronchoscopy

If performing bronchoscopy in positive-pressure rooms (such as operating rooms) is unavoidable, TB should be ruled out before the procedure. If bronchoscopy is being performed for diagnosis of pulmonary disease that may include TB, it should be performed in a room that meets TB isolation ventilation requirements.

3. Special Considerations for the Administration of Aerosolized Pentamidine (AP)

All patients should be screened for active TB before prophylactic AP therapy is initiated. Screening should include medical history, PPD test, and a chest radiograph.

Before each subsequent AP treatment, patients should be screened for symptoms suggestive of TB, such as development of a productive cough. If such symptoms are elicited, a diagnostic evaluation for TB should be initiated.

For patients with suspected or confirmed active TB, it is preferable to use oral prophylaxis for PCP if clinically practical.

I. EDUCATION AND TRAINING OF HEALTH-CARE WORKERS

All HCWs should receive education about TB that is appropriate to their job category. Training should be conducted before initial assignment and subsequently on a periodic basis (e.g., annually). Although the level and detail of this education may vary according to job description, the following elements should be included in the education of all HCWs:

The basic concepts of TB transmission, pathogenesis, and diagnosis, including the difference between latent TB infection and active TB disease, the signs and symptoms of TB, and the possibility of reinfection in persons with a positive PPD test. The potential for occupational exposure to persons with infectious TB in the health-care facility, including the prevalence of TB in the community and facility, the ability of the facility to appropriately isolate patients with active TB, and the situations with increased risk of exposure to TB.

The principles and practices of infection control that reduce the risk of transmission of TB, including the hierarchy of TB infection control measures and the written policies and procedures of the facility. Site-specific control measures should be provided to personnel in areas needing measures in addition to the basic control program.

The purpose of PPD testing, the significance of a positive result, and the importance of participation in the skin test program.

The principles of preventive therapy for latent TB infections. Indications, use, and effectiveness, including the potential adverse effects of the drugs (Part III.B).

The responsibility of the HCW to seek medical evaluation promptly if symptoms develop that may be due to TB or if PPD test conversion occurs in order to receive appropriate evaluation and therapy and to prevent transmission of TB to patients and other HCWs. The principles of drug therapy for active TB.

The importance of notifying the facility if diagnosed with active TB so appropriate contact investigation can be instituted. The responsibilities of the facility to maintain the confidentiality of the HCW while assuring that the HCW with TB receives appropriate therapy and is noninfectious before returning to duty.

The higher the risk posed by TB to individuals with HIV infection or other cause of severely impaired cell-mediated immunity including (1) the more frequent and rapid development of clinical TB after infection with *M. tuberculosis*, (2) the differences in the clinical presentation of disease, and (3) the high mortality rate associated with MDR-TB disease in such individuals.

The potential development of cutaneous energy as immune function, measured by CD4 + T-lymphocyte counts, declines.

The facility's policy on voluntary work reassignment options for immunocompromised HCWs.

J. HEALTH-CARE WORKER COUNSELING, SCREENING, AND EVALUATION

A TB screening and prevention program for HCWs should be established for protection of both HCWs and patients. Personnel with positive PPD tests, PPD test conversions, or symptoms suggestive of TB should be identified, evaluated to rule out active TB, and started on therapy or preventive therapy if indicated (3). In addition, the results of the HCW PPD screening program will permit evaluation of the effectiveness of current infection control practices. Recommendations for PPD testing and interpretation can be found in Part III.B.

1. Counseling the HCW Regarding TB

Because of the increased risk of rapid progression from latent TB infection to active TB in HIV-positive or otherwise severely immunocompromised persons, all HCWs should know if they have a medical condition or are receiving a medical treatment that may lead to severely impaired cell-mediated immunity. HCWs who may be at risk for HIV infection should know their HIV status, i.e., they should be encouraged to voluntarily seek counseling and testing for HIV antibody status. Existing guidelines for counseling and testing should be routinely followed (49). Knowledge of these conditions will allow for the HCW to seek appropriate preventive measures, as outlined in this document, and consider voluntary work reassignments. It is particularly important that HCWs who may be at risk for HIV infection and who work in settings where there is increased prevalence of MDR-TB among patients know their HIV status.

Though implementation of guidelines greatly reduces risk of occupational infection, all HCWs should be counseled about the potential risks, in severely immunocompromised persons, associated with taking care of patients with some infectious diseases, including TB. They should also be counseled about the need to follow existing recommendations for infection control to minimize the risk of exposure to infectious agents (50). As the best protection against becoming infected, severely immunosuppressed HCWs should avoid exposure to *M. tuberculosis*. HCWs with severely impaired cell-mediated immunity (due to HIV infection or other causes) who may be exposed to *M. tuberculosis* should consider a change in job setting. Therefore, HCWs should be advised of options for severely immunocompromised HCWs to voluntarily transfer to areas and activities in which there is the lowest possible risk of exposure to *M. tuberculosis*. This should be a personal decision for HCWs after being informed of the risk to themselves and evaluating their own job commitment and satisfaction.

Employers should make reasonable attempts to offer alternative job assignments to an employee with a documented condition compromising cell-mediated immunity who works in a high-risk setting for TB. Immunocompromised HCWs should be referred to an employee health professional who can counsel the employee on an individual basis regarding his or her risk of TB. Upon the request of the immunocompromised HCW, the facility should offer, but not compel, a work setting in which the HCW would have the lowest possible risk of occupational exposure to *M. tuberculosis*. Evaluation of these situations should also include consideration of the provisions of the Americans with Disabilities Act (ADA) of 1990 (51) and other applicable federal, state, and local laws.

All HCWs should be informed that immunosuppressed HCWs need to have appropriate follow-up and screening for infectious diseases, including TB. HCWs who are known to be HIV-infected or otherwise severely immunosuppressed should be tested for cutaneous anergy at the time of PPD testing (Part III.B). Consideration should be given to retesting immunocompromised HCWs with PPD and anergy tests at least every 6 months because of the high risk of rapid progression to active TB should infection occur.

Information provided to HCWs regarding their immune status should be treated confidentially. If the HCW requests voluntary job reassignment, the confidentiality of the worker should be maintained. Facilities should have written procedures on confidential handling of such information.

2. Screening of HCWs for Active TB

Any HCW with persistent cough (>2 weeks duration), especially in the presence of other symptoms or signs compatible with TB, such as weight loss, night sweats, bloody sputum, anorexia, or fever, should be evaluated promptly for TB. The HCW should not return to work until TB is excluded or the HCW is on therapy and documented to be noninfectious.

3. Screening HCWs for Latent TB Infection

At the time of employment, all HCWs, including those with a history of vaccination with bacillus Calmette-Guérin (BCG), should receive a Mantoux PPD (Part III.B). On the initial test, two-step testing should be performed to detect boosting phenomena that might be misinterpreted as skin test conversions. HCWs with a documented history of a positive PPD test, adequate treatment for disease, or adequate preventive therapy for infection, should be exempt from further PPD screening unless they develop signs or symptoms suggestive of TB.

All PPD-negative HCWs should undergo repeat PPD testing at intervals determined by the risk assessment (Part II.A). It may be advantageous to stagger the testing of HCWs in a given area or occupational group (e.g., do testing on employment anniversary date or birthdate) rather than testing all HCWs in the area or group at one time, since staggering may lead to earlier detection of transmission.

Initial and follow-up PPD tests should be administered, read, and interpreted according to current guidelines (Part III.A). At the time of testing, HCWs should be informed about the interpretation of PPD test results, whether positive or negative, including the possible variable interpretations of induration of ≥ 5 mm, depending on immune status and exposure to persons with infectious TB.

If PPD test conversions are identified, other HCWs assigned to the same work area or group should be tested to determine if there is additional evidence of transmission in the area. When HCWs not regularly assigned to a single work area have PPD conversions, an effort should be made to identify the areas where the HCW worked during the time when infection was likely to have occurred, so those areas can be evaluated.

In any area of the facility where transmission of TB is known to have recently occurred, PPD testing should be repeated every 3 months until no additional conversions have been detected for two consecutive 3-month intervals. This will allow detection of additional PPD conversions and rapid institution of preventive therapy, and documentation of the effectiveness of the control interventions that have been implemented.

Results of PPD tests should be recorded both in the individual HCWs employee health record and in a retrievable aggregate database of all HCW PPD test results, so that they can be periodically analyzed to estimate the risk of acquiring infection in each area or group of the facility.

4. EVALUATION AND MANAGEMENT OF HEALTH-CARE WORKERS WITH POSITIVE PPD TESTS

a. Evaluation.   All HCWs with newly recognized positive PPD tests or PPD test conversions should be promptly evaluated for clinically active TB with a chest radiograph and clinical evaluation. Those without clinical TB should be evaluated for preventive therapy according to published guidelines (Part III.B).

If a HCWs PPD test converts to positive, a history of possible exposure should be obtained in an attempt to determine the potential source of TB exposure. When the source of exposure is known, the drug susceptibility pattern of the *M. tuberculosis* isolated from the source should be determined in order to determine appropriate preventative therapy for the HCW with the PPD test conversion.

All HCWs, including those with a history of a positive PPD, should be reminded periodically that they should be evaluated promptly for any pulmonary symptoms suggestive of TB.

b. Routine and Follow-up Chest Radiographs.   Routine chest radiographs are not required for asymptomatic, PPD-negative HCWs. HCWs with positive PPD tests should have a chest radiograph as part of the initial evaluation of their PPD test; if negative, repeat chest radiographs are not needed unless symptoms develop that may be due to TB (52).

c. Work Restrictions

Active TB.   HCWs with pulmonary or laryngeal TB pose a risk to patients and other HCWs while they are infectious; therefore, they should be excluded from work until they are no longer infectious. The same work restrictions applicable for immunocompetent HCWs apply to HCWs with active TB and HIV infection or other conditions resulting in severely impaired cell-mediated immunity.

Before the HCW returns to work, the health-care facility needs to ensure that the HCW with TB is receiving adequate therapy, cough is resolved, and that the HCW has three consecutive daily sputum AFB smears that are negative. After work duties are resumed and while the HCW remains on antituberculosis therapy, facility staff should ensure that the HCW is maintained on effective drug therapy for the appropriate time period and remains AFB sputum smear negative.

HCWs with TB at sites other than the lung or larynx usually do not need to be excluded from work if concurrent pulmonary TB has been excluded.

HCWs with TB who discontinue treatment before the recommended course of therapy has been completed should be excluded from work until treatment is resumed, an adequate response to therapy is documented, and they again have negative sputum smears on 3 consecutive days.

Even if a HCW is treated for TB by a private physician, a knowledgeable professional in the health-care facility employee health service should be advised confidentially of the diagnosis and should verify the appropriateness of the treatment and monitor symptoms and job duties.

Latent TB Infection.   HCWs receiving preventive treatment for latent TB infection should be allowed to continue usual work activities.

HCWs with TB infection who cannot take or do not accept or complete a full course of preventive therapy do not need to be excluded from work, but they should be counseled about the risk of developing active TB and should be instructed on a regular basis to seek evaluation promptly if symptoms develop that may be due to TB, especially if they have exposure to high-risk patients (i.e., patients at high risk for developing TB if they become infected with *M. tuberculosis*, such as patients who are HIV infected).

K. PROBLEM EVALUATION

1. Investigating PPD Conversions and Active TB in HCWs

If a skin test conversion is identified, the following steps should be taken:

The HCW should be promptly evaluated for active TB; the initial evaluation should include a thorough history, physical examination, and chest radiograph.

Other diagnostic procedures (e.g., sputum examination) may be indicated, based on the initial evaluation. The HCW should be placed on preventative or curative therapy, if appropriate, according to current guidelines (Part III.B) (3).

A history of possible exposure should be obtained in an attempt to determine the potential source of TB infection. When the source of exposure is known, the drug susceptibility pattern of the *M. tuberculosis* isolated from the source should be determined in order to select appropriate preventive therapy.

Other HCWs in the same area or group who may have had similar exposure should receive PPD tests to determine if there is additional evidence of transmission. The contact investigation should extend to possibly exposed patients, if indicated.

Initiate problem evaluation (Table 10.4), if indicated. If a problem with patient identification, TB isolation practices, or engineering controls is identified, implement the appropriate interventions and follow the high-risk protocol until there have been two consecutive 3-month periods with no evidence of transmission.

If no specific problem can be identified or the problem does not resolve after the apparent cause is corrected and no other cause can be identified, continue following the high-risk protocol in that area and consult with the public health department or other persons with expertise in TB control.

If transmission appears to be occurring in TB isolation or procedure rooms, engineering controls should be improved as needed. If a HCW develops TB, the following steps should be taken: contact investigation should be performed, including other HCWs, patients, and visitors who had significant exposure to the HCW. The public health department should immediately be notified for consultation and to allow for investigation of community contacts not exposed in the health-care facility.

The public health department should notify facilities when HCWs with TB are reported by physicians so that appropriate contact investigation can be done

Table 10.4. Examples of Potential Problems with Patient Identification or TB Isolation

Patient Identification	Potential Problem	Intervention
Triage	Patient with signs or symptoms not identified	Review triage procedures, facilities, and practices
	Patient had no "triage" symptoms	Reevaluate triage protocol
	Patient previously admitted for TB not readmitted to isolation	Review triage process, review discharge planning process
Laboratory	Positive smear—results available >24 hours[a] after submitted	Change lab practice, assess potential bottlenecks, explore alternatives
	Positive smear—results available but not acted upon in a timely fashion	Education of appropriate personnel, review protocol for management of positive smear results
	Positive culture—results not available for >3 weeks[a]	Change lab practices, assess potential bottlenecks
	Positive culture—results available but not acted upon in a timely fashion	Education of appropriate personnel, review protocol for management of positive culture result
	Positive culture—susceptibility results not available for >6 weeks[a]	Change lab practices, assess potential bottlenecks, explore alternatives
	Positive culture—susceptibility results available but not acted upon in a timely fashion	Education of appropriate personnel, review protocol for management of positive culture susceptibility results
Diagnosis	Patient with signs/symptoms of TB—appropriate tests not ordered in a timely fashion	Education of appropriate personnel, evaluate protocols for TB detection
TB isolation	Isolation room unavailable	Reassess need for number of rooms
	Isolation not ordered or discontinued too soon or isolation policy not followed properly (e.g., patients ambulating outside of room)	Education of patients and appropriate personnel, evaluate institutional barriers to implementation of isolation policy
	Personnel not using respiratory protection appropriately	Education of appropriate personnel, evaluation of regularly scheduled reeducation, and institutional barriers to respiratory protection use
	Isolation room or procedure room not negative pressure relative to rest of facility	Appropriate engineering modifications including regular monitoring and maintenance program
	Inadequate air circulation	Appropriate engineering modifications
	Door left open	Education of appropriate personnel and patients, evaluate self-closing doors, comfort in room, other measures to promote door closing

[a]Time intervals are used as examples and should not be considered absolute standards.

in the facility. Sharing of such information is by law strictly limited to a need to know basis in order to protect the confidentiality of the HCW.

2. Investigating Possible Patient-to-Patient Transmission of TB

Surveillance of active TB cases in patients should be conducted. If this surveillance suggests the possibility of patient-to-patient TB transmission (e.g., high proportion of TB patients have prior admission in past year, sudden increase in patients with drug-resistant TB, multiple patients with identical and characteristic drug-susceptibility or DNA fingerprint patterns) the following steps should be taken:

Review HCW PPD test and patient surveillance data for the suspected areas to detect additional patients or HCWs with PPD conversions or active disease.
Look for possible exposures of the new TB patients to other patients with TB during prior admissions (e.g., admitted to same room, area, received same procedure or were in same treatment area on the same day, etc.).

If the above steps suggest that transmission has occurred, the following steps should be taken:

Conduct a problem evaluation (Fig. 10.2 and Table 10.4) to determine possible causes of the transmission (e.g., problem with patient detection, institutional barriers to implementation of appropriate TB isolation practices, or engineering controls).
Determine which additional patients or HCWs may have been exposed and evaluate with PPD tests.
Consult with the public health department for assistance in community contact investigation.

3. Investigating Contacts of Persons with TB Who Were Not Recognized and Isolated Appropriately

When a patient is seen in the institution without being recognized as having TB and promptly isolated, but is subsequently diagnosed as having infectious TB, the following steps should be taken:

Identify HCWs and other patients who were exposed to the TB patient by interviewing the patient and appropriate personnel and by reviewing the patient's medical record to determine which areas and persons may have been exposed to the patient prior to appropriate isolation (e.g., outpatient clinics; hospital rooms; treatment, radiology and procedure areas; patient lounges; persons providing direct care; other personnel such as therapists, clerks, transportation personnel, housekeepers, social workers, etc.). Contact investigation should follow a concentric circle, expanding from closest to less close contacts, if transmission to the former is found.
Administer a PPD test to all HCWs and patients with documented exposure as soon as possible after exposure. If the initial test is negative, a second test should be administered 12 weeks after the exposure was terminated.

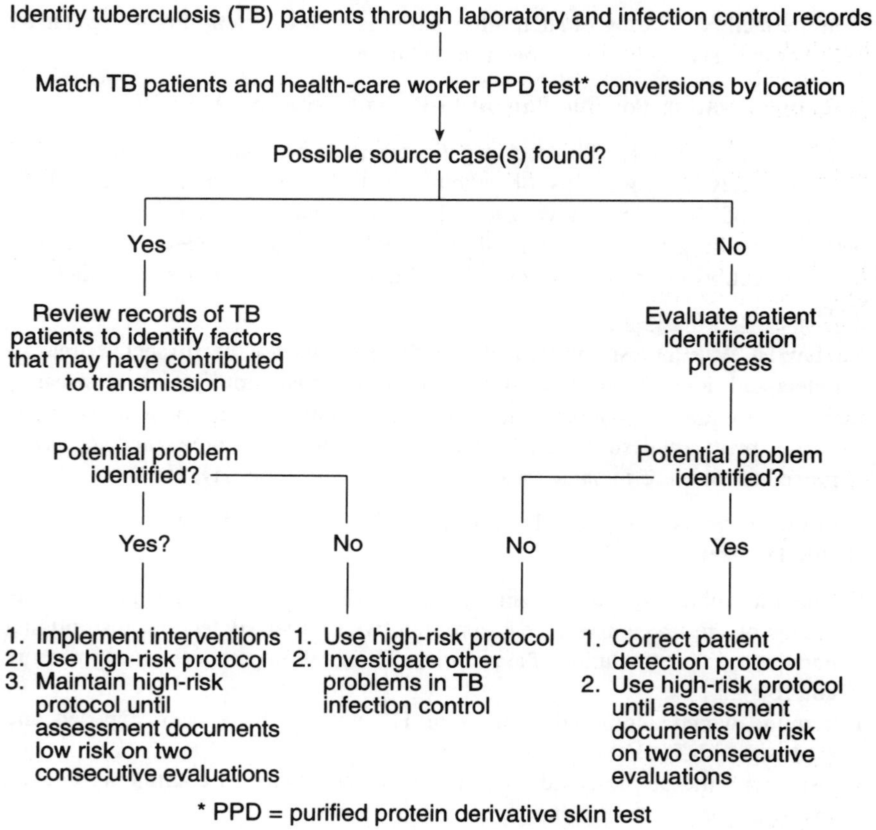

Identify tuberculosis (TB) patients through laboratory and infection control records

Match TB patients and health-care worker PPD test* conversions by location

Possible source case(s) found?

Yes

Review records of TB
patients to identify factors
that may have contributed
to transmission

Potential problem
identified?

Yes?

No

1. Implement interventions
2. Use high-risk protocol
3. Maintain high-risk
   protocol until
   assessment documents
   low risk on two
   consecutive evaluations

1. Use high-risk protocol
2. Investigate other
   problems in TB
   infection control

No

Evaluate patient
identification
process

Potential problem
identified?

No

Yes

1. Correct patient
   detection protocol
2. Use high-risk protocol
   until assessment
   documents low risk
   on two consecutive
   evaluations

* PPD = purified protein derivative skin test

Figure 10.2. Problem evaluation.

Exposed persons with PPD conversion or with symptoms suggestive of TB should
be evaluated clinically and with chest radiographs promptly. Persons with
previously known positive PPDs who have been exposed to an infectious
patient do not require a repeat PPD or a chest radiograph unless they have
symptoms suggestive of TB.

In addition to PPD testing of exposed HCWs and patients, an investigation should
be conducted to determine why TB was not recognized in the patient or, if
recognized, why the patient was not isolated promptly so that appropriate
corrective actions may be taken.

L. COORDINATION WITH THE PUBLIC HEALTH DEPARTMENT

As soon as a patient or HCW is known or suspected to have TB, the patient or
HCW should be reported to the health department so that appropriate community
contact investigation and follow-up can be performed. The health department
should be notified well before patient discharge to facilitate follow-up and contin-

uation of therapy. A discharge plan coordinated with the patient or HCW, the health department, and the inpatient facility should be implemented.

The public health department should protect the confidentiality of the HCW as prescribed by state and local law.

Health-care facilities and health departments should coordinate their efforts to perform appropriate contact investigations on patients and HCWs with active TB.

Results of all AFB-positive sputum smears, cultures positive for *M. tuberculosis*, and drug-susceptibility results on *M. tuberculosis* isolates should be forwarded to the health department as soon as they become available, in accordance with state and local laws and regulations.

The health department may be able to provide assistance to facilities for various aspects of planning and implementing a TB infection control program, such as surveillance, screening activities, and outbreak investigations. In addition, the state health department may be able to provide names of experts for the engineering aspects of TB control.

M. ADDITIONAL CONSIDERATIONS FOR SELECTED AREAS

The following comments do not apply to all areas or types of facilities, but should be incorporated into the TB control plan for the specific area discussed.

1. Operating Rooms

Elective operative procedures on patients with TB should be delayed until the patient is no longer infectious.

If procedures must be performed, they should be done in operating rooms with anterooms if possible. For operating rooms without anterooms, the doors to the operating room should be closed and traffic in and out of the room should be kept to a minimum to reduce the frequency of opening and closing the door. Attempts should be made to perform the procedure at a time when other patients are not present in the operative suite (i.e., end of day) and when a minimum number of personnel are present.

A bacterial filter placed on the patient's endotracheal tube or at the expiratory side of the breathing circuit of the anesthesia machine when general anesthesia is being administered to a patient with possible TB may be useful in reducing the risk of contamination of the anesthesia equipment or discharge of tubercle bacilli into the ambient air. The cost-benefit ratio of bacterial filter use is unknown, as no transmission of airborne pathogens has ever been traced to this route.

The patient should be monitored during recovery in an individual room meeting TB isolation room ventilation recommendations.

Personnel present when operative procedures are performed on patients who may have infectious TB should wear respiratory protection rather than standard surgical masks alone. Valved or positive-pressure respirators are not appropriate for use during procedures requiring surgical masks.

2. Autopsy Rooms

Due to the probability of the presence of infectious aerosols, autopsy rooms should be at negative pressure with respect to adjacent areas, with room air exhausted directly to the outside of the building. ASHRAE recommends that autopsy rooms have ventilation that provides 12 ACH (41). However, the effectiveness of this level of ventilation for reducing the risk of TB transmission has not been evaluated. Autopsy rooms should be designed to achieve the best possible air flows; substantially higher levels of ventilation than 12 ACH would be expected to provide greater dilution of droplet nuclei.

Respiratory protection should be worn by personnel while performing autopsies on patients who may have had TB (Part III.C).

In-duct, HEPA-filtered air recirculation or UVGI may be used as a supplement to the recommended ventilation.

3. Emergency Medical Services

When emergency medical response personnel or others must transport patients with confirmed or suspected active TB, a surgical mask should be placed on the patient, if possible. Because of the inability to ensure administrative and engineering controls in emergency transport situations and vehicles, the HCW should wear respiratory protection.

Emergency-response personnel should be included in a comprehensive PPD screening program and receive a PPD at least annually. They should also be included in the follow-up of contacts of a patient with infectious TB.

4. Laboratories

Laboratories processing specimens for mycobacterial studies (e.g., AFB smears and cultures) should conform to criteria previously specified by the Centers for Disease Control and Prevention (CDC) and the National Institutes of Health (NIH) (53).

5. Hospices

Hospice patients with confirmed or suspected TB should be managed in the manner described in this document for hospitals. General-use and special areas, such as treatment or TB isolation rooms, should be ventilated in the same manner as described for similar hospital areas.

6. Nursing Homes

Published recommendations for prevention and control of TB in nursing homes should be followed (54). TB isolation procedures described in this document should be followed.

7. Correctional Facilities

Published recommendations for prevention and control of TB in correctional facilities should be followed (55).

Prison medical facilities should follow the recommendations outlined in this document. Ventilation should be designed and maintained to reduce the risk of TB transmission. General and special areas, such as treatment or TB isolation rooms, should be ventilated in the same manner as described for similar hospital areas. If appropriate TB isolation rooms are not available, persons with suspected or known TB should be transferred to facilities with those provisions.

8. Dental Offices

During dental procedures, patients and dental workers share the same airspace for varying lengths of time. Aerosols of oral fluids and materials may be generated, and, on occasion, coughing may be stimulated by oral manipulations. No specific dental procedures have been classified as "cough-inducing." In light of these observations, the following additional considerations appear prudent in dental settings:

During initial medical history taking and periodic updates, dental HCWs should routinely ask all patients about a history of TB disease and symptoms suggestive of TB.

Patients with history and symptoms suggestive of active TB should be promptly referred for evaluation for possible infectiousness. Elective dental treatment should be delayed until a physician confirms that the patient does not have infectious TB. If the patient is determined to have infectious TB, elective dental treatment should be deferred until the patient is no longer infectious.

If urgent dental care must be provided for a patient who has, or is strongly suspected of having, infectious TB, TB isolation practices should be implemented (Parts II.E and G). Dental HCWs should use respiratory protection while performing procedures on such patients. Dental HCWs who work in a facility where there is a likelihood of exposure to patients with infectious TB should be included in an employer-sponsored PPD testing program.

9. Home-Health Services

For HCWs visiting the home of patients with suspected or confirmed infectious TB, precautions may be necessary if the patient is likely to be infectious. These precautions include instructing the patient to cover his or her mouth and nose with a tissue when coughing or sneezing and offering the patient a surgical mask. The worker should wear respiratory protection when entering the home or the patient's room until the patient is no longer infectious (Part III.A).

Precautions in the home may be discontinued when the patients is no longer infectious (Part III.A).

Home health-care personnel can assist in preventing TB transmission by educating the patient about the importance of taking medications as prescribed and by administering directly observed therapy.

If immunocompromised persons or young children live in the home with a patient who has infectious TB, they should be temporarily relocated until the patient is no longer infectious (Part III.A).

Cough-inducing procedures should be performed on patients with infectious TB only if absolutely necessary. When necessary cough-inducing procedures, such as AFB sputum collection for evaluation of therapy, must be performed on a patient who may have infectious TB, they should be performed in a well-ventilated area of the home away from other household members. Opening a window to improve ventilation or specimen collection outside should be considered, when feasible. The HCW collecting these specimens should wear respiratory protection during the procedure (Part III.C).

Home HCWs should be included in a comprehensive employer-sponsored TB screening and prevention program.

Home health-care personnel and patients who are at risk for contracting active TB should be reminded periodically of the importance of having pulmonary symptoms promptly evaluated to permit early detection and treatment of persons with TB.

III. Supplemental Information
A. DETERMINING THE INFECTIOUSNESS OF A TB PATIENT

The infectiousness of a person with TB correlates with the number of organisms expelled into the air, which, in turn, probably correlates with the following factors: (1) Presence of pulmonary, laryngeal, or oral involvement; (2) presence of cough or other forceful expirational maneuvers, including procedures that stimulate coughing; (3) AFB positive sputum smear; (4) willingness or ability of the patient to cover his or her mouth when coughing or sneezing; (5) presence of cavitation on chest radiograph; and (6) length of time the patient has been on adequate chemotherapy.

The most infectious persons are thought to be those untreated persons with pulmonary or laryngeal TB who have a cough or are undergoing cough-inducing procedures, who are AFB sputum smear positive, or who have cavitation on chest radiograph. Persons with extrapulmonary TB are usually not infectious, with the following exceptions: (1) concomitant pulmonary disease; (2) nonpulmonary disease located in the respiratory tract or oral cavity; or (3) extrapulmonary disease that includes an open abscess or lesion in which the concentration of organisms is high, especially if drainage from the abscess is extensive (17, 19). Although data are limited, some studies suggest that TB patients with acquired immunodeficiency syndrome (AIDS), if smear-positive, have infectiousness similar to that of smear-positive TB patients without AIDS (56–58).

Young children with TB are less likely than are adults to be infectious; however, transmission from children can occur. Therefore, children with TB should be evaluated for infectiousness using the same parameters as for adults (i.e., pulmonary or laryngeal TB, presence of cough or cough-inducing procedures, positive sputum AFB smear (or gastric aspirate), cavitation on chest radiograph, and adequacy and duration of therapy). Children with pulmonary or laryngeal TB should be placed on TB isolation until they are determined to be noninfectious.

Infection is most likely to result from exposure to persons with unsuspected pulmonary TB who are not receiving antituberculosis therapy or from persons with diagnosed TB who are not receiving adequate therapy. Administering effective antituberculous medications has been shown to be associated with decrease infectiousness among persons with TB (59). Effective chemotherapy reduces coughing, the amount of sputum, and the number of organisms in the sputum. However, the length of time a patient must be on effective medication before becoming noninfectious varies (60); some patients are never infectious, whereas those with unrecognized or inadequately treated drug-resistant TB may remain infectious for weeks or months (21). Thus, decisions about infectiousness should be made on a case-by-case basis.

In general, persons suspected or confirmed to have active TB should be considered infectious if (1) cough is present, (2) they are undergoing cough-inducing procedures, or (3) sputum AFB smears are positive, and (4) they are not on chemotherapy, have just started chemotherapy, or have a poor clinical or bacteriological response to chemotherapy. A person with drug-susceptible TB who is on adequate chemotherapy and has had a significant clinical and bacteriologic response to therapy (reduction in cough, resolution of fever, and progressively decreasing quantity of bacilli on smear) is probably no longer infectious. However, since drug-susceptibility results are usually not known when the decision to discontinue isolation is made, all TB patients should remain in TB isolation while hospitalized until three consecutive sputum smears are negative and they demonstrate clinical improvement.

B. DIAGNOSIS AND TREATMENT OF TB

1. Diagnostic Procedures for TB

a. Purified Protein Derivative (PPD) Skin Testing and Anergy Testing. The PPD skin test is the only method available for demonstrating infection with *M. tuberculosis*. Although currently available PPD tests are less then 100% sensitive and specific for detection of infection of *M. tuberculosis*, no better diagnostic methods have yet been devised. Interpretation of PPD test results requires a knowledge of the antigen used, the immunologic basis for the reaction to this antigen, the technique of administering and reading the test, and the results of epidemiologic and clinical experience with the test (2–4). The PPD test, like all medical tests, is subject to variability, but many of the inherent variations in administration and reading of tests can be avoided by proper training and careful attention to details.   The intracutaneous (Mantoux) administration of a measured amount of purified protein derivative tuberculin is the best means of detecting infection with *M. tuberculosis*. One-tenth milliliter of PPD (5 TU) is injected into either the volar or dorsal surface of the forearm. The tuberculin should be injected just beneath the surface of the skin. A discrete, pale elevation of the skin (a wheal) 6 to 10 mm in diameter should be produced.

PPD tests should be read by designated, trained personnel between 48 and 72 hours after injection. Patient or HCW self-reading tests of PPDs should not be accepted. The basis of the reading is the presence or absence of induration. Redness or erythema should not be measured. The transverse diameter of induration should be recorded in millimeters. The interpretation of a PPD reaction should be influenced by the purpose for which the test was given (e.g., epidemiologic versus diagnostic purposes), by the prevalence of TB infection in the population being tested, and by the consequences of false classification. Errors in classification can be minimized by establishing an appropriate definition of a positive reaction (Table 10.5).

The positive predictive value of PPD tests (i.e., the probability that a person with a positive PPD is truly infected with *M. tuberculosis*) is dependent on the prevalence of TB infection in the population being tested (61). In populations with a low prevalence of TB infection, the probability that a positive PPD represents true infection with *M. tuberculosis* is very low. In populations with a high prevalence of TB infection, the probability that a positive PPD represents true infection with *M. tuberculosis* is much higher. In order to ensure that very few persons infected with *M. tuberculosis* will be classified as having negative reactions and few persons not infected with tubercle bacilli will be classified as

---

Table 10.5. Summary of Interpretation of Skin Tests

1. A reaction of ≥5 mm is classified as positive in:
   Persons with HIV infection or risk factors for HIV infection with unknown HIV status
   Persons who have had recent close contact[a] with persons with active TB
   Persons who have abnormal chest radiographs consistent with old healed TB
2. A reaction of ≥10 mm is classified as positive in all persons who do not meet any of the criteria above, but who have other risk factors for TB including:
   High-risk groups
   Intravenous drug users known to be HIV seronegative
   Persons with other medical conditions that have been reported to increase the risk of progressing from latent TB infection to active TB, including silicosis, gastrectomy, jejunoileal bypass surgery, being 10% or more below ideal body weight; chronic renal failure, diabetes mellitus, high-dose corticosteroid and other immunosuppressive therapy, some hematologic disorders (e.g., leukemias and lymphomas), and other malignancies
   High-prevalence groups
   Foreign-born persons from high-prevalence countries in Asia, Africa, and Latin America
   Persons from medically underserved low income populations
   Residents of long-term care facilities (e.g., correctional institutions, nursing homes)
   Persons from high-risk populations in their communities, as determined by local public health authorities
3. Induration of ≥15 mm is classified as positive for persons who do not meet any of the above criteria.
4. Recent converters are defined on the basis of both induration and age:
   ≥10 mm increase within a 2-year period is classified as positive for persons <35 years of age
   ≥15 mm increase within a 2-year period is classified as positive for persons ≥35 years of age
   ≥5 mm increases under certain circumstances (item #1, above)

---

[a] Recent close contact implies household contact or unprotected occupational exposure similar in intensity and duration to household contact.

having positive reactions, different cut-points are used to separate positive reactions from negative reactions for different groups, depending on the risk of TB in that group.

A lower cut-point (i.e., 5 mm) is used for the highest risk groups, including HIV-infected persons, recent close contacts (recent close contact implies household contact or unprotected occupation exposure similar in intensity and duration to household contact), or persons with abnormal chest radiographs consistent with old TB. A higher cut-point (i.e., 10 mm) is used for persons who are not in the highest risk group but who have other risk factors, such as injecting drug users known to be HIV seronegative; persons with certain medical conditions that increase the risk of progression from latent TB infection to active TB (Table 10.5); medically underserved, low-income populations; foreign-born persons from countries with a high prevalence of TB; and residents of correctional institutions and nursing homes. An even higher cut-point (i.e., 15 mm) is used for all other persons with none of the above risk factors.

Recent PPD converters are considered a high-risk group. An increase of induration of $\geq$10 mm within a 2-year period is classified as a conversion to a positive test among persons <35 years of age. An increase of induration of $\geq$15 mm within a 2-year period is classified as a conversion for persons $\geq$35 years of age (3). Increases of induration $\geq$5 mm may be indicative of new infection in certain circumstances (4).

Persons with HIV infection may have suppressed reactions to skin tests because of anergy, particularly when CD4 + T-lymphocyte counts decline (62, 63). Persons with anergy will have a negative PPD whether or not they are infected with *M. tuberculosis*. Persons with HIV infection should be evaluated for anergy in conjunction with PPD testing. Two companion antigens (e.g., *Candida* antigen and tetanus toxoid) should be used in addition to PPD. Persons with >2 mm of induration to any of the skin tests (including tuberculin) are considered not anergic. Reactions of $\geq$5 mm to PPD are considered to be evidence of TB infection in HIV-infected persons regardless of the reaction to the companion antigens. If there is no reaction (i.e., <3 mm induration) to any of the antigens, the person being tested is considered anergic. In such persons, determining whether or not the person is likely to be infected with *M. tuberculosis* must be decided on the basis of other epidemiologic factors, such as the proportion of other persons with the same level of exposure who have positive PPDs and the intensity or duration of exposure to infectious TB patients that the anergic person experienced.

BCG vaccination may produce a PPD reaction that cannot be reliably distinguished from a reaction due to infection with *M. tuberculosis*. In a person who was vaccinated with BCG, the probability that a PPD test reaction results from infection with *M. tuberculosis* increases (1) as the size of the reaction increases, (2) when the patient is a contact of a person with TB, (3) when the patient's country of origin has a high prevalence of TB, and (4) as the length of time between vaccination and PPD testing increases. For example, a PPD test reaction of $\geq$10 mm can be attributed to infection with *M. tuberculosis* in an adult who was vaccinated with BCG as a child and who is from a country with a high prevalence of TB (64).

In persons with TB infection, the ability to react to PPD may gradually wane over time. If tested with PPD, persons who were remotely infected may have a negative reaction. However, the PPD may boost the hypersensitivity, and the size of the reaction may be larger on a subsequent test. This boosted reaction may be misinterpreted as a PPD test conversion from a new infection. The occurrence of the booster phenomenon increases with increasing age.

When PPD testing of adults is to be repeated periodically (as in HCW skin testing programs), two-step testing can be used to reduce the likelihood that a boosted reaction is misinterpreted as a new infection. Two-step testing should be done on all newly employed HCWs who have an initial negative PPD at the time of employment. A second test should be performed 1–3 weeks later. If the second test is positive, this is most likely a boosted reaction, and the person should be classified as previously infected. If the second test remains negative, the person is classified as uninfected. A positive reaction to a subsequent test is likely to represent a new infection with *M. tuberculosis* in the interval.

b. Chest Radiograph.   Persons with symptoms suggestive of TB should receive a chest radiograph regardless of PPD test results. Abnormalities strongly suggestive of active TB include upper lobe infiltration, particularly if cavitation is seen (65). Patchy or nodular infiltrates in the apical or subapical posterior upper lobes or the superior segment of the lower lobe are also suggestive of active TB. If abnormalities are noted or if the person has symptoms suggestive of extrapulmonary TB, additional diagnostic studies should be undertaken.

The radiographic presentation of pulmonary TB in patients with HIV infection may be unusual (66). Typical apical cavitary disease is less common among persons with HIV infection. They may have infiltrates in any lung zone, often associated with mediastinal and/or hilar adenopathy or rarely they may have a normal chest radiograph.

c. Bacteriology.   Smear and culture examination of three sputum specimens collected on different days is the main diagnostic procedure for pulmonary TB (4). Sputum smears that fail to demonstrate AFB do not exclude the diagnosis of TB. Nationwide, approximately 60% of patients with positive sputum cultures have positive AFB sputum smears. Sputum smears from patients with HIV infection and pulmonary TB may be less likely to reveal AFB then those from immunocompetent patients, a finding believed to be consistent with the lower frequency of cavitary pulmonary disease observed among HIV-infected persons (35, 37).

It is important that specimens for smear and culture have adequate volume of expectorated sputum and contain little saliva. In patients with negative sputum smears, bronchoscopy may produce positive results (33, 34). In young children who cannot adequately produce sputum, gastric aspirates may provide an adequate specimen.

A positive culture of sputum or other clinical specimens, with organisms identified as *M. tuberculosis*, provides a definitive diagnosis of TB. Conventional laboratory methods may require 4 to 8 weeks for species identification; however, the use of radiometric culture techniques and nucleic acid probes facilitates more rapid detection and identification of mycobacteria (67, 68). Mixed mycobacterial infection, either simultaneous or sequential, may occur and may obscure the recognition of *M. tuberculosis* clinically and in the laboratory (38). The use of nucleic acid probes of both *Mycobacterium avium* complex and *M. tuberculosis* may be useful for identifying mixed mycobacterial infections in clinical specimens.

2. Preventive Therapy for Latent TB Infection and Treatment of Active TB

a. Preventive Therapy for Latent TB Infection.   Determining whether or not a person with a positive PPD reaction or conversion is a candidate for preventive therapy must be based on (1) the likelihood that the reaction represents true infection with *M. tuberculosis* (as determined by the cut-points), (2) the estimated risk of progression from latent infection to active TB, and (3) the risk of hepatitis with isoniazid preventive therapy (as determined by age and other factors).

HCWs with positive PPD tests should be evaluated for preventive therapy, regardless of age if they are a recent converter, a close contact of a person with active TB, have a medical condition that increases the risk for TB, have HIV infection, or use injecting drugs (3). HCWs without those risk factors should be evaluated for preventive therapy if they are younger than age 35.

Preventive therapy should be considered for anergic persons who are known contacts of infectious TB patients and for those from groups in which the prevalence of TB infection is high (i.e., ≥10%).

Because of some reports of an increased risk of isoniazid hepatitis in the peripartum period, the decision to use preventive therapy during pregnancy should be made on a case-by-case basis, depending on the patient's estimated risk of progression to active disease (69–72). Although testing in animals has demonstrated a risk of cancer (73), there are no data to suggest that isoniazid (INH) poses a carcinogenic risk for humans (74–76).

The usual preventive therapy regimen is oral isoniazid 300 mg daily for adults and 10 mg/kg/day for children (77). The recommended duration of therapy is 12 months for persons with HIV infection and persons with abnormal chest radiographs consistent with old healed TB; other persons should receive 6 months of therapy. For persons likely to be infected with MDR-TB, alternative multidrug preventive therapy regimens should be considered (78).

All persons placed on preventive therapy should be educated about the possible adverse reactions associated with isoniazid and should be monitored at least monthly by appropriately trained personnel (69–72, 79, 80). Persons with asymptomatic TB infection should be advised of the possibility of reinfection with another strain of *M. tuberculosis* (81).

b. Treatment for Active TB.   Drug susceptibility test should be performed on all initial isolates from patients with TB. However, since test results may not be available for several weeks, selection of an initial regimen can be difficult, especially in areas where there is drug-resistant TB. Tables 10.6 and 10.7 summarize current recommendations for initial therapy and dosage schedules for the treatment of drug-susceptible TB (39). In areas or facilities in which there is a high prevalence of MDR-TB, the initial treatment regimen used (while results of drug-susceptibility test are pending) may need to be expanded. This decision should be based on analysis of surveillance data.

When drug susceptibility results become available, the regimen should be adjusted appropriately (82–85). If drug resistance is present, clinicians unfamiliar with the management of patients with drug-resistant TB should seek expert consultation.

In order for any regimen to be effective, adherence to the regimen must be assured. The most effective method of assuring adherence is the use of DOT following discharge (39, 80). This should be coordinated with the public health department.

C. RESPIRATORY PROTECTION

Personal respiratory protection should be used by persons entering rooms where patients with known or suspected infectious TB are being isolated, during cough-inducing or aerosol-generating procedures on patients with known or suspected infectious TB, and in other settings where administrative and engineering controls are not likely to protect persons from inhaling infectious airborne droplet nuclei.

The precise level of effectiveness of respiratory protection in protecting HCWs from transmission of *M. tuberculosis* in health-care settings cannot be determined with currently available data. Studies have provided data about the effectiveness of respiratory protection from many hazardous airborne materials, but not from *M. tuberculosis*. There are gaps in the understanding of the transmission of *M. tuberculosis* that limit the ability to conduct the appropriate studies to determine the effectiveness of respiratory protection against transmission of *M. tuberculosis*. Neither the smallest infectious dose of *M. tuberculosis* nor the highest level of exposure to *M. tuberculosis* at which transmission will not occur have been conclusively defined (53, 86, 87). Furthermore, the size, size distribution, and number of particles containing viable *M. tuberculosis* that are generated by infectious TB patients have not been adequately studied, and it is not possible to measure accurately with currently available methods the concentration of infectious droplet nuclei in a room.

Nevertheless, there are certain settings where administrative and engineering controls may not fully protect HCWs from airborne droplet nuclei, such as in TB isolation rooms, during cough-inducing or aerosol-producing procedures, and in certain other settings (e.g., transportation of an infectious TB patient in an ambulance). Respiratory protective devices used in these settings should have characteristics that are suitable for the organism they are protecting against (i.e., *M. tuberculosis*) and the settings in which they are used (i.e., health-care settings). The recommendations in this document are based on the available data about

Table 10.6. Options for the Initial Treatment of TB in Children and Adults

Option 1	Option 2	Option 3
Initial Phase: Daily isoniazid, rifampin, pyrazinamide, and either ethambutol or streptomycin for 8 weeks. Ethambutol or streptomycin may be discontinued if susceptibility to isoniazid and rifampin is demonstrated. Ethambutol or streptomycin may not be necessary for patients in areas where the primary isoniazid resistance rate is documented to be less than 4%. *Continuation Phase:* Isoniazid and rifampin for 16 weeks, either daily, two times weekly, or three times weekly.[a] Consult a TB medical expert if drug susceptibility results show resistance to any of the first-line drugs or if the patient remains smear positive after 3 months.	*Initial Phase:* Isoniazid, rifampin, pyrazinamide, and either ethambutol or streptomycin daily for 2 weeks, then two times weekly[a] for 6 weeks. *Continuation Phase:* Isoniazid and rifampin two times weekly[a] for 16 weeks. Consult a TB medical expert if drug susceptibility results show resistance to any of the first-line drugs or if the patient remains smear positive after 3 months.	Treat with directly observed therapy 3 times weekly[a] with isoniazid, rifampin, pyrazinamide, and ethambutol or streptomycin for 6 months. The strongest evidence from clinical trials is for the effectiveness of all four drugs administered for the full 6 months. There is weaker evidence that streptomycin can be discontinued after 4 months if the isolate is susceptible to all drugs. The evidence for stopping pyrazinamide before the end of 6 months is equivocal for the three times weekly regimen and there is no evidence on the effectiveness of this regimen with ethambutol for less than the full 6 months. Consult a TB medical expert if drug susceptibility results show resistance to any of the first-line drugs or if the patient remains smear positive after 3 months.

From CDC. Initial therapy for tuberculosis in the era of multidrug resistance: recommendations of the Advisory Council for the Elimination of Tuberculosis. MMWR 1993;42 no. RR-7.
[a] All regimens given two times weekly or three times weekly should be administered by directly observed therapy.

Table 10.7. Dosage Recommendations for the Initial Treatment of TB among Children[a] and Adults

Drugs	Dosage					
	Daily Dose		Two Times Weekly Dose		Three Times Weekly Dose	
	Children[a]	Adults	Children[a]	Adults	Children	Adults
Isoniazid	10–20 mg/kg Max 300 mg	5 mg/kg Max 300 mg	20–40 mg/kg Max 900 mg	15 mg/kg Max 900 mg	20–40 mg/kg Max 900 mg	15 mg/kg Max 900 mg
Rifampin	10–20 mg/kg Max 600 mg	10 mg/kg Max 600 mg	10–20 mg/kg Max 600 mg	10 mg/kg Max 600 mg	10–20 mg/kg Max 600 mg	10 mg/kg Max 600 mg
Pyrazinamide	15–30 mg/kg Max 2 gm	15–30 mg/kg Max 2 gm	50–70 mg/kg Max 4 gm	50–70 mg/kg Max 4 gm	50–70 mg/kg Max 3 gm	50–70 mg/kg Max 3 gm
Ethambutol	15–25 mg/kg Max 2.5 gm	15–25 mg/kg Max 2.5 gm	50 mg/kg	50 mg/kg	25–30 mg/kg	25–30 mg/kg
Streptomycin	20–40 mg/kg Max 1 gm	15 mg/kg Max 1 gm	20–40 mg/kg Max 1.5 gm	20–40 mg/kg Max 1.5 gm	20–40 mg/kg Max 1 gm	20–40 mg/kg Max 1 gm

[a]12 years of age or under.

the effectiveness of respiratory protection against noninfectious hazardous materials in work places other than health-care settings and in an interpretation of how these data can be applied to respiratory protection against *M. tuberculosis*. Although the following recommendations do not offer the maximum available protection, they probably exceed the minimum level of protection needed to prevent occupational exposure.[c]

These are interim recommendations. As new data and devices become available, and if new certification procedures are developed and implemented, these recommendations may be changed.

1. Performance Criteria for Personal Respirators for Protection against Transmission of *M. tuberculosis*

Based on the limited data currently available and the considerations stated above, it is recommended that respiratory protective devices used in health-care settings for protection against *M. tuberculosis* meet the following criteria. These criteria are based on estimated characteristics of respirators that were used in conjunction with administrative and engineering controls in outbreak settings where transmission to HCWs and patients appeared to cease.

1. The ability to filter particles 1 μm in size in the unloaded[d] state with a filter efficiency of ≥95% (i.e., filter leakage of ≤5%), given flow rates of up to 50 liters/min. Available evidence suggests that infectious droplet nuclei are in the 1- to 5-μm size range; therefore, respirators used in health-care settings should be able to filter the smallest particles in this range efficiently. Fifty liters per minute is a reasonable estimate of the higher flow rate a HCW is likely to achieve during breathing even with strenuous work activities.
2. The ability to be qualitatively or quantitatively fit tested in a reliable way (47) to obtain a face-seal leakage of no more that 10% for most workers.[e]
3. The ability to fit HCWs with different facial sizes and characteristics, which can usually be met by the availability of at least three sizes of respirators.
4. To ensure proper protection, the facepiece fit should be checked by the wearer each time he or she puts on the respirator, in accordance with OSHA's standard and good industrial hygiene practice.

---

[c] The Occupational Safety and Health Act of 1970 (PL 91-596) requires that NIOSH develop recommendations so that no worker will suffer impaired health or function or diminished life expectancy as a result of his or her work. In September 1992, NIOSH recommended the use of NIOSH-certified, powered half-mask respirators equipped with HEPA filters by all workers potentially exposed to TB in conjunction with an effective respiratory protection program (48, 88). NIOSH concluded that, because the amount of infectious droplet nuclei in the air cannot currently be measured and because an exposure limit to *M. tuberculosis* has not yet been established, a high level of respiratory protection should be recommended.

[d] Some filters become more efficient as they become loaded with dust. Health-care settings do not have enough dust in the air to "load" a filter on a respirator. Therefore, the filter efficiency for respirators used in health-care settings must be determined in the unloaded state.

[e] If quantitative fit testing is conducted, because of the well-documented deterioration of protection provided by respirators in the actual workplace compared to that obtained during a fit test, it is established industrial hygiene practice to require a fit test protection factor that is 10 times the assigned protection factor (APF) rating of the testing respirator. Thus, a quantitative fit test would require a fit factor of 100 to guarantee no more than 10% face-seal leakage for most workers in the workplace.

2. Specific Respirators

The OSHA respiratory protection standard requires that all respiratory protective devices be certified by NIOSH (88). Respirators with HEPA filters are the only currently available certified respirators that meet or exceed the performance criteria stated above. Although DM and DFM filters are certified, these criteria are not evaluated. Current NIOSH certification procedures require that DM and DFM filters filter 99% of silica dust, but the certification process does not include adequate tests for filter efficacy against low-concentration aerosols in the size range of droplet nuclei. There is evidence that some respirators with DM and DFM filters do meet these criteria. However, at the present time, there is no way to determine which NIOSH-certified DM and DFM filters meet these performance criteria.

In some settings, the risk of TB transmission may be estimated in the risk assessment or the best judgment of infection control staff to be so high that respiratory protection exceeding these criteria may be considered appropriate. In such settings, consideration may be given to the use of higher levels of protection (Table 10.3). Characteristics of a variety of currently available respiratory protection devices are summarized in Table 10.3.

3. The Efficacy of Respiratory Protective Devices

The following information summarizes the available data about the effectiveness of respiratory protection against hazardous airborne materials and is based on experience with respiratory protection in the industrial setting. Data for protection against transmission of *M. tuberculosis* are not available. Table 10.3 summarizes the differences among the categories of respirators. Table 10.8 summarizes the advantages and disadvantages for available categories of respirators.

The parameters used to determine the efficacy of a respiratory protective device are face-seal efficacy and filter efficacy.

a. Face-Seal Leakage.   Face-seal leakage compromises the ability of particulate respirators to protect the worker from airborne material (89–91). A proper seal between a respirator's sealing surface and a wearer's face is essential for effective and reliable performance of any negative-pressure respirator. It is less critical, but still important, for a positive-pressure respirator. Face-seal leakage can result from factors such as incorrect facepiece size or shape, incorrect or defective facepiece sealing-lip, beard growth on the wearer, perspiration or facial oils that can result in facepiece slippage, failure to use all the headstraps, incorrect positioning of a facepiece on a wearer's face, incorrect headstrap tension or position, improper mask maintenance, and mask damage.

The mechanism of action of negative-pressure (nonpowered) particulate respirators is based on the same principle. During each inhalation by a wearer, a negative pressure (relative to the workplace air) is created inside the facepiece of this type of respirator. Due to this negative pressure, air containing contaminants can take a path of least resistance into the respirator—through leaks at the face-seal interface—thus avoiding the higher-resistance filter material. Currently

Table 10.8. Advantages and Disadvantages of Different Types of Respirators

Type of Respirator	Advantages	Disadvantages, Limitations
Negative-pressure, particulate air-purifying respirators Disposable Dust-mist (DIM) Dust-fume-mist (DM) HEPA Replaceable filter Half facepiece with HEPA	General Lightweight Small size Ease of maintenance Little physiological stress to wearer Mobility is not restricted Simple design, easily understood by wearer Disposable respirators Require no maintenance, cleaning, or disinfecting Low breathing resistance	General Negative pressure may allow leakage, particularly if not fitted properly Negative pressure cannot be achieved if HCW is not clean-shaven Disposable respirators Measuring face-seal in the field may be difficult DM and DFM respirators May degrade if not stored properly Replaceable filter masks Require maintenance, cleaning, disinfection
Positive-pressure particulate air-purifying respirators Half facepiece with HEPA filter Full facepiece with HEPA filter Loose-fitting with HEPA filter	General Decreased inhalation resistance may make respirator more comfortable to wear Mobility is not restricted Loose-fitting devices No large sealing surfaces on the face allows some people with facial scars or facial hair to achieve an adequate fit	General Weight and bulk makes respirator more difficult to wear than nonpowered respirators Need for continued maintenance May compromise communication May be intimidating to some patients Motor and airflow will create noise, which may hamper wearer's ability to hear

available, cup-shaped, disposable particulate respirators have 0 to 10% (89) to 20% (92, 93) face-seal leakage. This leakage through the face-seal results from limitations in the design, construction, number or sizes available of these masks, and the variability of the human face. The face-seal leakage is assumed to be even higher if the respirators are not properly fitted to the wearer's face, tested for an adequate fit by a qualified individual, and then checked for fit by the wearer every time these masks are donned. Face-seal leakage may be reduced to less than 10% with improvements in design and more available sizes, combined with appropriate fit testing and fit checking.

In contrast to nonpowered filter respirators, powered air-purifying respirators (PAPRs) produce a positive pressure inside the facepiece under most conditions of use. The blower forcibly draws ambient air through HEPA filters and then delivers the filtered air to the facepiece. This air is blown into the facepiece at flow rates that generally exceed the expected inhalation flow rates. The small positive pressure inside the facepiece reduces face-seal leakage to low levels, particularly during the relatively low inhalation rates expected in health-care settings. Powered air-purifying respirators with a tight-fitting facepiece have less than 2% face-seal leakage under routine conditions (92). Powered-air respirators with loose-fitting facepieces, hoods, or helmets have less than 4% face-seal leakage under routine conditions (92). Thus, a powered air-purifying respirator may offer lower levels of face-seal leakage than nonpowered, half-mask respirators (full facepiece, nonpowered respirators have the same leakage, i.e., 2%, as PAPRs). However, a surgical mask should also be worn during procedures where a sterile field is maintained.

Another problem that can contribute to face-seal leakage of cup-shaped, disposable masks is that currently most of these masks are available in only one size. The single size in which most cup-shaped, disposable masks are available may produce higher leakage for wearers with small face sizes (94). The facepieces used for some reusable (including HEPA and replaceable filter, negative-pressure) and all positive-pressure particulate air-purifying respirators are available in up to three different sizes.

b. Filter Leakage.   Aerosol leakage through the respirator filter is dependent on at least five types of independent variables (95): (1) the filtration characteristics for each type of filter, (2) the size distribution of the droplets in the aerosol, (3) the linear velocity through the filtering material, (4) the filter loading (i.e., amount of contaminant deposited on the filter), and (5) any electrostatic charges on the filter and on the droplets in the aerosol.

DM and DFM filters have widely varying efficiencies against particles ≤ 2 μm (96–99) with filter leakage ranging from 0 to 40%. Current NIOSH certification procedures require DM and DFM filters to filter 99% silica dust,[f] but the certification process does not include adequate tests for filter efficacy against low-concentration aerosols in the size range of droplet nuclei. In contrast, the NIOSH

---

[f]In order to be certified, a filter is allowed a maximum penetration of 1.5 mg after the silica test. The total amount of dust that contacts the filter during the test is 144 mg. Therefore, a maximum allowable leakage is about 1%.

certification performance standard for HEPA filters requires HEPA filters to be at least 99.97% efficient (i.e., leakage must be less than or equal to 0.03%) against the most filter-penetrating aerosol size (approximately 0.3 μm), although these filters are not tested against biological aerosols (100).

When HEPA filters are used in a particulate air-purifying respirator, filter efficiency is so high (effectively 100%) that filter leakage is not a consideration. Hence, for all HEPA-filter respirators, the potential for inward leakage of droplet nuclei is essentially that which occurs at a mask's face-seal. In contrast, many currently available disposable, negative-pressure respirators with DM or DFM filters are likely to have some leakage through the filter that adds to the leakage at the face-seal.

c. Fit Testing.   A fit test is used to determine whether a respiratory protective device adequately fits a particular HCW. The HCW may need to be fit tested with several devices in order to determine which device offers the best fit for that HCW. However, fit tests can detect only the face-seal leakage that exists at the time of the fit testing. Also, fit tests do not distinguish face-seal leakage from filter leakage.

Determination of facepiece fit can involve qualitative or quantitative tests (101) (Table 10.9). A qualitative test relies on the wearer's subjective response. A quantitative test uses detectors to measure inward leakage.

Disposable, negative-pressure particulate respirators can be qualitatively fit tested with substances that can be tasted, although the results may not be reliable since they depend on the subjective response of the person being tested. Quantitative fit testing of disposable negative-pressure particulate respirators with DM or DFM filters can be performed only if the manufacturer provides a test respirator with a probe for this purpose and cannot be performed using the usual test aerosols of 0.6 to 0.7 μm, due to filter penetration. The reliability of quantitative fit testing of these devices is not known. Qualitative fit tests can also be performed on disposable negative-pressure particulate respirators with HEPA filters using irritant smoke. Quantitative fit testing can be performed on disposable, negative-pressure particulate respirators with HEPA filter devices using a test respirator with a probe.

Replaceable filter, negative-pressure particulate respirators, and all positive pressure particulate respirators can be reliably fit tested both qualitatively and quantitatively when fitted with HEPA filters.

d. Fit Checking.   A fit check is a maneuver that a HCW performs before each use of the respiratory protective device to check the fit. The fit check can be performed according to the manufacturer's facepiece fitting instructions or using a negative pressure test of a positive pressure test (Table 10.9).

Some currently available cup-shaped, disposable negative-pressure particulate respirators with DM, DFM, or HEPA filters cannot be reliable fit checked by wearers (93) because it is difficult to occlude the entire surface of the filter. Strategies for overcoming these limitations are under development by respirator manufacturers but have not been evaluated.

Table 10.9. Procedures for Qualitative Fit Testing and Fit Checking

---

Fit Testing

    A fit test is used to determine whether a respirator adequately fits a particular HCW. The HCW may need to be fit tested with several respirators in order to determine which respirator offers the best fit.

Qualitative (irritant or odorous chemical agent)

    The wearer is exposed to an irritant smoke, isoamyl acetate vapor, or other suitable test agent easily detectable by irritation, odor, or taste. If the wearer is unable to detect penetration of the test agent, the respirator is probably tight enough. DM and DFM filters do not filter irritant smoke, therefore they may not be tested with this agent. Isoamyl acetate vapor is not suitable for fit testing particulate respirators.

Quantitative (probe)

    A quantitative fit test uses a probe inserted through the device to determine the concentration of a substance inside the respirator compared to the concentration of the substance outside the respirator.

    Quantitative respirator fit testing procedures may be found in the NIOSH document, Guide to Industrial Respiratory Protection (151—NIOSH1987).

Advantages and disadvantages

    Usually qualitative tests are fast, require no complicated expensive equipment, and are easily performed in the field. However, most qualitative tests rely on the wearer's subjective response, so they may not be entirely reliable. The tests are unable to rank two or more adequately fitting respirators, due to the subjective nature of the test.

    One advantage of a quantitative test is that it does not rely on a subjective response and therefore may be more reliable. Quantitative fitting tests require expensive equipment that can be operated only by highly trained personnel. Each test respirator must be equipped with a sampling probe to allow removal of a continuous air sample from the facepiece, so the same facepiece cannot be worn in actual service. New tests are available that allow the HCW to wear the actual respirator. Filter elements contain the probe and are changed.

Fit checking

    HCWs should check the facepiece fit of a respirator before each use. They should be instructed how to adjust the respirator and to determine if it fits properly. This may be done following the manufacturer's facepiece fitting instructions. This may also be done in one of the following ways:

Negative pressure test

    To perform a negative-pressure fit check, the HCW dons the respirator and adjusts the straps. The HCW then occludes any portion of the respirator through which air may enter (i.e., wherever there is filter). The HCW then inhales deeply. Suction created by the inhalation should compress the respirator against the face, if the mask fits properly; no leakage should be detected.

Positive pressure test

    To perform a positive-pressure fit check, the HCW dons the device with the straps adjusted correctly and exhales with moderate force while occluding the exhalation valve. Leakage of air at the face seal indicates an inadequate fit.

---

    e. Reuse of Respirators. In use against nonbiological aerosols, filters must be changed when the filter becomes loaded with airborne material such that breathing resistance becomes uncomfortable or physical damage occurs to a filter. However, in health-care settings, there should be fewer particles in the air. In addition, once particles impact on a filter, they are not readily reaerosolized. Thus, in theory, respirator filters could remain functional for weeks to months, and one HCW could use the same respirator for that period of time. Before each use, the outside of each filter should be inspected for physical damage. Standard operating procedures should be developed by infection control personnel for the reuse of respirators designated as disposable and for disinfection and disposal of replaceable filter elements, according to published guidelines (101).

4. Implementing a Personal Respiratory Protection Program

Whenever personal respiratory protection is used for protection of HCWs, an effective personal respiratory protection program must be developed, implemented, administered, and periodically reevaluated (47, 92, 102).

All HCWs who enter TB isolation rooms or who are present when cough-inducing procedures are performed on patients with known or suspected TB must be included in the respiratory protection program. Visitors, such as family members, should be required to wear respiratory protection and should be given instruction on how to use it while in TB isolation rooms. However, they need not be included in the respiratory protection program.

The number of HCWs included in the program will vary in each facility according to the size of the facility and the number of potentially infectious TB patients in the facility. The program should include enough HCWs to provide adequate care for a patient with known or suspected TB should such a patient be admitted to the facility. Respiratory protection programs in facilities with a low prevalence of TB may include only a limited number of HCWs.

Information on how to develop and manage a respiratory protection program is available in technical training courses covering the basics of personal respiratory protection, which are offered by organizations such as NIOSH, OSHA, and the American Industrial Hygiene Association. In addition, similar short courses are available from private contractors and universities.

In order to be effective and reliable, any respiratory protection program must contain at least the following elements (89, 92, 102):

a. Assignment of Responsibility.   Supervisory responsibility for the respiratory protection program should be assigned to designated persons with expertise in issues relevant to the program, including occupational health.

b. Standard Operating Procedures.   Written standard operating procedures should contain information on all aspects of the respiratory protection program.

c. Medical Screening.   HCWs should not be assigned a task requiring use of respirators unless they are physically able to do the work while wearing the respirator. HCWs should be screened for pertinent medical conditions upon employment and periodically rescreened (92). The recommended periodicity varies according to several factors but could be as infrequent as every 5 years. The screening process should begin with a general screening (e.g., a questionnaire) for pertinent medical conditions. The results can then be used to identify HCWs who need further evaluation. The extent of the evaluation should be determined by what is medically indicated. Routine testing with chest roentgenograms or spirometry is not necessary or required.

Qualified personnel should determine what medical conditions are pertinent for each type of respiratory protection device that is used in the facility. There are very few medical conditions that would preclude the use of most negative-pressure particulate respirators. HCWs who have mild pulmonary or cardiac conditions may report some discomfort with breathing when wearing negative-pressure particulate respirators, but these respirators would not be expected to have any adverse health effect on the HCW. HCWs who have cardiac or pulmonary conditions that are more severe may have more difficulty performing their duties wearing negative-pressure respirators. These HCWs may be unable to use some powered air-purifying respirators because of the added weight of these respirators.

d. Training.   Respirator wearers and supervisors should receive training in the reasons for the need for wearing their respirator and the potential risks of not doing so. This training should also include at a minimum:

The nature, extent, and specific hazards of TB transmission in their health-care facility;
A description of specific risks of infection to each exposed individual, of any subsequent treatment with isoniazid or other chemoprophylactic agents, and of the possibility of active disease;
A description of why engineering controls may not be adequate to eliminate the need for personal respiratory protection;
An explanation of why a particular type of respirator has been selected for a specific location;
An explanation of the operation, capabilities, and limitations of the respirator provided;
Instruction in how the respirator wearer should inspect, don, fit check, and correctly wear their provided respirator;
An opportunity for each wearer to handle the respirator, learn how to don and wear it properly (i.e., achieve a proper face-seal fit on the wearer's face) and check important parts;
An explanation of why a particular type of respirator was chosen, how the respirator is properly maintained and stored, and the capabilities and limitations of the respirator provided;
Instruction in how to recognize an inadequately functioning respirator.

e. Face-Seal Fit Testing and Fit Checking.   HCWs should undergo fit testing to identify a respirator with an adequate fit for that HCW. The HCW should receive fitting instructions including demonstrations and practice in how the respirator should be worn, how to adjust it, and how to determine if it fits properly. The HCW should be instructed to check the facepiece fit before each use.

f. Respirator Inspection, Cleaning, Maintenance, and Storage.   Scrupulous respirator maintenance should be made an integral part of the overall respirator program. This applies to both replaceable filter respirators and respirators that are classified as disposable but that are reused. Manufacturer's instructions for inspection, cleaning, and maintenance of respirators should be followed to ensure that the respirator continues to function properly.

g. Periodic Evaluation of the Personal Respiratory Protection Program. The program should be completely evaluated at least annually, and both the written operating procedures and program administration should be modified as necessary based on the results. Elements of the program that should be evaluated include work practices and acceptance of respirators, including comfort and interference with duties.

D. DECONTAMINATION: CLEANING, DISINFECTING, AND STERILIZING OF PATIENT-CARE EQUIPMENT

Equipment used on patients with TB is unlikely to be involved in the transmission of the organism, although transmission of the organism by contaminated bronchoscopes has been demonstrated (103–105). The rationale for cleaning, disinfecting, or sterilizing patient-care equipment can be understood more readily if medical devices, equipment, and surgical materials are divided into three general categories (critical items, semicritical items, and noncritical items) based on the potential risk of infection involved in their use (107, 108).

Critical items are instruments such as needles, surgical instruments, cardiac catheters, or implants that are introduced directly into the bloodstream or into other normally sterile areas of the body. These items should be sterile at the time of use.

Semicritical items are items such as noninvasive flexible and rigid fiberoptic endoscopes or bronchoscopes, endotracheal tubes, or anesthesia breathing circuits, which may come in contact with mucous membranes but do not ordinarily penetrate body surfaces. Although sterilization is preferred for these instruments, high-level disinfection that destroys vegetative microorganisms; most fungal spores; tubercle bacilli; and small, nonlipid viruses may be used. Meticulous physical cleaning before sterilization or high-level disinfection is essential.

Noncritical items are those that either do not ordinarily touch the patient or touch only intact skin. Such items include crutches, bedboards, blood pressure cuffs, and various other medical accessories. These items are not associated with transmission of pathogens, including *M. tuberculosis*. Consequently, washing with a detergent is usually sufficient.

Generally, critical items should be sterilized, and semicritical items should be sterilized or subjected to high-level disinfection.

Health-care facility policies should identify whether cleaning, disinfecting, or sterilizing an item is indicated to decrease the risk of infection. Decisions about decontamination processes should be based on the intended use of the item and not on the diagnosis of the patient for whom the item was used. Selection of chemical disinfectants depends on the intended use, the level of disinfection required, and the structure and material of the item to be disinfected.

Although microorganisms are normally found on walls, floors, and other surfaces, these environmental surfaces are rarely associated with transmission of infections of patients or HCWs. This is particularly true with organisms such as *M. tuberculosis*, which generally require inhalation by the host for infection to occur.

Therefore, extraordinary attempts to disinfect or sterilize environmental surfaces are not indicated. If a detergent germicide is used for routine cleaning, a hospital-grade, Environmental Protection Agency-approved germicide/disinfectant that is not tuberculocidal can be used. The same routine daily cleaning procedures used in other rooms in the facility should be used to clean rooms of patients who are on TB isolation, and personnel cleaning the room should follow TB isolation practices.

GLOSSARY

This glossary contains many of the terms used in the guidelines, as well as others that are frequently encountered by those who work in TB infection control programs. The definitions given are not dictionary definitions but are the ones most applicable to usage relating to TB.

acid-fast bacilli—bacteria that retain certain dyes even when washed with an acid solution. Most acid-fast organisms are mycobacteria. When seen on a stained smear of sputum or other clinical specimen, a diagnosis of TB should be considered; however, the diagnosis is not confirmed until a culture is grown and identified as *M. tuberculosis*.

acquired drug resistance—resistance to one or more antituberculosis drugs which develops while a patient is on therapy, usually the result of nonadherence on the part of the patient or inadequate therapy prescribed by a health-care provider.

adherence—refers to the completion by patients of all aspects of the treatment regimen as prescribed by the medical provider; also refers to HCWs and employers following all guidelines pertaining to infection control.

aerosol, aerosolization—In TB, it refers to the infectious droplet nuclei that are expelled from a person and that can be transmitted to other people.

AIA—American Institute of Architects, a professional body that develops standards for building ventilation.

air changes—air flow quantity to a space measured in terms of the room volume, i.e., volume of air delivered ÷ room volume; usually expressed as number of air changes per hour.

alveoli—the small air sacs in the lungs that lie at the end of the bronchial tree; the site where carbon dioxide is replaced by oxygen in the lungs, and the site where TB infection usually begins.

anergy—the inability of a person to react to skin-test antigens because of defects in the immune system, even if the person is infected with the organisms tested.

anteroom—a small room located between an isolation room and a corridor that acts as an airlock, preventing escape of room contaminants into the corridor.

ASHRAE—American Society of Heating, Refrigerating and Air Conditioning Engineers, a professional body that develops standards for building ventilation.

asymptomatic—showing or causing no symptoms.

Bactec®—one of the most widely used radiometric methods to detect early growth of mycobacteria in culture. It provides rapid growth (average of 9 days), specific identification of *M. tuberculosis* (5 days), and rapid drug susceptibility testing (6 days).

bactericidal—capable of killing bacteria. Isoniazid and rifampin are the two most potent bactericidal antituberculosis drugs. (*See* bacteriostatic.)

bacteriostatic—capable of preventing bacterial growth but not necessarily capable of killing bacteria. Drugs such as ethambutol and *para*-aminosalicylic acid are primarily bacteriostatic. (*See* bactericidal.)

BCG (Bacillus Calmette-Guérin)—a TB vaccine widely used in some parts of the world.

booster phenomenon—seen when an individual with infection does not react to tuberculin because his or her body's cell responses to tuberculin have gradually waned over the years. An initial tuberculin test may stimulate (boost) the immune system so that the next test will be positive. This phenomenon is important in infection control in order to distinguish between recent converters and people who have been infected for a long time and to determine if in fact transmission is taking place. Although the booster phenomenon may occur at any age, it is most frequent among persons over 55 years.

bronchoscopy—a procedure for examining the respiratory tract by inserting an instrument (bronchoscope) through the mouth or nose into the trachea. Diagnostic specimens can be obtained during bronchoscopy.

capreomycin—an injectable second-line antituberculosis drug related to streptomycin. Used primarily for drug-resistant TB.

cavity—a hole in the lung resulting from destruction of pulmonary tissue; may be caused by TB, but also by other pulmonary infections and conditions. TB patients with cavities in their lungs are said to have "cavitary disease" and are often more infectious than patients without cavities.

chemotherapy—treatment of an infection or disease by means of oral or injectable drugs.

chest radiograph—In patients showing signs or symptoms of TB, a radiograph of the chest is taken to view the respiratory system. Abnormalities, such as lesions or cavities in the lungs and enlarged lymph nodes, may indicate the presence of TB.

contact—an individual who has shared the same air as a person with infectious TB for a sufficient amount of time so that there is a probability that transmission of TB has occurred.

conversion, PPD—(*See* purified protein derivative (PPD) test conversion.)

culture—the process of growing bacteria in the laboratory so that organisms can be identified.

cycloserine (CS)—a second-line oral antituberculosis drug, used primarily for treating drug-resistant TB and disease caused by nontuberculous mycobacteria.

dilution ventilation—an engineering control technique to dilute and remove airborne contaminants by the flow of air into and out of the area. Air that contains droplet nuclei is removed and replaced by air that is free of contaminants. If the flow is sufficient, droplet nuclei become dispersed, and their concentration in the air is diminished.

directly observed therapy—an adherence-enhancing strategy in which each dose of medication is ingested by the patient under the supervision of a health-care worker.

DNA probe—a technique that allows precise identification of mycobacterium such as *M. tuberculosis* and *M. bovis* that are grown in culture. The identification can be completed in as little as 2 hours.

droplet nuclei—microscopic particles (1 to 5 μm in diameter) produced when a person coughs, sneezes, shouts, or sings. The droplets can carry tubercle bacilli and remain in the air by normal air currents in the room.

drug susceptibility pattern—antituberculosis drugs to which a tubercle bacillus is susceptible and those to which it is resistant based on susceptibility tests.

drug susceptibility tests—laboratory tests that determine if the tubercle bacilli cultured from a patient is susceptible or resistant to various antituberculosis drugs.

ethambutol—an oral antituberculosis drug sometimes used with isoniazid and/or rifampin.

ethionamide—a second-line oral antituberculosis drug.

exposure—the condition of being subjected to something, such as infectious agents, which may have a harmful effect. A person exposed to TB does not necessarily become infected. (*See* transmission.)

fluorochrome stain—a technique for staining a clinical specimen with dyes that fluoresce, in order to perform a microscopic examination (smear) for mycobacteria. This technique is preferable to other staining techniques because the mycobacteria can be easily seen.

fomites—linens, books, dishes, or other objects used or touched by a patient. They are not involved in the transmission of TB.

gastric aspirates—procedure sometimes used to obtain mycobacteria for culture when a patient cannot produce adequate sputum. A tube inserted into the stomach is used to recover any bacilli that may have been coughed up and then swallowed. This procedure is particularly useful for diagnosis in children.

HEPA (high-efficiency particulate air) filter—specialized filter that is capable of removing 99.97% of particles 0.3 μm in diameter. It may be of assistance in control of TB transmission. It requires expertise in installation and maintenance.

human immunodeficiency virus or HIV infection—infection with the virus that causes the acquired immunodeficiency syndrome (AIDS). It is the most potent risk factor for progression from TB infection to active TB.

immunosuppressed—persons with severe cellular immunosuppression (e.g., HIV-infected or organ transplant patients on immunosuppressive therapy). These patients are at greatly increased risk for developing TB once infected. There are no data available on whether they are also at risk of becoming infected with *M. tuberculosis*, if exposed.

induced sputum—sputum obtained from a patient unable to cough up a spontaneous specimen. The patient inhales a mist of saline (salt water), which stimulates a cough from deep within the lungs.

induration—the area of swelling that surrounds the site of injection of tuberculin. The diameter of the indurated area is measured (in millimeters) 48 to 72 hours after the injection and is recorded as the result of the PPD test.

infection—the condition in which organisms capable of causing disease (e.g., *M. tuberculosis*) multiply within the body and cause a response from the host's immune defenses. Infection may or may not lead to clinical disease.

infectious—capable of causing infection. In TB, a person is infectious only if he or she has clinically active TB. TB patients whose sputum is AFB smear positive are often infectious.

intermittent therapy—therapy given on a twice weekly or three times weekly basis under direct supervision of a health-care worker.

intradermal—within the layers of the skin.

isoniazid (INH)—an oral drug used either alone to treat TB infection or in combination with one or more other drugs to treat TB disease.

kanamycin—injectable secondary antituberculosis drug related to streptomycin. It is used primarily for treatment of streptomycin-resistant TB.

local exhaust ventilation—used as a source control technique to capture and remove airborne contaminants by enclosing the contaminant source or by means of a hood placed very near the contaminant source.

Mantoux test—a tuberculin test given by injecting a measured amount of liquid tuberculin into the dermis (second layer of the skin) with a needle and syringe. It is the most reliable and best standardized technique for tuberculin testing. (*See* tuberculin skin test and purified protein derivative (PPD) test.)

mixing—the degree to which air supplied to a room mixes with the air already in the room. It is generally expressed in terms of a mixing value. A low value (i.e., 1) indicates good mixing; a higher value (i.e., 10) indicates poor mixing.

Mycobacterium tuberculosis *complex*—the complex of mycobacterial species that causes TB; it includes *M. tuberculosis*, *M. bovis*, and *M. africanum*.

negative pressure—a term used to describe the relative air pressure difference between two areas of the health-care facility. Air will flow from the higher pressure area into the lower pressure area.

para-*aminosalicylic acid (PAS)*—an oral antituberculosis drug used for drug-resistant TB.

pathogenesis—the natural development of a disease in the body without intervention (i.e., without treatment).

portable filtration units—portable devices that provide contaminant dilution by recirculating air within a room through a HEPA filter.

positive PPD reaction—a reaction to the purified protein derivative (PPD) test that suggests the individual tested is infected with tubercle bacilli. Determination of the reaction is largely dependent on interpretation by the person evaluating the test, given the patient's or HCWs medical history and risk factors.

preventive therapy—chemotherapy of TB infection, primarily used to prevent progression of infection to clinically active disease.

primary drug resistance (PDR)—resistance of bacteria to drugs that exists before the beginning of treatment. (*See* acquired drug resistance.)

primary drugs—term sometimes used to refer to the most commonly used antituberculosis drugs: isoniazid, rifampin, pyrazinamide, ethambutol, and streptomycin.

purified protein derivative (PPD)—a type of purified tuberculin preparation derived from old tuberculin (OT) and developed in the 1930s. The standard Mantoux test uses 5 tuberculin units (TU) of PPD.

purified protein derivative (PPD) test—a method to determine whether a person is infected with *M. tuberculosis*. A small dose of the antigen from *M. tuberculosis* is injected just beneath the surface of the skin, and the area is examined 48 to 72 hours after the injection. A positive reaction is measured according to the size of the induration. The classifications for positive reactions depend on the patient's medical history and various risk factors. (*See* Mantoux test.)

purified protein derivative (PPD) test conversion—growth in induration within a 2-year period after an initial negative reaction with a difference of 10 or more millimeters of induration. Such "conversion" may present new infection, which is associated with a high risk of developing disease, or may occur as a result of the booster phenomenon.

pyrazinamide (PZA)—an oral antituberculosis drug. It is important as a primary drug in short-course treatment regimens.

radiometric methods—a rapid method for culturing TB allowing identification of *M. tuberculosis* in 5 to 10 days.

recirculation—ventilation where all or most of the air exhausted from an area is returned to the area.

regimen—any particular treatment plan for TB specifying which drugs are used, in what doses, according to what schedule, and for how long.

registry—a record-keeping method to collect clinical, laboratory, and radiographic data on TB or any other pathological field so the data can be organized and properly processed to be made available for epidemiologic study.

resistance—the ability of some strains of bacteria (including *M. tuberculosis*) to grow and multiply even in the presence of certain drugs that normally kill them. (Such strains are referred to as "drug-resistant strains.")

rifampin—an oral antituberculosis drug that, when used along with isoniazid, provides the basis for short-course therapy.

secondary drugs—antituberculosis drugs used in difficult cases (such as for retreatment or when there is resistance to primary drugs). Examples are cycloserine, ethionamide, capreomycin.

single-pass ventilation—ventilation in which 100% of the air supplied to an area is exhausted to the outside.

smear (AFB smear)—a laboratory technique for visualizing mycobacteria. The specimen is smeared onto a slide, stained, and then placed under the microscope for examination. Smear results should be available within 24 hours. A large amount of mycobacteria usually indicates infectiousness; however, a "positive" result is not definitive for TB.

source case—an infectious individual who has transmitted tubercle bacilli to another person or persons.

source control—control of a contaminant at the source of generation rather than permitting it to enter the general work space.

specimen—any body fluid, secretion, or tissue sent to the laboratory where smears and cultures for tubercle bacilli will be performed. The specimen may consist of sputum, urine, spinal fluid, material obtained at biopsy, etc.

sputum—material coughed up from deep within the lungs. If a patient has a pulmonary infection, an examination of the sputum by smear and culture can indicate what organism is responsible for the infection. It should not be confused with saliva or with nasal secretions.

sputum smear positive—AFB are visible after staining when viewed under a microscope. Individuals with sputum smear positive for AFB are considered more infectious than those with smear-negative sputum.

streptomycin (SM)—the most commonly used injectable antituberculosis drug.

symptomatic—having symptoms that may be clues to the presence of TB or another disease. (*See* asymptomatic.)

transmission—the spread of an infectious agent like *M. tuberculosis* from one individual to another. The duration and intensity of exposure to TB is directly related to the likelihood that transmission will occur and a person will become infected. (*See* exposure.)

treatment failures—refers to individuals who fail to improve even after a course of chemotherapy is begun and to individuals whose disease worsens after having initially improved.

tubercle bacilli—the term often used to refer to the organism *M. tuberculosis*.

tuberculin skin test—a method to determine whether a person is infected with *M. tuberculosis*. A small dose of the antigen from *M. tuberculosis* is injected just beneath the surface of the skin and the area is examined 48 to 72 hours after the injection. A positive reaction is measured according to the size of the swelling. The classifications for positive reactions depend on the patient's medical history and various risk factors. (*See* Mantoux test, PPD test.)

tuberculosis (TB)—a clinically apparent active disease process caused by *M. tuberculosis* complex (usually *M. tuberculosis* or, rarely, *M. bovis* or *M. africanum*).

tuberculosis case—a particular instance of clinically active TB. It is sometimes used incorrectly to designate the individual with the disease.

tuberculosis infection—a condition in which living tubercle bacilli are present in the body, without producing clinically active disease. Although the infected individual has a positive tuberculin reaction, he or she has no symptoms related to the infection and is not infectious. However, the infected individual remains at lifelong risk of developing disease unless preventive therapy is given.

tuberculosis (TB) isolation precautions—infection control procedures that should be applied when persons with known or suspected infectious TB are hospitalized or residing in other inpatient facilities. These precautions include the use of a private room with negative pressure in relation to surrounding air and removal of air from the room directly to the outside. Not the same as ''respiratory isolation,'' which calls for a private room, but does not require negative pressure and exhaust of room air to the outside.

two-step testing—a procedure used among people who receive tuberculin skin tests periodically (such as health-care workers) to reduce the likelihood of mistaking a boosted reaction for a recent infection. If the initial tuberculin test is classified as negative, a second test is repeated 1 week later. If the reaction to the second test is positive, it probably represents a boosted reaction. If the second test result remains negative, the person is classified as being uninfected.

ultraviolet (UV) lamps—lamps that destroy germs by emitting radiation predominantly at a wavelength of 254 nm (intermediate between visible light and x-rays). They can be used in ceiling or wall fixtures or within air ducts of ventilation systems. The effectiveness in killing tubercle bacilli for infection control in health-care facilities is not yet proven.

ultraviolet germicidal irradiation (UVGI)—a form of radiation intermediate between visible light and x-rays. UVGI is effective in killing many bacteria including tubercle bacilli.

virulence—refers to the ability of a microorganism, such as *M. tuberculosis*, to produce serious disease. *M. tuberculosis* is a virulent organism. Some nontuberculous mycobacteria are virulent (e.g., *M. kansasii*), while others (e.g., *M. gordonae*) are not. (Pathogenicity is a related, though not identical, concept.)

REFERENCES

1. CDC. Draft guidelines for preventing the transmission of tuberculosis in health-care facilities. Federal Register, October 12, 1993. Atlanta: Department of Health and Human Services. 1993;Part II:52810-54.
2. CDC. Guidelines for preventing the transmission of tuberculosis in health-care settings, with special focus on HIV-related issues. MMWR 1990;39:RR-17.
3. CDC. Screening for tuberculosis and tuberculous infection in high-risk populations, and the use of preventive therapy for tuberculous infection in the United States: recommendations of the Advisory Committee for Elimination of Tuberculosis. MMWR 1990;39:RR-8.
4. ATS/CDC-American Thoracic Society, CDC. Diagnostic standards and classification of tuberculosis. Am Rev Respir Dis 1990;142:725–735.
5. Wells WF. Aerodynamics of droplet nuclei in airborne contagion and air hygiene. Cambridge: Harvard University Press, 1955:13–19.
6. Selwyn PA, Hartel D, Lewis VA, et al. A prospective study of the risk of tuberculosis among intravenous drug users with human immunodeficiency virus infection. N Engl J Med 1989;320:545–550.
7. Di Perri G, Cruciani M, Danzi MC, et al. Nosocomial epidemic of active tuberculosis among HIV-infected patients. Lancet 1989;2330:1502–1504.
8. Daley CL, Small PM, Schecter GF, et al. An outbreak of tuberculosis with accelerated progression among persons infected with the human immunodeficiency virus. An analysis using restriction-fragment-length polymorphisms. N Engl J Med 1992;326:231–235.
9. Edlin BR, Tokars JL, Grieco MH, et al. An outbreak of multidrug-resistant tuberculosis among hospitalized patients with the acquired immunodeficiency syndrome. N Engl J Med 1992;326:1514–1521.
10. Dooley SW, Villarino E, Lawrence M, et al. Nosocomial transmission of tuberculosis in a hospital unit for HIV-infected patients. JAMA 1992;267:2632–2634.
11. Barrett-Connor E. The epidemiology of tuberculosis in physicians. JAMA 1979;241:33–38.
12. Brennen C, Muder RR, Muraca PW. Occult endemic tuberculosis in a chronic care facility. Infect Control Hosp Epidemiol 1988;9:548–552.
13. Goldman KP. Tuberculosis in hospital doctors. Tubercle 1988;69:237–240.
14. Catanzaro A. Nosocomial tuberculosis. Am Rev Respir Dis 1982;125:559–562.

15. Ehrenkranz NJ, Kicklighter JL. Tuberculosis outbreak in a general hospital: evidence of airborne spread of infection. Ann Intern Med 1972;77:377–382.
16. Haley CE, McDonald RC, Rossi L, et al. Tuberculosis epidemic among hospital personnel. Infect Control Hosp Epidemiol 1989;10:204–210.
17. Hutton MD, Stead WW, Cauthen GM, et al. Nosocomial transmission of tuberculosis associated with a draining tuberculous abscess. J Infect Dis 1990;161:286-295.
18. Kantor HS, Poblete R, Pusateri SL. Nosocomial transmission of tuberculosis from unsuspected disease. Am J Med 1988;84:833–838.
19. Lundgren R, Norrman E, Asberg I. Tuberculous infection transmitted at autopsy. Tubercle 1987;68:147–150.
20. CDC. *Mycobacterium tuberculosis* transmission in a health clinic—Florida, 1988. MMWR 1989;38:256–264.
21. Beck-Sagué C, Dooley SW, Hutton MD, et al. Outbreak of multidrug-resistant *Mycobacterium tuberculosis* infections in a hospital: transmission to patients with HIV infection and staff. JAMA 1992:268:1280–1286.
22. CDC. Nosocomial transmission of multidrug-resistant tuberculosis to health-care workers and HIV-infected patients in an urban hospital—Florida. MMWR 1990;39:718–722.
23. CDC. Nosocomial transmission of multidrug-resistant tuberculosis among HIV-infected persons—Florida and New York, 1988–1991. MMWR 1991;40:585–591.
24. Pearson ML, Jereb JA, Frieden TR, et al. Nosocomial transmission of multidrug-resistant *Mycobacterium tuberculosis*. A risk to patients and health care workers. Ann Intern Med 1992;117:191–196.
25. Dooley SW, Jarvis WR, Martone WJ, Snider DE Jr. Multidrug-resistant tuberculosis [Editorial]. Ann Intern Med 1992;117:257–258.
26. CDC. Unpublished data.
27. Wenger P, Beck-Sagué C, Otten J, et al. Efficacy of control measures in preventing nosocomial transmission of multidrug-resistant tuberculosis among patient and health-care workers [Abstract 53A]. World Congress on Tuberculosis. Bethesda, MD: November 16–19, 1992.
28. Otten J, Chen J, Cleary T. Successful control of an outbreak of multidrug-resistant tuberculosis in an urban teaching hospital [Abstract 51D]. In: Program and abstracts of World Congress on Tuberculosis. Bethesda, MD: November 16–19, 1992.
29. Maloney S, Pearson M, Gordon M, et al. The efficacy of recommended infection control measures in preventing nosocomial transmission of multidrug-resistant TB [Abstract 51C]. In: Program and abstracts of the World Congress on Tuberculosis. Bethesda, MD: November 16–19, 1992.
30. Stroud C, Tokars J, Grieco M, Gilligan M, Jarvis W. Abstract A1-3. Third Annual Meeting of the Society for Hospital Epidemiologists of America. Chicago, IL: April 18–20, 1993.
31. Strong BE, Kubica GP. Isolation and identification of *Mycobacterium tuberculosis*. Atlanta: U.S. Department of Health and Human Services, Public Health Service. CDC, 1981; HHS publication no. CDC 81-8390.
32. CDC. Tuberculosis and human immunodeficiency virus infection: recommendations of the Advisory Committee for the Elimination of Tuberculosis (ACET). MMWR 1989;38:236–238, 243–250.
33. Willcox PA, Benator SR, Potgieter PD. Use of flexible fiberoptic bronchoscope in diagnosis of sputum-negative pulmonary tuberculosis. Thorax 1982;37:598–601.
34. Willcox PA, Potgieter PD, Bateman ED, Benator SR. Rapid diagnosis of sputum-negative military tuberculosis using the flexible fiberoptic bronchoscope. Thorax 1986;41:681–684.
35. Pitchenik AE, Cole C, Russell BW, et al. Tuberculosis, atypical mycobacteriosis, and the acquired immunodeficiency syndrome among Haitian and non-Haitian patients in South Florida. Ann Intern Med 1984;101:641–645.
36. Maayan S, Wormser GP, Hewlett D, et al. Acquired immunodeficiency syndrome (AIDS) in an economically disadvantaged population. Arch Intern Med 1985;145:1607–1612.
37. Klein NC, Duncanson FP, Lenox TH III, et al. Use of mycobacterial smears in the diagnosis of pulmonary tuberculosis in AIDS/ARC patients. Chest 1989;95:1190–1192.
38. Burnens AP, Vurma-Rapp U. Mixed mycobacterial cultures—occurrence in the clinical laboratory. Zbl Bakt 1989;271:85–90.
39. CDC. Initial therapy for tuberculosis in the era of multidrug-resistance: recommendations of the Advisory Council for the Elimination of Tuberculosis. MMWR 1993;42:no. RR-7.
40. Riley RL. Airborne infection. Am J Med 1974;57:466–475.

41. ASHRAE—American Society of Heating, Refrigeration, and Air Conditioning Engineers. Chapter 7: Health facilities. In: 1991 application handbook. Atlanta: American Society of Heating, Refrigeration, and Air Conditioning Engineers, Inc., 1991.
42. AIA—American Institute of Architects AIA, Committee on Architecture for Health. Chapter 7: General hospital. In: Guidelines for construction and equipment of hospital and medical facilities. Washington, DC: The American Institute of Architects Press, 1987.
43. HRSA—Health Resources and Services Administration. Guidelines for construction and equipment of hospital and medical facilities. Rockville, MD: U.S. Department of Health and Human Services, Public Health Service, 1984; PHS publication no. HRSA 84-14500.
44. Riley RL, O'Grady F. Airborne infection: transmission and control. New York: Macmillan, 1961:47, 134.
45. Galson E, Goddard KR. Hospital air conditioning and sepsis control. ASHRAE J July 1968:33–41.
46. Kethley TW. Air: its importance and control. In: Proceedings of the National Conference on Institutionally Acquired Infections. Washington, DC: PHS publication no. 1188. September 1963:35–46.
47. ANSI. American national standard practices for respiratory protection. New York: American National Standards Institute, 1992.
48. 29 CFR Part 1910.134.
49. Recommendations for HIV testing services for inpatients and outpatients in acute-care hospital settings and technical guide on HIV counseling. MMWR 1993;42:no. RR-2.
50. Williams WW. Guideline for infection control in hospital personnel. Infect Control 1983;4(suppl):326–349.
51. ADA—Americans with Disabilities Act. 1990. Public Law 101-336, 104 Stat. 327, 42.V.S.C. 12101 et seq. 101st Congress.
52. Barrett-Connor E, The periodic chest roentgenogram for the control of tuberculosis in health-care personnel. Am Rev Respir Dis 1980;122:153–155.
53. CDC, NIH. Agent: *Mycobacterium tuberculosis, M. bovis.* In: Biosafety in microbiological and biomedical laboratories. U.S. Department of Health and Human Services, Public Health Service. Washington, DC: U.S. Government Printing Office, May 1993:95.
54. CDC. Prevention and control of tuberculosis in facilities providing long-term care to the elderly. MMWR 1990;39:no. RR-10.
55. CDC. Prevention and control of tuberculosis in correctional institutions: recommendations of the Advisory Committee for the Elimination of Tuberculosis. MMWR 1989;38:313–320, 325.
56. Manoff SB, Cauthen GM, Stoneburner RL, Bloch AB, Schultz S, Snider DE Jr. TB patients with AIDS: Are they more likely to spread TB? Presented at the IVth International Conference on AIDS. Stockholm, Sweden: June 12–16, 1988.
57. Cauthen GM, Dooley SW, Gibler W, Burr J, Ihle W. Tuberculosis (TB) transmission by HIV-associated TB cases. Presented at the VIIth International Conference on AIDS. Florence, Italy: June 16–21, 1991.
58. Klausner JD, Ryder RW, Baende E, et al. *Mycobacterium tuberculosis* in household contacts of human immunodeficiency virus type 1-seropositive patients with active pulmonary tuberculosis in Kinshasa, Zaire. J Infect Dis 1993;168:106–111.
59. Riley RL, Mills CC, O'Grady F, Sultan LU, Wittstadt F, Shivpuri DN. Infectiousness of air from a tuberculosis ward. Am Rev Respir Dis 1962;85:511–525.
60. Noble RC. Infectiousness of pulmonary tuberculosis after starting chemotherapy: review of the available data on an unresolved question. Am J Infect Control 1981;9:6–10.
61. Snider DE Jr. The tuberculin skin test. Am Rev Respir Dis 1982 (Koch Centennial Issue) 1982;125:108–118.
62. CDC. Purified protein derivative (PPD)—tuberculin anergy and HIV infection: guidelines for anergy testing and management of anergic persons at risk of tuberculosis. MMWR 1991;40:no. RR-5.
63. Canessa PA, Fasano L, Lavecchia MA, Torraca A, Schiattone ML. Tuberculin skin test in asymptomatic HIV seropositive carriers [Letter]. Chest 1989;96:1215–1216.
64. Snider DE Jr. Bacille Calmetta-Guérin vaccinations and tuberculin skin test. JAMA 1985;253:3438–3439.
65. DesPrez RM, Heim CR. *Mycobacterium tuberculosis.* In: Mandell GL, Douglas RG, Bennett JE, eds. Principles and practice of infectious diseases. 3rd ed. New York: 1990:1877–1906.

66. Pitchenik AE, Rubinson HA. The radiographic appearance of tuberculosis in patients with the acquired immune deficiency syndrome (AIDS) and pre-AIDS. Am Rev Respir Dis 1985;131:393–396.

67. Kiehn TE, Cammarata R. Laboratory diagnosis of mycobacterial infection in patients with acquired immunodeficiency syndrome. J Clin Microbiol 1986;24:708-711.

68. Crawford JT, Eisenach KD, Bates JH. Diagnosis of tuberculosis: present and future. Semin Respir Infect 1989;4:171–181.

69. Moulding TS, Redeker AG, Kanel GC. Twenty isoniazid-associated deaths in one state. Am Rev Respir Dis 1989;140:700–705.

70. Snider DE Jr, Layde PM, Johnson MW, Lyle MA. Treatment of tuberculosis during pregnancy. Am Rev Respir Dis 1980;122:65–79.

71. Snider DE Jr. Pregnancy and tuberculosis. Chest 1984;86:130–135.

72. Hamadeh MA, Glassroth J. Tuberculosis and pregnancy. Chest 1992;101:1112–1120.

73. IARC monographs on the evaluation of the carcinogenic risk of chemicals to man: some aromatic amines, hydrazine and related substances. N-nitroso compounds and miscellaneous alkylating agents. vol 4. Lyon, France: 1974.

74. Glassroth JL, White MC, Snider DE Jr. An assessment of the possible association of isoniazid with human cancer deaths. Am Rev Respir Dis 1977;116(6):1065–1074.

75. Glassroth JL, Snider DE Jr, Comstock GW. Urinary tract cancer and isoniazid. Am Rev Respir Dis 1977;116(2):331–333.

76. Costello HD, Snider DE Jr. The incidence of cancer among participants in a controlled, randomized isoniazid preventive therapy trial. Am J Epidemiol 1980;111(1):67–74.

77. CDC. The use of preventive therapy for tuberculosis infection in the United States. MMWR 1990;39:(no. RR-8):9–12.

78. CDC. Management of persons exposed to multidrug-resistant tuberculosis. MMWR 1992;41:(no. RR-11):61–71.

79. American Thoracic Society, CDC. Treatment of tuberculosis and tuberculosis infection in adults and children, 1986. Am Rev Respir Dis 1986;134:355–363.

80. American Thoracic Society, CDC. Control of tuberculosis in the United States. Am Rev Respir Dis 1992;146:1624–1635.

81. Small PM, Shafer RW, Hopewell PC, et al. Exogenous infection with multidrug-resistant *Mycobacterium tuberculosis* in patients with advanced HIV infection. N Engl J Med 1993;86:128–135.

82. Iseman MD, Madsen LA. Drug-resistant tuberculosis. Clin Chest Med 1989;10:341–353.

83. Goble M. Drug-resistant tuberculosis. Semin Respir Infect 1986;1:220–225.

84. Goble M, Iseman MD, Madsen LA, et al. Treatment of 171 patients with pulmonary tuberculosis resistant to isoniazid and rifampin. N Engl J Med 1993;328:527–532.

85. Simone PM, Iseman MD. Drug-resistant tuberculosis: a deadly—and growing—danger. J Respir Dis 1992;13:960–971.

86. Bloom BR, Murray CJL. Tuberculosis: Commentary on a reemergent killer. Science 1992;257:1055–1064.

87. Nardell EA. Dodging droplet nuclei: reducing the probability of nosocomial tuberculosis transmission in the AIDS area. Am Rev Respir Dis 1990;142:501–503.

88. 29 CFR Part 1910.134.

89. American national standard practices for respiratory protection. New York: American National Standards Institute, 1980.

90. Hyatt EC. Current problems and new developments in respiratory protection. Am Ind Hyg Assoc J 1963; 24:295–304.

91. ANSI. American national standard practices for respiratory protection. New York: American National Standards Institute, 1969.

92. NIOSH. Guide to industrial respiratory protection. Cincinnati, OH: U.S. Department of Health and Human Services, Public Health Service, Centers for Disease Control, National Institute for Occupational Safety and Health. 1987; DHHS NIOSH publication no. 87-116.

93. National Cottonseed Products Association v. Brock and Minnesota Mining and Manufacturing v. Occupational Safety and Health Administration. 825 F.2d 482 D.C. Cir. 1987.

94. Lowry PL, Hesch PR, Revoir WH. Performance of single-use respirators. Am Ind Hyg Assoc J 1977;38:462–467.

95. Hyatt EC et al. Respiratory studies for the National Institute for Occupational Safety and Health—July 1, 1972, through June 3, 1973. Los Alamos, NM: Los Alamos Scientific Laboratory, Progress Report no. LA-5620-PR, May 1974.

96. Hinds WC, Kraske G. Performance of dust respirators with facial seal leaks: I. Experimental. Am Ind Hyg Assoc J 1987;48(10):836–841, Figures 5 and 6.
97. Liu BYH, Fardi B. A fundamental study of respiratory air filtration. Chapter 6: Experimental results. Final report for NIOSH Grant #R01 OHO1485-O1A1. University of Minnesota, Particle Technology Laboratory Publication no. 680, Minneapolis, MN: 1988:250–307.
98. Chen CC, Ruuskanen J, et al. Filter and leak penetration characteristics of a dust and mist filtering facepiece. Am Ind Hyg Assoc J 1990;51(12):632–639.
99. Chen CC, Lehtimaki M, Willeke K. Aerosol penetration through filtering facepieces and respirator cartridges. Am Ind Hyg Assoc J 1992;53(9):566–574.
100. NIOSH. 30 CFR Part 11—Respiratory protective devices; tests for permissibility, fees. Code of Federal Regulations. Washington, DC: U.S. Government Printing Office. Office of the Federal Register.
101. NIOSH. Guide to industrial respiratory protection. Morgantown, WV: U.S. Department of Health and Human Services, Public Health Service, Centers for Disease Control, National Institute for Occupational Safety and Health, DHHS (NIOSH) Publication no. 87-116. January 1991.
102. OSHA. 29 CFR 1910.134—Occupational safety and health standards, personal protective equipment, respiratory protection. Code of Federal Regulations. Washington, DC: U.S. Government Printing Office, Office of the Federal Register.
103. Nelson KE, Larson PA, Schraufnagel DE, Jackson J. Transmission of tuberculosis by fiber bronchoscopes. Am Rev Respir Dis 1983;127:97–100.
104. Leers WD. Disinfecting endoscopes: how not to transmit *Mycobacterium tuberculosis* by bronchoscopy. Can Med Assoc J 1980;123:275–283.
105. Garner JS, Simmons BP. Guideline for isolation precautions in hospitals. Infect Control 1983;4(suppl):245–325.
106. Rutala WA. APIC guidelines for selection and use of disinfectants. Am J Infect Control 1990;18:99–117.
107. Favero MS, Bond WW. Chemical disinfection of medical and surgical materials. In: Block SS, ed. Disinfection, sterilization, and preservation. 4th ed. Philadelphia: Lea & Febiger, 1991:617–641.
108. Garner JS, Favero MS. Guideline for handwashing and hospital environmental control. Atlanta: U.S. Department of Health and Human Services, Public Health Service, CDC, 1985.

SECTION 11
Sexually Transmitted Diseases

Diseases Characterized by Genital Ulcers

Management of the Patient with Genital Ulcers

In the United States, most patients with genital ulcers have genital herpes, syphilis, or chancroid. The relative frequency of each varies by geographic area and patient population, but in most areas of the United States genital herpes is the most common of these diseases. More than one of these diseases may be present among at least 3 to 10% of patients with genital ulcers. Each disease has been associated with an increased risk for human immunodeficiency virus (HIV) infection.

A diagnosis based only on history and physical examination is often inaccurate. Therefore, evaluation of all persons with genital ulcers should include a serologic test for syphilis and possibly other tests. Although ideally all of these tests should be conducted for each patient with a genital ulcer, use of such tests (other than a serologic test for syphilis) may be based on test availability and clinical or epidemiologic suspicion. Specific tests for the evaluation of genital ulcers are listed below:

Darkfield examination or direct immunofluorescence test for *Treponema pallidum*;
Culture or antigen test for HSV;
Culture for *Haemophilus ducreyi*.

HIV testing should be considered in the management of patients with genital ulcers, especially for those with syphilis or chancroid.

A health-care provider often must treat a patient before test results are available (even after complete testing, at least one quarter of patients with genital ulcers have no laboratory-confirmed diagnosis). In that circumstance, the clinician should treat for the diagnosis considered most likely. Many experts recommend treatment for both chancroid and syphilis if the diagnosis is unclear or if the patient resides in a community in which chancroid morbidity is notable (especially when diagnostic capabilities for chancroid and syphilis are not ideal).

CHANCROID

Chancroid is endemic in many areas of the United States and also occurs in discrete outbreaks. Chancroid has been well established as a cofactor for HIV transmission, and a high rate of HIV infection among patients with chancroid has been reported in the United States and in other countries. As many as 10% of patients with chancroid may be coinfected with *T. pallidum* or herpes simplex virus (HSV).

Definitive diagnosis of chancroid requires identification of *H. ducreyi* on special culture media that are not commercially available; even using these media, sensitivity is no higher than 80% and is usually lower. A probable diagnosis, for both clinical and surveillance purposes, may be made if the person has one or more painful genital ulcers and (1) no evidence of *T. pallidum* infection by Darkfield examination of ulcer exudate or by a serologic test for syphilis performed at least 7 days after onset of ulcers, and (2) either the clinical presentation of the ulcer(s) is not typical of disease caused by HSV or the HSV test results are negative. The combination of a painful ulcer with tender inguinal adenopathy (which occurs among one third of patients) is suggestive of chancroid and, when accompanied by suppurative inguinal adenopathy, is almost pathognomonic.

Treatment. Successful treatment cures infection, resolves clinical symptoms, and prevents transmission to others. In extensive cases, scarring may result despite successful therapy.

Recommended Regimens

Azithromycin 1 gm orally in a single dose
or
Ceftriaxone 250 mg intramuscularly in a single dose or **Erythromycin** base 500 mg orally 4 times a day for 7 days.

All three regimens are effective for the treatment of chancroid among patients without HIV infection. Azithromycin and ceftriaxone offer the advantage of single-dose therapy. Antimicrobial resistance to ceftriaxone and azithromycin has not been reported. Although two isolates resistant to erythromycin were reported from Asia a decade ago, similar isolates have not been reported.

Alternative Regimens

Amoxicillin 500 mg plus **clavulanic acid** 125 mg orally 3 times a day for 7 days
or
Ciprofloxacin 500 mg orally 2 times a day for 3 days.

NOTE: Ciprofloxacin is contraindicated for pregnant and lactating women, children, and adolescents ≤17 years of age.

These regimens have not been evaluated as extensively as the recommended regimens: neither has been studied in the United States.

Other Management Considerations. Patients should be tested for HIV infection at the time of diagnosis. Patients also should be tested 3 months later for both syphilis and HIV, if initial results are negative.

Follow-Up. Patients should be reexamined 3 to 7 days after initiation of therapy. If treatment is successful, ulcers improve symptomatically within 3 days and improve objectively within 7 days after therapy. If no clinical improvement is evident, the clinician must consider whether (1) the diagnosis is correct, (2) coinfection with another sexually transmitted disease (STD) agent exists, (3) the patient is infected with HIV, (4) treatment was not taken as instructed, or (5) the *H. ducreyi* strain causing infection is resistant to the prescribed antimicrobial. The time required for complete healing is related to the size of the ulcer; large ulcers may require 22 weeks. Clinical resolution of fluctuant lymphadenopathy is slower than that of ulcers and may require needle aspiration through adjacent intact skin—even during successful therapy.

Management of Sex Partners. Persons who had sexual contact with a patient who has chancroid within the 10 days before onset of the patient's symptoms should be examined and treated. The examination and treatment should be administered even in the absence of symptoms.

Special Considerations

Pregnancy. The safety of azithromycin for pregnant and lactating women has not been established. Ciprofloxacin is contraindicated during pregnancy. No adverse effects of chancroid on pregnancy outcome or on the fetus have been reported.

HIV Infection. Patients coinfected with HIV should be closely monitored. These patients may require courses of therapy longer than those recommended in this report. Healing may be slower among HIV-infected persons, and treatment failures do occur, especially after shorter-course treatment regimens. Since data on therapeutic efficacy with the recommended ceftriaxone and azithromycin regimens among patients infected with HIV are limited, those regimens should be used among persons known to be infected with HIV only if follow-up can be assured. Some experts suggest using the erythromycin 7-day regimen for treating HIV-infected persons.

GENITAL HERPES SIMPLEX VIRUS INFECTIONS

Genital herpes is a viral disease that may be recurrent and has no cure. Two serotypes of HSV have been identified: HSV-1 and HSV-2; most cases of genital herpes are caused by HSV-2. On the basis of serologic studies, approximately 30 million persons in the United States may have genital HSV infection.

Most infected persons never recognize signs suggestive of genital herpes; some will have symptoms shortly after infection and then never again. A minority of the total infected U.S. population will have recurrent episodes of genital lesions. Some cases of first clinical episode genital herpes are manifested by extensive disease that requires hospitalization. Many cases of genital herpes are acquired from persons who do not know that they have a genital infection with HSV or who were asymptomatic at the time of the sexual contact.

Randomized trials show that systemic acyclovir provides partial control of the symptoms and signs of herpes episodes when used to treat first clinical episodes or when used as suppressive therapy. However, acyclovir neither eradicates latent virus nor affects subsequent risk, frequency, or severity of recurrences after administration of the drug is discontinued. Topical therapy with acyclovir is substantially less effective than the oral drug and its use is discouraged. Episodes of HSV infection among HIV-infected patients may require more aggressive therapy. Immunocompromised persons may have prolonged episodes with extensive disease. For these persons, infections caused by acyclovir-resistant strains require selection of alternate antiviral agents.

First Clinical Episode of Genital Herpes

Recommended Regimen

Acyclovir 200 mg orally 5 times a day for 7 to 10 days or until clinical resolution is attained.

First Clinical Episode of Herpes Proctitis

Recommended Regimen

Acyclovir 400 mg orally 5 times a day for 10 days or until clinical resolution is attained.

Recurrent Episodes

When treatment is instituted during the prodrome or within 2 days of onset of lesions, some patients with recurrent disease experience limited benefit from therapy. However, since early treatment can seldom be administered, most immunocompetent patients with recurrent disease do not benefit from acyclovir treatment, and it is not generally recommended.

Recommended Regimen

Acyclovir 200 mg orally 5 times a day for 5 days,
Acyclovir 400 mg orally 3 times a day for 5 days,
or
Acyclovir 800 mg orally 2 times a day for 5 days.

Daily Suppressive Therapy.   Daily suppressive therapy reduces the frequency of HSV recurrences by at least 75% among patients with frequent recurrences (i.e., six or more recurrences per year). Suppressive treatment with oral acyclovir does not totally eliminate symptomatic or asymptomatic viral shedding or the potential for transmission. Safety and efficacy have been documented among persons receiving daily therapy for as long as 5 years. Acyclovir-resistant strains of HSV have been isolated from some persons receiving suppressive therapy, but these strains have not been associated with treatment failure among immunocompetent patients. After 1 year of continuous suppressive therapy, acyclovir should be discontinued to allow assessment of the patient's rate of recurrent episodes.

Recommended Regimen

Acyclovir 400 mg orally 2 times a day.

Alternative Regimen

Acyclovir 200 mg orally 3 to 5 times a day.

The goal of the alternative regimen is to identify for each patient the lowest dose that provides relief from frequently recurring symptoms.

Severe Disease

Intravenous therapy should be provided for patients with severe disease or complications necessitating hospitalization (e.g., disseminated infection that includes encephalitis, pneumonitis, or hepatitis).

Recommended Regimen

Acyclovir 5 to 10 mg/kg body weight intravenously every 8 hours for 5 to 7 days or until clinical resolution is attained.

Other Management Considerations.   Other considerations for managing patients with genital HSV infection are as follows:

Patients should be advised to abstain from sexual activity while lesions are present.

Patients with genital herpes should be told about the natural history of the disease, with emphasis on the potential for recurrent episodes, asymptomatic viral shedding, and sexual transmission. Sexual transmission of HSV has been documented to occur during periods without evidence of lesions. Many cases are transmitted during such asymptomatic periods.

The use of condoms should be encouraged during all sexual exposures. The risk for neonatal infection should be explained to all patients—male and female—with genital herpes. Women of childbearing age who have genital herpes should be advised to inform health-care providers who care for them during pregnancy about their HSV infection.

Management of Sex Partners.   Sex partners of patients who have genital herpes are likely to benefit from evaluation and counseling. Symptomatic sex partners should be managed in the same manner as any patient with genital lesions. However, the majority of persons with genital HSV infection do not have a history of typical genital lesions. These asymptomatic persons may benefit from evaluation and counseling; thus, even asymptomatic partners should be queried about histories of typical and atypical genital lesions and encouraged to examine themselves for lesions in the future.

Commercially available HSV type-specific antibody tests have not demonstrated adequate performance characteristics; their use is not currently recommended. Sensitive and specific type-specific serum antibody assays now utilized in research settings might contribute to future intervention strategies. Should tests with adequate sensitivity and specificity become commercially available, it might be possible to accurately identify asymptomatic persons infected with HSV-2, to focus counseling on how to detect lesions by self-examination, and to reduce the risk for transmission to sex partners.

Special Considerations

Allergy, Intolerance, or Adverse Reactions.   Effective alternatives to therapy with acyclovir are not available.

HIV Infection.   Lesions caused by HSV are relatively common among patients infected with HIV. Intermittent or suppressive therapy with oral acyclovir may be needed.

The acyclovir dosage for HIV-infected persons is controversial, but experience strongly suggests that immunocompromised patients benefit from increased dosage. Regimens such as 400 mg orally 3 to 5 times a day, as used for other immunocompromised persons, have been found useful. Therapy should be continued until clinical resolution is attained.

For severe disease, intravenous acyclovir therapy may be required. If lesions persist among patients undergoing acyclovir treatment, resistance to acyclovir should be suspected. These patients should be managed in consultation with an expert. For severe disease because of proven or suspected acyclovir-resistant strains, hospitalization should be considered. Foscarnet, 40 mg/kg body weight intravenously every 8 hours until clinical resolution is attained, appears to be the best available treatment.

Pregnancy.   The safety of systemic acyclovir therapy among pregnant women has not been established. Burroughs Wellcome Co., in cooperation with CDC, maintains a registry to assess the effects of the use of acyclovir during pregnancy. Women who receive acyclovir during pregnancy should be reported to this registry (Telephone: (800) 722-9292, extension 58465).

Current registry findings do not indicate an increase in the number of birth defects identified among the prospective reports when compared with those expected in the general population. Moreover, no consistent pattern of abnormalities emerges among retrospective reports. These findings provide some assurance in counseling women who have had inadvertent prenatal exposure to acyclovir. However, accumulated case histories comprise a sample of insufficient size for reaching reliable and definitive conclusions regarding the risks of acyclovir treatment to pregnant women and to their fetuses.

In the presence of life-threatening maternal HSV infection (e.g., disseminated infection that includes encephalitis, pneumonitis, or hepatitis), acyclovir administered intravenously is indicated. Among pregnant women without life-threatening disease, systemic acyclovir should not be used to treat recurrences nor should it be used as suppressive therapy near-term (or at other times during pregnancy) to prevent reactivation.

Perinatal Infections.   Most mothers of infants who acquire neonatal herpes lack histories of clinically evident genital herpes. The risk for transmission to the neonate from an infected mother appears highest among women with first episode genital herpes near the time of delivery and is low (1 to 3%) among women with recurrent herpes. The results of viral cultures during pregnancy do not predict viral shedding at the time of delivery, and such cultures are not routinely indicated.

At the onset of labor, all women should be carefully questioned about symptoms of genital herpes and should be examined. Women without symptoms or signs of genital herpes infection or prodrome may deliver their babies vaginally. Among women who have a history of genital herpes or who have a sex partner with genital herpes, cultures of the birth canal at delivery may aid in decisions relating to neonatal management.

Infants delivered through an infected birth canal proven by virus isolation or presumed by observation of lesions should be followed carefully, including virus cultures obtained 24 to 48 hours after birth. Available data do not support the routine use of acyclovir as anticipatory treatment for asymptomatic infants delivered through an infected birth canal. Treatment should be reserved for infants who develop evidence of clinical disease and for those with positive postpartum cultures.

All infants with evidence of neonatal herpes should be treated with systemic acyclovir or vidarabine; refer to the Report of the Committee on Infectious Diseases, American Academy of Pediatrics. For ease of administration and to lower toxicity, acyclovir (30 mg/kg/day for 10 to 14 days) is the preferred drug. The care of these infants should be managed by consultation with an expert.

LYMPHOGRANULOMA VENEREUM

Lymphogranuloma venereum (LGV), a rare disease in the United States, is caused by serovars L_1, L_2, or L_3 of *Chlamydia trachomatis*. The most common clinical manifestation of LGV among heterosexuals is tender inguinal lymphadenopathy that is most commonly unilateral. Women and homosexually active men may have proctocolitis or inflammatory involvement of perirectal or perianal lymphatic tissues resulting in fistulas and strictures. When patients seek care, most no longer have the self-limited genital ulcer that sometimes occurs at the site of inoculation. The diagnosis is usually made serologically and by exclusion of other causes of inguinal lymphadenopathy or genital ulcers.

Treatment. Treatment cures infection and prevents ongoing tissue damage, although tissue reaction can result in scarring. Buboes may require aspiration or incision and drainage through intact skin. Doxycycline is the preferred treatment.

Recommended Regimen

Doxycycline 100 mg orally 2 times a day for 21 days.

Alternative Regimens

Erythromycin 500 mg orally 4 times a day for 21 days
or

Sulfisoxazole 500 mg orally 4 times a day for 21 days or equivalent sulfon-amide course.

Follow-Up.   Patients should be followed clinically until signs and symptoms have resolved.

Management of Sex Partners.   Persons who have had sexual contact with a patient who has LGV within the 30 days before onset of the patient's symptoms should be examined, tested for urethral or cervical chlamydial infection, and treated.

Special Considerations

Pregnancy.   Pregnant and lactating women should be treated with the erythro-mycin regimen.

HIV Infection.   Persons with HIV infection and LGV should be treated following the regimens previously cited.

SYPHILIS

Background.   Syphilis is a systemic disease caused by *T. pallidum*. Patients with syphilis may seek treatment for signs or symptoms of primary infection (ulcer or chancre at site of infection), secondary infection (manifestations that include rash, mucocutaneous lesions, and adenopathy), or tertiary infection (cardiac, neurologic, ophthalmic, auditory, or gummatous lesions). Infections also may be detected during the latent stage by serologic testing. Patients with latent syphilis who are known to have been infected within the preceding year are considered to have early latent syphilis; others have late latent syphilis or syphilis of unknown duration. Theoretically, treatment for late latent syphilis (as well as tertiary syphilis) requires therapy of longer duration because organisms are dividing more slowly; however, the validity of this division and its timing are unproven.

Diagnostic Considerations and Use of Serologic Tests.   Darkfield examinations and direct fluorescent antibody tests of lesion exudate or tissue are the definitive methods for diagnosing early syphilis. Presumptive diagnosis is possible with the use of two types of serologic tests for syphilis: (1) nontreponemal (e.g., Venereal Disease Research Laboratory (VDRL) and rapid plasma reagin (RPR), and (2) treponemal (e.g., fluorescent treponemal antibody absorbed (FTA-ABS) and microhemagglutination assay for antibody to *T. pallidum* (MHA-TP)). The use of one type of test alone is not sufficient for diagnosis. Nontreponemal test antibody titers usually correlate with disease activity, and results should be reported quantitatively. A 4-fold change in titer, equivalent to a change of two dilutions (e.g., from 1:16 to 1:4, or from 1:8 to 1:32), is necessary to demonstrate a substantial difference between two nontreponemal test results that were obtained using the same serologic test. A patient who has a reactive treponemal test usually will have a reactive test for a lifetime, regardless of treatment or disease activity (15 to 25% of patients treated during the primary stage may revert to being serologically nonreactive after 2 to 3 years). Treponemal test antibody titers correlate poorly with disease activity and should not be used to assess response to treatment.

Sequential serologic tests should be performed using the same testing method (e.g., VDRL or RPR) by the same laboratory. The VDRL and RPR are equally valid, but quantitative results from the two tests cannot be directly compared because RPR titers are often slightly higher than VDRL titers.

Abnormal results of serologic testing (unusually high, unusually low, and fluctuating titers) have been observed among HIV-infected patients. For such patients, use of other tests (e.g., biopsy and direct microscopy) should be considered. However, serologic tests appear to be accurate and reliable for the diagnosis of syphilis and for evaluation of treatment response for the vast majority of HIV-infected patients.

No single test can be used to diagnose neurosyphilis among all patients. The diagnosis of neurosyphilis can be made based on various combinations of reactive serologic test results, abnormalities of cerebrospinal fluid (CSF) cell count or protein, or a reactive VDRL-CSF (RPR is not performed on CSF) with or without clinical manifestations. The CSF leukocyte count is usually elevated (>5 white blood cells (WBC)/mm^3) when active neurosyphilis is present, and it is also a sensitive measure of the effectiveness of therapy. The VDRL-CSF is the standard serologic test for CSF; when reactive in the absence of substantial contamination of the CSF with blood, it is considered diagnostic of neurosyphilis. However, the VDRL-CSF may be nonreactive when neurosyphilis is present. Some experts recommend performing an FTA-ABS test on CSF. The CSF FTA-ABS is less specific (i.e., yields more false positives) for neurosyphilis than the VDRL-CSF; however, the test is believed to be highly sensitive.

Treatment.   Parenteral penicillin G is the preferred drug for treatment of all stages of syphilis. The preparation(s) used (i.e., benzathine, aqueous procaine, or aqueous crystalline), the dosage, and the length of treatment depend on the stage and clinical manifestations of disease.

The efficacy of penicillin for the treatment of syphilis was well established through clinical experience before the value of randomized controlled clinical trials was recognized. Therefore, nearly all the recommendations for the treatment of syphilis are based on expert opinion reinforced by case series, open clinical trials, and 50 years of clinical experience.

Parenteral penicillin G is the only therapy with documented efficacy for neurosyphilis or for syphilis during pregnancy. Patients with neurosyphilis and pregnant women with syphilis in any stage who report penicillin allergy should almost always be treated with penicillin, after desensitization, if necessary. Skin testing for penicillin allergy may be useful for some patients and in some settings (see Management of the Patient with a History of Penicillin Allergy). However, minor determinants needed for penicillin skin testing are not available commercially.

The **Jarisch-Herxheimer reaction** is an acute febrile reaction—accompanied by headache, myalgia, and other symptoms—that may occur within the first 24 hours after any therapy for syphilis; patients should be advised of this possible adverse reaction. The Jarisch-Herxheimer reaction is common among patients with early syphilis. Antipyretics may be recommended, but there are no proven methods for preventing this reaction. The Jarisch-Herxheimer reaction may induce early labor or cause fetal distress among pregnant women. This concern should not prevent or delay therapy (see Syphilis during Pregnancy).

Management of Sex Partners.   Sexual transmission of *T. pallidum* occurs only when mucocutaneous syphilitic lesions are present; such manifestations are uncommon after the first year of infection. However, persons sexually exposed to a patient with syphilis in any stage should be evaluated clinically and serologically according to the following recommendations:

Persons who were exposed to a patient with primary, secondary, or latent (duration <1 year) syphilis within the preceding 90 days might be infected even if seronegative and therefore should be treated presumptively.

Persons who were sexually exposed to a patient with primary, secondary, or latent (duration <1 year) syphilis >90 days before examination should be treated presumptively if serologic test results are not available immediately and the opportunity for follow-up is uncertain.

For purposes of partner notification and presumptive treatment of exposed sex partners, patients who have syphilis of unknown duration and who have high nontreponemal serologic test titers (>1:32) may be considered to be infected with early syphilis.

Long-term sex partners of patients with late syphilis should be evaluated clinically and serologically for syphilis.

The time periods before treatment used for identifying at-risk sex partners are 3 months plus duration of symptoms for primary syphilis, 6 months plus duration of symptoms for secondary syphilis, and 1 year for early latent syphilis.

PRIMARY AND SECONDARY SYPHILIS

Treatment.   Four decades of experience indicate that parenteral penicillin G is effective in achieving local cure (healing of lesions and prevention of sexual transmission) and in preventing late sequelae. However, no adequately conducted comparative trials have been performed to guide the selection of an optimal penicillin regimen (i.e., dose, duration, and preparation). Substantially fewer data on nonpenicillin regimens are available.

Recommended Regimen for Adults.   Nonallergic patients with primary or secondary syphilis should be treated with the following regimen:

Benzathine penicillin G, 2.4 million units intramuscularly in a single dose.

NOTE: Recommendations for treating pregnant women and HIV-infected persons for syphilis are discussed in separate sections.

Recommended Regimen for Children.   After the newborn period, children diagnosed with syphilis should have a CSF examination to exclude a diagnosis of neurosyphilis, and birth and maternal medical records should be reviewed to assess whether the child has congenital or acquired syphilis. (See Congenital Syphilis.) Children with acquired primary or secondary syphilis should be evaluated (including consultation with child-protection services) and treated using the following pediatric regimen. (See Sexual Assault or Abuse of Children.)

Benzathine penicillin G, 50,000 units/kg intramuscularly, up to the adult dose of 2.4 million units in a single dose.

Other Management Considerations.   All patients with syphilis should be tested for HIV. In areas with high HIV prevalence, patients with primary syphilis should be retested for HIV after 3 months.

Patients who have syphilis and who also have symptoms or signs suggesting neurologic disease (e.g., meningitis) or ophthalmic disease (e.g., uveitis) should be fully evaluated for neurosyphilis and syphilitic eye disease (including CSF analysis and ocular slit-lamp examination). Such patients should be treated appropriately according to the results of this evaluation.

Invasion of CSF by *T. pallidum* with accompanying CSF abnormalities is common among adults who have primary or secondary syphilis. However, few patients develop neurosyphilis after treatment with the regimens described in this report. Therefore, unless clinical signs or symptoms of neurologic involvement are present (e.g., auditory, cranial nerve, meningeal, or ophthalmic manifestations), lumbar puncture is not recommended for routine evaluation of patients with primary or secondary syphilis.

Follow-Up.   Treatment failures can occur with any regimen. However, assessing response to treatment is often difficult, and no definitive criteria for cure or failure exist. Serologic test titers may decline more slowly among patients with a prior syphilis infection. Patients should be reexamined clinically and serologically at 3 months and again at 6 months.

Patients with signs or symptoms that persist or recur or who have a sustained 4-fold increase in nontreponemal test titer compared with either the baseline titer or a subsequent result can be considered to have failed treatment or to be reinfected. These patients should be re-treated after evaluation for HIV infection. Unless reinfection is likely, lumbar puncture also should be performed.

Failure of nontreponemal test titers to decline 4-fold by 3 months after therapy for primary or secondary syphilis identifies persons at risk for treatment failure. Those persons should be evaluated for HIV infection. Optimal management of such patients is unclear if they are HIV negative. At a minimum, these patients should have additional clinical and serologic follow-up. If further follow-up cannot be assured, re-treatment is recommended. Some experts recommend CSF examination in such situations.

When patients are re-treated, most experts recommend re-treatment with 3 weekly injections of benzathine penicillin G 2.4 million units intramuscularly, unless CSF examination indicates that neurosyphilis is present.

Management of Sex Partners.   Refer to General Principles, Management of Sex Partners.

Special Considerations

Penicillin Allergy.   Nonpregnant penicillin-allergic patients who have primary or secondary syphilis should be treated with the following regimen.

Doxycycline 100 mg orally 2 times a day for 2 weeks

or

Tetracycline 500 mg orally 4 times a day for 2 weeks.

There is less clinical experience with doxycycline than with tetracycline, but compliance is likely to be better with doxycycline. Therapy for a patient who cannot tolerate either doxycycline or tetracycline should be based upon whether the patient's compliance with the therapy regimen and with follow-up examinations can be assured.

For nonpregnant patients whose compliance with therapy and follow-up can be assured, an alternative regimen is erythromycin 500 mg orally 4 times a day for 2 weeks. Various ceftriaxone regimens also may be considered.

Patients whose compliance with therapy or follow-up cannot be assured should be desensitized, if necessary, and treated with penicillin. Skin testing for penicillin allergy may be useful in some situations. (See Management of the Patient with a History of Penicillin Allergy.)

Erythromycin is less effective than other recommended regimens. Data on ceftriaxone are limited, and experience has been too brief to permit identification of late failures. Optimal dose and duration have not been established for ceftriaxone, but regimens that provide 8 to 10 days of treponemicidal levels in the blood should be used. Single-dose ceftriaxone therapy is not effective for treating syphilis.

Pregnancy.   Pregnant patients who are allergic to penicillin should be treated with penicillin, after desensitization, if necessary (See Management of the Patient with a History of Penicillin Allergy and Syphilis during Pregnancy.)

HIV Infection.   Refer to Syphilis among HIV-Infected Patients.

LATENT SYPHILIS

Latent syphilis is defined as those periods after infection with *T. pallidum* when patients are seroreactive, but show no other evidence of disease. Patients who have latent syphilis and who have acquired syphilis within the preceding year are classified as having early latent syphilis. Patients can be demonstrated to have acquired syphilis within the preceding year on the basis of documented seroconversion, a 4-fold or greater increase in titer of a nontreponemal serologic test, history of symptoms of primary or secondary syphilis, or if they had a sex partner with primary, secondary, or latent syphilis (documented independently as duration <1 year). Nearly all others have latent syphilis of unknown duration and should be managed as if they had late latent syphilis.

Treatment.   Treatment of latent syphilis is intended to prevent occurrence or progression of late complications. Although clinical experience supports belief in the effectiveness of penicillin in achieving those goals, limited evidence is available for guidance in choosing specific regimens. There is very little evidence to support the use of nonpenicillin regimens.

Recommended Regimens for Adults.   These regimens are for nonallergic patients with normal CSF examination (if performed).

Early Latent Syphilis

Benzathine penicillin G, 2.4 million units intramuscularly in a single dose.

Late Latent Syphilis or Latent Syphilis of Unknown Duration

Benzathine penicillin G, 7.2 million units total, administered as 3 doses of 2.4 million units intramuscularly each, at 1-week intervals.

Recommended Regimens for Children. After the newborn period, children diagnosed with syphilis should have a CSF examination to exclude neurosyphilis, and birth and maternal medical records should be reviewed to assess whether the child has congenital or acquired syphilis. (See Congenital Syphilis.) Older children with acquired latent syphilis should be evaluated as described for adults and treated using the following pediatric regimens (See Sexual Assault or Abuse of Children.) These regimens are for nonallergic children who have acquired syphilis and who have had a normal CSF examination.

EARLY LATENT SYPHILIS. Benzathine penicillin G, 50,000 units/kg intramuscularly, up to the adult dose of 2.4 million units in a single dose.

LATE LATENT SYPHILIS OR LATENT SYPHILIS OF UNKNOWN DURATION. Benzathine penicillin G, 50,000 units/kg intramuscularly, up to the adult dose of 2.4 million units, for 3 total doses (total 150,000 units/kg up to adult total dose of 7.2 million units).

Other Management Considerations. All patients with latent syphilis should be evaluated clinically for evidence of tertiary disease (e.g., aortitis, neurosyphilis, gumma, and iritis). Recommended therapy for patients with latent syphilis may not be optimal therapy for the persons with asymptomatic neurosyphilis. However, the yield from CSF examination, in terms of newly diagnosed cases of neurosyphilis, is low.

Patients with any one of the criteria listed below should have a CSF examination before treatment:

Neurologic or ophthalmic signs or symptoms;
Other evidence of active syphilis (e.g., aortitis, gumma, iritis);
Treatment failure;
HIV infection;
Serum nontreponemal titer ≥1:32, unless duration of infection is known to be <1 year; or
Nonpenicillin therapy planned, unless duration of infection is known to be <1 year.

If dictated by circumstances and patient preferences, CSF examination may be performed for persons who do not meet the criteria listed above. If a CSF examination is performed and the results show abnormalities consistent with CNS syphilis, the patient should be treated for neurosyphilis. (See Neurosyphilis.)

All syphilis patients should be tested for HIV.

Follow-Up. Quantitative nontreponemal serologic tests should be repeated at 6 months and again at 12 months. Limited data are available to guide evaluation of the response to therapy for a patient with latent syphilis. If titers increase 4-fold, or if an initially high titer ($\geq$1:32) fails to decline at least 4-fold (two dilutions) within 12 to 24 months, or if the patient develops signs or symptoms attributable to syphilis, the patient should be evaluated for neurosyphilis and re-treated appropriately.

Management of Sex Partners.   Refer to General Principles, Management of Sex Partners.

Special Considerations

Penicillin Allergy.   For patients who have latent syphilis and who are allergic to penicillin, nonpenicillin therapy should be used only after CSF examination has excluded neurosyphilis. Nonpregnant, penicillin-allergic patients should be treated with the following regimens.

> **Doxycycline 100** mg orally 2 times a day
> or
> **Tetracycline** 500 mg orally 4 times a day.

Both drugs are administered for 2 weeks if duration of infection is known to have been <1 year; otherwise, for 4 weeks.

Pregnancy.   Pregnant patients who are allergic to penicillin should be treated with penicillin, after desensitization, if necessary. (See Management of the Patient With a History of Penicillin Allergy and Syphilis during Pregnancy.)

HIV Infection.   Refer to Syphilis among HIV-Infected Patients.

LATE SYPHILIS

Late (tertiary) syphilis refers to patients with gumma and patients with cardio-vascular syphilis, but not to neurosyphilis. Nonallergic patients without evidence of neurosyphilis should be treated with the following regimen.

Recommended Regimen

> **Benzathine penicillin G**, 7.2 million units total, administered as 3 doses of 2.4 million units intramuscularly, at 1-week intervals.

Other Management Considerations.   Patients with symptomatic late syphilis should undergo CSF examination before therapy. Some experts treat all patients who have cardiovascular syphilis with a neurosyphilis regimen. The complete management of patients with cardiovascular or gummatous syphilis is beyond the scope of these guidelines. These patients should be managed in consultation with experts.

Follow-Up.   There is minimal evidence regarding follow-up of patients infected with late syphilis. Clinical response depends partly on the nature of the lesions.

Management of Sex Partners.   Refer to General Principles, Management of Sex Partners.

Special Considerations

Penicillin Allergy.   Patients allergic to penicillin should be treated according to treatment regimens recommended for late latent syphilis.

Pregnancy.   Pregnant patients who are allergic to penicillin should be treated with penicillin, after desensitization, if necessary. (See Management of the Patient with a History of Penicillin Allergy and Syphilis during Pregnancy.)

HIV Infection.   Refer to Syphilis among HIV-Infected Patients.

NEUROSYPHILIS

Treatment.   Central nervous system disease can occur during any stage of syphilis. A patient with clinical evidence of neurologic involvement (e.g., ophthalmic or auditory symptoms, cranial nerve palsies) with syphilis warrants a CSF examination. Although four decades of experience have confirmed the effectiveness of penicillin, the evidence to guide the choice of the best regimen is limited.

Syphilitic eye disease is frequently associated with neurosyphilis, and patients with this disease should be treated according to neurosyphilis treatment recommendations. CSF examination should be performed on all such patients to identify those patients with CSF abnormalities who should have follow-up CSF examinations to assess response to treatment.

Patients who have neurosyphilis or syphilitic eye disease (e.g., uveitis, neuroretinitis, or optic neuritis) and who are not allergic to penicillin should be treated with the following regimen.

Recommended Regimen.   12 to 24 million units **aqueous crystalline penicillin G** daily, administered as 2 to 4 million units intravenously every 4 hours, for 10 to 14 days.

If compliance with therapy can be assured, patients may be treated with the following alternative regimen.

Alternative Regimen.   2.4 million units **procaine penicillin** intramuscularly daily, plus **probenecid** 500 mg orally 4 times a day, both for 10 to 14 days.

The durations of these regimens are shorter than that of the regimen used for late syphilis in the absence of neurosyphilis. Therefore, some experts administer benzathine penicillin, 2.4 million units intramuscularly after completion of these neurosyphilis treatment regimens to provide a comparable total duration of therapy.

Other Management Considerations.   Other considerations in the management of the patient with neurosyphilis are the following:

All patients with syphilis should be tested for HIV.

Many experts recommend treating patients with evidence of auditory disease caused by syphilis in the same manner as for neurosyphilis, regardless of the findings on CSF examination.

Follow-Up.   If CSF pleocytosis was present initially, CSF examination should be repeated every 6 months until the cell count is normal. Follow-up CSF examinations also may be used to evaluate changes in the VDRL-CSF or CSF protein in response to therapy, though changes in these two parameters are slower and persistent abnormalities are of less certain importance. If the cell count has not decreased at 6 months, or if the CSF is not entirely normal by 2 years, re-treatment should be considered.

Management of Sex Partners.   Refer to General Principles, Management of Sex Partners.

Special Considerations

Penicillin Allergy.   No data have been collected systematically for evaluation of therapeutic alternatives to penicillin for treatment of neurosyphilis. Therefore, patients who report being allergic to penicillin should be treated with penicillin, after desensitization if necessary, or should be managed in consultation with an expert. In some situations, skin testing to confirm penicillin allergy may be useful. (See Management of the Patient with a History of Penicillin Allergy.)

Pregnancy.   Pregnant patients who are allergic to penicillin should be treated with penicillin, after desensitization if necessary. (See Syphilis during Pregnancy.)

HIV Infection.   Refer to Syphilis among HIV-Infected Patients.

Syphilis among HIV-Infected Patients

Diagnostic Considerations.   Unusual serologic responses have been observed among HIV-infected persons who also have syphilis. Most reports involved serologic titers that were higher than expected, but false-negative serologic test results or delayed appearance of seroreactivity have also been reported. Nevertheless, both treponemal and nontreponemal serologic tests for syphilis are accurate for the majority of patients with syphilis and HIV coinfection.

When clinical findings suggest that syphilis is present, but serologic tests are nonreactive or confusing, it may be helpful to perform such alternative tests as biopsy of a lesion, Darkfield examination, or direct fluorescent antibody staining of lesion material.

Neurosyphilis should be considered in the differential diagnosis of neurologic disease among HIV-infected persons.

Treatment.   Although adequate research-based evidence is not available, published case reports and expert opinion suggest that HIV-infected patients with early syphilis are at increased risk for neurologic complications and have higher rates of treatment failure with currently recommended regimens. The magnitude of these risks, although not precisely defined, is probably small. No treatment regimens have been demonstrated to be more effective in preventing development of neurosyphilis than those recommended for patients without HIV infection. Careful follow-up after therapy is essential.

Primary and Secondary Syphilis among HIV-Infected Patients

Treatment.   Treatment with benzathine penicillin G, 2.4 million units intramuscularly, as for patients without HIV infection, is recommended. Some experts recommend additional treatments, such as multiple doses of benzathine penicillin G, as suggested for late syphilis, or other supplemental antibiotics in addition to benzathine penicillin G, 2.4 million units intramuscularly.

Other Management Considerations.   CSF abnormalities are common among HIV-infected patients who have primary or secondary syphilis, but these abnormalities are of unknown prognostic significance. Most HIV-infected patients respond appropriately to currently recommended penicillin therapy; however, some experts recommend CSF examination before therapy and modification of treatment accordingly.

Follow-Up.   Patients should be evaluated clinically and serologically for treatment failure at 1 month and at 2, 3, 6, 9, and 12 months after therapy. Although of unproven benefit, some experts recommend performing CSF examination after therapy (i.e., at 6 months).

HIV-infected patients who meet the criteria for treatment failure should undergo CSF examination and be re-treated just as for patients without HIV infection. CSF examination and re-treatment also should be strongly considered for patients in whom the suggested 4-fold decrease in nontreponemal test titer does not occur within 3 months for primary or secondary syphilis. Most experts would re-treat patients with benzathine penicillin G, 7.2 million units (as 3 weekly doses of 2.4 million units each), if the CSF examination is normal.

Special Considerations

Penicillin Allergy.   Penicillin regimens should be used to treat HIV-infected patients in all stages of syphilis. Skin testing to confirm penicillin allergy may be used (see Management of the Patient with a History of Penicillin Allergy), but data on the utility of that approach among immunocompromised patients are inadequate. Patients may be desensitized, and then treated with penicillin.

Latent Syphilis among HIV-Infected Patients

Diagnostic Considerations.   Patients who have both latent syphilis (regardless of apparent duration) and HIV infection should undergo CSF examination before treatment.

Treatment.   A patient with latent syphilis, HIV infection, and a normal CSF examination can be treated with benzathine penicillin G, 7.2 million units (as 3 weekly doses of 2.4 million units each).

Special Considerations

Penicillin Allergy.   Penicillin regimens should be used to treat all stages of syphilis among HIV-infected patients. Skin testing to confirm penicillin allergy may be used (see Management of the Patient with a History of Penicillin Allergy), but data on the utility of that approach in immunocompromised patients are inadequate. Patients may be desensitized and then treated with penicillin.

Syphilis during Pregnancy.   All women should be screened serologically for syphilis during the early stages of pregnancy. In populations in which utilization of prenatal care is not optimal, RPR-card test screening and treatment, if that test is reactive, should be performed at the time a pregnancy is diagnosed. In communities and populations with high syphilis prevalence or for patients at high risk, serologic testing should be repeated during the third trimester and again at delivery. (Some states mandate screening at delivery for all women.) Any woman who delivers a stillborn infant after 20 weeks gestation should be tested for syphilis. No infant should leave the hospital without the serologic status of the infant's mother having been determined at least once during pregnancy.

Diagnostic Considerations. Seropositive pregnant women should be considered infected unless treatment history is clearly documented in a medical or health department record and sequential serologic antibody titers have appropriately declined.

Treatment. Penicillin is effective for preventing transmission to fetuses and for treating established infection among fetuses. Evidence is insufficient, however, to determine whether the specific, recommended penicillin regimens are optimal.

Recommended Regimens. Treatment during pregnancy should be the penicillin regimen appropriate for the woman's stage of syphilis. Some experts recommend additional therapy (e.g., a second dose of **benzathine penicillin** 2.4 million units intramuscularly) 1 week after the initial dose, particularly for those women in the third trimester of pregnancy and for women who have secondary syphilis during pregnancy.

Other Management Considerations. Women who are treated for syphilis during the second half of pregnancy are at risk for premature labor or fetal distress, or both, if their treatment precipitates the Jarisch-Herxheimer reaction. These women should be advised to seek medical attention following treatment if they notice any change in fetal movements or if they have contractions. Stillbirth is a rare complication of treatment; however, since therapy is necessary to prevent further fetal damage, that concern should not delay treatment. All patients with syphilis should be tested for HIV.

Follow-Up. Serologic titers should be checked monthly until adequacy of treatment has been assured. The antibody response should be appropriate for the stage of disease.

Management of Sex Partners. Refer to General Principles, Management of Sex Partners.

Special Considerations

Penicillin Allergy. There are no proven alternatives to penicillin. A pregnant woman with a history of penicillin allergy should be treated with penicillin, after desensitization, if necessary. Skin testing may be helpful for some patients and in some settings (See Management of the Patient with a History of Penicillin Allergy.)

Tetracycline and doxycycline are contraindicated during pregnancy. Erythromycin should not be used because it cannot be relied upon to cure an infected fetus.

CONGENITAL SYPHILIS

Diagnostic Considerations

Who Should Be Evaluated. Infants should be evaluated for congenital syphilis if they were born to seropositive (nontreponemal test confirmed by treponemal test) women who meet the following criteria:

Have untreated syphilis;[a] or

---

[a] A woman treated with a regimen other than those recommended for treatment of syphilis (for pregnant women or otherwise) in these guidelines should be considered untreated.

Were treated for syphilis during pregnancy with erythromycin; or

Were treated for syphilis ≤1 month before delivery; or

Were treated for syphilis during pregnancy with the appropriate penicillin regimen, but nontreponemal antibody titers did not decrease sufficiently after therapy to indicate an adequate response (>4-fold decrease); or

Do not have a well-documented history of treatment for syphilis; or

Were treated appropriately before pregnancy but had insufficient serologic follow-up to assure that they had responded appropriately to treatment and are not currently infected (>4-fold decrease for patients treated for early syphilis; stable or declining titers ≤1:4 for other patients).

No infant should leave the hospital without the serologic status of the infant's mother having been documented at least once during pregnancy. Serologic testing also should be performed at delivery in communities and populations at risk for congenital syphilis. Serologic tests can be nonreactive among infants infected late during their mother's pregnancy.

Evaluation of the Infant.   The clinical and laboratory evaluation of infants born to women described above should include the following:

A thorough physical examination for evidence of congenital syphilis;

A quantitative nontreponemal serologic test for syphilis performed on the infant's sera (not on cord blood);

CSF analysis for cells, protein, and VDRL;

Long bone x-rays;

Other tests as clinically indicated (e.g., chest x-ray, complete blood count, differential and platelet count, liver function tests);

For infants who have no evidence of congenital syphilis on the above evaluation, determination of presence of specific antitreponemal IgM antibody by a testing method recognized by CDC as having either provisional or standard status;

Pathologic examination of the placenta or amniotic cord using specific fluorescent antitreponemal antibody staining.

Treatment

Therapy Decisions.   Infants should be treated for presumed congenital syphilis if they were born to mothers who, at delivery, had untreated syphilis or who had evidence of relapse or reinfection after treatment. (See Congenital Syphilis, Diagnostic Considerations.) Additional criteria for presumptively treating infants with congenital syphilis are as follows:

Physical evidence of active disease;

X-ray evidence of active disease;

A reactive VDRL-CSF or, for infants born to seroreactive mothers, an abnormal[b] CSF white blood cell count or protein, regardless of CSF serology;

---

[b] In the immediate newborn period, interpretation of CSF test results may be difficult; normal values vary with gestational age and are higher in preterm infants. Other causes of elevated values also should be considered when an infant is being evaluated for congenital syphilis. Though values as high as 25 WBC/1 mm³ and 150 mg of protein/dl occur among normal neonates, some experts recommend that lower values (5 WBC/1 mm³ and 40 mg/dl) be considered the upper limits of normal. The infant should be treated if test results cannot exclude infection. The absence of a 4-fold greater titer for an infant cannot be used as evidence against congenital syphilis.

A serum quantitative nontreponemal serologic titer that is at least 4-fold greater than the mother's titer;

Specific antitreponemal 1 gm antibody detected by a testing method that has been given provisional or standard status by CDC;

If they meet the previously cited criteria for "Who Should Be Evaluated," but have not been fully evaluated. (See Congenital Syphilis, Diagnostic Considerations.)

NOTE: Infants with clinically evident congenital syphilis should have an ophthalmologic examination.

Recommended Regimens

Aqueous crystalline penicillin G, 100,000 to 150,000 units/kg/day (administered as 50,000 units/kg intravenously every 12 hours during the first 7 days of life and every 8 hours thereafter) for 10 to 14 days,

or

Procaine penicillin G, 50,000 units/kg intramuscularly daily in a single dose for 10 to 14 days.

If more than 1 day of therapy is missed, the entire course should be restarted for an infant whose complete evaluation was normal and whose mother was (1) treated for syphilis during pregnancy with erythromycin; or (2) treated for syphilis <1 month before delivery; or (3) treated with an appropriate regimen before or during pregnancy, but did not yet have an adequate serologic response. These infants should be treated with benzathine penicillin G, 50,000 units/kg intramuscularly in a single dose. In some cases, infants with a normal complete evaluation for whom follow-up can be assured can be followed closely without treatment.

Treatment of Older Infants and Children with Congenital Syphilis.   After the newborn period, children diagnosed with syphilis should have a CSF examination to exclude neurosyphilis and records should be reviewed to assess whether the child has congenital or acquired syphilis. (See Primary and Secondary Syphilis and Latent Syphilis.) Any child who is thought to have congenital syphilis (or who has neurologic involvement) should be treated with aqueous crystalline penicillin G, 200,000 to 300,000 units/kg/day intravenously or intramuscularly (administered as 50,000 units/kg every 4 to 6 hours) for 10 to 14 days.

Follow-Up.   A seroreactive infant (or an infant whose mother was seroreactive at delivery) who is not treated for congenital syphilis during the perinatal period should receive careful follow-up examinations at 1 month and at 2, 3, 6, and 12 months after therapy. Nontreponemal antibody titers should decline by 3 months of age and should be nonreactive by 6 months of age if the infant was not infected and the titers were the result of passive transfer of antibody from the mother. If these titers are found to be stable or increasing, the child should be reevaluated, including CSF examination, and fully treated. Passively transferred treponemal antibodies may be present for as long as 1 year. If they are present >1 year, the infant should be reevaluated and treated for congenital syphilis.

Treated infants also should be followed every 2 to 3 months to assure that nontreponemal antibody titers decline; these infants should have become nonreactive by 6 months of age (response may be slower for infants treated after the neonatal period). Treponemal tests should not be used to evaluate response to treatment because test results can remain positive despite effective therapy if the child was infected. Infants with CSF pleocytosis should undergo CSF examination every 6 months, or until the cell count is normal. If the cell count is still abnormal after 2 years or if a downward trend is not present at each examination, the child should be re-treated. The VDRL-CSF also should be checked at 6 months; if still reactive, the infant should be re-treated.

Follow-up of children treated for congenital syphilis after the newborn period should be the same as that prescribed for congenital syphilis among neonates.

Special Considerations

Penicillin Allergy. Children who require treatment for syphilis after the newborn period, but who have a history of penicillin allergy, should be treated with penicillin after desensitization, if necessary. Skin testing may be helpful in some patients and settings. (See Management of the Patient with a History of Penicillin Allergy.)

HIV Infection. Mothers of infants with congenital syphilis should be tested for HIV. Infants born to mothers who have HIV infection should be referred for evaluation and appropriate follow-up.

No data exist to suggest that infants with congenital syphilis whose mothers are coinfected with HIV require different evaluation, therapy, or follow-up for syphilis than is recommended for all infants.

Management of the Patient with a History of Penicillin Allergy

No proven alternatives to penicillin are available for treating neurosyphilis, congenital syphilis, or syphilis among pregnant women. Penicillin also is recommended for use, whenever possible, with HIV-infected patients. Unfortunately, 3 to 10% of the adult population in the United States have experienced urticaria, angioedema, or anaphylaxis (upper airway obstruction, bronchospasm, or hypotension) with penicillin therapy. Re-administration of penicillin can cause severe immediate reactions among these patients. Because anaphylactic reactions to penicillin can be fatal, every effort should be made to avoid administering penicillin to penicillin-allergic patients, unless the anaphylactic sensitivity has been removed by acute desensitization.

However, only approximately 10% of persons who report a history of severe allergic reactions to penicillin are still allergic. With the passage of time after an allergic reaction to penicillin, most persons who have experienced a severe reaction stop expressing penicillin-specific IgE. These persons can be treated safely with penicillin. Many studies have found that skin testing with the major and minor determinants can reliably identify persons at high risk for penicillin reactions. Although these reagents are easily generated and have been available in academic centers for >30 years, currently only penicilloyl-poly-L-lysine (Pre-Pen, the major determinant) and penicillin G are available commercially. Experts estimate that testing with only the major determinant and penicillin G detects 90 to 97% of the currently allergic patients. However, because skin testing without the minor determinants would still miss 3 to 10% of allergic patients, and serious or fatal reactions can occur among these minor determinant positive patients, experts suggest caution when the full battery of skin test reagents listed in the table is not available.

Recommendations. If the full battery of skin-test reagents is available, including the major and minor determinants (see Penicillin Allergy Skin Testing), patients who report a history of penicillin reaction and are skin-test negative can receive conventional penicillin therapy. Skin-test positive patients should be desensitized.

If the full battery of skin-test reagents, including the minor determinants, is not available, the patient should be skin tested using penicilloyl (the major determinant, Pre-Pen) and penicillin G. Those with positive tests should be desensitized. Some experts believe that persons with negative tests, in that situation, should be regarded as probably allergic and should be desensitized. Others suggest that those with negative skin tests can be test-dosed gradually with oral penicillin in a monitored setting in which treatment for anaphylactic reaction is possible.

Penicillin Allergy Skin Testing. Patients at high risk for anaphylaxis (i.e., a history of penicillin-related anaphylaxis, asthma or other diseases that would make anaphylaxis more dangerous, or therapy with β-adrenergic blocking agents) should be tested with 100-fold dilutions of the full-strength skin-test reagents before testing with full-strength reagents. In these situations, patients should be tested in a monitored setting in which treatment for an anaphylactic reaction is possible. If possible, the patient should not have taken antihistamines (e.g., chlorpheniramine maleate or terfenadine during the past 24 hours, diphenhydramine HCl or hydroxyzine during the past 4 days, or astemizole during the past 3 weeks).

Reagents[c,d]

MAJOR DETERMINANT. Benzylpenicilloyl poly-L-lysine (Pre-Pen (Taylor Pharmacal Co., Decatur, IL) (6×10^{-5} M).

MINOR DETERMINANT PRECURSORS. Benzylpenicillin G (10^{-2} M, 3.3 mg/ml, 6000 U/ml); benzylpenicilloate (10^{-2} M, 3.3 mg/ml); benzylpenilloate (or penicilloyl propylamine)(10^{-2} M, 3.3 mg/ml).

POSITIVE CONTROL. Commercial histamine for epicutaneous skin testing (1 mg/ml).

NEGATIVE CONTROL. Diluent used to dissolve other reagents, usually phenol saline.

---

[c] Adapted with permission from Beall GN. Penicillins. In: Saxon A, moderator. Immediate hypersensitivity reactions to beta-lactam antibiotics. Ann Intern Med 1987;107;204–215.

[d] Aged penicillin is not an adequate source of minor determinants. Penicillin G should be freshly prepared or should come from a fresh-frozen source.

PROCEDURES. Dilute the antigens 100-fold for preliminary testing if the patient has had a life-threatening reaction or 10-fold if the patient has had another type of immediate, generalized reaction within the past year.

Epicutaneous (Prick) Tests. Duplicate drops of skin-test reagent are placed on the volar surface of the forearm. The underlying epidermis is pierced with a 26-gauge needle without drawing blood.

An epicutaneous test is positive if the average wheal diameter after 15 minutes is 4 mm larger than that of negative controls; otherwise, the test is negative. The histamine controls should be positive to assure that results are not falsely negative because of the effect of antihistaminic drugs.

Intradermal Test. If epicutaneous tests are negative, duplicate 0.02-ml intradermal injections of negative control and antigen solutions are made into the volar surface of the forearm using a 26- or 27-gauge needle on a syringe. The crossed diameters of the wheals induced by the injections should be recorded.

An intradermal test is positive if the average wheal diameter 15 minutes after injection is 2 mm or larger than the initial wheal size and also is at least 2 mm larger than the negative controls. Otherwise, the tests are negative.

Desensitization. Patients who have a positive skin test to one of the penicillin determinants can be desensitized. This is a straightforward, relatively safe procedure that can be done orally or intravenously. Although the two approaches have not been compared, oral desensitization is thought to be safer, simpler, and easier. Patients should be desensitized in a hospital setting because serious IgE-mediated allergic reactions, although unlikely, can occur. Desensitization can usually be completed in about 4 hours, after which the first dose of penicillin is given (Table 11.1). STD programs should have a referral center where patients with positive skin tests can be desensitized. After desensitization, patients must be maintained on penicillin continuously for the duration of the course of therapy.

Diseases Characterized by Urethritis and Cervicitis

Management of the Patient with Urethritis

Urethritis, or inflammation of the urethra, is caused by an infection characterized by the discharge of mucoid or purulent material and by burning during urination. However, asymptomatic infections are common. The two bacterial agents primarily responsible for urethritis among men are *Neisseria gonorrhoeae* and *C. trachomatis.* Testing to determine the specific diagnosis is recommended because both of these infections are reportable to state health departments and because, with a specific diagnosis, treatment compliance may be better and the likelihood of partner notification may be improved. If diagnostic tools (e.g., Gram stain and microscope) are unavailable, health-care providers should treat patients for both infections. The added expense of treating a person with nongonococcal urethritis (NGU) for both infections also should encourage the health-care provider to make a specific diagnosis. (See Nongonococcal Urethritis, Chlamydial Infections, and Gonococcal Infections.)

Table 11.1. Oral Desensitization Protocol for Patients with a Positive Skin Test[a]

Penicillin V Suspension Doses[b]	Amount[c] (units/ml)	ml	Units	Cumulative Dose (units)
1	1,000	0.1	100	100
2	1,000	0.2	200	300
3	1,000	0.4	400	700
4	1,000	0.8	800	1,500
5	1,000	1.6	1,600	3,100
6	1,000	3.2	3,200	6,300
7	1,000	6.4	6,400	12,700
8	10,000	1.2	12,000	24,700
9	10,000	2.4	24,000	48,700
10	10,000	4.8	48,000	96,700
11	80,000	1.0	80,000	176,700
12	80,000	2.0	160,000	336,700
13	80,000	4.0	320,000	656,700
14	80,000	8.0	640,000	1,296,700

Reprinted with permission from the *New England Journal of Medicine*. Oral desensitization protocol for patients with a positive skin test. N Engl J Med 1985;312:1229–1232.

[a] Observation period: 30 minutes before parenteral administration of penicillin.

[b] Interval between doses, 15 minutes; elapsed time, 3 hours and 45 minutes; cumulative dose, 1.3 million units.

[c] The specific amount of drug was diluted to approximately 30 ml of water and then administered orally.

NONGONOCOCCAL URETHRITIS

NGU, or inflammation of the urethra not caused by gonococcal infection, is characterized by a mucoid or purulent urethral discharge. In the presence or absence of a discharge, NGU may be diagnosed by >5 polymorphonuclear leukocytes per oil immersion field on a smear of an intraurethral swab specimen. Increasingly, the leukocyte esterase test (LET) is being used to screen urine from asymptomatic males for evidence of urethritis (either gonococcal or nongonococcal). The diagnosis of urethritis among males tested with LET should be confirmed with a Gram-stained smear of a urethral swab specimen. *C. trachomatis* is the most frequent cause of NGU (23 to 55% of cases); however, prevalence varies among age groups, with lower prevalence found among older men. Urea plasma urealyticum causes 20 to 40% of cases, and *Trichomonas vaginalis* 2 to 5%. HSV is occasionally responsible for cases of NGU. The etiology of the remaining cases of NGU is unknown.

Complications of NGU among men infected with *C. trachomatis* include epididymitis and Reiter's syndrome. Female sex partners of men who have NGU are at risk for chlamydial infection and associated complications.

Recommended Regimen

Doxycycline 100 mg orally 2 times a day for 7 days.[e]

Alternative Regimens

Erythromycin base 500 mg orally 4 times a day for 7 days
or
Erythromycin ethylsuccinate 800 mg orally 4 times a day for 7 days.

If a patient cannot tolerate high-dose erythromycin schedules, one of the following regimens may be used:

Erythromycin base 250 mg orally 4 times a day for 14 days
or
Erythromycin ethylsuccinate 400 mg orally 4 times a day for 14 days.

Treatment with the recommended regimen has been demonstrated in most cases to result in alleviation of symptoms and in microbiologic cure of infection. If the etiologic organism is susceptible to the antimicrobial agent used, sequelae specific to that organism will be prevented, as will further transmission; this is especially important for cases of NGU caused by *C. trachomatis*.

Follow-Up.   Patients should be instructed to return for evaluation if symptoms persist or recur after completion of therapy. Patients with persistent or recurrent urethritis should be re-treated with the initial regimen if they failed to comply with the treatment regimen or if they were reexposed to an untreated sex partner. Otherwise, a wet mount examination and culture of an intraurethral

---

[e] Azithromycin 1 gm in a single dose, according to manufacturer's data, is equivalent to doxycycline. However, this study has not been published in a peer-reviewed journal. For a discussion comparing azithromycin and doxycycline, refer to Chlamydial Infections.

swab specimen for *T. vaginalis* should be performed; if negative, the patient should be re-treated with an alternative regimen extended to 14 days (e.g., erythromycin base 500 mg orally 4 times a day for 14 days). The use of alternative regimens ensures treatment of possible tetracycline-resistant *Ureaplasma urealyticum*.

Effective regimens have not been identified for treating patients who experience persistent symptoms or frequent recurrences following treatment with doxycycline and erythromycin. Urologic examinations do not usually reveal a specific etiology. Such patients should be assured that, although they have persistent or frequently recurring urethritis, the condition is not known to cause complications among them or their sex partners and is not known to be sexually transmitted. However, men exposed to a new sex partner should be reevaluated. Symptoms alone, without documentation of signs or laboratory evidence of urethral inflammation, are not a sufficient basis for re-treatment.

Management of Sex Partners.   Patients should be instructed to refer sex partners for evaluation and treatment. Since exposure intervals have received limited evaluation, the following recommendations are somewhat arbitrary. Sex partners of symptomatic patients should be evaluated and treated if their last sexual contact with the index patient was within 30 days of onset of symptoms. If the index patient is asymptomatic, sex partners whose last sexual contact with the index patient was within 60 days of diagnosis should be evaluated and treated. If the patient's last sexual intercourse preceded the time intervals previously described, the most recent sex partner should be treated. A specific diagnosis may facilitate partner referral and partner cooperation. Therefore, testing for both gonorrhea and chlamydia is encouraged.

Patients should be instructed to abstain from sexual intercourse until patient and partners are cured. In the absence of microbiologic test-of-cure, this means when therapy is completed and patient and partners are without symptoms or signs.

Special Considerations

HIV Infection.   Persons with HIV infection and NGU should receive the same treatment as patients without HIV infection.

Management of the Patient with Mucopurulent Cervicitis

Mucopurulent cervicitis (MPC) is characterized by a yellow endocervical exudate visible in the endocervical canal or in an endocervical swab specimen. Some experts also make the diagnosis on the basis of an increased number of polymorphonuclear leukocytes on cervical Gram stain. The condition is asymptomatic among many women, but some may experience an abnormal vaginal discharge and abnormal vaginal bleeding (e.g., following intercourse). The condition can be caused by *C. trachomatis* or *N. gonorrhoeae*, although in most cases neither organism can be isolated. Patients with MPC should have cervical specimens tested for *C. trachomatis* and cultured for *N. gonorrhoeae*. MPC is not a sensitive predictor of infection; however, most women with *C. trachomatis* or *N. gonorrhoeae* do not have MPC.

Treatment.   The results of tests for *C. trachomatis* or *N. gonorrhoeae* should determine the need for treatment, unless the likelihood of infection with either organism is high or unless the patient is unlikely to return for treatment. Treatment for MPC should include the following:

Treatment for gonorrhea and chlamydia in patient populations with high prevalence of both infections, such as patients seen at many STD clinics;

Treatment for chlamydia only, if the prevalence of *N. gonorrhoeae* is low but the likelihood of chlamydia is substantial;

Await test results if the prevalence of both infections are low and if compliance with a recommendation for a return visit is likely;

Follow-Up.   Follow-up should be as recommended for the infections for which the woman is being treated.

Management of Sex Partners.   Management of sex partners of women with MPC should be appropriate for the STD (*C. trachomatis* or *N. gonorrhoeae*) identified. Partners should be notified, examined, and treated on the basis of test results. However, partners of patients who are treated presumptively should receive the same treatment as the index patient.

Special Considerations

HIV Infection.   Persons with HIV infection and MPC should receive the same treatment as patients without HIV infection.

CHLAMYDIAL INFECTIONS

Chlamydial genital infection is common among adolescents and young adults in the United States. Asymptomatic infection is common among both men and women. Testing sexually active adolescent girls for chlamydial infection should be routine during gynecologic examination, even if symptoms are not present. Screening of young adult women 20 to 24 years of age also is suggested, particularly for those who do not consistently use barrier contraceptives and who have new or multiple partners. Periodic surveys of chlamydial prevalence among these groups should be conducted to confirm the validity of using these recommendations in specific clinical settings.

Chlamydial Infections among Adolescents and Adults

The following recommended treatment regimens or the alternative regimens relieve symptoms and cure infection. Among women, several important sequelae may result from *C. trachomatis* infection, the most serious among them being pelvic inflammatory disease (PID), ectopic pregnancy, and infertility. Some women with apparently uncomplicated cervical infection already have subclinical upper reproductive tract infection. Treatment of cervical infection is believed to reduce the likelihood of sequelae, although few studies have demonstrated that antimicrobial therapy reduces the risk of subsequent ascending infections or decreases the incidence of long-term complications of tubal infertility and ectopic pregnancy.

Treatment of infected patients prevents transmission to sex partners, and for infected pregnant women may prevent transmission of *C. trachomatis* to infants during birth. Treatment of sex partners will help to prevent reinfection of the index patient and infection of other partners.

Because of the high prevalence of coinfection with *C. trachomatis* among patients with gonococcal infection, presumptive treatment for chlamydia of patients being treated for gonorrhea is appropriate, particularly if no diagnostic test for *C. trachomatis* infection will be performed. (See Gonococcal Infections.)

Recommended Regimens

Doxycycline 100 mg orally 2 times a day for 7 days
or
Azithromycin 1 gm orally in a single dose.

Alternative Regimens

Ofloxacin 300 mg orally 2 times a day for 7 days
or
Erythromycin base 500 mg orally 4 times a day for 7 days
or
Erythromycin ethylsuccinate 800 mg orally 4 times a day for 7 days
or
Sulfisoxazole 500 mg orally 4 times a day for 10 days (inferior efficacy to other regimens).

Doxycycline and azithromycin appear similar in efficacy and toxicity; however, the safety and efficacy of azithromycin for persons <15 years of age have not been established. Doxycycline has a longer history of extensive use, safety, efficacy, and the advantage of low cost. Azithromycin has the advantage of single-dose administration. Ofloxacin is similar in efficacy to doxycycline and azithromycin, but is more expensive than doxycycline, cannot be used during pregnancy or with persons <17 years of age, and offers no advantage in dosing. Ofloxacin is the only quinolone with proven efficacy against chlamydial infection. Sulfisoxazole is the least desirable treatment because of inferior efficacy.

Follow-Up. Patients do not need to be retested for chlamydia after completing treatment with doxycycline or azithromycin unless symptoms persist or reinfection is suspected. Retesting may be considered 3 weeks after completion of treatment with erythromycin, sulfisoxazole, or amoxicillin. This is usually unnecessary if the patient was treated with doxycycline, azithromycin, or ofloxacin. The validity of chlamydial culture testing performed at <3 weeks following completion of therapy among patients failing therapy has not been established. False-negative results may occur because of small numbers of chlamydial organisms. In addition, nonculture tests conducted at <3 weeks following completion of therapy for patients successfully treated may sometimes be false-positive because of the continued excretion of dead organisms.

Some studies have demonstrated high rates of infection among women retested several months following treatment, presumably because of reinfection. Rescreening women several months following treatment may be an effective strategy for detecting further morbidity in some populations.

Management of Sex Partners.   Patients should be instructed to refer their sex partners for evaluation and treatment. Because exposure intervals have received limited evaluation, the following recommendations are somewhat arbitrary. Sex partners of symptomatic patients with *C. trachomatis* should be evaluated and treated for chlamydia if their last sexual contact with the index patient was within 30 days of onset of the index patient's symptoms. If the index patient is asymptomatic, sex partners whose last sexual contact with the index patient was within 60 days of diagnosis should be evaluated and treated. Health-care providers should treat the last sex partner even if last sexual intercourse took place before the foregoing time intervals. Patients should be instructed to avoid sex until they and their partners are cured. In the absence of microbiologic test-of-cure, this means until therapy is completed and patient and partner(s) are without symptoms.

Special Considerations

Pregnancy.   Doxycycline and ofloxacin are contraindicated for pregnant women, and sulfisoxazole is contraindicated for women during pregnancy near-term and for women who are nursing. The safety and efficacy of azithromycin among pregnant and lactating women have not been established. Repeat testing, preferably by culture, after completing therapy with the following regimens is recommended because there are few data regarding the effectiveness of these regimens, and the frequent gastrointestinal side effects of erythromycin may discourage a patient from complying with the prescribed treatment.

Recommended Regimen for Pregnant Women

  Erythromycin base 500 mg orally 4 times a day for 7 days.

Alternative Regimens for Pregnant Women

  Erythromycin base 250 mg orally 4 times a day for 14 days
  or
  Erythromycin ethylsuccinate 800 mg orally 4 times a day for 7 days
  or
  Erythromycin ethylsuccinate 400 mg orally 4 times a day for 14 days
  or
  If erythromycin cannot be tolerated:
  Amoxicillin 500 mg orally 3 times a day for 7 to 10 days.

NOTE: Erythromycin estolate is contraindicated during pregnancy because of drug-related hepatotoxicity. Few data exist concerning the efficacy of amoxicillin.

HIV Infection.   Persons with HIV infection and chlamydial infection should receive the same treatment as patients without HIV infection.

Chlamydial Infections among Infants

Prenatal screening of pregnant women can prevent chlamydial infection among neonates. Pregnant women <25 years of age and those with new or multiple sex partners should, in particular, be targeted for screening. Periodic surveys of chlamydial prevalence can be conducted to confirm the validity of using these recommendations in specific clinical settings.

C. trachomatis infection of neonates results from perinatal exposure to the mother's infected cervix. The prevalence of C. trachomatis infection generally exceeds 5% among pregnant women, regardless of race/ethnicity or socioeconomic status. Neonatal ocular prophylaxis with silver nitrate solution or antibiotic ointments is ineffective in preventing perinatal transmission of chlamydial infection from mother to infant. However, ocular prophylaxis with those agents does prevent gonococcal ophthalmia and should be continued for that reason. (See Prevention of Ophthalmia Neonatorum.)

Initial C. trachomatis perinatal infection involves mucous membranes of the eye, oropharynx, urogenital tract, and rectum. C. trachomatis infection among neonates can most often be recognized because of conjunctivitis developing 5 to 12 days after birth. Chlamydia is the most frequent identifiable infectious cause of ophthalmia neonatorum. C. trachomatis also is a common cause of subacute, afebrile pneumonia with onset from 1 to 3 months of age. Asymptomatic infections of the oropharynx, genital tract, and rectum among neonates also occur.

Ophthalmia Neonatorum Caused by C. trachomatis

A chlamydial etiology should be considered for all infants with conjunctivitis through 30 days of age.

Diagnostic Considerations. Sensitive and specific methods to diagnose chlamydial ophthalmia for the neonate include isolation by tissue culture and nonculture tests, direct fluorescent antibody tests, and immunoassays. Giemsa-stained smears are specific for C. trachomatis, but are not sensitive. Specimens must contain conjunctival cells, not exudate alone. Specimens for culture isolation and nonculture tests should be obtained from the everted eyelid using a Dacron-tipped swab or the swab specified by the manufacturer's test kit. A specific diagnosis of C. trachomatis infection confirms the need for chlamydial treatment not only for the neonate, but also for the mother and her sex partner(s). Ocular exudate from infants being evaluated for chlamydial conjunctivitis should also be tested for N. gonorrhoeae.

Recommended Regimen

Erythromycin 50 mg/kg/day orally divided into 4 doses for 10 to 14 days.

Topical antibiotic therapy alone is inadequate for treatment of chlamydial infection and is unnecessary when systemic treatment is undertaken.

Follow-Up. The possibility of chlamydial pneumonia should be considered. The efficacy of erythromycin treatment is approximately 80%; a second course of therapy may be required. Follow-up of infants to determine resolution is recommended.

Management of Mothers and Their Sex Partners. The mothers of infants who have chlamydial infection and the mother's sex partners should be evaluated and treated following the treatment recommendations for adults with chlamydial infections. (See Chlamydial Infections among Adolescents and Adults.)

Infant Pneumonia Caused by *C. trachomatis*

Characteristic signs of chlamydial pneumonia among infants include a repetitive staccato cough with tachypnea, and hyperinflation and bilateral diffuse infiltrates on a chest roentgenogram. Wheezing is rare, and infants are typically afebrile. Peripheral eosinophilia, documented in a complete blood count, is sometimes observed among infants with chlamydial pneumonia. Because variation from this clinical presentation is common, initial treatment and diagnostic tests should encompass *C. trachomatis* for all infants 1 to 3 months of age who have possible pneumonia.

Diagnostic Considerations.   Specimens should be collected from the nasopharynx for chlamydial testing. Tissue culture remains the definitive standard for chlamydial pneumonia; nonculture tests can be used with the knowledge that nonculture tests of nasopharyngeal specimens produce lower sensitivity and specificity than nonculture tests of ocular specimens. Tracheal aspirates and lung biopsy specimens, if collected, should be tested for *C. trachomatis*.

The microimmunofluorescence test for *C. trachomatis* antibody is useful but not widely available. An acute IgM antibody titer 21:32 is strongly suggestive of *C. trachomatis* pneumonia. Because of the delay in obtaining test results for chlamydia, inclusion of an agent active against *C. trachomatis* in the antibiotic regimen must frequently be decided on the basis of the clinical and radiologic findings. Conducting tests for chlamydial infection is worthwhile, not only to assist in the management of an infant's illness, but also to determine the need for treatment of the mother and her sex partners.

Recommended Regimen

Erythromycin 50 mg/kg/day orally divided into 4 doses for 10 to 14 days.

Follow-Up.   The effectiveness of erythromycin treatment is approximately 80%; a second course of therapy may be required. Follow-up of infants is recommended to determine that the pneumonia has resolved. Some infants with chlamydial pneumonia have had abnormal pulmonary function tests later in childhood.

Management of Mothers and Their Sex Partners.   Mothers of infants who have chlamydial infection and the mother's sex partners should be evaluated and treated according to the recommended treatment of adults with chlamydial infections. (See Chlamydial Infections among Adolescents and Adults.)

Infants Born to Mothers Who Have Chlamydial Infection

Infants born to mothers who have untreated chlamydia are at high risk for infection and should be evaluated and treated as for infants with ophthalmia neonatorum caused by *C. trachomatis*.

Chlamydial Infections among Children

Sexual abuse must be considered a cause of chlamydial infection among preadolescent children, although perinatally transmitted *C. trachomatis* infection of the nasopharynx, urogenital tract, and rectum may persist beyond 1 year. (See Sexual Assault or Abuse of Children.) Because of the potential for a criminal investigation and legal proceedings for sexual abuse, diagnosis of *C. trachomatis* among preadolescent children requires the high specificity provided by isolation in cell culture. The cultures should be confirmed by microscopic identification of the characteristic intracytoplasmic inclusions, preferably by fluorescein-conjugated monoclonal antibodies specific for *C. trachomatis*.

Diagnostic Considerations.   Nonculture chlamydia tests should not be used because of the possibility of false-positive test results. With respiratory tract specimens, false-positive test results can occur because of cross-reaction of test reagents with *Chlamydia pneumoniae*; with genital and anal specimens, false-positive test results occur because of cross-reaction with fecal flora.

Recommended Regimen
CHILDREN WHO WEIGH <45 KG:

Erythromycin 50 mg/kg/day divided into four doses for 10 to 14 days.

NOTE: The effectiveness of erythromycin treatment is approximately 80%; a second course of therapy may be required.
CHILDREN WHO WEIGH 245 KG BUT WHO ARE <8 YEARS OF AGE:

Use the same treatment regimens for these children as the adult regimens of **erythromycin**. (See Chlamydial Infections among Adolescents and Adults).

CHILDREN ≤8 YEARS OF AGE:

Use the same treatment regimens for these children as the adult regimens of **doxycycline** or **tetracycline**. (See Chlamydial Infections among Adolescents and Adults.) Adult regimens of **azithromycin** also may be considered for adolescents.

Other Management Considerations.   See Sexual Assault or Abuse of Children.

Follow-Up.   Follow-up cultures are necessary to ensure that treatment has been effective.

GONOCOCCAL INFECTIONS

Gonococcal Infections among Adolescents and Adults

An estimated 1 million new infections with *N. gonorrhoeae* occur in the United States each year. Most infections among men produce symptoms that cause the person to seek curative treatment soon enough to prevent serious sequelae—but not soon enough to prevent transmission to others. Many infections among women do not produce recognizable symptoms until complications such as PID have occurred. PID, whether symptomatic or asymptomatic, can cause tubal scarring leading to infertility or ectopic pregnancy. Because gonococcal infections among women are often asymptomatic, a primary measure for controlling gonorrhea in the United States has been the screening of high-risk women.

Uncomplicated Gonococcal Infections

Recommended Regimens

    Ceftriaxone 125 mg intramuscularly in a single dose
    or
    Cefixime 400 mg orally in a single dose
    or
    Ciprofloxacin 500 mg orally in a single dose
    or
    Ofloxacin 400 mg orally in a single dose

PLUS: A regimen effective against possible coinfection with *C. trachomatis*, such as **doxycycline** 100 mg orally 2 times a day for 7 days.

Many antibiotics are safe and effective for treating gonorrhea, eradicating *N. gonorrhoeae*, ending the possibility of further transmission, relieving symptoms, and reducing the chances of sequelae.

Selection of a treatment regimen for *N. gonorrhoeae* infection requires consideration of the anatomic site of infection, resistance of *N. gonorrhoeae* strains to antimicrobials, the possibility of concurrent infection with *C. trachomatis*, and the side effects and costs of the various treatment regimens.

Because coinfection with *C. trachomatis* is common, persons treated for gonorrhea should be treated presumptively with a regimen that is effective against *C. trachomatis*. (See Chlamydial Infections.)

Most experts agree that other regimens recommended for the treatment of *C. trachomatis* infection are also likely to be satisfactory for the treatment of coinfection. (See Chlamydial Infections.) However, studies have not been conducted to investigate possible interactions between other treatments for *N. gonorrhoeae* and *C. trachomatis*, including interactions influencing the effectiveness and side effects of cotreatment.

In clinical trials, these recommended regimens cured >95% of anal and genital infections; any of the regimens may be used for uncomplicated anal or genital infection. Published studies indicate that ceftriaxone 125 mg and ciprofloxacin 500 mg can cure ≥90% of pharyngeal infections. If pharyngeal infection is a concern, one of these two regimens should be used.

Ceftriaxone in a single dose of either 125 mg or 250 mg provides sustained, high bactericidal levels in the blood. Extensive clinical experience indicates that both doses are safe and effective for the treatment of uncomplicated gonorrhea at all sites. In the past, the 250-mg dose has been recommended on the supposition that the routine use of a higher dose may forestall the development of resistance. However, on the basis of ceftriaxone's activity against *N. gonorrhoeae*, its pharmacokinetics, and the results in clinical trials of doses as low as 62.5 mg, the 125-mg dose appears to have a therapeutic reserve at least as large as that of other accepted treatment regimens. No ceftriaxone-resistant strains of *N. gonorr-hoeae* have been reported. The drawbacks of ceftriaxone are that it is expensive, currently unavailable in vials of <250 mg, and must be administered by injection. Some health-care providers believe that the discomfort of the injection may be reduced by using 1% lidocaine solution as a diluent. Ceftriaxone also may abort incubating syphilis, a concern when gonorrhea treatment is not accompanied by a 7-day course of doxycycline or erythromycin for the presumptive treatment of chlamydia.

Cefixime has an antimicrobial spectrum similar to that of ceftriaxone, but the 400-mg oral dose does not provide as high nor as sustained a bactericidal level as does 125 mg of ceftriaxone. Cefixime appears to be effective against pharyngeal gonococcal infection, but few patients with pharyngeal infection have been included in studies. No gonococcal strains resistant to cefixime have been reported. The advantage of cefixime is that it can be administered orally. It is not known if the 400-mg dose can cure incubating syphilis.

Ciprofloxacin at a dose of 500 mg provides sustained bactericidal levels in the blood. Clinical trials have demonstrated that both 250- and 500-mg doses are safe and effective for the treatment of uncomplicated gonorrhea at all sites. Most clinical experience in the United States has been with the 500-mg dose. Ciprofloxacin can be administered orally and is less expensive than ceftriaxone. No resistance has been reported in the United States, but strains with decreased susceptibility to some quinolones are becoming common in Asia and have been reported in North America. The 500-mg dose is recommended, rather than the 250-mg dose, because of the trend toward decreasing susceptibility to quinolones and because of rare reports of treatment failure. Quinolones are contraindicated for pregnant or nursing women and for persons <17 years of age on the basis of information from animal studies. Quinolones are not active against *T. pallidum*.

Ofloxacin is active against *N. gonorrhoeae* and has favorable pharmacokinetics, and the 400-mg dose has been effective for the treatment of uncomplicated anal and genital gonorrhea. In published studies, a 400-mg dose cured 22 (88%) of 25 pharyngeal infections.

Alternative Regimens

Spectinomycin 2 gm intramuscularly in a single dose.

Spectinomycin has the disadvantages of being injectable, expensive, inactive against *T. pallidum*, and relatively ineffective against pharyngeal gonorrhea. In addition, resistant strains have been reported in the United States. However, spectinomycin remains useful for the treatment of patients who can tolerate neither cephalosporins nor quinolones.

Injectable cephalosporin regimens other than ceftriaxone 125 mg that have demonstrated efficacy against uncomplicated anal or genital gonococcal infections include these injectable cephalosporins: ceftizoxime 500 mg intramuscularly in a single dose; cefotaxime 500 mg intramuscularly in a single dose; cefotetan 1 gm intramuscularly in a single dose; and cefoxitin 2 gm intramuscularly in a single dose.

None of these injectable cephalosporins offers any advantage compared with ceftriaxone, and there is less clinical experience with them for the treatment of uncomplicated gonorrhea. Of these four regimens, ceftizoxime 500 mg appears to be the most effective according to cumulative experience in published clinical trials.

Oral cephalosporin regimens other than cefixime 400 mg include cefuroxime axetil 1 gm orally in a single dose and cefpodoxime proxetil 200 mg orally in a single dose. These two regimens have antigonococcal activity and pharmacokinetics less favorable than the 400-mg cefixime regimen, and there is less clinical experience with them in the treatment of gonorrhea. They have not been very effective against pharyngeal infections among the few patients studied.

Quinolone regimens other than ciprofloxacin 500 mg and ofloxacin 400 mg include enoxacin 400 mg orally in a single dose; lomefloxacin 400 mg orally in a single dose; and norfloxacin 800 mg orally in a single dose. They appear to be safe and effective for the treatment of uncomplicated gonorrhea, but none appears to offer any advantage over ciprofloxacin at a dose of 500 mg or ofloxacin at 400 mg.

Enoxacin and norfloxacin are active against *N. gonorrhoeae*, have favorable pharmacokinetics, and have been effective in clinical trials, but there is minimal experience with their use in the United States. Lomefloxacin is effective against *N. gonorrhoeae* and has very favorable pharmacokinetics, but there are few published clinical studies to support its use for the treatment of gonorrhea, and there is little experience with its use in the United States.

Many other antimicrobials are active against *N. gonorrhoeae*. These guidelines are not intended to be a comprehensive list of all effective treatment regimens.

Other Management Considerations.   Persons treated for gonorrhea should be screened for syphilis by serology when gonorrhea is first detected. Gonorrhea treatment regimens that include ceftriaxone or a 7-day course of either doxycycline or erythromycin may cure incubating syphilis, but few data relevant to this topic are available.

Follow-Up.   Persons who have uncomplicated gonorrhea and who are treated with any of the regimens in these guidelines need not return for a test-of-cure. Those persons with symptoms persisting after treatment should be evaluated by culture for *N. gonorrhoeae*, and any gonococci isolated should be tested for antimicrobial susceptibility. Infections detected after treatment with one of the recommended regimens more commonly occur because of reinfection rather than treatment failure, indicating a need for improved sex partner referral and patient education. Persistent urethritis, cervicitis, or proctitis also may be caused by *C. trachomatis* and other organisms.

Management of Sex Partners.   Patients should be instructed to refer sex partners for evaluation and treatment. Sex partners of symptomatic patients who have *N. gonorrhoeae* infection should be evaluated and treated for *N. gonorrhoeae* and *C. trachomatis* infections, if their last sexual contact with the patient was within 30 days of onset of the patient's symptoms. If the index patient is asymptomatic, sex partners whose last sexual contact with the patient was within 60 days of diagnosis should be evaluated and treated. Health-care providers should treat the most recent sex partner, if last sexual intercourse took place before those time periods.

Patients should be instructed to avoid sexual intercourse until patient and partner(s) are cured. In the absence of microbiologic test-of-cure, this means until therapy is completed and patient and partner(s) are without symptoms.

Special Considerations

Allergy, Intolerance, or Adverse Reactions.   Persons who cannot tolerate cephalosporins should, in general, be treated with quinolones. Those who can take neither cephalosporins nor quinolones should be treated with spectinomycin, except for those patients who are suspected or known to have pharyngeal infection. For pharyngeal infections among persons who can tolerate neither a cephalosporin nor quinolones, some studies suggest that trimethoprim-sulfamethoxazole may be effective at a dose of 720 mg of trimethoprim/3600 mg of sulfamethoxazole orally once a day for 5 days.

Pregnancy.   Pregnant women should not be treated with quinolones or tetracyclines. Those infected with *N. gonorrhoeae* should be treated with a recommended or alternate cephalosporin. Women who cannot tolerate a cephalosporin should be administered a single dose of 2 gm of spectinomycin intramuscularly. Erythromycin is the recommended treatment for presumptive or diagnosed *C. trachomatis* infection during pregnancy. (See Chlamydial Infections.)

HIV Infection.   Persons with HIV infection and gonococcal infection should receive the same treatment as persons not infected with HIV.

Gonococcal Conjunctivitis

Only one North American study of the treatment of gonococcal conjunctivitis among adults has been published in recent years. In that study, 12 of 12 patients responded favorably to a single 1-gm intramuscular injection of ceftriaxone. The recommendations that follow reflect the opinions of expert consultants.

Treatment

Recommended Regimen.   A single, 1-gm dose of **ceftriaxone** should be administered intramuscularly, and the infected eye should be lavaged with saline solution once.

Management of Sex Partners.   As for uncomplicated infections, patients should be instructed to refer sex partner(s) for evaluation and treatment. (See Uncomplicated Gonococcal Infections, Management of Sex Partners.)

Disseminated Gonococcal Infection

Disseminated gonococcal infection (DGI) results from gonococcal bacteremia, often resulting in petechial or pustular acral skin lesions, asymmetrical arthalgias, tenosynovitis, or septic arthritis—and is occasionally complicated by hepatitis and, rarely, by endocarditis or meningitis. Strains of *N. gonorrhoeae* that cause DGI tend to cause little genital inflammation. These strains have become uncommon in the United States during the past decade. No North American studies of the treatment of DGI have been published recently. The recommendations that follow reflect the opinions of expert consultants.

Treatment.   Hospitalization is recommended for initial therapy, especially for patients who cannot be relied on to comply with treatment, for those for whom the diagnosis is uncertain, and for those who have purulent synovial effusions or other complications. Patients should be examined for clinical evidence of endocarditis and meningitis. Patients treated for DGI should be treated presumptively for concurrent *C. trachomatis* infection.

Recommended Initial Regimen

Ceftriaxone 1 gm intramuscularly or intravenously every 24 hours.

Alternative Initial Regimens

Cefotaxime 1 gm intravenously every 8 hours
or
Ceftizoxime 1 gm intravenously every 8 hours
or
For persons allergic to β-lactam drugs:
Spectinomycin 2 gm intramuscularly every 12 hours.

All regimens should be continued for 24 to 48 hours after improvement begins, and then therapy may be switched to one of the following regimens to complete a full week of antimicrobial therapy.

Recommended Subsequent Regimen

Cefixime 400 mg orally 2 times a day
or
Ciprofloxacin 500 mg orally 2 times a day.

NOTE: Ciprofloxacin is contraindicated for children, adolescents <17 years of age, and pregnant and lactating women.

Management of Sex Partners.   Gonococcal infection is often asymptomatic in sex partners of patients with DGI. As for uncomplicated infections, patients should be instructed to refer sex partner(s) for evaluation and treatment. (See Uncomplicated Gonococcal Infections, Management of Sex Partners.)

Gonococcal Meningitis and Endocarditis

Recommended Initial Regimen

1 to 2 gm of **ceftriaxone** intravenously every 12 hours.

Therapy for meningitis should be continued for 10 to 14 days and for endocarditis for at least 4 weeks. Treatment of complicated DGI should be undertaken in consultation with an expert.

Management of Sex Partners.   As for uncomplicated infections, patients should be instructed to refer sex partners for evaluation and treatment. (See Uncomplicated Gonococcal Infections, Management of Sex Partners.)

Gonococcal Infections among Infants

Gonococcal infection among neonates usually results from peripartum exposure to infected cervical exudate of the mother. Gonococcal infection among neonates is usually an acute illness beginning 2 to 5 days after birth. The incidence of *N. gonorrhoeae* among neonates varies in U.S. communities and depends on the prevalence of infection among pregnant women, on whether pregnant women are screened for gonorrhea, and on whether newborns receive ophthalmia prophylaxis. The prevalence of infection is <1% in most prenatal patient populations, but may be higher in some settings.

Of greatest concern are complications of ophthalmia neonatorum and sepsis, including arthritis and meningitis. Less serious manifestations at sites of infection include rhinitis, vaginitis, urethritis, and inflammation at sites of intrauterine fetal monitoring.

Ophthalmia Neonatorum Caused by *N. gonorrhoeae*

In most patient populations in the United States, *C. trachomatis* and nonsexually transmitted agents are more common causes of neonatal conjunctivitis than *N. gonorrhoeae*. However, *N. gonorrhoeae* is especially important because gonococcal ophthalmia may result in perforation of the globe and in blindness.

Diagnostic Considerations.   Infants at high risk for gonococcal ophthalmia in the United States are those who do not receive ophthalmia prophylaxis, whose mothers have had no prenatal care, or whose mothers have a history of STDs or substance abuse. The presence of typical Gram-negative diplococci in a Gram-stained smear of conjunctival exudate suggests a diagnosis of *N. gonorrhoeae* conjunctivitis. Such patients should be treated presumptively for gonorrhea after obtaining appropriate cultures for *N. gonorrhoeae*; appropriate chlamydial testing should be done simultaneously. The decision not to treat presumptively for *N. gonorrhoeae* among patients without evidence of gonococci on a Gram-stained smear of conjunctival exudate, or among patients for whom a Gram-stained smear cannot be performed, must be made on a case-by-case basis after considering the previously described risk factors.

A specimen of conjunctival exudate also should be cultured for isolation of *N. gonorrhoeae*, since culture is needed for definitive microbiologic identification and for antibiotic susceptibility testing. Such definitive testing is required because of the public health and social consequences for the infant and mother that may result from the diagnosis of gonococcal ophthalmia. *Moraxella catarrhalis* and other *Neisseria* species are uncommon causes of neonatal conjunctivitis that can mimic *N. gonorrhoeae* on Gram-stained smear. To differentiate *N. gonorrhoeae* from *M. catarrhalis* and other *Neisseria* species, the laboratory should be instructed to perform confirmatory tests on any colonies that meet presumptive criteria for *N. gonorrhoeae*.

Recommended Regimen

Ceftriaxone 25 to 50 mg/kg intravenously or intramuscularly in a single dose, not to exceed 125 mg.

NOTE: Topical antibiotic therapy alone is inadequate and is unnecessary if systemic treatment is administered.

Other Management Considerations. Simultaneous infection with *C. trachomatis* has been reported and should be considered for patients who do not respond satisfactorily. The mother and infant should be tested for chlamydial infection at the same time that gonorrhea testing is done. (See Ophthalmia Neonatorum Caused by *C. trachomatis*.) Ceftriaxone should be administered cautiously among infants with elevated bilirubin levels, especially premature infants.

Follow-Up. Infants should be admitted to the hospital and evaluated for signs of disseminated infection (e.g., sepsis, arthritis, and meningitis). One dose of ceftriaxone is adequate for gonococcal conjunctivitis, but many pediatricians prefer to maintain infants on antibiotics until cultures are negative at 48 to 72 hours. The decision on duration of therapy should be made with input from experienced physicians.

Management of Mothers and Their Sex Partners. The mothers of infants with gonococcal infection and the mothers' sex partners should be evaluated and treated following the recommendations for treatment of gonococcal infections in adults. (See Gonococcal Infections among Adolescents and Adults.)

Disseminated Gonococcal Infection among Infants

Sepsis, arthritis, meningitis, or any combination thereof are rare complications of neonatal gonococcal infection. Gonococcal scalp abscesses also may develop as a result of fetal monitoring. Detection of gonococcal infection among neonates who have sepsis, arthritis, meningitis, or scalp abscesses requires cultures of blood, CSF, and joint aspirate on chocolate agar. Cultures of specimens from the conjunctiva, vagina, oropharynx, and rectum onto gonococcal selective medium are useful to identify sites of primary infection, especially if inflammation is present. Positive Gram-stained smears of exudate, CSF, or joint aspirate provide a presumptive basis for initiating treatment for *N. gonorrhoeae*. Diagnoses based on positive Gram-stained smears or presumptive isolation by cultures should be confirmed with definitive tests on culture isolates.

Recommended Regimen

Ceftriaxone 25 to 50 mg/kg/day intravenously or intramuscularly in a single daily dose for 7 days, with a duration of 10 to 14 days, if meningitis is documented;
or
Cefotaxime 25 mg/kg intravenously or intramuscularly every 12 hours for 7 days, with a duration of 10 to 14 days, if meningitis is documented.

Prophylactic Treatment for Infants Whose Mothers Have Gonococcal Infection. Infants born to mothers who have untreated gonorrhea are at high risk for infection.

Recommended Regimen in the Absence of Signs of Gonococcal Infection

Ceftriaxone 25 to 50 mg/kg intravenously or intramuscularly, not to exceed 125 mg, in a single dose.

Other Management Considerations.   If simultaneous infection with *C. trachomatis* has been reported, mother and infant should be tested for chlamydial infection.

Follow-Up.   Follow-up examination is not required.

Management of Mothers and Their Sex Partners.   The mothers of infants with gonococcal infection and the mother's sex partners should be evaluated and treated following the recommendations for treatment of gonococcal infections among adults. (See Gonococcal Infections.)

Gonococcal Infections among Children

After the neonatal period, sexual abuse is the most common cause of gonococcal infection among preadolescent children. (See Sexual Assault or Abuse of Children.) Vaginitis is the most common manifestation of gonococcal infection among preadolescent children. PID following vaginal infection appears to be less common than among adults. Among sexually abused children, anorectal and pharyngeal infections with *N. gonorrhoeae* are common and are frequently asymptomatic.

Diagnostic Considerations.   Because of the potential medical/legal use of the test results for *N. gonorrhoeae* among children, only standard culture systems for the isolation of *N. gonorrhoeae* should be used to diagnose *N. gonorrhoeae* for these children. Nonculture gonococcal tests, including Gram-stained smear, DNA probes, or enzyme immunoassay (EIA) tests should not be used; none of these tests have been approved by the FDA for use in the oropharynx, rectum, or genital tract of children. Specimens from the vagina, urethra, pharynx, or rectum should be streaked onto selective media for isolation of *N. gonorrhoeae*. All presumptive isolates of *N. gonorrhoeae* should be confirmed by at least two tests that involve different principles, e.g., biochemical, enzyme substrate, or serologic. Isolates should be preserved to permit additional or repeated analysis.

Recommended Regimen for Children
CHILDREN WHO WEIGH ≥45 KG:

Children who weigh ≥45 kg should be administered the same treatment regimens as those recommended for adults. (See Gonococcal Infections).

CHILDREN WHO WEIGH <45 KG:

The following treatment recommendations are for children with uncomplicated gonococcal vulvovaginitis, cervicitis, urethritis, pharyngitis, or proctitis.

Ceftriaxone 125 mg intramuscularly in a single dose.

Alternative Regimen

Spectinomycin 40 mg/kg (maximum 2 gm) intramuscularly in a single dose.

CHILDREN WHO WEIGH <45 KG AND WHO HAVE BACTEREMIA, ARTHRITIS, OR MENINGITIS:

Ceftriaxone 50 mg/kg (maximum 1 gm) intramuscularly or intravenously in a single dose daily for 7 days.

NOTE: For meningitis, increase the duration of treatment to 10 to 14 days and the maximum dose to 2 gm.

Follow-Up. Follow-up cultures of specimens from infected sites are necessary to ensure that treatment has been effective.

Other Management Considerations. Only parenteral cephalosporins are recommended for use among children. Ceftriaxone is approved for all gonococcal indications among children; cefotaxime is approved for gonococcal ophthalmia only. Oral cephalosporins (cefixime, cefuroxime axetil, cefpodoxime) have not received adequate evaluation in the treatment of gonococcal infections among pediatric patients to recommend their use. The pharmacokinetic activity of these drugs among adults cannot be extrapolated to children.

All children with gonococcal infections should be evaluated for coinfection with syphilis and *C. trachomatis*. For a discussion of issues regarding sexual assault, refer to Sexual Assault or Abuse of Children.

Ophthalmia Neonatorum Prophylaxis

Instillation of a prophylactic agent into the eyes of all newborn infants is recommended to prevent gonococcal ophthalmia neonatorum and is required by law in most states. Although all the regimens that follow effectively prevent gonococcal eye disease, their efficacy in preventing chlamydial eye disease is not clear. Furthermore, they do not eliminate nasopharyngeal colonization with *C. trachomatis*. Treatment of gonococcal and chlamydial infections among pregnant women is the best method for preventing neonatal gonococcal and chlamydial disease. However, ocular prophylaxis should continue because it can prevent gonococcal ophthalmia, and in some populations, >10% of pregnant women may receive no prenatal care.

Prophylaxis

Recommended Preparations

Silver nitrate (1%) aqueous solution in a single application
or
Erythromycin (0.5%) ophthalmic ointment in a single application
or
Tetracycline ophthalmic ointment (1%) in a single application.

One of the above preparations should be instilled into the eyes of every neonate as soon as possible after delivery. If prophylaxis is delayed (i.e., not administered in the delivery room), hospitals should establish a monitoring system to see that all infants receive prophylaxis. All infants should be administered ocular prophylaxis, whether delivery is vaginal or caesarian. Single-use tubes or ampules are preferable to multiple-use tubes. Bacitracin is not effective.

Diseases Characterized by Vaginal Discharge

Management of the Patient with Vaginitis

Vaginitis is characterized by a vaginal discharge (usually) or vulvar itching and irritation; a vaginal odor may be present. The three common diseases characterized by vaginitis include trichomoniasis (caused by *T. vaginalis*), bacterial vaginosis (BV) (caused by a replacement of the normal vaginal flora by an overgrowth of anaerobic microorganisms and *Gardnerella vaginalis*), and candidiasis (usually caused by *Candida albicans*). MPC caused by *C. trachomatis* or *N. gonorrhoeae* may uncommonly cause a vaginal discharge. Although vulvovaginal candidiasis is not usually transmitted sexually, it is included here because it is a common infection among women being evaluated for STDs.

The diagnosis of vaginitis is made by pH and microscopic examination of fresh samples of the discharge. The pH of the vaginal secretions can be determined by narrow-range pH paper for the elevated pH (>4.5) typical of BV or trichomoniasis. One way to examine the discharge is to dilute a sample in 1 to 2 drops of 0.9% normal saline solution on one slide and 10% potassium hydroxide (KOH) solution on a second slide. An amine odor detected immediately after applying KOH suggests either BV or trichomoniasis. A cover slip is placed on each slide, and they are examined under a microscope at low- and high-dry power. The motile *T. vaginalis* or the clue cells of BV are usually easily identified in the saline specimen. The yeast or pseudohyphae of *Candida* species are more easily identified in the KOH specimen. The presence of objective signs of vulvar inflammation in the absence of vaginal pathogens, along with a minimal amount of discharge, suggests the possibility of mechanical or chemical irritation of the vulva. Culture for *T. vaginalis* or *Candida* species is more sensitive than microscopic examination, but the specificity of culture for *Candida* species to diagnose vaginitis is less clear. Laboratory testing fails to identify a cause among a substantial minority of women.

BACTERIAL VAGINOSIS

BV is a clinical syndrome resulting from replacement of the normal H_2O_2-producing *Lactobacillus* spp. in the vagina with high concentrations of anaerobic bacteria (e.g., *Bacteroides* spp., *Mobiluncus* spp.), *G. vaginalis*, and *Mycoplasma hominis*. This condition is the most prevalent cause of vaginal discharge or malodor. However, half the women who meet clinical criteria for BV have no symptoms. The cause of the microbial alteration is not fully understood. Although BV is associated with sexual activity in that women who have never been sexually active are rarely affected and acquisition of BV is associated with having multiple sex partners, BV is not considered exclusively an STD. Treatment of the male sex partner has not been found beneficial in preventing the recurrence of BV.

Diagnostic Considerations.   BV may be diagnosed by the use of clinical or Gram stain criteria. Clinical criteria require three of the following symptoms or signs:

A homogeneous, white, noninflammatory discharge that adheres to the vaginal walls;

The presence of clue cells on microscopic examination;

pH of vaginal fluid >4.5;

A fishy odor of vaginal discharge before or after addition of 10% KOH (whiff test).

When Gram stain is used, determining the relative concentration of the bacterial morphotypes characteristic of the altered flora of BV is an acceptable laboratory method for diagnosing BV. Culture of *G. vaginalis* is not recommended as a diagnostic tool because it is not specific. *G. vaginalis* can be isolated from vaginal cultures among half of normal women.

Treatment. The principal goal of therapy is to relieve vaginal symptoms and signs. Therefore, only women with symptomatic disease require treatment. Because male sex partners of women with BV are not symptomatic and because treatment of male partners has not been shown to alter either the clinical course of BV in women during treatment or the relapse/reinfection rate, preventing transmission to men is not a goal of therapy.

Many bacterial flora characterizing BV have been recovered from the endometrium or salpinx of women with PID. BV has been associated with endometritis, PID, or vaginal cuff cellulitis following invasive procedures such as endometrial biopsy, hysterectomy, hysterosalpingography, placement of an intrauterine device (IUD), cesarean section, or uterine curettage. A randomized controlled trial found that treatment of BV with metronidazole substantially reduced postabortion PID. Based on these data, it may be reasonable to consider treatment of BV (symptomatic or asymptomatic) before performing surgical abortion procedures. However, more data are needed to consider treatment of asymptomatic patients with BV when performing other invasive procedures.

Recommended Regimen

Metronidazole 500 mg orally 2 times a day for 7 days.

NOTE: Patients should be advised to avoid using alcohol during treatment with metronidazole and for 24 hours thereafter.

Alternative Regimens

Metronidazole 2 gm orally in a single dose.

The following alternative regimens have been effective in clinical trials, although experience with these regimens is limited:

Clindamycin cream, 2%, one full applicator (5 gm) intravaginally at bedtime for 7 days;

or

Metronidazole gel, 0.75%, one full applicator (5 gm) intravaginally 2 times a day for 5 days;

or

Clindamycin 300 mg orally 2 times a day for 7 days.

Oral metronidazole has been shown in numerous studies to be efficacious for the treatment of BV, resulting in relief of symptoms and improvement in clinical course and flora disturbances. Based on efficacy data from four randomized-controlled trials, the overall cure rates are 95% for the 7-day regimen and 84% for the 2-gm single-dose regimen.

Some health-care providers remain concerned about the possibility of metronidazole mutagenicity, which has been suggested by experiments on animals using extremely high and prolonged doses. However, there is no evidence for mutagenicity in humans. Some health-care providers prefer the intravaginal route because of lack of systemic side effects such as mild-to-moderate gastrointestinal upset and unpleasant taste (mean peak serum concentrations of metronidazole following intravaginal administration are <2% those of standard 500-mg oral doses, and mean bioavailability of clindamycin cream is about 4%).

Follow-Up.   Follow-up visits are not necessary if symptoms resolve. Recurrence of BV is common. The alternative treatment regimens suitable for BV treatment may be used for treatment of recurrent disease. No long-term maintenance regimen with any therapeutic agent is currently available.

Management of Sex Partners.   Treatment of sex partners in clinical trials has not influenced the woman's response to therapy, nor has it influenced the relapse or recurrence rate. Therefore, routine treatment of sex partners is not recommended.

Special Considerations

Allergy or Intolerance to the Recommended Therapy.   Clindamycin cream is preferred in case of allergy or intolerance to metronidazole. Metronidazole gel can be considered for patients who do not tolerate systemic metronidazole, but patients allergic to oral metronidazole should not be administered metronidazole vaginally.

Pregnancy.   Because metronidazole is contraindicated during the first trimester of pregnancy, clindamycin vaginal cream is the preferred treatment for BV during the first trimester of pregnancy (clindamycin cream is recommended instead of oral clindamycin because of the general desire to limit the exposure of the fetus to medication). During the second and third trimesters of pregnancy, oral metronidazole can be used, although the vaginal metronidazole gel or clindamycin cream may be preferable.

BV has been associated with adverse outcomes of pregnancy (e.g., premature rupture of the membranes, preterm labor, preterm delivery), and the organisms found in increased concentration in BV are also commonly present in postpartum or postcesarean endometritis. Whether treatment of BV among pregnant women would reduce the risk of adverse pregnancy outcomes is unknown; randomized controlled trials have not been conducted.

HIV Infection.   Persons with HIV and BV should receive the same treatment as persons without HIV.

TRICHOMONIASIS

Trichomoniasis is caused by the protozoan *T. vaginalis*. The majority of men infected with *T. vaginalis* are asymptomatic, but many women are symptomatic. Among women, *T. vaginalis* typically causes a diffuse, malodorous, yellow-green discharge with vulvar irritation. There is recent evidence of a possible relationship between vaginal trichomoniasis and adverse pregnancy outcomes, particularly premature rupture of the membranes and preterm delivery.

Recommended Regimen

Metronidazole 2 gm orally in a single dose.

Alternative Regimen

Metronidazole 500 mg twice daily for 7 days.

Only metronidazole is available in the United States for the treatment of trichomoniasis. In randomized clinical trials, both of the recommended metronidazole regimens have resulted in cure rates of approximately 95%. Treatment of the patient and sex partner results in relief of symptoms, microbiologic cure, and reduction of transmission. Metronidazole gel has been approved for the treatment of BV, but it has not been studied for the treatment of trichomoniasis. Earlier preparations of metronidazole for topical vaginal therapy demonstrated low efficacy against trichomoniasis.

Follow-Up.   Follow-up is unnecessary for men and for women who become asymptomatic after treatment. Infections by strains of *T. vaginalis* with diminished susceptibility to metronidazole occur. However, most of these organisms respond to higher doses of metronidazole. If failure occurs with either regimen, the patient should be retreated with metronidazole 500 mg 2 times a day for 7 days. If repeated failure occurs, the patient should be treated with a single 2-gm dose of metronidazole once daily for 3 to 5 days.

Patients with culture-documented infection who do not respond to the regimens described in this report and in whom reinfection has been excluded should be managed in consultation with an expert. Evaluation of such cases should include determination of the susceptibility of *T. vaginalis* to metronidazole.

Management of Sex Partners.   Sex partners should be treated. Patients should be instructed to avoid sex until patient and partner(s) are cured. In the absence of microbiologic test-of-cure, this means when therapy has been completed and patient and partner(s) are without symptoms.

Special Considerations

Allergy, Intolerance, or Adverse Reactions.   Effective alternatives to therapy with metronidazole are not available.

Pregnancy.   The use of metronidazole is contraindicated in the first trimester of pregnancy. Patients may be treated after the first trimester with 2 gm of metronidazole in a single dose.

HIV Infection.   Persons with HIV infection and trichomoniasis should receive the same treatment as persons without HIV.

VULVOVAGINAL CANDIDIASIS

Vulvovaginal candidiasis (VVC) is caused by *C. albicans* or, occasionally, by other *Candida* spp., *Torulopsis* sp., or other yeasts. An estimated 75% of women will experience at least one episode of VVC during their lifetime, and 40 to 45% will experience two or more episodes. A small percentage of women (probably <5%) experience recurrent VVC (RVVC). Typical symptoms of VVC include pruritus and vaginal discharge. Other symptoms may include vaginal soreness, vulvar burning, dyspareunia, and external dysuria. None of these symptoms is specific for VVC. VVC usually is not sexually acquired or transmitted.

Diagnostic Considerations.   A diagnosis of *Candida* vaginitis is suggested clinically by pruritus in the vulvar area together with erythema of the vagina or vulva; a white discharge may occur. The diagnosis can be made when a woman has signs and symptoms of vaginitis and when a wet preparation or Gram stain of vaginal discharge demonstrates yeasts or pseudohyphae or when a culture or other test yields a positive result for a yeast species. Vaginitis solely because of *Candida* infection is associated with a normal vaginal pH (<4.5). Use of 10% KOH in wet preparations improves the visualization of yeast and mycelia by disrupting cellular material that may obscure the yeast or pseudohyphae. Identifying *Candida* in the absence of symptoms should not lead to treatment, because approximately 10 to 20% of women normally harbor *Candida* spp. and other yeasts in the vagina. VVC may be present concurrently with STDs.

Treatment.   Topical formulations provide effective treatment for VVC. The topically applied azole drugs are more effective than nystatin. Treatment with azoles results in relief of symptoms and negative cultures among 80 to 90% of patients after therapy is completed.

Recommended Regimens.   The following intravaginal formulations are recommended for the treatment of VVC.

> **Butoconazole** 2% cream 5 gm intravaginally for 3 days[f];
> or
> **Clotrimazole** 1% cream 5 gm intravaginally for 7 to 14 days;
> or
> **Clotrimazole** 100 mg vaginal tablet for 7 days;
> or
> **Clotrimazole** 100 mg vaginal tablet, two tablets for 3 days;
> or
> **Clotrimazole** 500 mg vaginal tablet, one tablet single application;
> or
> **Miconazole** 2% cream 5 gm intravaginally for 7 days[f];
> or
> **Miconazole** 200 mg vaginal suppository, one suppository for 3 days[f];
> or

---

[f]These creams and suppositories are oil-based and may weaken latex condoms and diaphragms. Refer to product labeling for further information.

Miconazole 100 mg vaginal suppository, one suppository for 7 days[f];
or
Tioconazole 6.5% ointment 5 gm intravaginally in a single application[f];
or
Terconazole 0.4% cream 5 gm intravaginally for 7 days;
or
Terconazole 0.8% cream 5 gm intravaginally for 3 days;
or
Terconazole 80 mg suppository, 1 suppository for 3 days.[f]

OVER-THE-COUNTER (OTC) PREPARATIONS.   Although information is not conclusive, single-dose treatments should probably be reserved for cases of uncomplicated mild-to-moderate VVC. Multiday (3- and 7-day regimens) are the preferred treatment for severe or complicated VVC.

Preparations for intravaginal administration of both miconazole and clotrimazole are now available OTC (nonprescription), and women with VVC can choose one of those preparations. The duration for treatment with either preparation is 7 days. Self-medication with OTC preparations should be advised only for women who have been diagnosed previously with VVC and who experience a recurrence of the same symptoms. Any woman whose symptoms persist after using an OTC preparation or who experiences a recurrence of symptoms within 2 months should seek medical care.

Alternative Regimens.   Several trials have demonstrated that oral azole agents such as fluconazole, ketoconazole, and itraconazole may be as effective as topical agents. The optimum dose and duration of oral therapy have not been established, but a range of 1 to 5 days of treatment, depending on the agent, has been effective in clinical trials. The ease of administration of oral agents is an advantage over topical therapies. However, the potential for toxicity associated with using a systemic drug, particularly ketoconazole, must be considered. No oral agent is approved currently by the FDA for the treatment of acute VVC.

Follow-Up.   Patients should be instructed to return for follow-up visits only if symptoms persist or recur. Women who experience three or more episodes of VVC per year should be evaluated for predisposing conditions. (See Recurrent Vulvovaginal Candidiasis.)

Management of Sex Partners.   VVC is not acquired through sexual intercourse; treatment of sex partners has not been demonstrated to reduce the frequency of recurrences. Therefore, routine notification or treatment of sex partners is not warranted. A minority of male sex partners may have balanitis, which is characterized by erythematous areas on the glans in conjunction with pruritus or irritation. These partners may benefit from treatment with topical antifungal agents to relieve symptoms.

Special Considerations

Allergy or Intolerance to the Recommended Therapy.   Topical agents are usually free of systemic side effects, although local burning or irritation may occur. Oral agents occasionally cause nausea, abdominal pain, and headaches.

Therapy with the oral azoles has been associated rarely with abnormal elevations of liver enzymes. Hepatotoxicity secondary to ketoconazole therapy has been estimated to appear in 1:10,000 to 1:15,000 exposed persons. Clinically important interactions may occur when these oral agents are administered with other drugs, including terfenadine, rifampin, astemizole, phenytoin, cyclosporine, coumarin-like agents, or oral hypoglycemic agents.

Pregnancy.   VVC is common during pregnancy. Only topical azole therapies should be used for the treatment of pregnant women. The most effective treatments that have been studied for pregnant women are clotrimazole, miconazole, butoconazole, and terconazole. Many experts recommend 7 days of therapy during pregnancy.

HIV Infection.   Acute VVC occurs frequently among women with HIV infection and may be more severe for these women than for other women. However, insufficient information exists to determine the optimal management of VVC in HIV-infected women. Until such information becomes available, women with HIV infection and acute VVC should be treated following the same regimens as for women without HIV infection.

RECURRENT VULVOVAGINAL CANDIDIASIS

RVVC, usually defined as three or more episodes of symptomatic VVC annually, affects a small proportion of women (probably <5%). The natural history and pathogenesis of RVVC are poorly understood. Risk factors for RVVC include diabetes mellitus, immunosuppression, broad-spectrum antibiotic use, corticosteroid use, and HIV infection, although the majority of women with RVVC have no apparent predisposing conditions. Clinical trials addressing the management of RVVC have involved continuing therapy between episodes.

Treatment.   The optimal treatment for RVVC has not been established. Ketoconazole 100 mg orally once daily for up to 6 months reduces the frequency of episodes of RVVC. Current studies are evaluating weekly intravaginal administration of clotrimazole, as well as oral therapy with itraconazole and fluconazole, in the treatment of RVVC. All cases of RVVC should be confirmed by culture before maintenance therapy is initiated.

Although patients with RVVC should be evaluated for predisposing conditions, routinely performing HIV testing for women with RVVC who do not have HIV risk factors is unwarranted.

Follow-Up.   Patients who are receiving treatment for RVVC should receive regular follow-up to monitor the effectiveness of therapy and the occurrence of side effects.

Management of Sex Partners.   Treatment of sex partners does not prevent recurrences, and routine therapy is not warranted. However, partners with symptomatic balanitis or penile dermatitis should be treated with a topical agent.

Special Considerations

HIV Infection.   Insufficient information exists to determine the optimal management of RVVC among HIV-infected women. Until such information becomes available, management should be the same as for other women with RVVC.

Pelvic Inflammatory Disease

PID comprises a spectrum of inflammatory disorders of the upper genital tract among women and may include any combination of endometritis, salpingitis, tubo-ovarian abscess, and pelvic peritonitis. Sexually transmitted organisms, especially *N. gonorrhoeae* and *C. trachomatis*, are implicated in the majority of cases; however, microorganisms that can be part of the vaginal flora, such as anaerobes, *G. vaginalis, H. influenzae*, enteric Gram-negative rods, and *Streptococcus agalactiae*, also can cause PID. Some experts also believe that *M. hominis* and *U. urealyticum* are etiologic agents of PID.

Diagnostic Considerations.   Because of the wide variation in many symptoms and signs among women with this condition, a clinical diagnosis of acute PID is difficult. Many women with PID exhibit subtle or mild symptoms that are not readily recognized as PID. Consequently, delay in diagnosis and effective treatment probably contributes to inflammatory sequelae in the upper reproductive tract. Laparoscopy can be used to obtain a more accurate diagnosis of salpingitis and a more complete bacteriologic diagnosis. However, this diagnostic tool is often neither readily available for acute cases nor easily justifiable when symptoms are mild or vague. Moreover, laparoscopy will not detect endometritis and may not detect subtle inflammation of the fallopian tubes. Consequently, the diagnosis of PID is usually made on the basis of clinical findings.

The clinical diagnosis of acute PID is also imprecise. Data indicate that a clinical diagnosis of symptomatic PID has a positive predictive value (PPV) for salpingitis of 65 to 90% when compared with laparoscopy as the standard. The PPV of a clinical diagnosis of acute PID varies depending on epidemiologic characteristics and the clinical setting, with higher PPV among sexually active young (especially teenage) women and among patients attending STD clinics or from settings with high rates of gonorrhea or chlamydia. In all settings, however, no single historical, physical, or laboratory finding is both sensitive and specific for the diagnosis of acute PID (i.e., can be used both to detect all cases of PID and to exclude all women without PID). Combinations of diagnostic findings that improve either sensitivity (detect more women who have PID) or specificity (exclude more women who do not have PID) do so only at the expense of the other. For example, requiring two or more findings excludes more women without PID but also reduces the number of women with PID who are detected.

Many episodes of PID go unrecognized. Although some women may have asymptomatic PID, others are undiagnosed because the patient or the health-care provider fails to recognize the implications of mild or nonspecific symptoms or signs, such as abnormal bleeding, dyspareunia, or vaginal discharge (''atypical PID''). Because of the difficulty of diagnosis and the potential for damage to the reproductive health of women even by apparently mild or atypical PID, experts recommend that providers maintain a low threshold of diagnosis for PID. Even so, the long-term outcome of early treatment of women with asymptomatic or atypical PID on important clinical outcomes is unknown. The following recommendations for diagnosing PID are intended to help health-care providers recognize when PID should be suspected and when they need to obtain additional information to increase diagnostic certainty. These recommendations are based in part on the fact that diagnosis and management of other common causes of lower abdominal pain (e.g., ectopic pregnancy, acute appendicitis, and functional pain) are unlikely to be impaired by initiating empiric antimicrobial therapy for PID.

Minimum Criteria.   Empiric treatment of PID should be instituted on the basis of the presence of all of the following three minimum clinical criteria for pelvic inflammation and in the absence of an established cause other than PID:

Lower abdominal tenderness;
Adnexal tenderness;
Cervical motion tenderness.

Additional Criteria.   For women with severe clinical signs, more elaborate diagnostic evaluation is warranted because incorrect diagnosis and management may cause unnecessary morbidity. These additional criteria may be used to increase the specificity of the diagnosis.

Listed below are the **routine criteria** for diagnosing PID:

Oral temperature >38.3°C;
Abnormal cervical or vaginal discharge;
Elevated erythrocyte sedimentation rate;
Elevated C-reactive protein;
Laboratory documentation of cervical infection with *N. gonorrhoeae* or *C. trachomatis*.

Listed below are the **elaborate criteria** for diagnosing PID:

Histopathologic evidence of endometritis on endometrial biopsy;
Tubo-ovarian abscess on sonography or other radiologic tests;
Laparoscopic abnormalities consistent with PID.

Although initial treatment decisions can be made before bacteriologic diagnosis of *C. trachomatis* or *N. gonorrhoeae* infection, such a diagnosis emphasizes the need to treat sex partners.

Treatment.   PID therapy regimens must provide empiric, broad-spectrum coverage of likely pathogens. Antimicrobial coverage should include *N. gonorrhoeae, C. trachomatis*, Gram-negative facultative bacteria, anaerobes, and streptococci. Although several antimicrobial regimens have proven effective in achieving clinical and microbiologic cure in randomized clinical trials with short-term follow-up, few studies have been done to assess and compare elimination of infection of the endometrium and fallopian tubes or the incidence of long-term complications such as tubal infertility and ectopic pregnancy.

No single therapeutic regimen has been established for persons with PID. When selecting a treatment regimen, health-care providers should consider avail-

ability, cost, patient acceptance, and regional differences in antimicrobial susceptibility of the likely pathogens.

Many experts recommend that all patients with PID be hospitalized so that
supervised treatment with parenteral antibiotics can be initiated. Hospitalization
is especially recommended when the following criteria are met:

The diagnosis is uncertain, and surgical emergencies such as appendicitis and
   ectopic pregnancy cannot be excluded;
Pelvic abscess is suspected;
The patient is pregnant;
The patient is an adolescent (among adolescents, compliance with therapy is
   unpredictable);
The patient has HIV infection;
Severe illness or nausea and vomiting preclude outpatient management;
The patient is unable to follow or tolerate an outpatient regimen;
The patient has failed to respond clinically to outpatient therapy;
Clinical follow-up within 72 hours of starting antibiotic treatment cannot be
   arranged.

Inpatient Treatment.   Experts have experience with both of the following
regimens. Also, there are multiple randomized trials demonstrating the efficacy
of each regimen.

REGIMEN A

Cefoxitin 2 gm intravenously every 6 hours or **cefotetan** 2 gm intravenously
every 12 hours,
   plus
Doxycycline 100 mg intravenously or orally every 12 hours.

NOTE: This regimen should be continued for at least 48 hours after the patient
demonstrates substantial clinical improvement, after which doxycycline 100 mg
orally 2 times a day should be continued for a total of 14 days. Doxycycline
administered orally has bioavailability similar to that of the intravenous formulation and may be administered if normal gastrointestinal function is present.

Clinical data are limited for other second- or third-generation cephalosporins
(e.g., ceftizoxime, cefotaxime, and ceftriaxone), which might replace cefoxitin
or cefotetan, although many authorities believe they also are effective therapy
for PID. However, they are less active than cefoxitin or cefotetan against anaerobic
bacteria.

REGIMEN B

Clindamycin 900 mg intravenously every 8 hours,
   plus
Gentamicin loading dose intravenously or intramuscularly (2 mg/kg body
weight) followed by a maintenance dose (1.5 mg/kg) every 8 hours.

NOTE: This regimen should be continued for at least 48 hours after the patient
demonstrates substantial clinical improvement, and then followed with doxycy-

cline 100 mg orally 2 times a day or clindamycin 450 mg orally 4 times a day to complete a total of 14 days of therapy. When tubo-ovarian abscess is present, many health-care providers use clindamycin for continued therapy rather than doxycycline, because it provides more effective anaerobic coverage. Clindamycin administered intravenously appears to be effective against *C. trachomatis* infection; however, the effectiveness of oral clindamycin against *C. trachomatis* has not been determined.

Alternative Inpatient Regimens.   Limited data support the use of other inpatient regimens, but two regimens have undergone at least one clinical trial and have broad-spectrum coverage. Ampicillin/sulbactam plus doxycycline has good anaerobic coverage and appears to be effective for patients with a tubo-ovarian abscess. Intravenous ofloxacin has been studied as a single agent. A regimen of ofloxacin plus either clindamycin or metronidazole provides broad-spectrum coverage. Evidence is insufficient to support the use of any single agent regimen for inpatient treatment of PID.

Outpatient Treatment.   Clinical trials of outpatient regimens have provided little information regarding intermediate and long-term outcomes. The following regimens provide coverage against the common etiologic agents of PID, but evidence from clinical trials supporting their use is limited. The second regimen provides broader coverage against anaerobic organisms but costs substantially more than the other regimen. Patients who do not respond to outpatient therapy within 72 hours should be hospitalized to confirm the diagnosis and to receive parenteral therapy.

REGIMEN A

Cefoxitin 2 gm intramuscularly plus **probenecid**, 1 gm orally in a single dose concurrently,
or
Ceftriaxone 250 mg intramuscularly
or
other parenteral third-generation **cephalosporin** (e.g., **ceftizoxime** or **cefotaxime**),
plus
Doxycycline 100 mg orally 2 times a day for 14 days.

REGIMEN B

Ofloxacin 400 mg orally 2 times a day for 14 days,
plus
Either **clindamycin** 450 mg orally 4 times a day, or **metronidazole** 500 mg orally 2 times a day for 14 days.

Clinical trials have demonstrated that the cefoxitin regimen is effective in obtaining short-term clinical response. Fewer data support the use of ceftriaxone or other third generation cephalosporins, but, based on their similarities to cefoxitin, they also are considered effective. No data exist regarding the use of oral cephalosporins for the treatment of PID.

Ofloxacin is effective against both *N. gonorrhoeae* and *C. trachomatis*. One clinical trial demonstrated the effectiveness of oral ofloxacin in obtaining short-term clinical response with PID. Despite results of this trial, there is concern related to ofloxacin's lack of anaerobic coverage; the addition of clindamycin or metronidazole provides this coverage. Clindamycin, but not metronidazole, further enhances the Gram-positive coverage of the regimen.

Alternative Outpatient Regimens.   Information regarding other outpatient regimens is limited. The combination of amoxicillin/clavulanic acid plus doxycycline was effective in obtaining short-term clinical response in one clinical trial, but many of the patients had to discontinue the regimen because of gastrointestinal symptoms.

Follow-Up.   Hospitalized patients receiving intravenous therapy should show substantial clinical improvement (e.g., defervescence, reduction in direct or rebound abdominal tenderness, and reduction in uterine, adnexal, and cervical motion tenderness) within 3 to 5 days of initiation of therapy. Patients who do not demonstrate improvement within this time period usually require further diagnostic workup or surgical intervention, or both. If the provider elects to prescribe outpatient therapy, follow-up examination should be performed within 72 hours, using the criteria for clinical improvement previously described.

Because of the risk for persistent infection, particularly with *C. trachomatis*, patients should have a microbiologic reexamination 7 to 10 days after completing therapy. Some experts also recommend rescreening for *C. trachomatis* and *N. gonorrhoeae* 4 to 6 weeks after completing therapy.

Management of Sex Partners.   Evaluation and treatment of sex partners of women who have PID is imperative because of the risk for reinfection and the high likelihood of urethral gonococcal or chlamydial infection of the partner.

Since nonculture, and perhaps culture, tests for *C. trachomatis* and *N. gonorrhoeae* are thought to be insensitive among asymptomatic men, sex partners should be treated empirically with regimens effective against both of these infections—regardless of the apparent etiology of PID or pathogens isolated from the infected woman.

Even in clinical settings in which only women are seen, special arrangements should be made to provide care for male sex partners of women with PID. When this is not feasible, health-care providers should ensure that sex partners are appropriately referred for treatment.

Special Considerations

Pregnancy.   Pregnant women with suspected PID should be hospitalized and treated with parenteral antibiotics.

HIV Infection.   Differences in the clinical manifestations of PID between HIV-infected women and noninfected women have not been described clearly. However, in one study, HIV-infected women with PID tended to have a leukopenia or a lesser leukocytosis than women who were not HIV-infected, and they were more likely to require surgical intervention. HIV-infected women who develop PID should be managed aggressively. Hospitalization and inpatient therapy with one of the intravenous antimicrobial regimens described in this report is recommended.

Epididymitis

Among men <35 years of age, epididymitis is most often caused by *N. gonorrhoeae* or *C. trachomatis*. Epididymitis caused by sexually transmitted *Escherichia coli* infection also occurs among homosexual men who are the insertive partners during anal intercourse. Sexually transmitted epididymitis is usually accompanied by urethritis, which is often asymptomatic. Nonsexually transmitted epididymitis associated with urinary tract infections caused by Gram-negative enteric organisms is more common among men <35 years of age and among men who have recently undergone urinary tract instrumentation or surgery.

Diagnostic Considerations.   Men with epididymitis typically have unilateral testicular pain and tenderness; palpable swelling of the epididymis is usually present. Testicular torsion, a surgical emergency, should be considered in all cases but is more frequent among adolescents. Emergency testing for torsion may be indicated when the onset of pain is sudden, pain is severe, or test results available during the initial visit do not permit a diagnosis of urethritis or urinary tract infection. The evaluation of men for epididymitis should include the following procedures:

A Gram-stained smear of urethral exudate or intraurethral swab specimen for *N. gonorrhoeae* and for NGU (>5 polymorphonuclear leukocytes per oil immersion field);
A culture of urethral exudate or intraurethral swab specimen for *N. gonorrhoeae*;
A test of an intraurethral swab specimen for *C. trachomatis*;
Culture and Gram-stained smear of uncentrifuged urine for Gram-negative bacteria.

Treatment.   Empiric therapy is indicated before culture results are available. Treatment of epididymitis caused by *C. trachomatis* or *N. gonorrhoeae* will result in microbiologic cure of infection, improve signs and symptoms, and prevent transmission to others.

Patients with suspected sexually transmitted epididymitis should be treated with an antimicrobial regimen effective against *C. trachomatis* and *N. gonorrhoeae*; confirmation of these agents by testing will assist in partner notification efforts, but current tests for *C. trachomatis* are not sufficiently sensitive to exclude infection with that agent.

Recommended Regimen

Ceftriaxone 250 mg intramuscularly in a single dose,
Doxycycline 100 mg orally 2 times a day for 10 days.

The effect of substituting the 125-mg dose of ceftriaxone recommended for treatment of uncomplicated *N. gonorrhoeae* or the azithromycin regimen recommended for treatment of *C. trachomatis* is unknown.

As an adjunct to therapy, bed rest and scrotal elevation are recommended until fever and local inflammation have subsided.

Alternative Regimen

Ofloxacin 300 mg orally 2 times a day for 10 days.

NOTE: Ofloxacin is contraindicated for persons <17 years of age.

Follow-Up.   Failure to improve within 3 days requires reevaluation of both the diagnosis and therapy and consideration of hospitalization. Swelling and tenderness that persist after completing antimicrobial therapy should be evaluated for testicular cancer and tuberculous or fungal epididymitis.

Management of Sex Partners.   Patients with epididymitis that is known or suspected to be caused by *N. gonorrhoeae* or *C. trachomatis* should be instructed to refer sex partners for evaluation and treatment. Sex partners of these patients should be referred if their contact with the index patient was within 30 days of onset of symptoms.

Patients should be instructed to avoid sexual intercourse until patient and partner(s) are cured. In the absence of microbiologic test-of-cure, this means until therapy is completed and patient and partner(s) are without symptoms.

Special Considerations

HIV Infection.   Persons with HIV infection and uncomplicated epididymitis should receive the same treatment as persons without HIV. Fungal and mycobacterial causes of epididymitis are more common, however, among patients who are immunocompromised.

Human *Papillomavirus* Infection

GENITAL WARTS

Exophytic genital and anal warts are benign growths most commonly caused by human *Papillomavirus* (HPV) types 6 or 11. Other types that may be present in the anogenital region (e.g., types 16, 18, 31, 33, and 35) have been strongly associated with genital dysplasia and carcinoma. These types are usually associated with subclinical infection, but occasionally are found in exophytic warts.

Treatment.   The goal of treatment is removal of exophytic warts and the amelioration of signs and symptoms—not the eradication of HPV. No therapy has been shown to eradicate HPV. HPV has been identified in adjacent tissue after laser treatment of HPV-associated cervical intraepithelial neoplasia and after attempts to eliminate subclinical HPV by extensive laser vaporization of the anogenital area.

Genital warts are generally benign growths that cause minor or no symptoms aside from their cosmetic appearance. Treatment of external genital warts is not likely to influence the development of cervical cancer. A multitude of randomized clinical trials and other treatment studies have demonstrated that currently available therapeutic methods are 22 to 94% effective in clearing external exophytic genital warts and that recurrence rates are high (usually at least 25% within 3 months) with all modalities. Several well-designed studies have indicated that treatment is more successful for genital warts that are small and that have been present <1 year. No studies have assessed if treatment of exophytic warts reduces transmission of HPV. Many experts speculate that exophytic warts may be more infectious than subclinical infection, and therefore, the risk for transmission might be reduced by "debulking" genital warts. Most experts agree that recurrences of genital warts more commonly result from reactivation of subclinical infection than from reinfection by a sex partner. The effect of treatment on the natural history of HPV is unknown. If left untreated, genital warts may resolve on their own, remain unchanged, or grow. In placebo-controlled studies, genital warts have cleared spontaneously without treatment in 20 to 30% of patients within 3 months.

Regimens. Treatment of genital warts should be guided by the preference of the patient. Expensive therapies, toxic therapies, and procedures that result in scarring should be avoided. A specific treatment regimen should be chosen with consideration given to anatomic site, size, and number of warts as well as the expense, efficacy, convenience, and potential for adverse effects. Extensive or refractory disease should be referred to an expert.

Carbon dioxide laser and conventional surgery are useful in the management of extensive warts, particularly for those patients who have not responded to other regimens; these alternatives are not appropriate for treatment of limited lesions. One randomized trial of laser therapy indicated efficacy of 43%, with recurrence among 95% of patients. A randomized trial of surgical excision demonstrated efficacy of 93%, with recurrences among 29% of patients. These therapies and more cost-effective treatments do not eliminate HPV infection.

Interferon therapy is not recommended because of its cost and its association with a high frequency of adverse side effects, and efficacy is no greater than that of other available therapies. Two randomized trials established systemic interferon-α to be no more effective than placebo. Efficacy of interferon injected directly into genital warts (intralesional therapy) during two randomized trials was 44 to 61%, with recurrences among none to 67% of patients.

Therapy with 5-fluorouracil cream has not been evaluated in controlled studies, frequently causes local irritation, and is not recommended for the treatment of genital warts.

EXTERNAL GENITAL/PERIANAL WARTS

Regimen

Cryotherapy with liquid nitrogen or cryoprobe,
or
Podofilox 0.5% solution for self-treatment (genital warts only). Patients may apply podofilox with a cotton swab to warts twice daily for 3 days, followed by 4 days of no therapy. This cycle may be repeated as necessary for a total of 4 cycles. Total wart area treated should not exceed 10 cm^2, and total volume of podofilox should not exceed 0.5 ml/day. If possible, the health-care provider

should apply the initial treatment to demonstrate the proper application technique and identify which warts should be treated. The use of podofilox is contraindicated during pregnancy.

or

Podophyllin 10 to 25%, in compound tincture of benzoin. To avoid the possibility of problems with systemic absorption and toxicity, some experts recommend that application be limited to ≤ 0.5 ml or ≤ 10 cm^2 per session. Thoroughly wash off in 1 to 4 hours. Repeat weekly if necessary. If warts persist after six applications, other therapeutic methods should be considered. The use of podophyllin is contraindicated during pregnancy.

or

Trichloroacetic acid (TCA) 80 to 90%. Apply only to warts; powder with talc or sodium bicarbonate (baking soda) to remove unreacted acid. Repeat weekly if necessary. If warts persist after six applications, other therapies should be considered.

or

Electrodesiccation or electrocautery. Electrodesiccation and electrocautery are contraindicated for patients with cardiac pacemakers or for lesions proximal to the anal verge.

Cryotherapy is relatively inexpensive, does not require anesthesia, and does not result in scarring if performed properly. Special equipment is required, and most patients experience moderate pain during and after the procedure. Efficacy during four randomized trials was 63 to 88%, with recurrences among 21 to 39% of patients.

Therapy with 0.5% podofilox solution is relatively inexpensive, simple to use, safe, and is self-applied by patients at home. Unlike podophyllin, podofilox is a pure compound with a stable shelf-life and does not need to be washed off. Most patients experience mild/moderate pain or local irritation after treatment. Heavily keratinized warts may not respond as well as those on moist mucosal surfaces. To apply the podofilox solution safely and effectively, the patient must be able to see and reach the warts easily. Efficacy during five recent randomized trials was 45 to 88%, with recurrences among 33 to 60% of patients.

Podophyllin therapy is relatively inexpensive, simple to use, and safe. Compared with other available therapies, a larger number of treatments may be required. Most patients experience mild to moderate pain or local irritation after treatment. Heavily keratinized warts may not respond as well as those on moist mucosal surfaces. Efficacy in four recent randomized trials was 32 to 79%, with recurrences among 27 to 65% of patients.

Few data on the efficacy of TCA are available. One randomized trial among men demonstrated 81% efficacy and recurrence among 36% of patients; the frequency of adverse reactions was similar to that seen with the use of cryotherapy. One study among women showed efficacy and frequency of patient discomfort to be similar to podophyllin. No data on the efficacy of bichloroacetic acid are available.

Few data on the efficacy of electrodesiccation are available. One randomized trial of electrodesiccation demonstrated an efficacy of 94%, with recurrences among 22% of patients; another randomized trial of diathermocoagulation demonstrated an efficacy of 35%. Local anesthesia is required, and patient discomfort is usually moderate.

CERVICAL WARTS

For women with (exophytic) cervical warts, dysplasia must be excluded before treatment is begun. Management should be carried out in consultation with an expert.

VAGINAL WARTS

Regimen

Cryotherapy with liquid nitrogen. The use of a cryoprobe in the vagina is not recommended because of the risk for vaginal perforation and fistula formation, or

TCA 80 to 90%. Apply only to warts; powder with talc or sodium bicarbonate (baking soda) to remove unreacted acid. Repeat weekly as necessary. If warts persist after six applications, other therapeutic methods should be considered. or

Podophyllin 10 to 25% in compound tincture of benzoin. Apply to the treatment area, which must be dry before removing the speculum. Treat <2 cm^2 per session. Repeat application at weekly intervals. Because of concern about potential systemic absorption, some experts caution against vaginal application of podophyllin. The use of podophyllin is contraindicated during pregnancy.

URETHRAL MEATUS WARTS

Regimen

Cryotherapy with liquid nitrogen.
Podophyllin 10 to 25% in compound tincture of benzoin. The treatment area must be dry before contact with normal mucosa. Podophyllin must be washed off in 1 to 2 hours. Repeat weekly if necessary. If warts persist after six applications, other therapeutic methods should be considered. The use of podophyllin is contraindicated during pregnancy.

ANAL WARTS

Regimen

Cryotherapy with liquid nitrogen.
TCA 80 to 90%. Apply only to warts; powder with talc or sodium bicarbonate (baking soda) to remove unreacted acid. Repeat weekly if necessary. If warts persist after six applications, other therapeutic methods should be considered.

SURGICAL REMOVAL

NOTE: Management of warts on rectal mucosa should be referred to an expert.

ORAL WARTS

Cryotherapy with liquid nitrogen
or
Electrodesiccation or electrocautery
or
Surgical removal

Follow-Up.   After warts have responded to therapy, follow-up is not necessary. Annual cytologic screening is recommended for women with or without genital warts. The presence of genital warts is not an indication for colposcopy.

Management of Sex Partners.   Examination of sex partners is not necessary for management of genital warts because the role of reinfection is probably minimal. Many sex partners have obvious exophytic warts and may desire treatment; also, partners may benefit from counseling. Patients with exophytic anogenital warts should be made aware that they are contagious to uninfected sex partners. The majority of partners, however, are probably already subclinically infected with HPV, even if they do not have visible warts. No practical screening tests for subclinical infection are available. Even after removal of warts, patients may harbor HPV in surrounding normal tissue, as may persons without exophytic warts. The use of condoms may reduce transmission to partners likely to be uninfected, such as new partners; however, the period of communicability is unknown. Experts speculate that HPV infection may persist throughout a patient's lifetime in a dormant state and become infectious intermittently. Whether patients with subclinical HPV infection are as contagious as patients with exophytic warts is unknown.

Special Considerations

Pregnancy.   The use of podophyllin and podofilox are contraindicated during pregnancy. Genital papillary lesions have a tendency to proliferate and to become friable during pregnancy. Many experts advocate removal of visible warts during pregnancy.

HPV types 6 and 11 can cause laryngeal papillomatosis among infants. The route of transmission (transplacental, birth canal, or postnatal) is unknown, and laryngeal papillomatosis has occurred among infants delivered by cesarean section. Hence, the preventive value of cesarean delivery is unknown. Cesarean delivery must not be performed solely to prevent transmission of HPV infection to the newborn. However, in rare instances, cesarean delivery may be indicated for women with genital warts if the pelvic outlet is obstructed or if vaginal delivery would result in excessive bleeding.

HIV Infection.   Persons infected with HIV may not respond to therapy for HPV as well as persons without HIV.

SUBCLINICAL GENITAL HPV INFECTION (WITHOUT EXOPHYTIC WARTS)

Subclinical genital HPV infection is much more common than exophytic warts among both men and women. Infection is often indirectly diagnosed on the cervix by Pap smear, colposcopy, or biopsy and on the penis, vulva, and other genital skin by the appearance of white areas after application of acetic acid. Acetowhitening is not a specific test for HPV infection, and false-positive tests are common. Definitive diagnosis of HPV infection relies on detection of viral nucleic acid (DNA or RNA) or capsid proteins. Pap smear diagnosis of HPV generally does not correlate well with detection of HPV DNA in cervical cells. Cell changes attributed to HPV in the cervix are similar to those of mild dysplasia and often regress spontaneously without treatment. Tests for the detection of several types of HPV DNA in cells scraped from the cervix are now widely available, but the clinical utility of these tests for managing patients is not known. Management decisions should not be made on the basis of HPV DNA tests. Screening for subclinical genital HPV infection using DNA tests or acetic acid is not recommended.

Treatment.   In the absence of coexistent dysplasia, treatment is not recommended for subclinical genital HPV infection diagnosed by Pap smear, colposcopy, biopsy, acetic acid soaking of genital skin or mucous membranes, or the detection of HPV nucleic acids (DNA or RNA) or capsid antigen, because diagnosis often is questionable and no therapy has been demonstrated to eradicate infection. HPV has been demonstrated in adjacent tissue after laser treatment of HPV-associated dysplasia and after attempts to eliminate subclinical HPV by extensive laser vaporization of the anogenital area of men and women.

In the presence of coexistent dysplasia, management should be based on the grade of dysplasia.

Management of Sex Partners.   Examination of sex partners is not necessary. The majority of partners are probably already infected subclinically with HPV. No practical screening tests for subclinical infection are available. The use of condoms may reduce transmission to partners likely to be uninfected, such as new partners; however, the period of communicability is unknown. Experts speculate that HPV infection may persist throughout a patient's lifetime in a dormant state and become infectious intermittently. Whether patients with subclinical HPV infection are as contagious as patients with exophytic warts is unknown.

Proctitis, Proctocolitis, and Enteritis

Sexually transmitted gastrointestinal syndromes include proctitis, proctocolitis, and enteritis. Proctitis occurs predominantly among persons who participate in anal intercourse, and enteritis occurs among those whose sexual practices include oral-fecal contact. Proctocolitis may be acquired by either route depending on the pathogen. Evaluation should include appropriate diagnostic procedures, such as anoscopy or sigmoidoscopy, stool examination, and culture.

Proctitis is an inflammation limited to the rectum (the distal 10 to 12 cm) that is associated with anorectal pain, tenesmus, and rectal discharge. *N. gonorrhoeae, C. trachomatis* (including LGV serovars), *T. pallidum*, and HSV are the most common sexually transmitted pathogens involved. Among patients coinfected with HIV, herpes proctitis may be especially severe.

Proctocolitis is associated with symptoms of proctitis plus diarrhea and/or abdominal cramps and inflammation of the colonic mucosa extending to 12 cm. Pathogenic organisms include *Campylobacter* spp., *Shigella* spp., *Entamoeba histolytica*, and, rarely, *C. trachomatis* (LGV serovars). CMV or other opportunistic agents may be involved among immunosuppressed patients with HIV infection.

Enteritis usually results in diarrhea and abdominal cramping without signs of proctitis or proctocolitis. In otherwise healthy patients, *Giardia lamblia* is most commonly implicated. Among patients with HIV infection, other infections that are not generally sexually transmitted may occur, including cytomegalovirus (CMV), *Mycobacterium avium-intracellulare, Salmonella* spp., *Cryptosporidium, Microsporidium*, and *Isospora*. Multiple stool examinations may be necessary to detect *Giardia*, and special stool preparations are required to diagnose cryptosporidiosis and microsporidiosis. Additionally, enteritis may be a primary effect of HIV infection.

When laboratory diagnostic capabilities are available, treatment should be based on the specific diagnosis. Diagnostic and treatment recommendations for all enteric infections are beyond the scope of these guidelines.

Treatment. Acute proctitis of recent onset among persons who have recently practiced receptive anal intercourse is most often sexually transmitted. Such patients should be examined by anoscopy and should be evaluated for infection with HSV, *N. gonorrhoeae, C. trachomatis*, and *T. pallidum*. If anorectal pus is found on examination, or if polymorphonuclear leukocytes are found on a Gram-stained smear of anorectal secretions, the following therapy may be prescribed pending results of further laboratory tests.

Recommended Regimen

Ceftriaxone 125 mg intramuscularly (or another agent effective against anal and genital gonorrhea) and

Doxycycline 100 mg orally 2 times a day for 7 days.

NOTE: For patients with herpes proctitis, refer to Genital Herpes Simplex Virus Infections.

Follow-Up. Follow-up should be based on specific etiology and severity of clinical symptoms. Reinfection may be difficult to distinguish from treatment failure.

Management of Sex Partners. Partners of patients with sexually transmitted enteric infections should be evaluated for any diseases diagnosed in the index patient.

Ectoparasitic Infections

PEDICULOSIS PUBIS

Patients with pediculosis pubis (pubic lice) usually seek medical attention because of pruritus. Commonly, they also notice lice on pubic hair.

Recommended Regimens

Lindane 1% shampoo applied for 4 minutes and then thoroughly washed off (not recommended for pregnant or lactating women or for children <2 years of age)
or
Permethrin 1% creme rinse applied to affected areas and washed off after 10 minutes
or
Pyrethrins with piperonyl butoxide applied to the affected area and washed off after 10 minutes.

The lindane regimen remains the least expensive therapy; toxicity (as indicated by seizure and aplastic anemia) has not been reported when treatment is limited to the recommended 4-minute period. Permethrin has less potential for toxicity in the event of inappropriate use.

Other Management Considerations. The recommended regimens should not be applied to the eyes. Pediculosis of the eyelashes should be treated by applying occlusive ophthalmic ointment to the eyelid margins two times a day for 10 days.

Bedding and clothing should be decontaminated (machine washed or machine dried using heat cycle or dry-cleaned) or removed from body contact for at least 72 hours. Fumigation of living areas is not necessary.

Follow-Up. Patients should be evaluated after 1 week if symptoms persist. Re-treatment may be necessary if lice are found or if eggs are observed at the hair-skin junction. Patients who are not responding to one of the recommended regimens should be retreated with an alternative regimen.

Management of Sex Partners. Sex partners within the last month should be treated.

Special Considerations

Pregnancy. Pregnant and lactating women should be treated with permethrin or pyrethrins with piperonyl butoxide.

HIV Infection. Persons with HIV infection and pediculosis pubis should receive the same treatment as those without HIV infection.

SCABIES

The predominant symptom of scabies is pruritus. For pruritus to occur, sensitization to *Sarcoptes scabiei* must occur. Among persons with their first infection, sensitization takes several weeks to develop, while pruritus may occur within 24 hours after reinfestation. Scabies among adults may be sexually transmitted, although scabies among children is usually not sexually transmitted.

Recommended Regimen

Permethrin cream (5%) applied to all areas of the body from the neck down and washed off after 8 to 14 hours, or

Lindane (1%) 1 oz. of lotion or 30 gm of cream applied thinly to all areas of the body from the neck down and washed off thoroughly after 8 hours.

NOTE: Lindane should not be used following a bath, and it should not be used by persons with extensive dermatitis, pregnant or lactating women, and children <2 years of age.

Alternative Regimen

Crotamiton (10%) applied to the entire body from the neck down nightly for 2 consecutive nights and washed off 24 hours after the second application.

Permethrin is effective and safe but costs more than lindane. Lindane is effective in most areas of the country, but lindane resistance has been reported in some areas of the world, including parts of the United States. Seizures have occurred when lindane was applied after a bath or used by patients with extensive dermatitis. Aplastic anemia following lindane use also has been reported.

Other Management Considerations.   Bedding and clothing should be decontaminated (machine washed or machine dried using hot cycle or dry-cleaned) or removed from body contact for at least 72 hours. Fumigation of living areas is not necessary.

Follow-Up.   Pruritus may persist for several weeks. Some experts recommend re-treatment after 1 week for patients who are still symptomatic; other experts recommend retreatment only if live mites can be observed. Patients who are not responding to the recommended treatment should be retreated with an alternative regimen.

Management of Sex Partners.   Both sexual and close personal or household contacts within the last month should be examined and treated.

Special Considerations

Pregnant Women, Infants, and Young Children.   Infants, young children, and pregnant and lactating women should not be treated with lindane. They may be treated with permethrin or crotamiton regimens.

HIV Infection.   Persons with HIV infection and uncomplicated scabies should receive the same treatment as persons without HIV infection. Persons with HIV infection and others who are immunosuppressed are at increased risk for Norwegian scabies, a disseminated dermatologic infection. Such patients should be managed in consultation with an expert.

SUGGESTED READINGS

American Academy of Pediatrics, American College of Obstetrics and Gynecology (ACOG). Guidelines for perinatal care. 3rd ed. 1992.

Beall GN. Penicillins. In: Saxon A, moderator. Immediate hypersensitivity reactions to beta-lactam antibiotics. Ann Intern Med 1987;107:204–215.

CDC. The use of preventive therapy for tuberculosis infection in the United States. MMWR 1990;39(no. RR-8):6–8.

CDC. Sexually transmitted diseases clinical practice guidelines. 1991.

CDC. Guidelines for prophylaxis against *Pneumocystis carinii* pneumonia for children infected with human immunodeficiency virus. MMWR 1991;40(no. RR-2):1–13.

CDC. Purified protein derivative (PPD-tuberculin anergy) and HIV infection: guidelines for anergy testing and management of anergic persons at risk of tuberculosis. MMWR 1991;40(no. RR-5):27–33.

CDC. Hepatitis B virus: a comprehensive strategy for eliminating transmission in the United States through universal childhood vaccination. Recommendations of the Advisory Committee on Immunization Practices (ACIP). MMWR 1991;40(no. RR-13):1–25.

CDC. Recommendations for prophylaxis against *Pneumocystis carinii* pneumonia for adults and adolescents infected with human immunodeficiency virus. MMWR 1992;41(no. RR-4):1–11.

CDC. Management of persons exposed to multidrug-resistant tuberculosis. MMWR 1992;41(no. RR-11):59–71.

CDC. Testing for antibodies to human immunodeficiency virus type 2 in the United States. MMWR 1992;41(no. RR-12):1–9.

CDC. Technical guidance on HIV counseling. MMWR 1993;42(no. RR-2):8–17.

CDC. Recommendations for the prevention and management of *Chlamydia trachomatis* infections, 1993. MMWR 1993;42(no. RR-12):1–39.

Committee on Infectious Diseases, American Academy of Pediatrics. Report of the Committee on Infectious Diseases. 22nd ed. 1991.

Guide to clinical preventive services. Report of the U.S. Preventive Services Task Force. Baltimore: Williams & Wilkins, 1989.

National Cancer Institute Workshop. The 1988 Bethesda System for reporting cervical/vaginal cytological diagnoses. JAMA 1989;262:931–934.

Oral desensitization protocol for patients with a positive skin test (Table 11.1). N Engl J Med 1985;312:1229–1232.

Recommendations of the Advisory Committee on Immunization Practices (ACIP): use of vaccines and immune globulins in persons with altered immunocompetence. MMWR 1993;42(no. RR-4):1–18.

INDEX

Page numbers followed by ''f'' denote figures; those followed by ''t'' denote tables.

A

A. calcoaceticus, 166t
A. hydrophila, 166t
Abdominal pain, with clofazimine, 32
Abdominal surgery, antibiotic prophylaxis for, 96t
Abortion, antibiotic prophylaxis for, 96t
Abscess(es)
 brain, 57t
 hepatic, 306t
 infected pancreatic, 74t
 liver, 74t
 lung, 60t, 77t
 perirectal, 58t, 73t
 tubo-ovarian, 446
Acanthamoeba
 drugs for, 306t
 from fatal granulomatous amebic encephalitis, 317t
Acetazolamide-methenamine interaction, 39
Acinetobacter
 antibacterial drugs for, 87t
 antibiotic therapy for, 68t
 antimicrobial susceptibility patterns of, 185t
 MICs for, 162f
Acquired immunodeficiency syndrome (AIDS)
 drugs for, 134–138t
 pneumococcal polysaccharide vaccine in, 259
 treatment of infections of, 129–147
 tuberculosis in, 367
Actinomyces
 antibiotic therapy for, 79t
 antimicrobial MICs for, 171t
 israelii, antibacterial drugs for, 90t
Actinomycetes, antibacterial drugs for, 90t
Actinomycosis, antibacterial drugs for, 90t
Acyclovir
 adult dosages and routes for, 3t

adverse reactions of, 22
allergic reaction to, 400
for dermatomal zoster, 136t
drug interactions of, 22
for genital herpes, 398
 recurrent, 398–399
for herpes simplex virus, 136t, 139
pharmacological characteristics of, 11t
for varicella-zoster virus, 136t, 139
Adenoidectomy, bacteremia with, 102
Adenovirus vaccine, 198t
Adherence, definition of, 384
Adjuvants, immunobiologic, 196
Adrenal suppression, ketoconazole-induced, 39
Advisory Committee on Immunization Practices (ACIP), recommendations of, 194–195
Advisory memoranda on vaccines, 230
Aeromonas, antibacterial drugs for, 87t
Aerosol, definition of, 384
Aerosolization, definition of, 384
AFB smear, 345
 definition of, 389
 in tuberculosis diagnosis, 371
Agranulocytosis
 with flucytosine, 36
 with trimethoprim-sulfamethoxazole, 51–52
Air change, definition of, 384
Air filtration, 335
Air mixing, definition of, 387
Albendazole, 304, 321t, 322
 adverse effects of, 322
 for ascariasis, 307t
 for capillariasis, 307t
 for cysticercosis, 326t
 for echinococcosis, 327t
 for hookworm, 310t
 for nematode intestinal infections, 327t–328t
 for pinworm, 308t

for strongyloidiasis, 315t
for taeniasis, 326t
for tapeworm infection, 315t
for tissue nematode infection, 328t
for toxocariasis, 329t
for trichinosis, 329t
for *Trichostrongylus* infection, 316t
for trichuriasis, 316t
Alcohol drug interactions
 with cefamandole, 28
 with metronidazole, 40
Alkaline phosphatase elevation, with netilmicin, 42
Alkalinizing agents-methenamine interaction, 39
Allergic reaction. *See also* Hypersensitivity reaction
 to gonococcal infection treatment, 430
 to rabies vaccine, 283
 to vaccine additives, 196
 to vulvovaginal candidiasis treatment, 441–442
Alveolus, definition of, 385
Amantadine
 adult dosages and routes for, 3t
 adverse reactions of, 23–24
 in children, 256
 drug interactions of, 24, 256
 in elderly persons, 254
 for health care workers, 251
 for immunodeficient persons, 251
 with impaired renal function, 254
 for influenza, 237–238
 for influenza A, 249–256
  after vaccination of high-risk persons, 250
  institutional outbreaks of, 252–253
 with liver disease, 255
 pharmacological characteristics of, 11t
 as prophylaxis, 250
 with seizure disorders, 255

Imipenem
  for *Acinetobacter*, 87t
  for *Aeromonas*, 87t
  antimicrobial activity against *Staphylococcus aureus*, 180t
  for *Bacillus*, 84t
  for *Bacteroides*, gastrointestinal strain, 84t
  for *Campylobacter fetus*, 84t
  for *Clostridium perfringens*, 84t
  E. faecalis and *E. faecium* susceptibility to, 182t
  for *Enterobacter*, 85t
  Enterobacteriaceae resistance to, 178t
  for *Escherichia coli*, 85t
  ganciclovir interaction with, 36
  for gastrointestinal infection, 73t–74t
  for *Haemophilus*, 157t
  for *Klebsiella pneumoniae*, 86t
  for melioidosis, 81t
  MICs for susceptible anaerobes, 170t
  MICs for susceptible mycobacteria, 172t
  MICs for susceptible organisms, 162t–163t
  for musculoskeletal infection, 56t, 68t
  for *Mycobacterium avium* complex, 89t
  for *Nocardia*, 81t, 90t
  pharmacological characteristics of, 17t
  for *Proteus*, 86t
  for *Providencia stuartii*, 86t
  for *Pseudomonas*, 88t–89t
  for *Serratia*, 87t
  for skin infections, 62t
  Streptococcus pneumoniae susceptibilities to, 184t
  tentative interpretive categories and MICs of, 160t
  for urinary tract infection, 59t, 76t
  zone diameter standards and equivalent MIC breakpoints for, 154t, 157t
Imipenem-cilastatin
  adult dosages and routes for, 5t
  adverse reactions to, 37
Imipenem/gentamicin, for gastrointestinal infection, 74t
Immune adherence hemagglutination (IAHA), 291–293

Immune globulin
  definition of, 232
  hepatitis B, 301–302t
  human rabies (HRIG), 273–275, 278
    adverse reactions to, 282
    outside U.S., 282
  indications for infectious disease prevention, 200–201t
  intravenous (IVIG), 211
    definition of, 232
    immunocompromise with, 217–218
  killed vaccine, 211–212
  live vaccine, 210–211
  preparations
    guidelines for spacing and administration of, 212t
    intervals between administration for, 213t
  rabies, 268–269
  specific, 232
  vaccinia, 287–288. *See also* Smallpox vaccine
  varicella-zoster, 289–299
Immune response, blood products and, 211
Immune thrombocytopenic purpura vaccine, intervals between administration for, 213t
Immunization. *See also* Vaccination
  active, 232
  breast-feeding and, 215–216
  during chemotherapy or radiation therapy, 218
  definition of, 232
  general recommendations on, 194–303
  of infants and children, 194–195
  passive, 232
  pediatric, standard practice of, 219–222
  during pregnancy, 194, 216–217
  for rabies, 273–275
  recommendations for, 126
  recommended accelerated schedule for infants and children, 206t
  recommended schedule for persons not vaccinated in early infancy, 207t
  for travelers, 123–126
  universal, 228–229

  versus vaccination, 232–233
Immunization Practices Advisory Committee, on pneumococcal polysaccharide vaccine, 257–258
Immunization records
  patient, 225
  for persons without vaccination documentation, 225
  provider, 224–225
  for vaccinations received outside U.S., 225–228
Immunobiologics, 196
  age at administration, 204–205t
  antigenic and antibody-containing components of, 231–232
  availability of from CDC, 187–190
  characteristics of, 195
  clinical use of, 187–303
  preservatives and stabilizers of, 196
  prophylactic, distributed by CDC, 188t
  routes of administration of, 197–204
  simultaneous administration of, 207–210
  spacing of, 204–214
  storage and handling of, 196–197
  suspending fluids for, 196
  therapeutic, distributed by CDC, 188t
Immunocompetence, altered, 217–218
Immunocompromise
  in children, varicella and, 294
  pneumococcal polysaccharide vaccination and, 261
  tuberculosis infection and, 333–334
  varicella and, 296
Immunosuppression
  congenital immunodeficiency and, 217
  definition of, 387
  with rabies vaccination, 283
Impetigo, 62t
Inactivated polio vaccine, 125
Inclusion conjunctivitis, 90t
Indomethacin-penicillin G interaction, 44
Induration, definition of, 387
Infants
  chlamydial infections among, 423–425

Pepto-Bismol, for travelers' diarrhea prophylaxis, 123
Peptococcus
  antimicrobial MICs for, 170t
  fluoroquinolone antimicrobial activity against, 167t
  third-generation cephalosporin activity against, 165t
Peptostreptococcus
  antibacterial drugs for, 82t
  antimicrobial MICs for, 170t
  fluoroquinolone antimicrobial activity against, 167t
Periapical infections, 101–102
Pericarditis, pyogenic, 55t
Periodontal infections, 101–102
Peripheral neuropathy
  with griseofulvin, 37
  with isoniazid, 38
  with metronidazole, 40
  with polymyxin B, 45
Peritonitis
  antibiotic therapy for, 58, 73t
  spontaneous bacterial, 73t
Permethrin, 305
  adverse effects of, 324
  for lice infestation, 311t
  for malaria prevention, 126
  for pediculosis pubis, 456
  for scabies, 314t
Permethrin cream, for scabies, 457
Personal respirators, performance criteria for, 375–376
Pertussis
  prevention in exposed persons, 120–121
  vaccination for with influenza vaccination, 243
  vaccine
    administration of, 198t
    storage and handling of, 196
Pharyngeal surgery, prophylaxis for, 96t
Pharyngitis
  antibiotics for, 60t, 77t
  group A streptococcal, 108–109
Phenobarbital-griseofulvin interaction, 37
Phenol saline, 416
Phenoxymethyl penicillin. *See also* Penicillin V
  daily dosage schedules for pediatric patients, 7t
  for skin infections, 62t
Phenytoin
  chloramphenicol inhibition of, 31

fluconazole interaction with, 35
isoniazid interactions with, 38
sulfisoxazole interaction with, 49
Phlebitis
  with azotreonam, 27
  with nafcillin, 41
Photosensitive metabolites, metronidazole, 40
Photosensitivity, tetracycline, 50
Phthirus pubis, 311t
PID. *See* Pelvic inflammatory disease
Pinworm, 308t, 327t
Piperacillin
  for *Acinetobacter*, 87t
  adult dosages and routes for, 5t
  for *Bacteroides*, gastrointestinal strain, 84t
  for *Enterobacter*, 85t
  Enterobacteriaceae resistance to, 178t
  for *Escherichia coli*, 85t
  for gastrointestinal infection, 58t
  for *Klebsiella pneumoniae*, 86t
  for meningitis, 70t
  MICs for susceptible organisms, 162–163t
  for musculoskeletal infection, 68t
  pharmacological characteristics of, 18t
  plus tobramycin/gentamicin, for infective endocarditis, 65t
  for *Proteus*, 86t
  for *Providencia stuartii*, 86t
  for *Pseudomonas aeruginosa*, 88t
  for respiratory infections, 61t, 78t
  for *Serratia*, 87t
  zone diameter standards and equivalent MIC breakpoints for, 154t
Piperacillin/tazobactam
  adult dosages and routes for, 5t
  for *Bacteroides*, gastrointestinal strain, 84t
  for *Escherichia coli*, 85t
  for gastrointestinal infection, 73t–74t
  for *Klebsiella pneumoniae*, 86t
  for *Proteus*, indole-positive, 86t
  for *Providencia stuartii*, 86t
  tentative interpretive categories and MICs of, 160t

Piperazine citrate, for nematode intestinal infections, 327t
Piperonyl butoxide, 305
  adverse effects of, 324
  for lice infestation, 311t
  for pediculosis pubis, 456
Plague
  antibacterial drugs for, 89t
  antibiotic therapy for, 81t
  vaccine
    administration of, 198t
    hypersensitivity to, 215
Plaquenil. *See* Hydroxychloroquine
Plasma concentration, antibiotic, 21
Plasmodium
  falciparum
    chloroquine-resistant, 312t, 319t
    drugs for, 311t
  ovale
    drugs for, 311–312t
    prevention of relapses, 312t
  vivax
    drugs for, 311–312t
    prevention of relapses, 312t
Platelet aggregation, decreased, 28
Platinum compound-amikacin interaction, 25
Pneumococcal disease
  high-risk population for, 258–259
  mortality from, 258
  prevention of in asplenic patient, 118–119
  vaccination for, 257–265
Pneumococcal polysaccharide vaccine, 257–259
  adverse reactions to, 262
  in children, 261–262
  cross-reactivity to, 259
  delivery strategies for, 264–265
  development of, 265
  distribution of in U.S., 264f
  efficacy of, 259–261
  precautions to, 262
  recommendations for use of, 261–262
  repeat of, 262–264
  simultaneous administration of, 209
  timing of, 262
Pneumococcal vaccination, 198t
  with influenza vaccination, 243
  repeated, 225
Pneumococcus
  antibacterial drugs for, 82t

TANGLED TONGUE

Tangled Tongue

LIVING WITH A STUTTER

JOCK A. CARLISLE

University of Toronto Press
Toronto Buffalo London

© University of Toronto Press 1985
Toronto Buffalo London
Printed in the U.S.A.

ISBN 0-8020-2558-7 (cloth)
ISBN 0-8020-6577-5 (paper)

Canadian Cataloguing in Publication Data
Carlisle, Jock A. (Jock Alan), 1924–
Tangled tongue: living with a stutter
Bibliography: p.
Includes index.
ISBN 0-8020-2558-7 (bound). – ISBN 0-8020-6577-5 (pbk.)
1. Carlisle, Jock A. (Jock Alan), 1924–
2. Stuttering. 3. Stuttering – Treatment. I. Title.
RC424.C37 1985   616.85'54   C85-098689-3

This book is dedicated to my much loved wife, Joan, who has helped me pick up the pieces of my life so many times.

Publication of this book has been assisted by the Ontario Arts Council under its block grant program.

Contents

Acknowledgments

This book could not have been written without the encouragement and help of my wife, Joan, who typed so many drafts that she more than earned her IBM word processor.

I shall always be grateful to the speech rehabilitation team led by Susan Carrol-Thomas at the Royal Ottawa Hospital's Regional Rehabilitation Centre, particularly to Ann Meltzer, Anne Godden, Carol Dixon, and Vicky Inns for their compassion, perceptiveness, and unswerving dedication. Dr Norman Ward of Ottawa deserves special thanks for his wise counsel and for placing his finger gently on so many tender truths.

I wish to thank all the people who reviewed the manuscript and made helpful, constructive criticisms, particularly Professor Einer Boberg, Susan Carrol-Thomas, and Ann Meltzer. The comments and encouragement of the 'dean' of Speech Pathology, Professor Charles Van Riper, made the struggle of revising the book worth while.

My thanks also go to my literary agent, Joanne Kellock of Edmonton, whose eagle eye and sense of balance saved me from drowning my readers in a deep well of words.

I wish to acknowledge the many store clerks, waitresses, hotel receptionists, car-hire clerks, airline booking clerks, telephone operators, and others who unwittingly played important roles as guinea pigs in testing various speech techniques and observing the responses.

Ann Dewar of Edinburgh University, Mike Hughes of St John, New Brunswick, and Findlay, Irvine Ltd., of Penicuik, Scotland, kindly provided information about the Edinburgh

Masker. I also wish to express my appreciation to those speech pathologists in North America, Europe, South Africa, Australia, and Japan who provided the data about stuttering and speech centres. The scientific attachés of the different embassies were most helpful in making the overseas contacts.

My thanks go to Virgil Duff and the other members of the editorial and marketing staff of the University of Toronto Press for their encouragement and advice. Their help was invaluable.

For permission to refer in the text to other published works, I am indebted to: the National Easter Seals Society and to Professor Oliver Bloodstein, author of the masterly *A Handbook on Stuttering* (1969, 1981); Pergamon Press (Oxford) for material from H.E. Beech and F. Fransella, *Research and Experiment in Stuttering*; Doubleday (New York) for material from Richard M. Restak, *The Brain: the Last Frontier*; Faber and Faber (London), Random House Inc. (New York), and Alfred A. Knopf, Inc. (New York) for the quotations from W.H. Auden and C. Isherwood's *The Ascent of F6*; William Morrow Co. Inc. (New York) for material from *Peter's Quotations*; and Prentice-Hall, Inc. (Englewood Cliffs, NJ) and Professor Charles Van Riper for material from *Speech Correction: Principles and Methods*.

Warm thanks go to the many patients of the Royal Ottawa Hospital Regional Rehabilitation Centre for their friendship, support, good humour, and courage in spite of the difficulties they face every day. They were the best possible companions on a difficult voyage.

I remember our therapy sessions as times of affection, laughter, adventure, and determination. They will never be forgotten. Particular thanks go to Bob and Dolly Smith who, besides brightening the day for every person they met, gave so freely of their time and experiences.

Last but not least, I wish to thank my three daughters – Kate, Sara, and Susan – for not being aware of the tangle in my tongue while they were growing up.

Preface

Six people patiently waited to order their burgers, french fries, and Cokes at Harvey's in Pembroke, Ontario. As my turn approached I felt the familiar tightening of my stomach muscles and adjusted my mind to handle the ordeal ahead. My wife, Joan, hovered in the background, encouraging but nervous.

I soon found myself facing the smiling, uniformed girl at her microphone, and said, 'Two chicken sandwiches, please, one with sauce, one without sauce, one portion of french fries, and two coffees. We'll eat them here.' The girl smiled, repeated the order over the intercom, took my money, and wished me a nice day. 'Next please!'

Joan joined me at the counter while the food was being prepared and, with a big smile and eyes flashing with pleasure, said, 'Terrific! You did it! Did you see her face and watch her eyes? They didn't change! It worked!' It was the best fast-food lunch we had ever eaten. This type of scene takes place millions of times every day in Canada and the United States, but for me it was a unique experience.

I had had difficulty speaking for about fifty-five years and, although at times I was more or less fluent, there were some situations I could never handle. Ordering food in a stand-up situation was one of them. By about the third word I always stuttered and went into a block of prolonged silence while the person behind the counter became embarrassed, nervous, or even hostile. Sometimes I couldn't start at all, and then eyes would glaze as the order-taker waited. When someone tittered in the background it took a tremendous effort to control both my feelings and my temper and to get my speech back on course. I always got there in the end, but ill feelings would crackle on both sides of the counter.

This type of experience happens nearly every time anybody with a severe stutter goes into a store, a restaurant, or any public place where he has to ask for something.

On that particular day I was trying out an electronic device, called the Edinburgh Masker, which stops you from hearing your own speech and makes speaking easier for some people.[1] The masker does not work equally well for everybody. Even when it works it isn't foolproof, and you need to think carefully about the technique when you speak. Nevertheless, on this day the snares and pitfalls in the sentences needed to order the sandwiches melted away, I slid slowly through the words, and the girl's face did not change to an expression of anxiety or hostility. I entered an unfamiliar world where people did not automatically react badly whenever I opened my mouth.

I tested the instrument in many situations for a week or more and found it surprisingly effective. Since then the masker has had varied effects on my stutter; but in general it has made life easier. I can seek telephone assistance without causing the operator to become abusive or insolent, ask for merchandise in stores, and chat to people in the street, all without the need for a tight rein on my feelings and articulation.

During fifty years of speech therapy I have often heard other patients say, 'If only I could speak perfectly for one day – just one bloody day – I'm sure I could control my stutter.' They have a point. Since the day I ordered the chicken sandwiches my speech has been much more controlled, with or without the masker.

Many years ago I stood on top of a mountain leaning on my ice axe. Looking at the sparkling-white, windswept world through my tinted snow goggles, I made a promise that if I could learn to control my speech, even for a short time, I would help other people who stutter by writing a book to explain their problems to the rest of the world. This book fulfils that promise.

My purpose in writing was to cast some light on the mystery surrounding the causes of stuttering; the kind of people who stutter, and the difficulties they face every day; the ways stuttering can be treated; and the responses of society to this strange, erratic way of speaking.

Although the book deals with a disability, above all it is about people – the kind of people who face life with a handicap that society finds hard to understand and accept.

Most writing about disabilities views the patient from the outside, but in this case the viewpoint is that of the patient looking outward at life.

The focus is stuttering, but many of the problems described relate to other disabilities, particularly those that interfere with communication. Deaf people may recognize parallels with their own situations.

People who stutter can be fluent one minute and completely speechless the next. The intermittence and apparent unpredictability of the speech make listeners nervous. The average person may know, more or less, how to deal with a blind or deaf person, a paraplegic, an amputee, or someone who is mentally handicapped; but very few people know what to do when faced by a stutterer. Do you help the guy begin his word? Do you look at him or look away as he struggles to speak? Do you smile encouragingly or sit there like a stuffed dummy? Most people look away, fidget, and think of ways to escape; or, if they happen to be holding a cup of coffee, stir it as though their lives depend upon it. Many just flee in alarm as the stutterer battles his way to the next word. Few know what to do, and uncertainty breeds fear with its attendant tension, rudeness, hostility, and anger. To make matters worse stutterers' own attitudes vary – some welcome help and others do not. All stutterers welcome a little patience.

Stutterers can exhibit such bizarre tics and grimaces when they try to speak that people think they are mad, or at best wildly eccentric. Some people feel, incorrectly, that anybody who loses control of his speech is mentally impaired and treat him accordingly. They may also wonder why someone will speak fluently on some occasions and stutter on others.

Stuttering interferes with the attribute that sets human beings apart from all the other animals – the aptitude for verbal communication. Other mammals – whales, for example – communicate by signals, but only humans have the gift of expressing complex thoughts in spoken words. Speech is the basis of our culture. The inability to communicate fluently affects every moment of a stutterer's life and tends to push him or her outside society.

W.H. Auden, in his dramatic poem *The Ascent of F6*, writes about 'the girl imprisoned in the tower of a stutter.' I prefer to think of people who stutter as living in a *glass* tower. The glass wall is placed there by society. Stutterers can see people and hear them, but cannot reach out and touch them physically or mentally. They would gladly walk out and mingle with people, but every time they speak the transparent, impenetrable wall closes around them.

It is hoped that this book will help to shatter or at least crack this glass wall and remove misconceptions about the disability. The book is not a scientific, in-depth study of the origins of stuttering and how to cure it, although these subjects are discussed in some detail. There are plenty of publications on the psychology, physiology, and treatment of stuttering; but few discuss a stutterer's relationships with other people.

I am not a speech therapist or a psychiatrist but, after fifty-five years of stuttering and fifty years of therapy, I am familiar with most forms of treatment and can claim to be an authority on *my* stutter. A hen may not be an expert on the physiology of eggs, but she knows better than anybody else what it feels like to lay an egg.

Although this book is not an autobiography, many of the incidents described were experienced or seen by me. Others I heard of from responsible people or read about in books written by reliable authors. Wherever possible the incidents are described unchanged, but in cases where participants would be embarrassed I have modified the circumstances, location, and personal descriptions to prevent identification.

Often, people who stutter have an acute appreciation of the absurd and face their problems with remarkable courage and good humour. Nevertheless, although they can laugh at the ludicrous situations they encounter, they take strong exception to being ridiculed or patronized. Some parts of this book describe funny situations, but this does not mean that stuttering is just an amusing aberration to be taken lightly. Far from it. Living with a stutter – dealing with its social effects every day – is no laughing matter.

Throughout the book the word 'stuttering' is used. This is the North American term for 'stammering' (British), *'begaiement'* (French), *'balbuzie'* (Italian), *'stottern'* (German), *'tartamudez'* (Spanish), and *'gagueira'* (Portuguese).[2] The disability has also been called 'spasmophemia,' 'laloneurosis,' and 'balbuties' in the scientific literature.[3]

Some writers group stuttering and cluttering[4] into the single category of 'clutter-stuttering.' In this text stuttering, with its complex, unclear origins, is considered separately from cluttering, a different type of disorder, which is apparently caused by neurological abnormality. It is recognized that some stutterers also clutter and that the borderline between the two disabilities is not clear.

Most speech therapists are women and they are referred to as 'she.' The masculine third person 'he' is used for stutterers, but no disrespect is meant to women, lib. or non-lib. Four out of five people with stutters are male, and a surfeit of 'he or she's' would be tedious. Ugly words such as 'chairperson' and 'salesperson' are widely used and I could have written 'stutterperson,' but that would have been absurd. So 'he' it is, and I'll just have to take my lumps. May the Creator, wherever she is, forgive me.

TANGLED TONGUE

'I wouldst thou couldst stammer, that thou mightst pour this concealed man out of thy mouth, as wine comes out of a narrow-mouthed bottle; either too much at once, or none at all.'

William Shakespeare

ONE

What is a stutter?

'A man is hid under his tongue.'

Ali-Ibn-Abi-Talib (seventh century)

During the 1950s a speech therapist asked me to write down a definition of a stutter, and I thought it would be easy. I wrote down all the key terms – 'blocking,' 'repetition,' 'lack of rhythm,' and so on – and had nearly finished my masterpiece when he leaned over my shoulder and said, 'While you're at it, tell me how a stutter differs from untidy normal speech and from the other speech disorders you've encountered.' After an hour all I had was a page full of notes, but my mentor said, 'Not to worry! I don't know either. I just thought you might come up with a bright idea!'

Everybody knows what a severe stutter looks and sounds like with its tics, blocks, and repetitions, but inarticulate people with normal speech also frequently pause and repeat. When one patient was asked to describe his stutter briefly he replied, 'Downright embarrassing! A darned nuisance!' The point was that he blocked and repeated to such an extent that his hesitations inconvenienced him, made him feel anxious and uncomfortable, and handicapped him in daily life. It is these sorts of consequences that distinguish a stutter from normal disfluency.

This is still a little vague, and the United States Health Service was cautious when it wrote: 'Stuttering remains an enigma while illustrating the type of disorder which does not have a clear organic cause or a clearly habitual basis.'[1] A cop-out, yes, but an honest cop-out.

Enigma or not, it is very clear to me what I am writing about. Most experts agree that, in general, a stutter is the interruption of the flow of speech by hesitations, prolongation of sounds, avoidance of difficult words, struggles to speak, and blockages sufficient to cause anxiety and impair verbal communication. Other symptoms may or may not be associated with the stutter. These include low self-esteem, grimacing, stamping the foot, clenching the hands, twisting the fingers, protruding the tongue, looking away, closing the eyes, and contorting the body in the enormous effort to move from one word to the next.

Speech disorders that are not stutters involve some of these symptoms. People suffering from aphasia following a stroke may have speech blockages in addition to difficulty in choosing the right words to form syntax that makes sense. They don't stutter. The hasty, sloppy, stumbling, jerky speech of a clutterer in some ways resembles a stutter, but is quite different.

People who stutter often detach themselves completely when they freeze into a prolonged block. While the listener and the stutterer wait for the locked lips or tongue to release for communication to continue, the stutterer may go into a kind of trance. His articulatory muscles seem to be carved from stone and, without therapy to provide him with a key to his lock, he is helpless and in danger of (literally) running out of air. The strange part is the depth of the detachment. While a stutterer is frozen in a block, people can slam doors, shout 'Fire,' or tell him that he has won a lottery, with no response whatsoever. I used to plan the next day's activities and remind myself to pay bills and complete my income tax return during long blocks, while my audience patiently or impatiently waited for speech to continue. A major speech block is hard to describe, but many stutterers feel completely out of touch as they wait for release.

It is difficult for the layman to differentiate between normal lack of fluency and the hesitations and repetitions of some stutterers. If you listen to any radio talk-show or analyse any political speech, you will notice that many speakers, besides mangling English grammar and syntax, include a remarkable number of hesitations in every spoken sentence. I remember hearing an opera singer interviewed on the radio. She paused, repeated, blocked, and said 'um,' 'ah,' and 'er' to such an extent that it was hard to understand her. She was not a stutterer, or a clutterer, nor did she have aphasia. She was just inarticulate. It is hoped that she sang better than she talked.

Even with children it is difficult to tell the difference between normal childish disfluency and the hesitations and repetitions that develop into a full-blown stutter. A parent may be unaware that the child has a stutter, or may think that the child is starting to stutter when he is only normally hesitant. Some children use highly abnormal repetitions of individual sounds, as many as forty, at an age of four or less. It seems likely that these children will develop stutters.

Lacking any clear definition, I shall describe the kind of stutter I am going to write about – my kind. My speech was, and still is to some extent, impaired by intermittent, unpredictable difficulty in progressing from one sound to the other, with repetition, stumbling, and debilitating blocking – sometimes lasting as long as thirty seconds – leading to a complete breakdown of verbal communication. In particular, the blocking type of stutter can be a major handicap to communication and social involvement.

A stutter can vary so much from day to day, or even from hour to hour, that people tend to underestimate its importance. It is not such an obvious, continual handicap as blindness, deafness, or paralysis of the limbs, all of which have received considerable attention from the medical profession and sympathy from the public. A person who stutters severely can usually manage his life fairly well and learns to cope with the fear, despair, humiliation, and frustration that accompany him every time he talks to strangers and sees their change of expression, asks for a meal and encounters rudeness, or tries to make a telephone call and meets impatience or worse.

A stutter is not just inarticulacy; it includes a whole syndrome of effects that feed back to the person who stutters and make his speech worse. Rebuffs and rejection are as much a part of stuttering as the speech blockages and interruptions. People who react badly to stuttering are not usually deliberately unkind. They respond to their fear that they cannot cope with the unfamiliar situation and tend to copy the behaviour of others toward people with noticeable disabilities. Stuttering is not part of their usual experience.

A small boy and his father watched a group of adults tormenting a beautiful green snake in a slippery plastic bucket. Tiring of the sport, the tormentors tipped the snake out and laughingly crushed its head underfoot. When the perplexed boy asked why they tormented and killed the harmless reptile, his father replied, 'A snake is just not part of their world.'

TWO

Questions people are afraid to ask – and things they shouldn't say

'He who asks a question is a fool for five minutes; he who does not ask a question is a fool for ever.'

Chinese Proverb

People who stutter can sometimes be prickly about their impediment, particularly when they are not willing to admit even to themselves that they have a handicap. Others will discuss their disability freely. When you first meet a stutterer you don't know what kind of person he is. If you ask him a question about his speech you may get short shrift with 'Mind your own business,' or you may launch your companion on his favourite topic – his stutter.

If you manage to start a conversation, you may want to ask questions about stuttering, but feel diffident about doing so in case you intrude upon the stutterer's privacy. People meeting a person with a stutter for the first time tend to be as wary in their conversation as though picking their way through a verbal minefield. The purpose of this chapter is to defuse some of the mines and correct some misconceptions.

Do you help a stutterer with his words, offer advice, or look away?

This trilogy of questions strikes at the core of the difficulties a stutterer encounters when dealing with people in stores, restaurants, and other social situations. People who meet a stutterer don't know what to do.

I accompanied a young man with a severe stutter into a store to try out his newly learned speech techniques by ordering some cigarettes. On the second word he blocked badly. Instead of using the speech techniques, he panicked and tried to push through the word with quivering, pursed lips. The eyes of the woman behind the counter went blank. She shrugged, walked away to serve another customer, and never returned.

The stutterer, without his cigarettes, was in a cold fury, but after he'd calmed down we tried again at another store. He blocked again, but the pleasant girl behind the counter gave him her full attention, maintained eye contact without staring, and patiently waited the few seconds he needed to collect himself and apply his techniques. There was no problem.

In the first situation the response of the ill-mannered, impatient woman was bad and made the stutter worse. The second case demonstrated how a little patience and pleasant, helpful feedback helped the stutterer recover from his block. The way you respond to a stutterer will greatly affect his speech. Don't look away or leave him as soon as you find a plausible excuse. Just act with normal good manners. Most stutterers dislike it intensely when people switch them off and walk away to spare their own feelings.

Whether you should help a stutterer complete a blocked word is best answered by, 'When in doubt, don't.' Some people who stutter severely welcome help, but if they are undergoing therapy their therapist won't thank you for finishing words or sentences. If your urge to help is overwhelming, ask the stutterer, 'Would you like me to complete your difficult words or not?' He'll probably say no, but at least you'll both know where you stand.

The majority of stutterers find it difficult when somebody ends their words and sentences for them because the completion is usually not what they wanted to say, which means that they need to start all over again. Some irritating people are compulsive sentence-finishers, even with people who have normal speech. One stutterer spoke longingly of consigning sentence-finishers to a syntactical hell where small devils interrupted their victims in the middle of each sentence and completed it with words meaning the complete opposite of what they wanted to say. Anybody can be forgiven for wanting to throttle a person who, as you struggle to say 'I went for my holiday in G____' fills in with the word 'Glasgow' when you really wanted to say exotic 'Guadeloupe.'

Stutterers may be pestered by well-meaning people asking tactless questions and offering bad advice. Winston Churchill is to be admired as a wartime leader, but he is the bane of stutterers' lives as far as speech is concerned. At social occasions over-familiar strangers may say challengingly, 'Churchill cured his stutter. Why can't you?' The implication is that your failure indicates a lack of moral fibre. I don't know how bad Churchill's stutter was, and I am not sure that he cured it. His articulacy in political oratory was amazing, but it is said that he still stuttered in conversation. I would like to lay Churchill and his stutter to rest a second time, and hope that his ghost will cease to haunt the stutterers of the world.

Another statement guaranteed to raise a stutterer's hackles is, 'I once stuttered very badly, but I worked at it and look at me now!' (Yes, look at him – the tactless so-and-so!) A variant of this is, 'I had a friend (aunt, uncle, girl-friend, mistress) who stuttered but he (she) overcame it by sheer determination!' These statements are usually followed by suggestions that you relax, take a deep breath, clench your left fist, say 'er' before every word, tap your foot, or have faith in yourself. These unofficial experts frequently end by saying, 'You can cure your stutter if you *really* want to,' implying that since you still have an impediment you are a weak-kneed jellyfish.

Then there are the purveyors of gloom and doom who urge you to be realistic and face facts. They say that they've read a great deal about stuttering and to them it is clear that you'll never get any better. One of these individuals tactfully left on my desk a large tome by a man with a German name so long I looked for the verb at the end. The heavy-faced author, pictured with a crew-cut, bushy moustache, black tails, and pin-stripe pants, ran a speech clinic somewhere in Bavaria where stutterers were bludgeoned into fluency by talking as they rhythmically marched up and down and clapped their hands.

When they failed to be fluent, they were consigned to guilt-ridden psychological purgatory. On the last page – which was flagged for my attention – the expert declared that if you stuttered after the age of forty the problem would get worse and worse and cast you into an inarticulate, lonely old age – unless you went to old crew-cut's clinic and paid his huge fees.

People who offer unsolicited advice may be well intentioned, but they can be a trial, like those people who knock on your door and give you religious tracts and a homily about how to achieve salvation. They seem to assume that you've never given the matter a moment's thought.

The person who stutters wants your full attention. For him, speaking is hard work, and nothing is more exasperating than someone who, as the stutterer tries to disentangle his speech, carries on a side-conversation with other people. One of my daughters used to do this. She still lives, which speaks well for my self-control.

Most people who stutter communicate remarkably well using their abnormally disfluent speech, plus the body language through which much is communicated even by people with normal speech. Words are only one way of conveying information. Albert Mehrabian found that only about 7 per cent of communication involves words. The rest consists of non-verbal vocal or paralinguistic cues (38 per cent) and facial expressions (55 per cent).[1] Non-verbal communication came before complex speech in the evolution of man. Even today babies learn to communicate long before they can talk.

In recent years, sociologists and anthropologists have shown increasing interest in the science of kinesics, which is concerned with the implications of patterns of behaviour in non-verbal communication. This new science caught the interest of the public under the 'body language' label as part of the wave of pop-psychology that swept the Western world during the 1970s.[2]

If a person who stutters doesn't get your attention, he cannot use his non-verbal skills, and this may be one of the reasons he finds it so hard to use the telephone.

What do you do when speaking to a stutterer? Be patient, don't look away, don't fill in words or end sentences, don't offer unsolicited advice. Just act with ordinary good manners. It's not very difficult.

What kind of people stutter?

During the 1970s I participated in group therapy sessions as both a patient and a hospital volunteer at the Royal Ottawa Hospital in Ottawa. On Thursday nights adult patients with stutters assembled in a room and discussed their problems and progress. It was a great challenge to speak in a controlled manner to twenty or more people under the watchful eyes of the therapists. Most of us were nervous, so I made a list of the age, sex, ethnic origin, and occupations of the patients in the room to calm my feelings.

The stutterers' ages ranged from about eighteen to sixty-four, and about a fifth of the group were girls. There were a few students, a teacher, a forester, a labourer, a scientist, four civil servants, a girl with a beaded headband and buckskins, a storekeeper, a pig farmer, an auto-mechanic, a fireman, a man and a woman in the restaurant business, a soldier, a recreation specialist, a political scientist, a statistician, a truck driver, a building contractor, and a novice priest from a seminary who had trouble saying grace.

The patients were Canadians with Chinese, Greek, Jewish, Italian, French, and British backgrounds. Many of them were doing well in their jobs, but had encountered difficulties while speaking to customers, making telephone calls, addressing meetings, or ordering cattle feed. They were there to ease the tension and anxiety in their lives by learning to control their erratic speech.

Some had already had a great deal of therapy, and they maintained reasonable fluency as they spoke to the group using the speech techniques they had been taught. Others were obviously tense. Their throat muscles involuntarily quivered, their lips trembled, and their faces twitched nervously as they slowly described their progress, prolonging every word and striving to keep in touch with their speech and maintain eye contact with the audience. There were people who were confident, insecure, shy, humorous, solemn, extroverted, introverted, aggressive, and timid. People of all races, professions, and characters have stutters. It is a myth that all people who stutter are shy, unsociable, moronic, and introverted.

Each person responds to having a stutter in his own way depending on his personality. There are braggarts and buffoons who wave their stutters in public like a flag, just as there are timid people driven into solitude and despair by their handicap. Some are totally crushed by the stress of trying to speak; but most cope from day to day and arrange their lives so that their stuttering interferes as little as possible.

The people in the group mixed remarkably well considering the differences in education, interest, occupation, age, and ethnic origin. Some were easier to get along with than others, but most were warm, friendly, and intelligent. Although they had all been stressed and battered by the daily need to cope with their disfluent speech, the majority were remarkably unsoured by their experiences. I enjoyed their company, even when the therapy frayed my nerves as I tried to do mundane but seemingly impossible tasks like making a collect telephone call.

The group had a boisterous sense of humour, and meetings were great fun, with bright repartee and kindly teasing punctuated by gusts of laughter. The patients trusted each other with their feelings, and their respect for the therapists was obvious. There was so little unkindness, bitchiness, selfishness, self-pity, and hostility that I looked forward to the sessions as a relief from the competitive work situation. They restored my wilting confidence in humanity. People who stutter have a great deal to offer if others have the patience and the good manners to listen to them.

About 1 per cent of school children in North America, Europe, and Australia stutter. The impediment seems to be less common in the United States (about 0.7 per cent) than in Europe (about 1.1 per cent); it is relatively common in Poland (1.7 per cent).

The data generally refer to school children rather than adults because young people are captive participants in school surveys. The figures reflect an equilibrium because some children recover from their impediment while others develop it.

Inventories of children and adults who either have stutters or at some time stuttered and recovered have given results far higher than 1 per cent. Oliver Bloodstein gives rates ranging from about 5 to 15 per cent and averaging about 10 per cent.[3] In North America about 2.5 million people are known to stutter; this number takes no account of people who successfully hide their stutters and adults who don't report their handicap or request therapy. The true figure is probably much higher.

A stutterer like myself, who has had many years of therapy, can spot another stutterer as soon as he opens his mouth, even when he is fluent. I can identify those who use speech techniques to keep fluent and spot those who hide their stutter by word substitution, changes in accent, and shifts in role. It becomes a sixth sense.

I unobtrusively surveyed two research establishments where I worked; 3 per cent of the staff of a laboratory in Britain had stutters, and 6 per cent of a research institute in Canada. Some of the stutterers who didn't have prolonged speech blockages seemed to be unconcerned about their problem. Others hid their disfluency nearly perfectly. Nevertheless, they stuttered – no doubt about it.

Do some types of people stutter more than others? Yes, more boys stutter than girls. The ratio of boys with stutters to girls varies between 2:1 and 6:1, but on average about four boys stutter for every girl with the same problem. This preponderance of male stutterers has caused a great deal of speculation, and some authorities feel it reflects the relatively slow speech development of boys and the congenital vulnerability of the male constitution compared with females. Others feel that boys encounter more competition and frustration in speaking than girls, while another school of thought feels that parents react differently to normal hesitations in a boy's speech than in a girl's.[4] It may be that girls just speak more easily than boys. At the age of five, all my minuscule girl-friends had the gift of gab. In a mixed group of children the only way for me to get a word in edgeways was to bat a girl with my teddy bear.

Whether people who stutter are more or less intelligent than people without stutters has been the subject of much debate. Many people feel that because a person cannot control his speech he must be stupid or mad. There are many stories about stutterers who, because they grimaced in their struggles to speak, were certified insane by ill-informed physicians and confined in mental institutions for many years. Even today there is a tendency to look upon people with severe stutters as mentally impaired. It is true that some people with severe mental handicaps stutter, but some of them also have deficiencies of vision and hearing. Nobody links these disabilities with mental impairment.

Stutterers and their families and friends often counter these unfounded accusations by saying that people with stutters are *more* intelligent than others. They refer to the many famous and intelligent people in history who had the disability. There is no doubt that some exceptionally bright people stutter, but the scientific evidence about the relationship between stuttering and intelligence is conflicting. The trouble is that stuttering can be confused with other speech disabilities such as cluttering, and even with normal inarticulacy. The main tool used to measure intelligence is the IQ test, which has been misused and misunderstood ever since it was invented. There does not seem to be any simple way of ranking human intelligence within the normal range. The IQ takes little account of a person's innate abilities to use intuitive thought and to adapt, both of which have been and still are vital in mankind's mental evolution. A person with a stutter may have such low self-esteem that it affects his performance in any test situation. Some people have an aversion to tests in general, and a person with perfectly normal intelligence may get a low test score.

The IQ test was designed by a Frenchman, Alfred Binet, in 1908, for a specific, limited purpose: to identify children with learning disabilities or mild retardation who needed special education. The IQ was modified by W. Stern in 1912 and in its final form is a person's mental age divided by his chronological age and multiplied by 100. The test consists of a series of graded questions, of increasing complexity, that average children of different ages can answer. It simply assesses mental age.

The test is useful for identifying definite mental abnormalities. Unfortunately, like many other good ideas, the IQ has been misused, particularly in the education systems of North America, where educators have tended to use it blindly as an index of relative intelligence of normal children, labelling a child as stupid or bright for the rest of his or her scholastic life. There are people with low IQ scores who are intelligent, effective citizens; and there are people with genius IQs who are ineffective ninnies. In the next century, the IQ test as an index of relative intelligence of normal people will probably join craniometry in the rag-bag of quaint and misused scientific ideas.

For the record, children with stutters at schools and speech clinics in the United States have IQs ranging from low (54) to very high (162) and averaging 95–100, which is similar to the average for the population as a whole. A few studies imply that stutterers are slightly more common among people with lower IQ scores, but these results have not withstood close scrutiny because of problems of sampling and lack of suitable experimental controls. There is some evidence that stuttering students at universities are more intelligent than the average student, but in general stutterers seem to be neither brighter nor more stupid than the average Joe on the street.[5]

The Clan of the Tangled Tongue includes the prophet Moses and the philosophers Demosthenes and Aristotle. Emperors and kings (Emperor Claudius of Rome, and kings Charles I and George VI of England) and statesmen (Thomas Jefferson, Winston Churchill, and Aneuran Bevan) stuttered, and some well-known scientists (Isaac Newton, Erasmus Darwin, and Charles Darwin) and authors (Virgil, Aesop, Charles Lamb, Nevil Shute, Arnold Bennett, and Somerset Maugham) had trouble with their speech. Some public figures, film stars, television personalities, and musicians (Lorne Green, Eric Roberts, Marilyn Monroe, Gary Moore, Jack Paar, Annie Glenn, and Mel Tillis) managed to cope in public in spite of their blocks and hesitations, and many professors of speech pathology, psychiatrists, and speech therapists have been troubled by tangled tongues, particularly the eminent Wendell Johnson, Charles Van Riper, Joseph Sheehan, Hugo Gregory, and Einer Boberg.

The list is endless. All these people rose to prominence by great effort and courage in spite of their stuttering. Some may feel that the challenging barriers imposed by the disability provided the impetus that drove them to the top.

Twins tend to be more prone to develop stutters than others, and estimates range from a nearly normal 1.9 per cent[6] to as high as 13 per cent.[7] Although this has genetic implications, the slowness of maturation and competitive pressure between the individuals in a twin pair have been suggested as possible causes of the high incidence of stuttering in twins.[8]

Unless you stutter yourself you can't tell if a person stutters just by looking at him, or even listening to him. A person can chat to you for an hour or so, and you may have no idea that he stutters. One attractive girl in her twenties had been married for several years. She worked in a government office and requested therapy because the stress of concealing her stutter from her employers was affecting her health. Her husband had no idea that she stuttered. When the therapists persuaded her to stutter openly to relieve the tension of concealment it was quite a surprise to her family. People with moderately severe stutters can get away with hiding it for years – but they pay a price.

The simple answer to the question about what kind of people stutter is that all kinds of people stutter. The impediment can affect kings as well as paupers.

Why don't you stutter when you sing, whisper, or speak in unison?

It is true that many stutterers can sing, whisper, or speak in unison fluently, but the degree of fluency tends to vary from person to person, and their speech can let them down when they least expect it. The reasons for fluency in these situations are far from clear.

At the age of eleven, when I had a moderate but not debilitating stutter, I had the misfortune to possess an exceptionally clear, well-pitched, soprano voice, which led to my being shanghaied into performing as soloist at many local concerts. I objected to singing solo carols and traditional songs in cavernous churches and dusty school halls. I loathed wearing a white robe and a starched collar that rubbed my neck raw. But the teachers were bigger than I was, so there was no use protesting.

I became blasé about the whole thing. It was all a bit of a bore, but I had done it before and could do it again. All I had to do was go on stage, sing, and go home for baked beans on toast.

My nemesis caught up with me in Blackpool, a town in northwestern England, where I was to sing 'Strawberry Fair.' With feelings of resignation and boredom, I stood on a wooden dais on a large dusty stage. The curtain went up and there was a burst of applause from a sea of faces before me. To my horror I found I was alone on the stage of the Blackpool Opera House being grilled to a clinker by bright lights. Instead of the usual scattering of parents and teachers, I faced a huge, packed auditorium.

The orchestra struck up the introduction, I opened my mouth, and there was dead silence. Not a squeak. The violins quaveringly petered out, the conductor rapped for my attention, and we tried again. Not a chirrup. I blocked completely on my easiest word, 'As.' The audience began to shuffle, and I fled, but the teachers bullied me back on to the platform. There I stood, plain mad and bloody-minded, sang like an angry lark, stumped scowling off the stage, and bashed a bigger boy in the wings who dared to giggle.

Singing can increase fluency, but it can also catch you bending. People often ask, 'Why don't you sing every time you speak?' (Tra, la, la.) I curb my inner reply of, 'Don't be daft!' and politely say that it just doesn't work. Singing for me is not communication; it seems to involve different mechanisms from those I use when I express thoughts and feelings in speech.

Unless one sings dirty lyrics in the wrong company or indulges in political satire in a totalitarian state, the content of a song doesn't have potentially dire consequences for the singer. Children and adults are well aware that words have power for good or bad and evoke responses and consequences. In common with most people with the same impediment, I am more likely to stutter the higher the message content of the words.

It seems possible that when a stutterer is singing, the fact that he is playing another role helps his fluency. This effect of role on speech is skimmed over by many textbooks on stuttering, although it is known that some adolescent stutterers have difficulty perceiving their own life roles.[9] I know several apparently fluent people who hide their stutters completely by changing their accents when they get into blocks. One man switches so swiftly from unaccented English to broad Scottish, to cockney, to Welsh, or to American that it leaves me bewildered and wondering which person he really is. He keeps perfectly fluent by switching his roles, but it is exhausting to listen to him.

One stutterer, who later became a therapist, completely controlled a moderate stutter at the age of twenty-five by participating in amateur theatricals. He was fluent when he played roles other than himself, and this improved his speech off the stage. It makes me wonder which role he played away from the theatre to maintain his fluency.

Some pundits say that stutterers can sing because their breathing is controlled, or because they are more concerned with voice pitch and volume than words, or because of a change in role, but these are all guesses.

Stutterers whisper fairly fluently as a rule. I could always talk *sotto voce* in churches and libraries where I was supposed to be silent. (Even so, the fluent whisper can collapse.)

Why whispering helps fluency is another mystery. The common explanations involving theories about speech concealment, role-playing, and distraction don't bear close examination. There may be something to the explanation that when the stutterer's lower speech frequencies are blanked out so that he can't hear them he is usually more fluent. These low frequencies seem to interfere with speech.[10] and whisperers don't use low frequencies, so there is less risk of speech interference. But the answer to the question of why stutterers can whisper fluently probably lies in the interaction of many factors.

The fact that stutterers can read poems in class in unison with other people but not alone is puzzling. I was fluent in unison, but would block completely when I tried to read aloud on my own, and this led to misunderstandings. Several teachers said, 'You see! You *can* speak fluently! You just don't *try*,' and penalties usually followed. This intermittent fluency leads to the belief that the stutterer can easily choose not to stutter, so that people may penalize him for selecting the wrong option. Absurd though this is, a stuttering child at school who shows that he can be fluent can make himself a bed of nails.

I used to think that I could speak in unison because I could hardly hear my voice, but this theory was scuttled by the fact that when I wanted to make a fluent tape recording of a speech or scientific paper, I could do so if my wife read in unison in a whisper so low that the microphone did not pick it up. Reading in unison made me feel more relaxed about my speech. Possibly, sharing the responsibility of communicating and having someone to fall back on when I got into trouble helped my fluency. Possibly, the presence of a distraction accounted for it. All of these theories hold about enough water to float a matchstick. The fact is that nobody really knows the answer.

When my speech was exceptionally bad it helped to read slowly in unison with somebody, but it was at best a crutch. No one can go around speaking in unison all the time unless he happens to be a Siamese twin with a co-operative partner, and then he has other problems.

People who stutter tend to be more fluent when they shadow another person's speech, and one form of therapy was based on this fact. The stutterer produces a running copy of somebody else's speech. I used to spend hours shadowing radio announcers, but unfortunately the beneficial effects ceased immediately when I spoke to anybody else. The shadowing may have temporarily improved my fluency because I was concentrating on another person's voice and had my attention distracted from the stutter, or because I was not communicating and did not need to synchronize my thoughts with my speech.

Distracting a stutterer's attention away from his speech often improves fluency and some therapies are based on this fact. During World War II there were moments when my thoughts were so distracted by the possibility of imminent extinction that I became noisily and vehemently fluent.

Do you stutter when you've had a few drinks?

Yes, I do! I stutter in my sleep, under narcotics, or filled to the gills with good Scotch whiskey – preferably pure malt. Several drinks make some stutterers fluent and others completely speechless.

I've experimented with many speech-improvement techniques, but the whiskey trials were the most fun. At the time, I was a student and had a bad cold, so I decided to kill two birds with one stone by combining the Scottish Bowler Hat Treatment for colds with research on the effects of alcohol on my stutter.

The Bowler Hat Treatment is an old and respected remedy whereby you go to bed with a bottle of good malt whiskey and a bowler hat. You hang the bowler hat at the foot of the bed and leisurely sip the whiskey until you see two, or preferably three, bowler hats. By this time you can be sure that either the cold is cured or you can't feel it. I tried this technique in my lodgings and, although the whiskey did wonders for my cold, it rendered me speechless. That does not mean that I was silent, because my landlady complained about my bawdy songs in the night and nearly showed me the door.

More seriously, alcohol relaxes people and affects their co-ordination – that's why we have breathalyser tests. Relaxation helps some stutterers to control their speech, but alcohol interferes with the co-ordination of most stutterers' systems and makes their speech worse. Theoretically, enough alcohol to relax the stutterer but not sufficient to interfere appreciably with his co-ordination should improve his fluency. The effects will vary from person to person and there's no harm in doing a few enjoyable experiments.

Do you stutter on your own?

I can read aloud and speak on my own fairly fluently if I am careful to keep my rate of speech below eighty words a minute, to prolong words, and to approach the first sounds of words gently. Nevertheless stress enters my speech after a while, and I have to watch techniques very carefully indeed or I start to block. Even talking to a dog or cat can increase the blocks, and when I tape my speech it is difficult to keep it under control for long.

Some stutterers have no difficulty at all speaking when alone, and some have more difficulty than I do. The fact that people stutter when freed from audience pressures is hard to explain, but it may be that some are so conditioned to connect speaking with anxiety that the stress builds up, feeds back to the speech, and disrupts co-ordination.

Some stutterers are said to have controlled their stuttering by standing on mountain tops or lonely beaches and declaiming loudly and at length to imaginary audiences. One winter I tried this on Ben Macdhui, a mountain in Scotland, and startled a flock of white ptarmigan, which crackled away to cries of, 'Go-back, go-back, go-back.' I followed their suggestion, but my speech was no better.

Why do you stutter in some situations and not in others?

Whenever a stutterer approaches a speech situation and begins to speak he must deal with the anxieties and uncertainties that affect his speech. Memories of penalties, frustrations, situation fears, and difficult words or sounds initiate and increase these anxieties. For decades I was as conditioned as Pavlov's dog to go into a major block whenever a taxi driver requested my destination or a telephone operator asked for my name and number. I was reacting to old memories of repeated speech failures in these situations. Some people with speech handicaps, battered by parental, teacher, and peer disapproval, develop feelings of guilt and low self-regard ('What a fool I am not to be able to speak!'). Others, shunned by society and bolted in their glass towers, become filled with frustration, anger, and hostility. All these emotions affect the speech.

The importance of the spoken message can affect a person's fluency. Many stutterers when faced by a life-or-death situation that can only be resolved verbally, are rendered mute. Others, like myself, become completely fluent. Most find that the more important the words, the worse the speech.

Fortunately, there are factors that improve the speech. A

stutterer with high self-regard, good morale, and confidence in himself can bulldoze his way through difficult speaking situations. Success breeds success, and the more fluent a stutterer feels, the more fluent he tends to become.

Charles Van Riper[11] of Western Michigan University combined these factors into a simple model:

$$S = \frac{PFAGH + SfWf + Cs}{M + Fl}$$

where S is the frequency and severity of stuttering, P is penalties; F, frustrations; A, anxiety; G, guilt; H, hostility; Sf, situation fears caused by old memories; Wf, word fear; Cs, communication content; M, morale or confidence; and Fl, amount of felt fluency.

This looks complicated, but all it means is that the factors on the top line increase the stutter and those below the line reduce the stutter. An individual may not feel that all of these factors apply to him, but most will admit that P, F, Sf, and Wf play a major part in their speech control. My main problems were always Sf and Cs, but I managed to develop a strong M which enabled me to communicate fairly well.

Different speaking situations bring different factors to bear on the speech, and a stutterer cannot always predict which emotions will develop and how powerful they will be. Sometimes he starts to speak sure that he is going to block and yet is remarkably fluent. At other times he feels confident and becomes speechless. Good therapy helps him to control his speech even when he is buffeted by conflicting influences and feelings; but without therapy his speech is vulnerable to even minor changes in circumstances or attitude. The answer to the question about why people stutter in some situations and not in others is locked in the labyrinths of our brains.

Will you always stutter? Won't it just go away?

In my case I can be fairly sure that my stutter will not just go away. Although I may learn to control it to the point of 90 per cent fluency, I shall always stutter. This does not apply to everybody. In many cases, particularly in young people, a stutter disappears of its own accord.

Stuttering usually begins in childhood, and between 42 and 81 per cent of children who develop the impediment spontaneously lose it.[12] The age of recovery varies, but some experts feel there is a tendency for stuttering to disappear between the ages of thirteen and twenty years. Studies in Britain suggested a far earlier recovery, and, in one town, a third of the children recovered from transient stuttering by the age of four.[13] The statistics are confused by differences in criteria of what constitutes stuttering. Some so-called early stuttering may have been within the range of normal childish disfluency. Nevertheless, it is safe to say that about half the stutters developed in early childhood more or less disappear, and that spontaneous recovery tends to occur with children who have the less severe speech problems, as you would expect.[14] The reasons for spontaneous recovery are far from clear.

Even stutterers who recover completely, or rapidly improve, can deteriorate in conditions of stress. My own stutter began to fade and caused me few inconveniences between the ages of thirteen and eighteen. However, three years of exposure to the stresses, bangs, and bumps of war caused a steady deterioration in my speech, until I was barely able to communicate at all.

Even in moments of intense anxiety a stutter can have its funny side. A colleague and I were crouching in a slit trench while the opposition noisily tried to turn us into a protein mulch. I kept saying, 'Oh sh____, sh____. Oh sh____, sh____,' until my friend yelled in my ear, 'Telling 'em to shush won't stop them, you idiot!'

'I'm not shushing,' I roared back, angrily and fluently. 'I'm trying to say "Oh shit!" '

Does forcing a left-handed child to use his right hand make him stutter?

My usual reply is that there is no solid evidence that forcing right-handedness on a left-handed child causes a stutter, but my position is undermined a little by the fact that I am ambidextrous, can write with both hands, and got into trouble at school when I held a mug in my left hand!

Early societies tended to look askance at left-handed people as abnormal members of society. The grim word 'sinister' means left. Even in the opening decades of this century there were campaigns in the United States to abolish left-handedness in public schools by compulsion. Early surveys of schools in London, England, revealed that 17 per cent of congenitally left-handed children forced to write with their right hands developed stutters, suggesting that shifting handedness caused the stuttering.[15] Results from later research conflicted with this view; some of the 'shifted' stutterers had developed the impediment before they learned to write.[16]

Since then, a great deal of conflicting information has been collected. The general conclusion reached by Bloodstein in his review of left-handedness and stuttering is that, although some scientists still feel that in some cases a shift of handedness may contribute to the onset of stuttering, stutterers do not differ from non-stutterers in their handedness.[17] Nevertheless, the asymmetry of the brain is still regarded by some scientists as one possible root of the complex problem.

How does a person with a severe stutter cope with life?

My response to this is 'Remarkably well considering the circumstances!' This is not true for people who stutter very severely and have no marketable skills or characteristics that society values. They can be very lonely and unhappy and usually find it hard to get jobs.

In order to survive and do well a person who stutters badly must be determined, skilful, and courageous. He must learn to deal several times a day with traumatic situations that would seriously impair the confidence, self-regard, and even mental health of many people with normal speech. The stutterer strives to maintain his self-esteem and to ignore the adverse responses of other people to his handicap. Some stutterers may appear to be arrogant, but it is usually a reflection of their survival equipment.

Although therapists deplore stutterers' attempts to avoid situations because of their disfluency, it is necessary to be realistic. A severe stutterer would be a fool (and a pauper) if he were to embark on a career as a criminal lawyer. Most of us choose our vocations with care, taking into account our interests, skills, and vocal capabilities; even so, it is not easy and can go awry. One stutterer trained to become an expert on Shakespeare, but found it impossible to get a job in his field and went into horticulture. Another qualified in economics and became a store clerk. The vocal demands of various professions may push stutterers into jobs they did not originally want.

Stutterers tend to plan their day's activities carefully. This is possible if you can allocate your own time and do things at your own pace in your own way, but few of us enjoy those luxuries. I used to go over all the speech situations I was likely to meet and design ways of dealing with them. Many people who stutter have told me how they begin every day with cold, stomach-churning fear of the many foreseeable situations they know they cannot handle. As one man said to me, 'You take your fear of speaking to bed with you, it greets you when you wake in the morning, and it walks beside you all the day.' Stutterers are experts at dealing with fear, anxiety, and rejection.

I was at a scientific conference in Spain where a Dutchman read an excellent scientific paper in English. He had a stutter and was nervous, but coped by using speech techniques effectively. There were a few fifteen-second pauses as he collected his speech and calmed his nerves, but they did not interfere unduly with the flow of information. It was an incredibly good performance. A couple of young Ivy League Americans were sitting beside me, the kind of born-again laboratory scientists who think that only they and their work are of any consequence. They began to laugh, and one of them said, 'The stuttering fool's wasting our time!'

I gave myself ten seconds to curb the flare of anger, then leaned across and burned their ears long and fluently. I pointed out that since neither of them had the professionalism to look beyond the stutter and listen to the useful paper, or the humanity to admire the way the speaker coped with his impediment, they were more handicapped than he was. They walked out of the meeting.

Someone once said, 'Show me a stutterer and I'll show you an angry man.' It is not true to say that stutterers are usually angry people, but they all have to learn to control their tempers when faced by rudeness and brutality. You can't go around modifying people's facial topography all the time.

Small boys who stutter severely are inclined to explode from frustration and punch the nearest tormentor. My father was understandably annoyed when a parent sent him a large dentist's bill for restructuring the front teeth of a son who had had the poor judgment to mimic my stuttering.

People who stutter develop extra keen senses in the same manner that blind people have acutely sensitive touch and hearing. Some stutterers tend to develop the non-verbal components of communication to such an extent that their acute interpretation of body language and synthesis of visual factors can be mistaken for telepathy. A few stuttering individuals can read eye, face, hand, and body signals so well that they have earned their living on the stage as so-called mind readers. This acute visual awareness makes some stutterers foresee people's needs and sense what is going to happen before it happens to an extent that can be disturbing.

Not many stutterers use their impediment deliberately to avoid situations. I did so once, to avoid being forced by the bilingual program in Canada to spend a year away from my research learning French, which I would seldom use. I knew a young soldier who in sheer desperation deliberately increased his stutter and tics to a grotesque degree to discourage a predatory woman with wedding bells ringing in her ears.

Fortunately people can carry on and live under unbelievable hardships. Some stutterers bend beneath the weight of their struggles to speak, while others look upon their stuttering as a challenge and become stronger than most people with normal speech. Nietzsche once wrote, 'That which does not kill me, makes me stronger.' Provided life, or even a handicap, has meaning, people can cope despite pain and deprivation.

Has the stutter held you back in life?

All the severe stutterers who discussed with me the extent to which their impediment controls their lives were unanimous in the view that stuttering hindered their progress more than anything else. I agreed with them until I was asked by my therapist to make a presentation to about forty people about how my stuttering had affected my life.

Before the presentation I drew up a flow-chart, like a good scientist, and examined the main factors that had determined my career decisions and my life's directions. To my great surprise I found that, although the stuttering had caused me many frustrations and problems, it had affected the direction of my life much less than a minor defect in my vision and my inherited personality. The defective eyesight prevented me from going to a naval academy at fourteen years of age and later barred me from becoming a fighter pilot. It probably saved my life. My personality is optimistic, and I more or less ignored my impediment when making career decisions. If people let me – which sometimes they don't – I just cope with the problems my stuttering causes as they crop up.

Although I more or less flunked my public-speaking test by getting the jitters, the presentation helped me to see my handicap objectively. This, I suspect, was the real intention of my crafty therapist.

Of course a stutter is important in a person's career, but it is only one of many influences. Personal skills and character can still be the main influences on lifestyle even when a person cannot communicate effectively.

Does a stutter affect your health?

I chaired a meeting on one of those days when my speech was in an unpredictable downswing. Afterwards a friend asked, 'Does a stutter hurt?' and I replied, 'No, of course not, although the tension can give me a headache.' This was followed by another question asking whether or not stuttering affects a person's health. I replied, 'Probably,' without any solid evidence to support me.

You don't have to be a physician to know that exposure to excessive stress for long periods can undermine your health. Stress is all very well in its place and can be the spice of life, but when it occurs too often and too strongly and is accompanied by frustration and anxiety, the spice tends to turn sour. The stresses caused by stuttering are not always of the healthy kind.

Early research on stuttering focused on physiological and psychological phenomena, but few reports discuss the possible effects on general health and longevity. During stuttering there can be antagonism between abdominal and thoracic breathing and irregularity of breathing cycles. When a stutterer blocks, breathing can cease.[18] I once saw a stutterer faint from a prolonged block; he just ran out of oxygen. During stuttering there is often an acceleration of the heart rate and a change in the distribution of the blood, as well as a decrease in the blood's total sugar and blood protein.[19] Surprisingly, little definitive information about the blood pressure of stutterers was located, although many of the middle-aged male stutterers I meet suffer to some extent from hypertension – which is to be expected in a frequently stressed person.

These symptoms arise in non-stutterers when they are excited or stressed, but people who stutter are exposed to excessive stress so often that it seems likely that their health will be affected in the long run. It would be interesting to see figures comparing the incidence of hypertension and heart complaint in middle-aged stutterers and non-stutterers. You are probably better off without a stutter as far as your general health is concerned.

Does it help to speak slowly?

Yes, it does. Most stutterers try to speak far too quickly as they try to get the words over with before they stumble and block. For a stutterer, speaking quickly is about as wise as running over ground strewn with jagged boulders in the dark instead of picking his way carefully step by step. He's likely to fall painfully on his fanny.

Most people speak at a rate of about 150 to 200 words per minute (wpm), although two of my daughters communicate in a verbal deluge of 200 to 300 wpm. Most untreated stutterers try to get out about 150 wpm or more when most of them can only cope with 60 wpm or less. The majority of speech pathologists start treatment by reducing the patient's speech rate to 30 to 40 wpm, and most stutterers can keep fluent in the clinic at these rates if they prolong their words. Unfortunately, prolonged speech at 30 wpm is a little bizarre and not really socially acceptable; although, as the therapists say, it's far better than going into a block, running out of breath, twitching, and closing your eyes as you fight to ask the way to the washroom.

Reducing speech rate is not as easy as it sounds. All people delude themselves about how fast they talk. I sat for days with a stop-watch and tape recorder before I managed to bring my speech rate down from a torrential 200 wpm to 60 wpm or less. The slow speech sounded like a 78 rpm record played at 33 rpm, but I was much more fluent. After a while I learned to feel my speech rate. When I felt tension entering my speech, I knew that I was exceeding my optimum speech rate of 80 wpm. The speech-rate control worked in the therapy sessions, but it was not the whole answer. Outside the clinic the slow speech was penalized by the startled expressions on listeners' faces and was not rewarded by the beams of approval the heavy-footed words earned in the clinic.

One bit of advice will help both stutterers and clutterers. Speak slowly and smoothly, on oiled wheels, as slowly as you can. It won't harm and it could be a great help.

Technology has entered the picture with an electronic speech-rate monitor called the Hector Speech Aid.[20] The principle is that when a person who stutters speaks too quickly, the gadget emits a warning tone. The aim is to help those who have difficulty feeling their speech rate to regulate their speech speed, and to remind people like myself to slow down when they begin to gabble. I am considering buying each of my fast-talking daughters one of these speech-rate monitors for Christmas.

Can a stutter be cured?

The simple answer is that it is unlikely that an adult with a severe, long-established stutter will ever be *completely* cured by the clinical methods available today. Young children and adolescents may be 'cured,' but not adults.

This is not as gloomy as it sounds, because most people who stutter can, if they co-operate fully, be taught to control their stuttering to the extent that it is no longer a social embarrassment or a handicap in the workplace. They can learn to communicate without major interruptions and express their thoughts and feelings much more freely. Every year scientists gain deeper insights into stuttering and more patients respond to better treatment. The sooner a person with a stutter comes for treatment, the more the clinicians can help him. The various treatments for stuttering are described in a later chapter. Here it suffices to say that a person with a very severe stutter (like mine) can be helped more than he imagines in his wildest dreams. The future is bright.

People will come up with other, more difficult questions. It is hoped that the rest of this book will provide a few of the answers.

THREE

The bending of the twig

' 'Tis education forms the common mind.
Just as the twig is bent, the tree's inclined.'

Alexander Pope

The roots of most stuttering reach down into early childhood.
The problem can begin when the child utters his first stumbling words and solicitous parents lean over the crib and
marvel at the cleverness of such a morsel of humanity in being able to speak so clearly. They may encourage or even
pressure the babe to say more words as clearly as possible as
soon as possible and lovingly marvel at his precocity, thereby
sowing the seeds of a stutter. These seeds may or may not ger-
minate and grow. It depends upon the child.

People are prone to jump to the conclusion that all stutters
were caused by unhappy childhoods. Many stutterers can
remember being unhappy when they were children, but so
can many people who don't have problems with their speech.
In any case, happiness is hard to define, and expecting early
childhood to be free from stress and frustration is unrealistic.

There are volumes of learned papers about the frequency
of stuttering in people of different ages, social levels, and
races. The findings of the scientists are contradictory, but
there is a common thread running through the reports. There
is good evidence that stuttering is frequent in societies that expect children to conform to rigid patterns of behaviour and to
develop and display speaking skills when very young. Stutters
seem to flourish where social pressures are brought to bear

early in life, and it is fair to say that stuttering is to some extent a social complaint.

Pressures on young children

If young children were to be freed from all social pressures and strictures there would be anarchy in the nursery. Little twigs need to be gently bent to grow in directions that will make them happy, useful, and acceptable members of society. The question is how to do so without creating fertile ground in which stuttering and other problems can develop.

Those of us who were raised in the first third of this century were encouraged to read worthy books designed to hammer into our heads the Victorian ideals of courage, honour, truth, duty, and other virtues now regarded as outmoded, while our teachers gave us ample opportunity to develop and demonstrate stoicism as they whacked the same values into our other ends. One of the best pictures of those days is found in Desmond Coke's *The Bending of the Twig*, a book that describes dispassionately how boys were painfully but effectively moulded into the form demanded by a strict society. It was the way things were. Few people, not even the children, regarded the process as unkind.

Books of this genre show that it was perfectly normal to force children to conform to clearly defined patterns of behaviour, and pressures like these persist to this day in different and less physical forms. Modern educators condemn the corporal disciplining of children in the earlier school systems as brutal and uncivilized, but some modern, so-called psychological methods of disciplining a child through peer pressure, ridicule, and guilt can be no less brutal. The application of intense emotional pressure can inflict lasting pain. In the old system, the person who was most feared and hated was not the teacher with the switch but the one with a sarcastic, cutting tongue who could shrivel a child's self-respect to the size of a peanut with a few carefully chosen words. Pressures are pressures whether they are physical or mental.

Competitive Western society has never been particularly kind to its children, and intense pressures to behave in certain ways are still brought to bear as soon as the umbilical cord has been cut. There are people who expose the developing foetus to high levels of oxygen in the hope that the child will become a genius. Pressures on a young child begin at home, but they immediately escalate when apprehensive small fry are thrown into the educational fish pond where they are urged to communicate well in public and to *Achieve* with a capital 'A.'

Contrary to what most school children think, teachers are ordinary people trying to do a job as best they can. Some are kind, some are indifferent, and a few are brutally sadistic. The majority mean well. It is curious, therefore, that a number of stuttering adults I have met felt that, although other children could be cruel, the ridicule and insensitivity of their teachers caused their worst problems. Even today I hear hair-raising stories about teachers' thoughtless cruelty to children slightly handicapped by impaired speech, or sight, or hearing but not enough to warrant special education. The cruelty most frequently takes the shape of ridicule. The stuttering child may be made the class scapegoat, or may thoughtlessly be asked to carry out tasks that, because of his partial handicap, are beyond his capabilities. 'Partial' is the key word; teachers can deal with someone who is completely mute, deaf, or blind. They simply send him to a specialist.

Most teachers who maltreat handicapped children are not vicious, cruel people. They merely suffer from insensitivity, impatience, and a shortage of time to think about and allow for a child's physical and mental shortcomings. I clearly remember being taken to task at the age of eight when I biffed an impatient, frustrated English teacher on her belly-button for mimicking my speech. She sat down on the floor and displayed to all the class her thick, dark-blue knickers, which were secured by yellow ribbons just above her knees. She was, in fact, a nice person, but she never forgave me.

If you have a stutter, a funny accent, a long nose, sticky-out teeth, big ears, a wandering eye, slightly webbed feet, a slight limp, or a facial lump, or are fat, skinny, or unusual in any way and have not been unduly penalized in the safe cocoon of home, you soon will be when you go to school. Young children are likely to chomp their milk teeth into any companion who has the misfortune to look strange or act differently from the herd. Sending a stuttering child to school is like throwing a kitten into the dog pound, but the kitten must take its chances in the mêlée of life and develop sufficient agility and sharp enough claws to survive.

School is tough even for children who speak normally. Those who stutter are under greater pressure than others in the school system, and this tends to make the stuttering worse. Today, teachers are more understanding and better trained than when I was at school, and there are often speech therapists (albeit overworked ones) to assist the school's staff. Nevertheless, the child must still cope with the classroom jungle. Some stuttering children accept defeat and leave school early. Those who remain must struggle to survive.

A therapist once asked me what I felt about my early days at school. I replied that it was one long fight. Most stutterers I have met feel the same.[1]

Stuttering in primitive societies

Some primitive societies provide a clue to the relationship between social pressures and the development of stuttering in young children. In some tribes stuttering is rare. There may not even be a word for the disorder in their languages. Investigations of 6,000 people in eight tribes in New Guinea revealed no stutterers, and the impediment appeared to be rare in Australian aborigines. Anthropologist Margaret Mead never saw stuttering in the people of New Guinea and the South Pacific, and in the first half of this century stuttering was unknown in certain groups of Eskimos.[2]

Studies of speech defects of North American Indians provided insights into the effects of social pressures on children. During the 1930s, the Bannock and Shoshone Indians lived on isolated reservations in southeastern Idaho where the impact of European social customs was minimal. John C. Snidecor, who studied these tribes from 1937 to 1939, once asked the tribal council if they knew any stuttering Indians. They didn't have a word for stuttering in their language and didn't know what the researcher was talking about. Snidecor had to demonstrate what stuttering looked and sounded like, and the chiefs thought his antics very funny indeed. Nevertheless, the scientist offered a reward to anybody who could find a *bona fide* stuttering Indian. The hunt was on.[3]

I like to imagine what happened when Snidecor interviewed 800 people and demonstrated stuttering by blocking and repeating to audiences who hadn't the faintest idea what it was all about. There must have been a few hilarious moments. Snidecor had great difficulty finding any Indians with definite stutters.

In these non-stuttering Indian societies there was little or no cultural pressure on children. They were not expected to speak and perform until adolescence and were permitted a great deal of freedom. They were not forced to conform with rigid cultural standards, and a child was not likely to be criticized for the way he spoke. The tribes looked upon speech development as a normal part of growing up, and interference in the process by solicitous parents for purposes of display was not encouraged.[4]

The Indians of the Northwest coast – for example, the Kwakiutl, the Nootka, and the Salish tribes – were just the opposite. Edwin Lemert, a social anthropologist from the University of California, observed large numbers of individuals with stutters in these tribes, which also had words for stuttering in their language and even rituals to treat the disability.[5] Speech defects of this kind were commonplace, and memories of stuttering ancestors went back to the first half of the nineteenth century, before European cultures had much impact.

These tribes, which lived by salmon fishing, were fiercely competitive communities and brought severe pressures to bear on very young children. There were bitter clan rivalries, and so the prestige and status of the clan and its families were of prime importance. People were valued when their prowess reflected favourably on the tribe, and weakness and nonconformity were frowned upon. Young children were expected to comply with clearly defined codes of behaviour and were rigorously taught to participate in public rituals under the critical eye of clan members. Poor verbal delivery, mistakes in procedure, and differences in appearance and behaviour were not acceptable.

People with such handicaps as left-handedness, obesity, smallness, lameness, and impaired speech were treated with scorn and rejected by the clan because they reflected badly on the group. Anybody with hesitant speech must have had a bad time in this competitive, intolerant society. Unfortunately, there are many parallels in modern Western society where competitive tribes tend to develop in the workplace.

Surveys of the stuttering Cowichan Indians of Vancouver Island in Canada and of the non-stuttering Ute Indians supported Lemert's results.[6] The Cowichans, with their stutterers, were competitive and less permissive in child raising than the fluent Utes, who allowed children to develop at their own rates. Stuttering was common in the Idoma and Ibo peoples of West Africa. As many as 2.6 per cent of the Ibos stuttered in a society where verbal communication and the ability to speak in public were important. Orators were greatly admired, and children who were not fluent were slapped and ridiculed by their parents. The people of this highly competitive tribe expected children to be successful in school and provided an environment where a child was likely to develop anxieties about his speech if he were at all disfluent.[7]

Stuttering is known in the Bantu tribe of South Africa and was present before the arrival of white settlers. Bantu and European societies have similar attitudes toward developing fluency, and it is interesting that the frequencies of stuttering (about 1 per cent) in the two societies are similar.[8]

Modern speech pathologists question that there are societies with no stutterers, but there is no doubt that stuttering is much more common in some groups than in others. It is often said that stuttering is more common in Japan than elsewhere, but there is little evidence to support this view. The idea may have originated in a misinterpretation of Lemert's averral that stuttering in Japan is relatively frequent compared with other Pacific societies, where it is rare.

The frequency of stuttering in Japan is an enigma, and estimates vary considerably. Although Japanese children are raised strictly in a conformist society, it has been estimated that about 0.82 per cent of the children stutter.[9] Surprisingly, this is a little less than the average 1 per cent. The Tokyo

Speech Clinic indicated that the data available suggest that only 0.05 per cent of the populace stutter, but felt that the reason for this very low estimate is that Japanese stutterers are ashamed of their hesitancy, tend to hide their problem, don't seek help, and hence are not recorded in the surveys.[10]

Surveys of children show considerable variation from nation to nation and even between towns in the same country. On average about 1 per cent stutter, but in Prague, Czechoslovakia, for example, only 0.55 per cent of 26,000 children stuttered, while 1.82 per cent of 875,384 children studied in Poland stuttered. About 0.93 per cent of the children of a Moslem nation such as Egypt stutter, which is about the same for the Christian society of Denmark (0.90 per cent). The American town of Tuscaloosa, Alabama, had a great many stuttering children (2.12 per cent) in 1973 compared to the Rocky Mountain region (0.30 per cent) in 1969. The stuttering male:female ratio is low in Tuscaloosa (2.7:1) and very high in the Rockies (6:1).[11]

What causes these differences and similarities? Is it the attitude of parents toward their children, the pressures of society, the phonetic complexity of language, or inherited abnormalities? Nobody knows. The answer probably lies in the interaction of many human and environmental factors. Perhaps some day a systems analyst will put it all together in a computer and provide the answer, or at least help us to ask the right questions.

A child is capable of bringing upon himself intense pressures to communicate that could affect his speech before he goes to school, quite apart from pressures from the family and society. I suspect that I was one of these self-starters, because, although my memory goes back to the age of two years, I have no memories of family demands to conform and perform. There was certainly sibling rivalry, and my father was a formidable figure whom we treated with huge respect and addressed with polite caution, but there were few strictures on how we spoke and no penalties for imperfect syntax. Nevertheless, I certainly stuttered when I went to school at the age of five. I couldn't answer my name at roll call on the first day and was soundly spanked for dumb insolence.

I know from my memories and checking with my family

that I was a mentally active child, spilling over with curiosity and wonder about my new world and constantly saying 'Why?' I don't remember anxiety about speaking, but I can still recall the intense frustration of not being able to put my childish thoughts, feelings, and questions into words because I had not yet mastered language and had such a limited vocabulary.

When a child learns that his parents and siblings don't understand what he says, this leads to fears about isolation from the family group. It takes a child time to learn to cope with frustration and isolation. Impeded communication can be as great a pressure as fear of speaking.

Western society, with its increasing emphasis on early achievement and with the high value it places on the spoken word, is a fertile breeding ground for stuttering. Impatience and intolerance are commonplace in the home and workplace. As people strive for material things they tend to ignore human values. An awareness by teachers and parents that early social pressures can damage a child who is only slightly impaired or a little slow to develop would be a start. Unfortunately, many parents and teachers were raised in the pressure-cooker of the Western educational system and, as they survived, cannot see much wrong with it. As the prophet Ezekiel said, when fathers eat sour grapes, the children's teeth are set on edge.

I know a tall husky man with a severe stutter who lives on the rolling farmlands of Ontario. He smiles a great deal and loves to meet people. His outgoing manner helps him to make friends easily. He plays the fiddle, revels in a party, and has great fun with singing roles in amateur theatricals. He enjoys life. As a child he walked a mile or two to school. For several years the bigger boys used to lie in wait for him and beat him up nearly every day, just because he stuttered. At school the busy teacher, impatient with the boy's slowness in answering questions and reading aloud, publicly labelled him stupid. How he managed to grow up into a warm and friendly adult is a mystery.

FOUR

What causes a stutter?

'To harmonize the pressures exerted by society and by the individuals' drives is the greatest problem of human life.'

Abraham Meyerson

Charles Van Riper described the origins of a stutter in terms of a river and its sources.[1] The river is there for all to see, but any attempt to trace it back to its source is complicated by the fact that high up in the hills it is fed by many small streams. It is impossible to say which one is the main source.

A child starts off with his inherited physical and mental equipment – his constitution – which, as the child grows older will be affected by what he experiences and learns. The tempo of life increases, and so does speech development. In these early stages any stuttering problems can be easily treated, but some children get swept along on emotional currents they find hard to control. Gradually, if the speech remains impeded, the child meets frustration and fear and by then is in real trouble. Without help he will be swept by life into the whirlpool of self-reinforcement, where stuttering breeds anxiety, which increases stuttering – a closed cycle that is the unenviable fate of many adults. They can only be rescued by well-designed therapy and great determination.

Although scientists have sought the single cause of a stutter for centuries, most modern experts accept that many factors are involved. Some psychologists still cling to the idea of a single neurotic origin; however, even if such neuroses exist, their effects are likely to be shaped by the pressures of life.

Most people have childhood problems of one kind or another, but most people don't stutter.

Numerous attempts have been made by scientists to find an organic cause for stuttering in, for example, abnormalities of brain structure and/or biochemistry, but the results of research are conflicting. Other authorities favour such so-called non-organic reasons as neuroses, fears of speaking, and faulty speech techniques.

Non-organic phenomena, like neuroses and fear, originate in our brain's chemistry, so that differentiating between organic and non-organic causes of stuttering is fundamentally questionable. Nevertheless, the two categories are useful in that they neatly separate the two therapeutic approaches: the one focusing on a person's physical make-up and the other on his attitudes and speech techniques. The second approach is the most common.

Whether a child is predisposed to stutter by a physical quirk of brain structure and chemistry, which may or may not be triggered by his life's experiences, is still a point in question. Many researchers speak of the 'syndrome' of stuttering, implying a set of symptoms; and this is perhaps the best way to think of a stutter – as a speech abnormality consisting of a set of interacting factors that vary from one person to another. Any attempt to attribute individual causes would be premature, although most speech pathologists have their own private and, so far, unprovable hunches.

There are so many factors that could contribute to the onset of a stutter and perpetuate the impediment that novice speech-therapy students tend to raise their hands in horror and take up some other profession. It is necessary, however, to be aware of these factors in order to understand their complexity and how difficult it is to treat the stutter as a whole.

If at times my tone is irreverent, I offer the plea that some of the theories tested on me did not fit my stutter when I participated as a guinea pig in speech research. Some of the ideas seemed very funny at the time. Nevertheless these theories may fit other stutters much better than mine. While I smile at these ideas, I do not mean to deride them.

According to H.R. Beech and Fay Fransella of the University of London, England, 'Stuttering theory, in general, does not reflect the kind of progressive change and refinement which one might expect from a developing science. To some extent the field may suffer as a result of being treated as one of the social sciences, and perhaps it is the case that the "hard facts" which are necessary to the foundation of a satisfactory science are lacking and difficult to discover.'[2] A friend who is a frustrated speech pathologist stated this much more succinctly: 'It's a can of worms!'

The labyrinth of the mind

Psychologists have theorized for nearly a century about the possibility that stuttering is an expression of urgent but unconscious needs with roots in the nursing and toilet-training stages of development and in the earliest and most primitive of a baby's satisfactions. The 'Repressed Need Theory' is that a stutterer unconsciously wishes to stutter in order to gratify these unconscious needs. This is probably the origin of the incautious layman's belief that a stutterer can choose not to stutter. He inflicts his stutter on himself because he wants to – so let him get on with it! Even if the repressed need theory were correct, the wish would be unconscious, and a stutterer would need lengthy psychotherapy to consciously control it. This theory *may* apply to *some* stutterers, since people stutter for such a variety of reasons, including psychological abnormality, abnormal brain structure and function, and physical injury.

Psychoanalysis of many stutterers has produced no conclusive evidence one way or the other that stuttering originates from a repression of infantile needs. For a while this theory was very much in vogue. It was the basis of treatment of stuttering and many other disabilities, but is less widely accepted today. We are all products of our genes, chemistry, experience, and environment. Events, emotions, and needs encountered during our early childhood affect us for the rest of our lives. Whether we like it or not, the small child exists within us even though we may not recognize it as such. We learn to live with it. As Nietzsche wrote, 'In every real man a child is hidden that wants to play.'

Memories of infantile needs may affect a stutter – since

practically every emotion and change in environment seem to do so – but labelling repressed need as the main or sole cause of stuttering seems to be unjustified. It may be one of the numerous tributaries feeding the mainstream of the stutter, but it is not likely to be the main source of the whole river.

Shortly after World War II a grateful government offered to pay psychoanalysts to seek out the cause of my severe stutter if I would act as a guinea pig for the mind-benders. An official made it quite clear that it would be good for me, like a dose of Epsom Salts. He left no doubt in my mind that he thought that anyone who stuttered was nuts. Since I was between jobs, as it were, and the expense allowance was attractive, I accepted.

My mentor was a serious, unsmiling young man, full to overflowing with the teachings of good old Sigmund Freud. It was a period when psychologists and psychiatrists tended to see everything you said, dreamed, or did in terms of Freudian symbolism. After the long period of Victorian taboos about mentioning any part of the anatomy lower than the chin, Freud gave people a marvellous reason to talk about their reproductive bits and pieces. Freud doubtless brought mental health out of the Dark Ages, but he would be horrified if he could see how many of his disciples have gone overboard in their interpretation of his theories when there is so little evidence to support their views.

North America adopted these ideas with such enthusiasm that every flag-pole, cigar, or linear object came under suspicion as a symbol of some dark and sexy motivation. Maybe that's why church steeples went out of fashion in most of Canada and the United States and were replaced by horrible, soulless triangles and cubes of no possible naughty significance. (The exception is, of course, Quebec. French Canadians kept their steeples, which will doubtless give Freudian sociologists something to write doctoral theses about.)

When I started the analysis I soon learned that the difference between a psychologist and a psychiatrist is that the latter can stick needles in you and the former can't. Within a short time I became a pincushion.

At one session my serious young man pumped me full of pentothal. As I floated on a warm, comfortable, carefree cloud, he asked me a strange question. I read the transcript later and I remember my replies clearly:

DOCTOR: Now just relax. *(I was already paralysed.)* Can you hear me?

ME: Mmmm.

DOCTOR: Tell me, now, which of your testicles is lower than the other?

ME: You're joking?

DOCTOR: No, this is serious. Please tell me.

ME: *(Silence)*

DOCTOR: What's wrong?

ME: I'm thinking. Wouldn't you?

DOCTOR: Come along now. Surely you know.

ME: I haven't the faintest idea.

DOCTOR: Nonsense! You must know. We *all* know.

ME: Do you know which of yours is lowest?

DOCTOR: That's beside the point.

ME: I couldn't put it better myself. *(Low chuckle)*

DOCTOR: *(Long silence)* Try to remember. Haven't you ever looked?

ME: I just don't know. I guess I've never looked that closely.

DOCTOR: You've never looked? Oh come now! Can you tell me if you have two of them?

ME: My God! Are you implying I've got more than two? I *demand* a recount!

End of session. In fact, it was the end of the experiment because he said that I was the only patient he knew who could crack jokes, argue, and tell downright lies when I was nearly unconscious. I was not a suitable guinea pig.

The real reason for my ignorance about my anatomy was that in the Armed Forces the only mirror I possessed was very small, bent, and made of scratched polished steel. I used it for shaving. It was not designed for wider surveys.

My young analyst was hot on the track of things like repressed needs and low self-awareness, but I was a grave disappointment to him because he found remarkably little wrong with my mental health. I learned a great deal about myself and the way the human mind works, and both have been invaluable. I shall always be grateful to him even when I chuckle at his expense.

Supporters of the repressed need theory have several arrows in their quiver. They feel that a stutter may satisfy an infantile need to recall the oral gratifications of breast-feeding; may attempt to satisfy anal erotic needs by recalling infantile satisfactions; or may hide hostile feelings that the person who stutters is scared to display. They hypothesize that the stutterer chews words in order symbolically to cannibalize his parents; or achieves silence in the face of social pressures to speak in order to avoid uttering obscenities.[3] However, many stutterers I know have no trouble at all uttering four-letter words when they are angry. Adults with anal obsessions apparently exhibit excessive moral rectitude, punctuality, stinginess, and orderliness, whereas most of the stutterers I know are messy, generous, not excessively moral, and not particularly punctual. The hat doesn't seem to fit. These anal characteristics are, however, a fair definition of what is generally required in a good public servant.

The scientific evidence suggests that the average stutterer is not unusually neurotic or severely maladjusted. He doesn't appear to have any special characteristics that set him apart from non-stutterers except his strange way of speaking. Some stutterers may not be so well adjusted to society as non-stutterers; and some do suffer from low self-esteem, anxiety, hostility, and an unwillingness to take risks. All these are to be expected considering the nature of the impediment and the frequently adverse responses of society to disfluency.

It is important to bear in mind that while no fundamental neurosis has been shown to be a general cause of stuttering, all people who stutter severely experience fear of speaking, anxiety, and frustration every day of their lives. These powerful emotions are integral parts of stuttering, and their control is of vital importance in therapy. It is here that the psychiatrists and psychologists have an important role to play.

In the previous chapter the relationship between stuttering and societies where children are expected to speak, perform, conform, and achieve at a very early age was discussed. There seems little doubt that social pressures and the fears arising from them are involved in the development of stuttering. This is, however, a matter of conscious fear and is not to be confused with such deeply rooted Freudian neuroses as unconscious repressed needs.

All of us are beset by mental problems every day. The important thing is how our problems manifest themselves and how we deal with them. Many seemingly normal people are handicapped by tremendous secret inner conflicts. The trouble with stuttering is that it is there for all to see whenever you speak.

Is stuttering inherited?

Stuttering parents often have stuttering offspring, but there is little concrete evidence that stuttering is inherited. Nevertheless, according to some scientists, recent evidence suggests that biological inheritance may play some role in stuttering. I know several stuttering parents with stuttering sons, but I also know many more stutterers, including myself, who have no other people with stutters in their family trees. Many non-stutterers have stuttering children. It is all too easy to jump to unsupported conclusions.

Parental attitudes and their effect on the way a child feels about speech may account for stuttering that runs in families. A parent who stutters is sure to be anxious about speaking. It goes with the territory. A stuttering parent is also likely to be apprehensive about a child's normal, early, stumbling speech as he learns to talk. There is always the fear that the child's minor disfluencies will develop into the stuttering that caused the parent so much anxiety and frustration. Unless the parent is sufficiently well-informed to be able to tell the difference between normal, childish disfluency and the tension, avoidance, and fear of words of a true stutter, he may try to correct the child, and punish him whenever he struggles to form words and sentences. There are many heartbreaking stories about stuttering parents slapping their children every time their speech stumbled in desperate attempts to spare the children their lifelong pain. Early association of fear, pain, disapproval, and anxiety with speaking is likely to increase a child's risk of becoming disfluent.

From 23 to 69 per cent of people who stutter have family histories of stuttering, while 1.3 to 42 per cent of non-stutterers have family histories of stuttering.[4] The two sets of percentages overlap considerably.

A detailed study was made of a family in Iowa in which 40 per cent of the family members stuttered. The family tree showed five generations of stutterers. The members were exceedingly conscious of their speech and believed their disorder was inherited. A genetic and social analysis indicated that the stuttering in the Iowa family arose from the fact that the family members themselves falsely diagnosed normal, early speech disfluencies as stuttering and acted accordingly. Twenty years after the stuttering family had been counselled about the problem only one in forty-four of the family stuttered.[5]

The fact that children develop stutters when raised away from their parents in communal institutions, such as *kibbutzim* in Israel, where they receive objective upbringing, has been interpreted as refuting the theory of environmental (i.e., parental) triggering of stuttering. Nevertheless, objective schooling away from the parents usually involves persuading the child to conform with institutional rather than parental standards in early life; the pressures may be different, but they are still there. Life in an institution is not usually warm-hearted and supportive. Even the word 'objective' has a cold ring to it.

If a predisposition to stuttering is inherited, it is likely to be controlled by many genes (polygenic inheritance) rather than by only one. Genes can interact with each other and with the environment. The factors that produce a stutter are exceedingly complex.

The occurrence of disorders in twins is a useful tool for probing whether a malady is controlled by the genes in our chromosomes. The classic case is schizophrenia. It has been known for many years that the average person has about a 1 per cent chance of developing schizophrenia, while the identical twin of a schizophrenic has a 50 per cent chance of developing the complaint. If a child is schizophrenic and has a non-identical twin, this twin has a 15 per cent chance of being schizophrenic. The same applies to non-twin brothers and sisters.[6]

Many studies of twins have been unsatisfactory because of small samples, inappropriate procedures, and differences in the way parents treat identical and non-identical twins. Seymour Kety and his colleagues in Massachusetts were aware of these shortcomings when they made a careful study of 5,000 adopted 20- to 45-year-old twins in Denmark.[7] Thirty-three of these people were schizophrenic and twenty-eight of the latter had been adopted as babies. The researchers located thirty-three non-schizophrenic adopters with similar backgrounds and surveyed the relatives of both schizophrenic and non-schizophrenic groups. None of the original, biological relatives of non-schizophrenic adopted children had schizophrenia, and the incidences of schizophrenia in the adoptive parents of adopted schizophrenics and non-schizophrenics were similar (2 to 4 per cent). As many as 10 per cent of the biological relatives of the schizophrenic adopters had schizophrenia. This carefully controlled experiment demonstrated that schizophrenia is genetically mediated.

It is well known that up to 13 per cent of individuals in twin pairs have stutters compared with about 1 per cent of the normal population. Conversely, 4.5 per cent of 461 stutterers studied had a twin, compared with 1.2 per cent in 500 non-stutterers. There is good reason to assume that stuttering and twinning are linked.

Although some researchers feel that this link between twinning and stuttering is genetic,[8] not all researchers are convinced that there is solid proof that stuttering is an inherited disorder. Stuttering develops in response to childhood pressures and stresses, whatever the initial cause. If one twin (particularly a close, identical twin) stutters severely, the other is likely to associate anxiety with speech and to be more likely to stutter than others. Identical twins are treated alike, and any censure of a stuttering member of the pair is likely to be felt by the other.

When a child is adopted and still develops a stutter, if he has a family history of stuttering it is easy to jump to the conclusion that, since he has been raised away from the influence of his stuttering parents or siblings, he is genetically predisposed to stutter and is responding to genes rather than to environment. Unfortunately, human nature again muddies the water. Not all people want to adopt a stuttering child or a child with a family history of stuttering. There is a tendency for people who stutter or who have stuttering relatives to be more sympathetic to a disfluent child and more ready to take him under their wing. Since such adoptive parents are aware of budding stuttering symptoms, they are also likely to check the child's speech, so that he may well develop a stutter in his new, sympathetic surroundings.

Bloodstein studied twelve adopted stutterers, and in only three cases was there stuttering in the adoptive family.[9] Again, this small sample suggests a possible hereditary basis, but genetic analysis of large stuttering families does not support this view. Conclusive evidence could be obtained from a rigorous, large-scale investigation of adopted, stuttering twins and their families similar to that carried out by Kety and his colleagues to confirm the genetic basis of schizophrenia. Perhaps the information already exists in Kety's files and just awaits analysis. His team studied 5,000 individuals and 4,967 of these were non-schizophrenic. In general about 1 per cent of people in Europe stutter, so about 50 of Kety's sample, including twins, would stutter. A survey of the incidence of stuttering in the biological and adoptive families of the stuttering twins and a comparable sample of non-stuttering twins would settle once and for all whether stuttering, or the predisposition to it, is mediated by genes.

The tools used to study whether stuttering is a genetic disorder have been relatively crude, and most of the discussions focus on how much of the stutter is genetically and how much environmentally caused. Even if stuttering is a genetic disorder, it is likely to be affected by the environment one way or the other. The gene effects could be very subtle, because chemicals (e.g., a steroid latched onto another molecule within our body) can effect the patterns by which ribonucleic acid (RNA, involved in our energy supply) and protein (e.g., enzyme) are produced without interfering with heredity. The influences of the genes are therefore liable to be blown on different courses by the winds of chemical mediation.[10]

When you consider how complex is the development of the nerve patterns in our brains during the growth of the human foetus, and how even minor defects – in the chemical gradients, in the attractions and rejections of our immune system, in the microscopic brain structures that guide the developing threadlike axons, and in the chemistry of the neurotransmitters at the synaptic connections – can cause major behavioural defects, it is a miracle that more of us don't suffer from major abnormalities of the nervous system.

Even when the nerve network is established, it can be changed by the environment. People used to think that human behaviour was quite distinct from genetics and that, although we can inherit eye and hair colour, the environment and how we react to it determines what we do. Many biologists now feel that this is incorrect and that minor differences in genes and their effects on the nervous system can strongly determine our behaviour.

Can anxiety be inherited?

There is little doubt that anxiety has a major effect on the fluency of an adult with a severe stutter, and it is fair to ask whether anxiety or fearfulness can be inherited. It appears that it can be – at least in dogs, which don't differ a great deal from people in their chemistry.

John P. Scott and John L. Fuller studied the genetics of behaviour in cocker spaniels and basenjis. Spaniels are bred for their responses to hand signals and for the soft mouths necessary for game retrieval. The dogs have a long history of benevolent association with man. Basenjis are tough hunting dogs that were used by pygmies and other Africans in a much less kindly manner.

Both types of dog were crossed and back-crossed and examined for the amount of aggression they showed in play and for their fearfulness. The evidence strongly indicated that both aggressive play and fearfulness were inherited, the former being controlled by two genes and the latter by one gene. The pure basenji pups were much more playfully aggressive at three to four months than the pure spaniels. While the spaniels were at ease with man, five-week-old basenji pups showed their fear of people by yelping, snapping, and running away. This fear subsided later, but the basenjis were always more restless than the spaniels.[11]

Since youthful anxiety appears to be heritable, how does this apply to a stutter? Anxiety about speaking could be genetically controlled, but if this is the case, why do so many stutters spontaneously disappear? In the case of the basenji pups, they lost most of their inherited fear when they learned to trust people and expect kindness from them. It is possible that stuttering children lose their stutters when the world treats them kindly, while those who feel the full weight of society's censure develop intractable, persistent, self-reinforcing stutters. This is, of course, sheer speculation, but the possibility of inherited speech-related anxiety and the development from it of an anxiety-conditioned speech disability cannot be ignored.

Would we expect speech to be conditioned by anxiety during man's evolution? Yes, we probably would. Ever since early man learned to speak and found that what he said to his peers could, if sufficiently ill-advised, get his hair parted by a Neanderthal club, he would be inclined to get hang-ups about speaking. He would be disposed to watch what he said and lapse into fractured speech the moment someone disapproved – unless, of course, he was the best club wielder in the tribe. Anxiety is closely associated with hesitant communication, even when people have normal speech. There remains the knotty problem of why more men stutter than vocally precocious females. Maybe our ancestors were reluctant to bash their breeding woman and learned to put up with their early verbosity.

All this speculation is on shaky foundations, and some scientists are sceptical about the sociobiologists' claim that behaviour can be inherited. Nevertheless, it is possible that whether a stutter is genetically mediated is not just a matter of abnormal genes directly affecting the stutterer's vocal motor system and musculature. It may be much more subtle – so subtle, in fact, that the elementary techniques used so far could not possibly recognize the defects. If a stutter proves to be genetically controlled, it would be as well for researchers to focus on how the genes affect the stutter at a chemical level, rather than debate how much is genetically and how much environmentally caused.

If we accept that anxiety and behaviour may be inherited, we need to buy a larger can to accommodate all the new, fat, and active worms.

Since a stutter is so complex, why bother to probe it in depth? Schizophrenia is a complex disability; but when it was discovered that it was controlled by genes, and when its processes were understood better, it was possible to help many schizophrenics with neuroleptic drugs to block the receptors of dopamine (a neurotransmitter) in the gaps between the nerve cells (synapses).

Nevertheless, I believe that the debate between the organic and non-organic schools of thought about the origins of stuttering is futile. Whether stuttering is an organic disorder is beside the point. All our anticipatory fears about speech and our avoidances are chemically controlled in the enzymatic stew of our brain's limbic system and its links with our speech and motor centres. How many times does a stuttering child face the choice between 'fight or flight' in a difficult speaking situation and respond blindly from his old brain inherited from reptilian ancestors? Are the sudden fear and response inorganic? They are not.

Although there is still no clear evidence that stuttering is inherited, modern science is leaning toward the idea that genetic factors are involved. Studies are hindered by the difficulty of distinguishing between childish disfluency and an early stutter, by the fact that many attributes of a stutter are hard to measure, and by the complex effects of emotional factors on fluency. If many genes are involved, and the environment can affect their expression, the researchers must cope with a maze of interactions.

Bugs in the brain's computer

One of my preparatory school teachers was an athletic disciplinarian as well as the school oracle. While the children in her class had a healthy respect for her effective follow-through with a rosewood hairbrush, they had less respect for her predictions. When she said it would rain, the sun shone.

Any politician she felt would win an election was doomed. When she was confident that we would win a football match we were certain to lose.

Her diagnosis of the cause of my stutter was one of her better efforts. She looked down my throat as though looking for a dislocated tonsil, shut my jaws with a neat snap, and said, 'It's just his nerves!'

Since all our actions, thoughts, and feelings are relayed by nerves, she couldn't be far wrong, and numerous scientists have tried to prove her right. A number of disabilities – for example, epilepsy, cluttering, and aphasia – are linked with abnormalities of the brain's nervous system caused by inheritance or injury. Many researchers have tried to link stuttering with brain structure and function, but most of them came up against the problem of distinguishing between cause and effect.

Although, as mentioned earlier, there is no solid evidence to support the long-held view that stuttering was caused by forcing left-handed children to use their right hands, the 'Cerebral Dominance Theory' was very popular in the 1920s and 1930s, and is being re-examined today. The theory was based on the assumption that normal speech occurs when one side (the left) of the cerebral cortex dominates the other (the right) for timing the nerve impulses controlling the muscles of those organs (lips, tongue, jaw, etc.) involved in speech. The supporters of the theory suggested that, if the left hemisphere is not sufficiently dominant, the co-ordination of the speech muscles will be poor, and the speech liable to break down. This theory lent credence to the idea that stuttering could be caused by forcing a left-handed child to become right-handed.

Like many other stutterers in the 1940s I sat with my head sprouting electrical terminals like a bionic man while some bright fellow watched the spikes on the chart of a machine trying to discover whether or not my brain waves were normal. Epileptics and people with brain damage have abnormal patterns, but mine seemed to be the common or garden, uninteresting type.

Nevertheless, studies in the 1940s produced evidence that,

compared to non-stutterers, some stutterers have a relatively high proportion of alpha rhythm (8 to 12 oscillations per second) in the cerebral cortex's left hemisphere. The stutterer's brain waves were sometimes out of phase if he was left-handed.[12]

One must realize, however, that the brain activity of a person who stutters is likely to be affected by the way he speaks; so that the problem of deciding what is cause and what is effect clouds the interpretation of these findings.

The early electroencephalographic (EEG) studies of stutterers were contradictory, partly because of rudimentary techniques. Modern research has demonstrated definite abnormalities in the cerebral cortex of some stutterers, but the relationships between these abnormalities and the predisposition to or the act of stuttering is far from clear.

Recent EEG studies by Einer Boberg, of the University of Alberta, Edmonton, and his colleagues at the Alberta Hospital in the same city support the view that stuttering is associated with abnormalities in the activity of the brain. Professor Boberg and his colleagues pointed out that, since Orton and Travis concluded in the 1920s that stutterers lacked the dominance of one side of the brain for speech functions, a great deal of evidence has been accumulated that people who stutter tend to lack the specialization of the left hemisphere of the brain that predominates in people with normal speech.[13] Quinn has suggested that people who stutter use the right hemisphere for speech and the left for non-verbal processing;[14] while other scientists have found that stutterers tend to process both speech and non-verbal activities in the right hemisphere, a reversal of the normal situation.[15]

Boberg and his colleagues examined the possibility that abnormal asymmetry of the brain's hemispheres was related to stuttering. They examined eleven stutterers, including two women, and measured their brain waves before and after three weeks of intensive speech therapy. In all cases the stutterers' speech improved, with two patients becoming almost totally fluent – at least in the clinic.

Before the speech therapy the stutterers showed abnormally high activity, during speech, in the posterior frontal region of the *right* hemisphere of the brain. After therapy the situation was reversed, the greatest activity being in the posterior frontal region of the *left* hemisphere of the brain.[16]

These findings indicate that treatment can shift the patterns of brain activity during speech from the 'abnormal' right to the 'normal' left. Once again, the problem of deciding what is cause and what is effect hovers in the background.

During a chat with one of the workers in this fascinating field I mentioned that I could write or draw mirror images with both hands simultaneously. His eyes lit up, and he cried, 'Aha! I know how your brain works!' I wish I did.

It was suggested that my right hemisphere may be unusually closely integrated with my left hemisphere. Because the billions of messages that cross my corpus callosum (the neurological telegraph line that links the two hemispheres) do so all too efficiently, the activity of my speech areas is mucked up. For years, I have consciously integrated my intuitive, creative, right-hemisphere activities with my logical left-hemisphere functions to boost my mental creativity. It worked remarkably well. I encouraged it, but maybe it made my stuttering worse. Anyway, I'm not going to change the habit. I'd rather stutter and be creative than be stutterless and lose those flashes of intuition and insight.

The muscle system, which is controlled by the motor tissues of the brain, has received a great deal of attention as a possible cause of stuttering. Control of the jaw muscles tends to be abnormal during stuttering, and it is well known that people who stutter have difficulty controlling their diaphragm, larynx, and breathing when they speak. Some feel that stutterers tend to lack co-ordination, but evidence is conflicting.[17] All of these differences are more likely to be the result of a person's struggle to speak rather than the cause of his disfluency.

One explanation was that stuttering is essentially a convulsion or muscular spasm similar to epilepsy: excitement, fear, and anxiety can trigger stuttering just as they do epilepsy. On this theory, stuttering is a series of small convulsions interfering with the speech.[18] Stuttering is sometimes associated with epilepsy, but there does not appear to be any strong, direct evidence to support this explanation.

The fact that stutterers find it difficult to move from one sound to the next gave rise to J. Eisenson's 'Perseveration Theory,' which attributes stuttering partly to an organic abnormality and partly to the stresses a stutterer is exposed to when he tries to speak.[19] Perseveration is simply the tendency for a pattern of behaviour to persevere. When it is applied to speech it refers to automatic and often involuntary abnormal continuation of speech behaviour. The stylus of your speech gets stuck in a rut.

According to this theory, when a stutterer speaks, the message or stimulus from the brain that orders the mind and muscles to adopt the conformation that produces a particular sound persists longer than is necessary. This prevents the speaker from moving to the next conformation needed for the next sound. The muscles switch on but do not switch off soon enough to permit fluency.

Eisenson proposed that people who stutter perseverate more than non-stutterers. He linked this constitutional or organic cause with the degree of meaning in the spoken words; the more meaningful the words, the more stutterers tend to stutter. He suggested that the temporary disruption of meaningful or propositional speech by perseveration could determine the degree of stuttering. He felt that only about 60 per cent of people who stutter perseverate for physical reasons; the others just perseverate (and stutter) according to the degree of significance they attach to their words and the difficulty of the speaking situation. These latter stutterers may not have a neurological problem.

Not all people who perseverate for physical reasons stutter. Some experts feel that the evidence supporting the theory is weak and that the relationships between the many factors involved are far from clear. Attempts to confirm the theory appear to have been unsuccessful, and at present the perseveration theory is not widely accepted. Nevertheless, the possibility of a link between physical and emotional origins of a stutter is interesting. Many stutterers, including myself, experience blocking in the middle of fluent speech with no change in situation and emotion, which makes them wonder if a physical switch turns off their fluency. It all serves to illustrate the difficulty of tracing a stutter to its source.

During the past two decades scientists trying to unravel the biology of the brain have created an information explosion. Melvin Konner, in his fascinating book *The Tangled Wing: Biological Constraints on the Human Spirit*,[20] describes how brain activity affects our feelings of fear, joy, grief, lust, and love, and how new knowledge and techniques are providing fresh insights into human behaviour. It is possible that new information will help us determine whether a child is physically predisposed to stutter. Recent investigations of brain abnormalities associated with dyslexia, a disorder of perception and communication, raise many questions.

The parallel of dyslexia

Dyslexia interferes with a person's ability to read, write, and spell. Not surprisingly, this makes learning difficult. Dyslexics vary in their symptoms, but most of them distort words and sentences and have difficulty distinguishing letters with similar shapes. They may have trouble writing down words they hear, may confuse left and right, may reverse series of numbers in calculations, and may even have difficulty pronouncing words.

Although dyslexia is very different from a stutter, there are striking parallels with stuttering. For example more boys than girls are dyslexic; the handicap seems to run in families; many dyslexics are left-handed or ambidextrous; the disability appears to be unpredictable, with the dyslexic being able to read correctly on some occasions and not on others; dyslexics' IQs are more or less normal; society (including impatient, uninformed parents and teachers) tends to label dyslexics as stupid or mentally retarded and to taunt and penalize them; and many dyslexics suffer from low self-esteem. All of these apply to stutterers. Even the early research on stuttering, with its emphasis on dominance of the brain's hemispheres, genetics, neuroses, and environmental pressures, parallels early research on dyslexia. Dyslexia, as with stuttering, is treated by teaching the patient how to control and live with his handicap rather than how to cure it. Both dyslexia and stuttering take a great deal of skill and effort to control because both involve many interacting factors.

Recent studies of the brains of dyslexics indicate that the handicap may be associated with abnormal patterns in the nerve cells in the 'speech zone' of the brain's left cerebral hemisphere. The evidence is still incomplete and the conclusions tentative, but the fact that the brains of some foetuses show similar aberrations suggests an early breakdown in the patterns of brain development, possibly caused by abnormal hormone levels.[21]

As with stutterers, early studies of dyslexics' brains revealed no abnormalities, but new techniques may show otherwise. What if both dyslexia and stuttering prove to be neurological disorders? Will this mean they can be treated more easily? Not necessarily; but it may at least permit early diagnosis and treatment before the handicaps produce emotional problems that are difficult to deal with in later life. If it turns out that stuttering and dyslexia are caused by abnormal neurotransmitter gradients, then medication could also be helpful. For the time being, we must wait and see what the scientists come up with next. The pendulum seems to be swinging again toward hypotheses of organic origins for stutters, after a long period of disfavour.

Whatever science uncovers, my school teacher was right. It's just nerves.

Stuttering and sound

The railway engines of my childhood were magnificent, smelly monsters that rumbled like flatulent elephants, hissed white clouds of steam, and belched volcanoes of grey, gritty smoke. On their black, gleaming sides they sported polished brass name plates with aristocratic titles like *The Duke of York*. They were quite different from the diesels that throb quietly along our modern tracks like faceless bureaucrats. When three or four of the old, noisy beasts were in a railway station and thunderous rumbles hammered at my ears, I was perfectly fluent.

Years later in the Armed Forces I welcomed the shattering roar when we warmed up the Rolls-Royce Merlin Spitfire engines during morning check-up. Nobody suggested that we should wear earguards, so, as one fitter said, we couldn't hear ourselves think. Every day for this short period I was fluent. Even though I had to shout to make myself understood, the respite from the stress of trying to speak was welcome.

The majority of people who stutter can speak more fluently when they can't hear themselves. Very few deaf people stutter. In my case I wasn't sure if the fluency was because I couldn't hear myself or because I had to shout, because stutterers are often more fluent when they speak loudly. During timber cruises I had no difficulty calling tree measurements to the record keeper. Speech pathologists share this uncertainty about what causes the fluency in noisy situations, but it seems that blocking out stutterers' lower speech frequencies by noise increases fluency whether they speak loudly or not. [22]

The effect of noise on fluency has led to a number of theories. Some scientists hold the view that noise is just a distraction; others feel that noise affects the perception of speech feedback. All people with normal hearing hear themselves speak and automatically monitor what they have said. The theory is that there is a delay in the feedback from a stutterer's speech caused by an organic difference in the hearing process.

The level of noise seems to be important. Ninety decibels produce almost normal fluency, 50 decibels reduce disfluency, and below 50 decibels there is little effect. Lower frequencies (less than 500 Hz) appear to be most effective in producing fluency, and this has been used in therapy.

The obvious inference is that the stutterer's response to sounds differs from the non-stutterer's. There is evidence that stutterers differ from non-stutterers in their perception of sound, but only at frequencies of 2,000 Hz, which is puzzling. [23] Another inference could be that since boys are more likely to stutter than girls, boys should differ from girls in their feedback of speech. A study of eight male and eight female non-stutterers showed that when the speech feedback was artificially delayed by about 0.2 to 0.8 second, the males developed speech patterns similar to a stutter, and the females did not. There is some doubt that this artificial stutter is the same as a real stutter, but females may deal with speech perception in a different way from males.

When the feedback of speech is delayed by about 0.2 second and amplified, the speech of normal speakers tends to disintegrate.[24] When stutterers are exposed to this delayed auditory feedback (DAF), the speech of the more severe stutterers tends to improve, while others have the same difficulty as non-stutterers.[25]

Some scientists feel that the effects of noise on fluency indicate that stuttering is a perceptual rather than a motor disorder. Shane suggested that noise removed the anxiety of people who stutter by obliterating their perception of their own stuttering.[26] Many experts still feel that sound helps the stutterer mainly because it is distracting.

There are still many questions to be answered. Do all stutterers respond to noise in the same way? Does the benefit fade when the novelty of noise wears off? Can some stutterers still perceive their speech in spite of noise and yet remain fluent? Is the frequency of a sound all that important?

Whenever somebody comes up with an idea of how something works, an engineer is sure to get in on the act. Stuttering is no exception. A great many of our bodily functions involve servomechanisms or automatic controls. When we get hot, the body's thermostat automatically controls our temperature (unless we are sick); when we run up a steep hill the body's controls stimulate the cardiovascular system to pump more oxygen to our flagging tissues; and when we are afraid, adrenalin is fed into the bloodstream to help us handle the situation. We possess sensor units that respond to our body's signals and send information to the controller units that compare what we need with what we have. If there is a deficiency or a surplus, a controller signals to the gland or tissue concerned to do something about it.

Normal speech appears to be an automatic process, regulated by feedback from many sources and involving a servomechanism with automatic controls. The ear acts as the sensor and hears the voice production from the vocal machinery. The controller, with its ability to compare what we want to say with what we have said, is somewhere in the brain. If what we have said does not complete what we want to say, an error signal goes out for the body to complete the communication.[27]

This feedback theory of speech was linked with the discovery that many stutterers become more fluent when the feedback of their speech to the ear's sensor is masked. The theory is that stuttering is a breakdown in the speech's automatic controls. The breakdown is caused by disruption of the feedback circuits that integrate thought and speech, or by responses to false error signals that arise from anticipated problems with fluency. Stuttering could also be caused by a fault in the sensor unit (conduction of sound to the ear), or by negative feedback from a listener ('I don't understand. Please repeat.'), which prompts the child to develop the habit of repeating himself.[28]

Cybernetic models like this are useful because they encourage the scientist to organize his thoughts in a logical manner, provide insights into interactions between speech components, and help the researcher to ask the right questions. They may not produce specific answers, but they do provide a valuable framework. The approach, which takes into account possible physical abnormalities as well as effects of feedback from listeners or from anticipated difficulty (anxiety), also, refreshingly, breaks down the artificial distinctions between organic and non-organic causes of stutters.

The effects on stuttering of delayed auditory feedback and masking with low-frequency noise are still the subject of debate. They are just two of the keys to the prison of a stutter, with its numerous locks and alarms.

Stutterers' physiology

The concept of human biorhythms is based on the fact that everyone's levels of vitality, clearness of thought, and coordination vary from day to day. Since ancient times people have believed that the phases of the moon affect mental activity, with werewolves, vampires, and other mythical nasties carrying out their dirty deeds when the moon is full. There are many who feel that atmospheric pressure affects mood; and, indeed, a succession of grey, rainy days does make me sluggish and irritable. Any change in mood, vitality, or coordination can affect the fluency of a stutterer. On those days when I wake with a brain that feels like cold rice pudding, clumsy fingers that drop the breakfast cereal packet, and a lack of concentration that makes me burn the bacon, my words seem to wade ankle deep in molasses. As Van Riper wrote, my mode of speech is gluency rather than fluency.

All of these daily changes are the result of shifts in our physiological processes. In spite of the fact that scientists have not found any clear physiological differences between stutterers and non-stutterers, completely to divorce stuttering from physiology would be absurd. Although the experimental results are inconclusive, it is useful to examine them, particularly those of relevance to therapy. All people who stutter hope that one day some genius will find out that stuttering is caused by a biochemical deficiency that can be cured by a magic pill, making unnecessary all the hard work and frustration of extended speech therapy. It doesn't seem likely that the complex syndrome of stuttering will respond to such simple treatment, but we can hope.

The trouble with studying the physiology of stuttering is that both stuttering and expecting to stutter cause physiological changes arising from associated stress and anxiety. This state can persist for some time after speaking – basically, until the speaker's frustration diminishes. When a silent stutterer is being studied by a scientist, the stutterer's attention is focused on his quiescent speech and he is likely to be nervous even when silent. Some scientists have been careful to allow for this and others have not, so results need to be scrutinized carefully.

Several early studies suggested that a stutterer's heartbeat is faster than a non-stutterer's; but other studies have indicated otherwise.[29] Even in carefully controlled conditions, stutterers had more variations in heart rate and faster heartbeats than others, and there were suggestions of sex differences. The pulse rate of females with normal speech tends to be faster than that of males; but, when the pulses of young male and female stutterers were examined, the opposite was true.[30] Other workers found that, although females usually have lower basal metabolic rates than males, these rates were relatively high in female stutterers.[31] The research results were interpreted by some scientists to mean that stuttering was associated with differences in metabolism and sex, but nobody was rash enough to use the word 'cause.' These conclusions were based on shaky experimental grounds and are not widely accepted. The vocal tension of a person who stutters is obvious. This led to the study of voice mechanisms, particularly the behaviour of the larynx, which was admirably reviewed by C. Woodruff Starkweather.[32] It is hard to sort out cause and effect, and research has been inconclusive.

Other studies have shown that, compared to non-stutterers, people who stutter have high levels of blood sugar, calcium, phosphorus, albumen, and globulin, high urinary creatinine, and a greater tendency to allergies, but later evidence has contradicted this.[33]

Because a person who stutters can get quite worked up about the act of speaking, you'd expect scientists to have looked at blood pressures carefully. However, there is remarkably little information in the literature on the subject. Early studies of the blood pressures of male stutterers and non-stutterers indicated that there were no differences, but later evidence suggests that a male stutterer's blood pressure increases when he tries to speak, which is to be expected.[34]

The reported high carbon-dioxide content of the stutterer's blood became the basis of a carbon-dioxide therapy that was popular for a few years.[35] The idea was that the relatively high acidity of the stutterer's blood was caused by high levels of carbon dioxide, although some scientists didn't agree. In spite of the doubts, carbon-dioxide gas was administered to thirty-three stutterers. A third of them (eleven) became much more fluent; others (twelve) showed a little improvement; and the rest did not respond at all. Other attempts were made to use carbon dioxide, sometimes with nitrous-oxide gas, but success was variable. Stutterers whose impediment began in adolescence or later seemed to respond better to carbon dioxide than stutterers who developed their problem when very young. The usefulness of carbon-dioxide therapy and the implications of carbon-dioxide levels in the blood are very much in doubt.[36]

Several attempts were also made to link stutters with endocrine malfunction. It was known in 1928 that when some non-stuttering patients were given a thyroid extract they started to stutter, and that the stuttering stopped when the dose ceased. Unfortunately, the recorded stuttering could have been cluttering, a different disorder, since cluttering can develop when thyroid extracts are administered.[37]

There are many physiological differences between stutterers and non-stutterers, but not one is beyond dispute or can be labelled as the cause of a stutter. People who stutter are notoriously hard to study in an objective way. All results tend to be clouded by physiological changes associated with the approach to speaking, the moment of stuttering, and its aftermath.

Anticipation, anxiety, conflicts, and cues

You never get used to a stutter no matter how long you have it. Those people who say they don't care are kidding themselves. Any stutterer who is honest with himself will admit that he feels a chilling fear whenever he anticipates speaking at length in front of a large audience. There are public speakers with severe stutters who manage to cope, and I asked one of them how he felt about blocking and grimacing in front of a large number of people. His reply was, 'It doesn't really bother me,' and he obviously believed it. He must have learned to anaesthetize his feelings so well that if he did care he didn't realize it. My next question was whether he found public speaking stressful and exhausting. He said, 'No, of course not,' but his eyes said the opposite.

Anticipation of stuttering can be unnerving, and there have been many times when I've wanted to take to the hills (and a few times when I have). The more you fear that your speech will break down, the worse the stutter becomes. It is not surprising that speech pathologists have looked closely at the effects of fearful anticipation on fluency. Their work was the basis of the 'Anticipatory Struggle Theory,' which, in spite of the fact that it is based on many intangibles, makes a great deal of sense to many stutterers, who find it seems to fit their disability.[38]

The hypothesis proposes that a person who stutters interferes with his own speech (i.e., stutters) because he believes, either consciously or unconsciously, that speaking is difficult. The stutterer becomes disfluent when he anticipates that he is going to stutter, which on the surface seems to be a chicken-or-egg situation. It can be argued that if he didn't stutter he wouldn't anticipate stuttering, and, consequently, that fearful anticipation can't be the cause of a stutter. This riddle is resolved when it is realized that speech experts distinguish between the factors affecting the *onset* of a stutter (i.e., its early beginnings) and the factors affecting the speech at or immediately before the *moment* of stuttering. A child may begin to stutter for one or more of the reasons discussed earlier in this chapter (neurosis, brain malfunction, auditory feedback, parental and social pressures, etc.); but the future development of the childish, hesitant stutter into a major, well-established stutter is affected by the memory of speech failure, with all its attendant humiliation, rejection, and frustration, and the anxiety that it will happen again. It is hard to allay such fears.

Many emotions and situations affect the fluency of an established stutterer, and anxiety plays a major role. If a person for many years experiences a sharp pain when he bends over, he will be a bit nervous and careful about bending – with good reason. Similarly, the stutterer has good reason to worry about speaking. He knows from experience that whenever he speaks it is highly likely that he will block, stutter, grimace, and get a bad response from his audience. He anticipates that he will struggle to speak. So he struggles and stutters.

The hypothesis involves the idea that a stutterer doesn't stutter if he doesn't think about his speech. If you think too hard about what you are doing and don't trust your automatic reflexes, you are likely to make a mess of anything, whether you are playing the piano, walking a tightrope, or doing the pole-vault.

I once climbed a razor-backed ridge with drops of a thousand feet or so on both sides. It was no great feat. The well-worn track was a yard wide, my boots were cleated, and I don't suffer from vertigo. I happily plodded upwards bouncing echoes off the black cliffs for fun until I came to a metal plaque in memory of someone who had stepped into the void. It made me more careful. Thereafter I watched my feet, assessed the chances of my cleats' skidding on the veins of hard quartz, and made sure that my centre of gravity didn't stray too far to one side or the other. To my dismay, I began to stumble and scrabble, and a flicker of apprehension soon blossomed into a sickening fear. The chasms looked horrifying and, for the first time, I froze on a mountain. I sat on a rock, ate some chocolate, calmed down, and reminded myself that, since my feet knew their job, I'd better let them get on with it. I switched onto automatic and contentedly bounced echoes all the way to the top.

Speech can be like that. When you think about all the lip, tongue, larynx, and word co-ordination involved you are liable to fall into the abyss of disfluency. Anybody with the tendency to stutter may well freeze from fear of speaking. The old story about the centipede who was crippled when ordered to explain how it walked has been refined by scientists who contend that the stutterer gets into trouble when he consciously tries to produce and synchronize all of the speech movements instead of relying on his automatic co-ordination.

Early students of stuttering were aware of the fears and doubts associated with disfluency and suggested that the impediment could be caused by faulty auto-suggestion, or a deep-seated neurotic conviction of speech failure, or the lack of automatic speech mentioned earlier.[39]

The anticipated struggle involves a large element of avoidance. Wendell Johnson and his colleagues felt that stuttering is an attempt to avoid an anticipated, feared breakdown of fluency. Rather than being caused by neuroses and brain abnormalities, it is a disorder of perception precipitated by society and its demands for verbal communication.[40] In this kind of situation stutterers are damned if they try to avoid stuttering and damned if they stutter. It's not surprising that some of them lapse into silence. They want to speak but at the same time don't want to speak. This conflict has led to the idea that stuttering results from the desire to avoid speech. Avoidance and anxiety rear their ugly heads again. The 'Approach-Avoidance Conflict Theory' developed by J.G. Sheehan is used a great deal in therapy. It differs a little from the idea of stuttering to avoid stuttering in that it implies that a person stutters to avoid speaking.[41]

Sheehan's theory also involves the idea that when a stutterer blocks, his block actually reduces his fear. In other words, much of the fear felt by a stutterer arises from an attempt to hide from his audience the fact that he stutters. When he blocks there is no need to try and hide the stutter. It is obvious to everybody that his speech has broken down. Consequently the fear associated with hiding the disfluency is reduced. Stutterers can put enormous emotional effort into hiding their stutters by switching roles and changing words. Teaching a stutterer to stop changing words is an important part of therapy.

Another facet of the anticipatory struggle theory is the 'preparatory set' developed by Charles Van Riper in the United States. That is, as the stutterer approaches a feared word, he directs his attention onto his speech organs and tensely approaches the word. He prepares for the first difficult sound with a fixed speaking posture and may even rehearse the dreaded sound, making it impossible for him to say the word normally. He approaches the word with a prepared set of muscular and psychological positions, and, as happened to me on the mountain, he stumbles. [42]

Oliver Bloodstein summarized the complex anticipatory struggle theory as a sequence. First there is a suggestion that speaking is difficult. Failure is therefore expected, and a need to avoid failure is felt. Normal automatic speech is replaced by a short-term speaking strategy. The physical and mental sets to carry out the strategy are mustered, and the result is tension and fragmented speech. [43]

During the early 1970s I found myself involved in work that required a great deal of telephoning. Although many of the numbers were on automatic dialling, I often had to request extension numbers or give my own number. Every time I asked for or gave a number I scanned digits looking for road blocks. 'Nine' was a nightmare; I would either block or 'nnnn' like a hornet. 'Two' was tricky, but not so bad. On 'six' and 'seven' I was liable to hiss like a viper, and on 'four' or 'five' my 'fffff' sounded like a slow puncture. 'Three' was fine and only tied my tongue in a knot occasionally. 'Eight' and 'zero' always slid out on well-oiled wheels. My own number was 589-2880. I slow-punctured my way through 'five,' blocked on 'nine' and 'two,' and breezed by the 'eights' and 'zero.' French numerals were terrible. Only *'un'* and *'huit'* stood a fair chance of coming out of my mouth untangled. I could easily predict on which sounds my speech would freeze. Stutterers are remarkably good at forecasting their troubles.

Stutterers' forecasts of speech blockages were found to be between 85 and 96 per cent correct. According to the anticipatory struggle theory, stutterers are not clairvoyant, but simply stutter when they expect to do so.[44]

The participants in these experiments were well aware of the speech blocks ahead, but conscious anticipation of stuttering does not inevitably fragment the speech. Many stutterers I know sometimes block completely on words they can usually say fluently. I do the same and, even during a phase of complete fluency when I am thinking about my research more than my speech, I can suddenly come to a dead halt, much to my surprise. I used to think that a neurological circuit had shorted out, but it may be that the anticipation of blocks is unconscious or subliminal, conditioned by past experience.

All of us, whether we have normal speech or stutter, suffer from delusions about our fluency. Normal speakers are usually unaware of their normal disfluencies and get quite a shock when they hear themselves on a tape recorder ('Is that me ...?'). I sometimes think that I have been fluent when in fact I blocked in a minor way about ten times each minute. I tend to notice the major, debilitating blocks and don't register the minor hesitations and repetitions.

I know very well that speaking to an audience of fifteen is harder for me than to an audience of four, and this has nothing to do with conventional stage fright. Standing and talking to a mike at a lecture is harder than talking when I sit in a chair. I am much more fluent when I can see my audience – that's why I never speak and show colour transparencies at the same time, and why the telephone is so difficult.

One of the speaking situations I try to forget occurred when I had just taken on a new job in Oxford. Within the first month I was told to visit the Meteorological Office. I was a little nervous about my speech. I anticipated trouble, and I got it! I was marched straight into an auditorium and asked to tell an audience of about fifty scientists and managers about my work. I started to block badly and nearly took to my heels, but controlled myself and called upon my personal wily devil that gets me out of that kind of mess. I changed my tactics and told them that I was new to the job and was there to ask them questions – which I did, stutter and all. It went very well. They did most of the talking.

The trouble with going to fortune tellers is that they might tell you something bad is going to happen, and that they might be right. Stutterers see their own speech future remarkably clearly. It is usually bad, and their predictions are nearly always right on the nail.

Although a stutterer can predict most of the sounds and some of the situations that will provoke his stutter, he finds it difficult to understand what triggers bad speech phases. He is bewildered when his speech collapses around him for no reason that he can perceive. Some scientists feel that the occurrence of stuttering, once it is firmly established, is fairly consistent and can be triggered by definite learned cues. This, of course, refers to events that precipitate the moment of stuttering after the impediment is established, not to the onset of disfluency in childhood. The alleged causes of the onset and of the moment of stuttering may be quite different.

It was noticed by Wendell Johnson and his co-workers that, when stutterers read a passage several times, the number of hesitations tended to decrease because they adapted to the situation, but the places on the page where a patient blocked were always more or less the same. About 65 per cent of the words stuttered in one reading were stuttered in the next. Either the position of the words or their meaning precipitated the blocks. Stuttering is not haphazard, whatever the bewildered stutterer may think.[45]

Several stutterers were tested to find out whether their memories of past difficult words cued further speech difficulty. All the subjects read a passage, and the words upon which they stuttered were blanked out on the script. They read the passage again, and, as before, the stuttered words were blanked out. This was repeated several times until most of the stuttering was removed. The few remaining stuttered words were next to blocked-out words that had given the stutterer difficulty in previous readings, so the stutterers appeared to respond to cues of past failure (the nearby blocked-out words) rather than to the form or meaning of the words. If the stuttered words were removed from the page and the text closed up to fill the gaps, stuttering was much less than when the blocked-out words remained on the page. People who stutter seem to respond to cues related to past difficulties.[46]

This led to the theory that the moment of stuttering involves a cue that evokes anticipation of trouble, and that this results in attempts to avoid stuttering. Of course, this fits in well with the idea of anticipated struggle. The struggle is the stutter. The cues may not even be words. Colours and light intervals associated with past stuttering have been used in experiments to condition stutterers to be more disfluent.[47]

Why I stuttered more on one word than another was a mystery until I read about Spencer Brown's research in the 1930s and early 1940s.

Brown found that in thirty-two adults with stutters, about 90 per cent of their stuttering was on the first sounds of words, and the rest of the hesitations were on sounds at the beginning of syllables, particularly the accented syllables in long words. Brown also observed that while the likelihood of stuttering was affected by the sounds of the words, this varied a great deal from one stutterer to another. Most of his subjects, however, stuttered more on consonants than on vowels. This may have been caused by the fact that consonants are more important in communication (some languages don't have vowels), by the greater tension of lip and tongue, by the interruption of air flow, or simply by the fact that there are more consonants than vowels.[48]

The sound doesn't appear to be completely responsible for triggering the stutter. Words starting with 'f' give me more trouble than those beginning with 'ph,' and 'ph' is easier for me than the plosive 'p,' which seems illogical. Bloodstein quotes the case of the New York City boy who, when he read aloud, blocked on words starting with 'th' and had no difficulty with 't' and 'd' in spite of the fact that with his accent he pronounced 'th' as 't' or 'd,' as in 'tink' and 'dis.' This sounds absurd until the principles of anticipated avoidance are applied. The 'th' cued anticipated failure, the stutterer tried to avoid disfluency, struggled, and blocked. The phonetics were secondary.[49]

Although many stuttering children have trouble with pronouns and conjunctions, when adults read aloud they stutter more on nouns, verbs, adjectives, and adverbs than on pronouns, conjunctions, articles, and prepositions. This suggests that the main problems are associated with the words that contain the most information. You can shorten the sentence 'The red cat sat on the woolly blue mat' to 'Red cat sat woolly blue mat' without losing much meaning. People who stutter get into trouble on important words. What could be more loaded than: 'John Smith; born 2 February 1934; Residence, 2 Maple Street, Felixville, Ontario; Telephone number: 613-576-2112.' No wonder a stutterer, faced by a battery of loaded nouns, falls apart when asked to give his basic data.

I am often fluent after a few blocks and repetitions in the first sentence or so. Like a car engine started at thirty below, my speech motor warms up – but it can conk out later, like a car when the gas line freezes. Brown found that stutterers have more trouble with the first and early words in sentences than with later words. I always find that the first words in a sentence look like a crag to be climbed as I prepare to relinquish anxiety-free silence for anxiety-loaded speech. Scientists feel that the conspicuousness of the early words are the stutterer's downfall, fitting in with the idea of anticipated struggle. The crag looms up, the struggle to climb it is anticipated, the struggle begins, and the speech falls apart.

I've always been nervous about long, hyphenated words with their double or even triple barrels pointing at my speech, making me all too conscious of my speech anxiety's hair trigger. Stutterers in general have more trouble with long words than short ones, possibly because it is harder to say them, or possibly because they stand out in the sentence.[50] Anything that looks hard to say to a stutterer is likely to give him trouble.

In order to simplify this tangled web of influences, Oliver Bloodstein summarized the conditions that appear to affect a stutterer's sometime fluency (as when singing, reciting, whispering, speaking in unison, or acting another role) or lack of fluency (as when talking to other people). Rather than seek the fundamental causes that precipitated the stutter in childhood, he concentrated on why the fluency of an established stutterer varies to such a large extent.

He supplemented the results of other workers with a survey of his own, in which he solicited views on the conditions affecting the fluency of young adults, and was able to define 115 situations that affected the stutter.[51] There was considerable variation from one individual to another according to the different meanings the situations had for each person. When asked 'Do you stutter when speaking to a parent?' the response would depend on whether or not the parent was supportive or antagonistic about the impediment. After allowing for such variables, Bloodstein was able to recognize the following eight broad classes of factors that either increased or decreased stuttering:

1 Communication content
2 Listener's reaction
3 Desire for approval
4 Distractions
5 Response to suggestion
6 Changes in physical tension
7 Period between planning to speak and speaking
8 Presence or absence of stuttering cues

The *communication content* of words plays an important role in stuttering. A person who stutters does so more when reading passages that have meaning than when reading meaningless words. He can usually sing, count, read in unison, shadow other speakers, swear, recite, talk to a dog, tease a baby, read lists that the audience can see, engage in banal social chit-chat at parties, and say 'Hello,' 'Goodbye,' 'Thank you,' and 'Have a nice day.' He can be fluent when he says anything that doesn't contain much meaning or involve the responsibility of communicating.

I even stuttered talking to my dog. He was very bright, understood many words, and seemed to know what I was saying. My experience with tape recording is a good example of the effect of meaningful communication on fluency. When I worked for the government I had sufficient speech control to make recordings with no effort at all when the only person who heard them later was myself. Nevertheless, when I dictated a letter to my secretary on the tape recorder, I had to use learned speaking techniques very carefully indeed or I soon lost control. It was the same audience – the tape recorder – but the communication content (and context) of the dictation differed.

I can say tongue-twisters quickly and fluently, so there's nothing wrong with my muscular co-ordination. My motor system and my brain's speech centres seem to fire on all their cylinders. Ask me to *describe* the phonetics of the tongue-twister, however, and I'm soon floundering in the quicksands of disfluency.

The *listener's reaction* plays another key role. I can usually tell whether a stranger and I are going to get along within a minute of meeting him. Even seeing photographs of certain types of people can jolt the stability of my speech. (Many others have found this, too.)[52] It seems to be a matter of the cues described earlier in this chapter. The speech can be disrupted by a particular type of person or even by a cue associated with the person. In general, when the listener shows (or seems to show, because people who stutter sometimes see reactions that aren't there) embarrassment, impatience, shock, hostility, amusement, or pity, a confirmed stutterer's fluency often scatters to the four winds. He may be completely fluent with a friend who sees him daily and is familiar with his strange way of speaking.

People who stutter tend to be visually acute, sometimes too acute for their own peace of mind. They seem to pick up vibes remarkably well. Even when well hidden, a person's surprise at hearing me stutter can affect my speech.

While some stutterers find it easy to talk at home, others find that their worst speaking situation. Many adolescents I have spoken to found that their parents' lack of sympathy about their stutter made it worse (a two-way street if one of the parents also stutters!). Audience reaction is important and may be one reason I find it hard to speak to audiences of more than five or six; the larger the audience, the more likely it is that some of them will respond badly to my hesitations. I used to describe listener response as audience interaction, because I would respond to the audience myself, quite apart from stuttering; in turn, my response would affect their response, and so on.

Desire for approval affects stutterers in many ways, and many need approval to keep fluent. Others, like myself, find out early in life that when a person stutters approval comes his way in small doses. These people learn to survive with very little. You have to speak and you know that people will react badly, so you tend to say 'To hell with it!' and get on with communicating, letting the audience think what they wish.

People who stutter are inclined to have trouble speaking to those in positions of authority, particularly when such individuals are formally dressed.[53] Conversely, a stutterer is often more fluent when he *is* the person in authority and is speaking to subordinates. Stutterers vary, though, and this didn't work in my case. I was relatively fluent talking to superiors (sometimes more fluent than they liked), and my stutter became worse as I rose in the government's scientific hierarchy and talked to more subordinates, probably because of increasing administrative frustration.

The idea that leaders stutter less when talking to the led didn't work for me in my school's Officers' Training Corps, either. I was fluently drilling a platoon when I blocked badly on the word 'Halt!' My soldiers determinedly marched straight into a wooden pavilion and ended up in a laughing heap of tangled arms, legs, and Lee-Enfield rifles.

The fluency of a male stutterer's conversation with a female, and vice versa, depends a great deal on approval. A pretty girl who feels that boys approve of her appearance may be more fluent in a girl-boy situation than when talking to girls. Some males who stutter, fearing and often getting rejection by girls, may well be more disfluent in boy-girl conversations. I never had much trouble talking to girls, although I had my fair share of 'Get lost.' Since I was educated in one of those monastic boys' schools where the boys don't talk to a girl for months on end, and spent years enthusiastically repairing the omission, I was spared the nastiness that adolescent girls show to white blackbirds in the flock.

Distractions that divert a stutterer's attention away from his fear of disfluency, his stuttering cues, the information content of his words, and the response of listeners are likely to help him to control his speech. The stronger the distraction, the greater the control. This has been the basis of several therapies, most of which help for only a short time. Any exposure to unusually stimulating situations tends to increase fluency. It is safe to guess that few people who stutter have major speech problems on their honeymoons.

Bloodstein wrote that 'speaking in a monotone, whispering, shouting, using an abnormally high pitch or an abnormally low pitch, adopting an unusual voice quality, speaking with exaggerated articulatory movements, or with slurred articulation, with objects in the mouth, at a slow rate, with altered breathing, or in time to rhythmical movements' all tend to improve fluency.[54] These all distract the speaker.

When I was about nine years old I heard that objects held in the mouth increased the fluency of people with tangled tongues. What could be more sensible than to experiment with one of my most treasured glass marbles, a large, opaque, blue-and-red beauty called a 'Mex,' which was worth ten transparent marbles in the school market. I popped it into my mouth and spoke fluently to a sceptical friend who unfortunately cracked a joke about losing my marbles. I laughed, choked, and swallowed my Mex so that it was necessary for me to stay in hospital on a diet of dry bread and sips of water until my Mex reappeared. It was gratifying to find that in subsequent games my Mex had increased in value by 300 per cent after its long and mysterious journey. I still have it.

A stuttering colleague of mine used the slurred speech technique with remarkable success, even on public platforms. Unfortunately it gave the wrong impression and he was approached on several occasions by advocates of Alcoholics Anonymous.

Any distraction seems to help a stutterer for a while, and dancing, piano-playing, swimming, and operating a machine have been cited as examples. I haven't tried swimming and talking at the same time, but it sure would focus my attention on timing my breathing.

The idea of *response to suggestion*, hypnotic or otherwise, has always fascinated stutterers, who have a mental image of a wise, old man swinging a shiny disc on a chain before their eyes and lulling them into a deep sleep from which they emerge completely fluent. This is, of course, wishful thinking. I do not hypnotize easily. The only time anybody succeeded, he cured me of hayfever instead of my stutter – which raised a few eyebrows among professional immunologists. Nevertheless, some stutterers respond to suggesions that they need not worry about their hesitations and become fluent for short periods. For example, a Frenchman used non-hypnotic powers of suggestion so effectively that a stutterer's fluency improved for a week until his speech collapsed to a state worse than before.[55] Stutterers, like most people, can be brainwashed to do a great many things, but suggesting that they speak fluently seems to be a little too much. It may help some people, but there are dangers, unless the treatment is handled with great care.

It has always been said that *changes in physical tension* affect the severity of a stutter. I have tried many relaxation tapes and auto-suggestion techniques that were supposed to relax me, but they had no effect at all. A great many stutterers feel that relaxation of physical tension helps their fluency and that they stutter more when scared or stressed, but the effect on fluency of physical relaxation seems to vary from one person to another. I have always wondered how you can relax deeply and expose yourself to tension-filled stuttering cues and bad stuttering situations at the same time. If somebody could have taught me how to relax my anxiety about speaking, that would have been much more useful.

The *period between planning to speak and speaking* used to have devastating effects on my speech until I achieved better control. Fortunately my surname begins with 'C', so my sojourn in purgatory before descending into the hell of having to read aloud in class was mercifully short.

Later in life I had terrible problems at round-table committee meetings of thirty or forty people when each participant had to stand up in turn and introduce himself. Not only were my name, position, organization, and occupation hard for a person with my kind of stutter to say, but the delay in saying it seemed to be interminable, and my anxiety mounted exponentially. Since the final result was always a disaster, I preferred to chair and control the meetings myself, or to arrive five minutes late.

The tendency for stutterers' speech to fall apart when they are forced to wait for periods as short as ten seconds before speaking has been confirmed experimentally.[56] Delays of three minutes used to bring me out in goose-bumps of apprehension. If I have to make a mess of something, I like to get it over with.

The eighth situation affecting fluency – *the presence or absence of stuttering cues* (e.g., the grammatical identity of words, their position in the sentence, their meaning and phonetics, the type of situation, and the response of the listener) – spills over into the other seven situations of Bloodstein's list. As he points out, the greater the number of these cues in the situation, the more chance there is that the stutterer's speech will fall apart.

Some cues can be removed by changing a stutterer's location, at least for a while. One stutterer was a virtual nomad. He stayed in a place until his speech deteriorated and then moved on.

Bloodstein's eight categories usefully organize the many factors affecting an established stutterer's speech and the paradoxes associated with it. As he says, all of these categories essentially boil down to anxiety about stuttering.

Although Bloodstein's categories refer mainly to the moment of stuttering associated with an established impediment, few will deny that anxiety about communication pervades a child's speech behaviour once he is conscious that he is different from others. All stutterers are anxious about their speech; those who deny it are either not aware of their anxieties or are not prepared to admit them.

Some speech pathologists do not accept these complex ideas about stuttering. They feel that, no matter what caused the stutter, most people with stutters just speak the wrong way and can be retrained to speak correctly – that there is no need to treat the whole person and his anxieties. R.L. Webster developed his program of fluency modification because he felt that so many of the theoretical notions about stuttering are 'cumbersome' and 'poorly defined.'[57]

The role of anxiety, word fear, and stuttering cues cannot be ignored, but neither can the more direct behavioural approaches. The answer probably lies between the two, and a great deal of good modern therapy uses both approaches in combinations best suited to individuals.

The impact of these ideas on therapy will be discussed in the next chapter. The stuttering syndrome and the human psyche are so complex that it is not surprising that stuttering is difficult to control. What is surprising is the amount of success speech pathologists have under the circumstances.

FIVE

How do you treat stuttering?

'There are no such things as incurables; there are only things for which man has not found a cure.'

Bernard M. Baruch

A few years ago I accidentally overheard one of our executives (a man noted more for his loud voice than for his tact; the kind of overbearing person who thinks that if you say something loudly enough and often enough it must be true) talking about me. He said, in a voice everybody in the building could hear, 'You'd think Carlisle would do something about that darned stuttering! If he made the effort he could speak as well as I can. I knew a kid who cured his stutter by the age of thirteen. You'd think an adult like Carlisle would make the effort.'

No doubt he heard my loud and scatological response (the walls were thin), because the conversation abruptly ceased. Nevertheless, he reflected the commonly held view that stuttering is easy to cure if the individual makes the effort. People can always cite examples of someone they know who overcame the disability when young. 'If one person can do it, why can't they all do it?' is the feeling.

Most people ignore the fact that stuttering varies from person to person. Many slight stutters spontaneously disappear in early childhood or adolescence for reasons that are not fully understood. Some stutterers are relatively easy to treat. Nevertheless, when a severe stutter persists in an adult, it is usually the self-reinforcing kind, where disfluency breeds anxiety and tension, which in turn make the stuttering worse, which creates still more stress, and so on. This type is usually difficult to treat, and cures are rare.

Responsible therapists treating adults with severe stutters don't promise a cure. They can help the adult stutterer get better control, reduce the silent, stressful blocks, improve fluency, and reduce anxiety about speaking, but they seldom cure the disability completely. Children with mild disfluencies and adults who stutter slightly with few associated anxieties can often be helped without too much difficulty, but full-blown, severe stuttering in adults poses real problems for the therapist and the patient.

People have been trying to find the cause of stuttering and the remedy for more than two thousand years, but until recently they didn't have much success. During the heyday of the Greek and Roman empires, attention focused on stutterers' speech machinery, particularly the tongue, and this approach persisted until the last half of the nineteenth century. It was widely assumed that stuttering was caused by a physical disability, but at the same time efforts were made to divert the stutterer's attention away from his speech by various devices.

By the end of the nineteenth century, the influence of Freud led clinicians to try to treat the alleged psychological abnormalities that they supposed were the cause of stuttering. During the present century, people who stutter have been subjected to a barrage of different treatments, among them breath control, elocution, relaxation, distraction, sound, pills, hypnosis, ventriloquism, conditioning, and speech training.

Since the 1930s the trend has been to treat the stutterer as a whole person, modifying his attitudes as well as his speech; modern conditioning techniques, too, have helped to deal with the problems. The current trend is to use the particular combination of techniques that seems best suited to an individual. Scientists are still looking for an organic cause that will respond to medication.

With all these treatments available to stutterers, you'd think that there would be something to help everybody. Unfortunately this is not quite the case. Treatments not only take a long time but can also be expensive and often make great demands on the patient's emotional stamina. Not all people are able to receive or persist with treatment. There is also still a tendency for those who become fluent in the clinic to relapse into disfluency in the outside world. Recent sophisticated approaches are reducing the number of relapses, but regression into disfluency is still common – and frustrating for both the therapist and the patient. Even after fifty-five years of therapy I still relapse when I am tired, careless, or anxious.

Historically, the treatment of stutters has been empirical, and it still is to a large extent; if a treatment worked it was used, even though the underlying reasons were not fully understood. Unfortunately, many treatments help only for a short time.

Although many of the early treatments look absurd today, the therapists of the past were doing their best to deal with a malady they did not understand. A great deal more is now known, although we still cannot fit together all the pieces in the jigsaw. Some are missing and others don't fit very well; but the outlines of the picture are gradually beginning to emerge. There is every reason to believe that stuttering will yield to modern science.

What follows describes the early gropings for solutions during the Dark Ages of speech therapy together with the methods used in the transition period before the 1930s, when many theories were tested, and most were found to be wrong. The emergence of modern therapy with its twin thrusts of treating the whole person and conditioning him to speak more fluently are then outlined. The attempt is made to describe a complex subject as simply as possible. If at times my descriptions stray from the solid path of fact and flounder in the mud of conjecture, I am in good company.

The Dark Ages of speech therapy

For centuries, treating stuttering has been a bonanza for quacks. Few treatments are likely to be lethal except for some of the more ill-advised surgical procedures, so a charlatan whose treatment fails isn't likely to be sued. He can always say the patient didn't co-operate or persevere with the treatment.

As early as the fifth century BC, the famous physician Hippocrates (460–400 BC) concluded that stuttering was caused by a dry tongue and prescribed substances to blister the tongue and remove the black bile responsible for the disfluency. Many stutterers have dry mouths because they are frequently anxious about speaking, and Hippocrates confused cause with effect.

A century later the Greek philosopher Aristotle (384–322 BC) agreed that stuttering (which he called 'ischnophonoi') had something to do with the tongue. He also felt that coldness impeded the speech, but had the wisdom not to prescribe treatments.

While Aristotle was acting as mentor to Alexander the Great in Macedonia, the great orator Demosthenes was making a great deal of trouble in Athens with his caustic tongue, stirring up opposition to Alexander's father, Philip of Macedon. Demosthenes seems to have been remarkably testy and articulate. Nevertheless historians tell us that he suffered from a speech defect, allegedly stuttering, and overcame his problem by placing pebbles under his tongue and shouting above the thunder of the waves pounding the coast of Greece. Modern therapists feel that he distracted his attention away from his speech, but the roaring waves may have masked his voice and made him more fluent. Speaking loudly helps some people with their stuttering for a short period, so his approach was triple-barrelled.

During the first century BC, the philosopher Celsus tried to treat stuttering as a physician and as a surgeon. His prescriptions were bad enough. He advised people plagued by stuttering to carry out breathing exercises, wash the head in cold water, eat horseradish, and vomit, which sounds socially messy. His surgical techniques at a time when anaesthesia and aseptic procedures were regarded as unnecessary sound horrendous. Following the guidelines of a doctor called Aetius, he lifted the tongue, stretched the membrane on the underside with a hook, and carefully cut the membrane all the way through with a sharp knife. The mouth was then rinsed with a mixture of vinegar and water, called *'posca'*, followed by powdered frankincense and manna, a solidified honeydew.

Some patients had their speech restored, but there was often profuse bleeding. An alternative was to perforate the membrane with a needle, draw a thread through the hole, and tie it into a knot. The thread was gradually tightened and slowly amputated the membrane. The wound was 'consumed' by Egyptian ointment and drying powders to prevent the membrane from forming again. As one commentator later wrote, 'this is a most agreeable method.' One wonders for whom.[1]

Persuasion and faith were also used to treat stuttering. A Greek prince named Batthus, who apparently stuttered very badly, consulted the famous Oracle at Delphi about what he should do to cure his handicap. The Oracle advised him to go abroad and never return, one of the earliest examples of brushing an intractable complaint under the medical carpet. Batthus gathered together an army and sailed to North Africa where he managed to control his stuttering enough to vanquish his enemies and become governor of Cyrene. Many stutterers find that a change of environment and success in life help their speech for a while. The Delphic Oracle was not all that far out of line.

Incidentally, Batthus (sometimes called Batarus) tended to repeat the first syllable of each word and lent his name to the speech defect known in medieval times as *'batarismus.'*[2]

During the Middle Ages, physicians' attention still focused on the tongue in the tradition of Hippocrates and Aristotle. Some unfortunates with stutters had their tongues burned to encourage fluency, and no doubt they made every effort to overcome their problem and avoid the treatment.

About this time doctors had another look at the idea that dryness of the body, particularly of the tongue, caused stuttering. Strange prescriptions were offered to stutterers, such as gargling with woman's milk or rinsing the mouth with an infusion of boiled water-lily leaves. Dampening the tongue with water mallow, oil of almonds, water lily, and saffron was also thought to help stutterers with their speech.[3]

In 1584 Hieronymous Mercurialis, a famous physician who based his work on Galen's idea that people's behaviour and

health were controlled by the four bodily humours (blood –
the sanguine; phlegm – the phlegmatic; bile – the choleric;
and water – the melancholic), wrote what was probably the
first complete overview of stuttering in a book on childhood
diseases. He recommended that a person with a stutter remain in warm, dry conditions, avoid outbreaks of anger, and
refrain from making love, drinking wine, and eating pastry,
nuts, or fish. Poultices were prescribed, and the patients were
told to speak loudly and forcefully, maintain bowel activity,
and engage in vigorous physical exercise. He advocated a
strenuous and boring life. I wonder how many of his patients
persisted with the treatment.[4]

Mercurialis's treatment was fairly benign. Much later, in
the middle of the nineteenth century, treatment of stutterers
was more drastic. In 1841, the famous Prussian surgeon, Dr
Dieffenbach, developed a surgical procedure to cure stuttering that was sheer butchery. Like Hippocrates and Celsus he
thought that the source of the trouble was the tongue, so he
cut large wedges from the tongues of many patients with stutters. His procedure was copied in both Europe and the
United States at a time before effective anaesthetics and
sterile procedures were widely used. Several patients died in
agony. The pain and distress of the victims do not bear thinking about, and the treatment is a dark blot on the history of
speech therapy.[5]

During the nineteenth century several surgical treatments
of the tongue, the tonsils, and the palate were used in attempts to relieve speech disorders. Cutting the tongue's
frenulum, which connects the underside of the tongue to the
floor of the mouth, was thought to be beneficial by allowing
more freedom of movement. Luchsinger and Arnold felt that
this surgery had as much value as clipping someone's toe-
nails to cure a walking disorder.[6]

I suspect that I was indirectly the victim of one of these
misguided procedures in the early 1930s when tonsillectomies
were almost a ritual for young boys aged about ten, like a second circumcision. The surgeons used the operation to maintain their cash flows. I'd had a sore throat for a while, and an
elderly surgeon, who wore a bow-tie, tails, and spats, decided
to whip out my tonsils, adding that it would 'probably cure

his stutter.' He was right. The ham-fisted fellow broke my jaw, and since I couldn't speak in more than a mumble, for a while I had no trouble with stuttering whatsoever.

Some wily entrepreneurs have lined their pockets by selling strange devices for stutterers to wear in their mouths while speaking. I never used these contraptions but saw one in London, England, that looked like a ferocious rat trap, all plates and springs. Even respected physicians have recommended gadgets like a golden fork attached to the teeth to exercise and strengthen the tongue.[7]

Anybody interested in the more macabre side of medicine should read Murray Katz's 1977 'Survey of patented anti-stuttering devices.'[8] The technical drawings of the devices are reminiscent of designs for the furnishing of medieval torture chambers, complete with enough gags, spikes, levers, clamps, nutcrackers, shafts, springs, grids, belts, and tubes to scare anybody into fluency. Most of these toys were registered in the first half of this century. Some kept the air passages open (to yell for help?), some prevented the stutterer from clenching his teeth, others exercised or immobilized the tongue muscles, and a few co-ordinated breathing and speaking. One little beauty consisted of a spiked reed attached to the roof of the mouth. When the stutterer breathed out it whistled and helped him to maintain his airflow. If he moved his tongue incorrectly, the spike pricked the offending member, goading the speaker along the paths of articulacy. The responses of stutterers to these devices is not recorded. My response is quite definite. Sheer terror!

A physician once advised me to clamp the stem of an unlit pipe between my teeth when I spoke to stabilize my lips. My jaws ached most of the time, and it made me sound like a stuttering ventriloquist. One lady, a Madame Leigh, persuaded the French government to pay her several hundred thousand francs for her secret cure for stuttering, which consisted of a pad of cotton wool beneath the tongue. It may have reduced some of the speech tremors and was far better than some of the junk that experts have told stutterers to stick in their mouths.

People afflicted by stuttering have suffered a great deal at the hands of physicians with little knowledge about stuttering who nevertheless administered drugs or therapy based on reports half remembered from their student days. Over a period of forty years, well-meaning practitioners have prescribed for me tranquillizers, stimulants, vitamins, pills to improve muscular co-ordination, purgatives (!), exercises, diets, learning French, and illicit love. Fortunately I knew enough about my speech not to comply with most of them, although the last one attracted my interest. It would not have surprised me in the least to have been offered leeches to relieve my system of surplus blood to take the pressure off my stuttering. People who stutter should look askance at any prescription that is not based on a thorough clinical assessment by a qualified speech pathologist. The Dark Ages of speech therapy ended all too recently.

A matter of faith

Faith is such a rare and precious commodity that it cannot be consigned to the rag-bag of unsuccessful stuttering remedies and pushed away out of sight. Any stutterer entering intensive therapy must have faith in himself, the therapist, and the treatment or he should stay at home and make room for a patient with better motivation. The faith healers and those practitioners outside the medical profession who use unorthodox suggestion and vibration techniques sometimes have remarkable results with sick people, particularly those whose conditions are complicated by emotional problems. A person with a stutter is a prime target for treatment by these methods.

One stuttering friend paid large sums of money to a well-known faith healer in Europe who assured him that the donations would be used for charitable purposes. This practitioner clearly hadn't taken a vow of poverty; after all, charity begins at home. In spite of my doubts, my friend's speech improved tremendously for the two years I knew him.

The only faith healer I ever met was staying at a small, unheated hotel in an isolated part of northern Europe in the middle of winter. We were drawn together more by a mutual need of body heat than by any intellectual affinity. He was a great man for vibrations and laying on of hands and insisted on trying them out on me after dinner one night. I suspect that his laying on of hands was an excuse to warm his finger tips, but he came up with the diagnosis that my problem lay in a bit of bone on my frontispiece called the sternum. He told me that if I had faith and rubbed the bone every night with a mixture of vinegar and honey, my stuttering would disappear. He didn't charge me a fee, which surprised me, because he was in the area to use his vibes to find hidden gold in a peat bog. I'm afraid I didn't test his method.

In spite of the encounter with my vibrating friend, it is possible that any therapy that results in a marked change in a person's attitude toward himself, his goals and philosophy, his speech, and the people around him could affect his fluency considerably. Anything that relieves some of his anxiety about speaking is sure to be beneficial. Some unorthodox practitioners hit the right spot by accident, others do it by building up real faith.

Stand and deliver: elocution

Prior to World War II, when speech therapists were still groping in the dark, a large number of people set up businesses in Britain as elocutionists to teach dramatic delivery, remove unfashionable accents, and overcome stuttering. The practitioners were usually retired actors and actresses (with names like James Mayhew, Esquire, and Madame Lear) who believed sincerely that any speech defect could be cured by breathing and enunciating correctly and by projecting the voice in the correct manner. They had been on the stage long before amplifiers, woofers, and tweeters were used, and were very keen on *projection*, because they had to be heard up in the *gods*, the upper, upper circle. As one good lady with a queen-sized operatic bust said, 'A parrot can speak, my dear, but he cannot PROJECT.' The windows rattled.

I passed through several elocutionists' hands, including those of one dragon lady who whomped our heads with her conductor's baton whenever we mangled our words. The finest of all was a blue-eyed, jolly, Falstaffian actor with pendulous jowls, long, white, silky hair, and a booming voice. His name was Ryder Boyes, and I met him when I was twelve years of age. He had been on the stage with Sir Henry Irving – he proudly showed me the silver-headed cane given to him by the great man – and his rooms were full of theatrical memorabilia and signed photographs of Victorian and Edwardian

thespians. He loved language, and even more he loved people.

For months he taught me how to 'breathe from the belly,'
'stand up and deliver,' and 'project,' until one day he asked
me to his home for tea and a man-to-man talk. He said it was
clear that he couldn't cure my stutter, so he would teach me
how to live with it. For one hour every week for a year he
taught me love of life, love of people, and love of words, supported by appropriate quotations from Shakespeare. He insisted that I should value myself and face the world with 'the
bright blade of honour, courage, and determination.' It was
hard for a small boy with a stutter to wield a bright blade
when most of his teachers called him a fool in spite of his
good grades, but old Ryder Boyes's jowls would quiver and
his voice boom with anger whenever he heard my resolution
falter. For the sum of one guinea a week I received Darjeeling
tea (with no milk), fruity Dundee cake, and the best counselling in the world. My speech steadily improved for several
years. Ryder Boyes – across the years I salute you!

The trouble with elocution was that it focused a stutterer's
attention on his speech and, because the teachers were largely
theatrical artists, rewarded perfection and performance.
Most of the teachers had little platforms for you to stand on
and *deliver*, while the other sufferers giggled at your inarticulacy. The classes tended to recreate the social pressures
that may have precipitated the stuttering in the first place.

Nevertheless, some of these elocutionists had success.
Charles Van Riper describes one woman who helped stutterers by drilling them in mental arithmetic.[9] The stutterers
were mostly poor, deprived children with low school grades
and even lower morale. The elocutionist ignored their stuttering and gave the children love, faith, and patience, as well as
a facility with mental arithmetic that amazed the other
children, the teachers, and the parents. The speech of some
of the children improved. Like Ryder Boyes, she increased
their self-confidence and self-regard.

The limp rag in a steel world: relaxation

When a stutterer speaks he often appears to be nervous, tense
and agitated. For centuries it was thought that the agitation

caused the stutter, when in fact the reverse seems to be true. During the nineteenth century the therapist Sandow taught stutterers how to relax when they spoke, and many found that their fluency greatly improved, although this improvement was only temporary.[10] Since anxiety and struggling to speak often disappear when a patient is deeply relaxed, this type of therapy works fairly well until the stutterer is thrust into competitive society where relaxation is difficult or even impossible. As Van Riper said, it is hard to be a limp rag in a steel world. Anxiety and struggles of one kind or another are just parts of normal life.

Relaxation therapy reached a peak of popularity during the 1930s, and for a short time I participated in a class in northern Britain. We assembled in a gymnasium smelling strongly of sweaty gymnasts and did relaxation exercises on dusty mats that made us sneeze. The teacher, a well-endowed young woman, taught us to think peaceful thoughts and achieve tranquillity by closing our eyes, breathing deeply, and exhaling slowly with a faint hissing sound. When relaxed we were urged to speak on any topic that came to our minds.

My problem was that the young teacher was so attractive that, like all the other young men in her class, I could not resist peeking at her magnificent endowments through my eyelashes. My thoughts were not particularly peaceful and my feelings were far from tranquil, so relaxation was out of the question.

On the few occasions when I managed to relax completely, I just fell asleep on the floor and had lurid dreams. Even when I managed to control my adolescent urges, relax, stay awake, and speak all at the same time, I still stumbled and bumbled over my words. Some of the older members of the class who stuttered less severely had some luck and became quite fluent in the clinic.

Relaxation therapy is still widely used. From my own experience it was most valuable as a part of a wider therapeutic approach involving complete speech rehabilitation. During such therapy the patients can become very tense, and relaxation helps to increase the effectiveness of the other therapies.

Many therapists look on relaxation techniques with scepticism, but anything that makes people relax a little without using drugs in the headlong dash of modern living has a place.

Distraction

Distractive methods direct the attention of the stutterer away from his speech. Many have been successful in the clinics, but there has been much less success in the conditions of everyday life. Distraction techniques include rhythmics, some forms of speech training, devices such as corks between the teeth or pads beneath the tongue, chewing, shrugging, whistling, counting, ventriloquism, and smoking a pipe. Delayed auditory feedback and use of speech maskers have also been regarded as distractions, but that is an over-simplification.

I first met distraction therapy in 1936. I had fallen in the school workshop and struck my head on the sharp edge of a large metal vise, neatly splitting my scalp and producing spectacular pools of gore. I was rushed to the doctor bleeding all over the teacher's Austin Seven, and endured the shaving of a freeway across my head, followed by the painful attachment of six metal clips like silvery hockey pucks along the incision. While he worked, the doctor chatted about my speech to take my mind off the pain.

When I returned for treatment a few days later he made me tap my foot and speak at the same time, with little success. On the next visit he had me speaking while I crawled all over his Persian carpet on all fours. This worked quite well, but, like any small boy, I couldn't help going off into fits of giggles at the thought of going back to school and asking questions on my hands and knees.

This treatment may sound like the height of medical absurdity, but the doctor had done his homework. I found out years later that at about that time a scientist called Geniesse[11] had discovered that timing stutterers' speech with their movements while they crawled around on all fours significantly increased their fluency. The physician was not as daft as I thought he was. The technique poses obvious social hazards, and if I were to go to a restaurant and order my meal on all fours the *mâitre d'hotel* could be forgiven for either calling the police or offering me a doggy-bag.

A well-meaning school teacher introduced me to an innovative therapy that he claimed would distract my attention from my speech, improve my breathing, and help my fluency. He was the Officers' Training Corps bandmaster and was short of buglers. What could be more sensible than to recruit me into the discordant brass and show me how to blow that strident and unlovely instrument, the bugle? I spent a week making wet, hissing noises down the coiled tube, with an apoplectic face and the imprint of the circular mouthpiece on my swollen lips. My breathing was a total disaster. I never did get the hang of blowing and speaking at the same time, so it didn't help the stutter at all. I was dismissed in disgrace from the wind section, and I have a feeling that if the band had needed a big bass drum thumper, the bass drum would have been prescribed as speech therapy.

One of the distractions that frequently improves fluency is intense fear. During World War II there were many instances of stutterers becoming fluent in moments of intense crisis. Some soldiers and air crew found that they spoke quite normally in action and stuttered badly when at home on leave. This appears to be illogical when fear is so closely associated with the roots of stuttering, but Bloodstein[12] makes the point that it is not just anxiety that precipitates stuttering, but anxiety about stuttering.

Rhythmics have played a major role in distractive stuttering therapy for more than a century. As early as 1837, Serre d'Alais used an instrument called an isochrome, which produced a rhythmic beat for the stutterer to follow when he spoke.[13] The well-known and sometimes infamous stuttering schools leaned heavily on rhythmics because they were fairly sure to get good short-term responses from most of the patients in the clinical situation. The stuttering would completely disappear while the patients spoke to a rhythm as they marched, swung their arms, tapped their feet and fingers, timed their speech syllables with metronomes, nodded their heads, and danced. I was told to march and swing my arms when I spoke, but this didn't work too well at formal dinner parties.

I learned to use my pulse as a metronome and measure my rate of speaking at the same time. My pulse rate was about seventy beats a minute, so it helped to keep my rate of speaking below 80 words a minute, which is my most controllable rate. When I speak faster than 120 words a minute my speech falls apart. The trouble was that everybody thought I was listening to my pulse in case I had a heart attack. The pulse monitor didn't work under pressure, but I still use it occasionally to time my speaking rate.

A portable rhythmic device, developed by Meyer and Mair in 1963,[14] looked like a hearing aid and delivered a rhythmic beat that enabled stutterers to time their speech without embarrassment. The patients slowly became less dependent on the device as their speech improved, but unfortunately they tended to relapse.

The effectiveness of the rhythmic beat depends upon its rate. About ninety beats per minute seems to be the best rate. Faster or more irregular beats are less effective.[15] Some feel that improvement in fluency from rhythmic therapy may not be caused merely by distraction. The rhythm reduces the rate of speaking to levels stutterers can manage, as with my heartbeat. There is also some evidence that rhythm itself, quite apart from its distraction and control of speech rate, can modify the speech by making the time of the speech sounds more predictable. Rhythmic therapy may be much more than distraction and is still used in some schools of stuttering.

Rhythmics and other tricks taught by the earlier therapists (tricks like articulating a glottal stop before a hard word) have the drawback that they are inclined to leave a legacy of undesirable tics and mannerisms. Any therapy that uses speech tricks, starters, or physical movements can have undesirable residual effects. I still tend to twitch my hand and leg when I stutter, a throwback to rhythmic therapy of thirty years ago when I was taught to tap my foot and hand to get through a block. One man was taught to clench his right hand when he stuttered 'to stimulate the left side of the brain' where right-handed people have their speech and language centre. He did this so well that he developed huge muscles on his right arm in contrast to his skinny left.

Phonation therapy (or resonance therapy) was used in some of the large hospitals in Britain during the 1930s and 1940s. In some ways this therapy was simply speech training, because it taught control of air flow and the vocal chords; but it also contained a large element of distraction.

Following World War II my speech was at a low ebb. I was not so bad as some stutterers whom the stresses of war had reduced to total mutes, but my ability to communicate was so limited that the Armed Forces sponsored my treatment at a large London hospital. The therapist was a man in his late fifties with a distinctly military, no-nonsense air. Treatment was on a one-to-one basis with no opportunity to compare notes with other patients. The therapist was a bully, and we didn't get on at all well. He started the therapy with a finger-wagging homily about how all his patients had recovered, so I had better maintain his record, and continued with the warning that I would become a social outcast, etc., etc., unless I stopped stuttering. It was all a bit threatening and discouraging.

The therapy had none of today's psychological frills. You established a fundamental, low-frequency, resonant tone by uttering the prolonged sound 'er,' and checking with your fingertips to see that your larynx was vibrating. You maintained this basic monotone, thereby keeping up the airflow, and superimposed your words. I tried this for a week with little success, because my speech was so bad that I blocked on the 'er' and couldn't resonate most of the time. When I could resonate, the words I tried to superimpose just wouldn't come out. The therapist became impatient and angry, and I protested (with a stutter) that asking me to say 'er' and superimpose my words on the sound was like telling a short-sighted person without glasses to read small-print instructions on how to improve his sight.

This miserable business went on for six months and my speech became worse and worse. I learned to say the 'er' and resonate, but nothing else, and my voice fixed on the monotone. The 'er' became a vocalized block that I couldn't go beyond. When I met people, instead of saying, 'Hello', I just said 'Er,' which limited further conversation, and I began to associate therapy and speaking with increased frustration and anger. The authoritarian therapist may have helped some patients, but for me the treatment was a disaster. It took me three years to recover from the conditioned 'er' block. The therapist retired before my treatment was completed, so he kept his score of 100 per cent success.

Very few therapists I met were bullies. Most were firm and demanding, but in a positive way. The only other bullies I met were young male trainees who, feeling their power over the patients, created superior-subordinate relationships. The patients soon let these young men know their displeasure. It was all part of the trainees' learning process. A rapport between patient and therapist is vital.

The clinician was not necessarily lying when he said that all his resonating patients recovered. They may have done so in the clinic, but it is doubtful that many maintained their fluency in the workplace and under social pressures.

This therapy, like many others, used one approach for all patients and did not take into account the different needs of individuals. My martinet created an atmosphere of anxiety, hostility, and guilt that modern therapists avoid at all costs, because these emotions are cues to stutter.

There are many other methods of distraction. The trouble with all of them is that the patient is delighted when he becomes fluent for a while and is shattered with disappointment when he later plunges back into disfluency. One man made me say tongue-twisters before every therapy session to distract me, saying that if I could focus on the difficult words the ordinary words would be easy. I could say 'Peggy Babcock' and 'Black Bug's Blood' five times quickly without hesitation, but saying 'Good morning' still defeated me. Distraction involves avoiding facing up to the stuttering squarely. It is a mere escape hatch. Like anybody else with a handicap, a person with a severe stutter cannot afford to run away from his problem.

Auditory feedback

Auditory feedback refers to the feedback of the sounds of speech to a person's ear. Delayed auditory feedback (DAF) tends to disrupt the speech, and when sound is used to prevent a stutterer from hearing his own speech his fluency often increases. Both of these facts have been used to treat stuttering.

The therapeutic use of DAF arose from research on effects of conditioning stutterers using reward and punishment. The stutterer was exposed to continuous delayed (0.2 second) auditory feedback of his speech. When he was relieved from the disruptive, delayed feedback for ten seconds each time he blocked, he responded by speaking in a slow, prolonged, and more fluent manner, so DAF was used to develop slow, prolonged speech. The delayed sound was slowly reduced and normal speech rates gradually restored. There seemed to be some carry-over of the improved speech from the clinic to ordinary life.[16]

It is not clear whether DAF is effective simply because it distracts the stutterer from his speech, but even if it is a distraction the carry-over seems to be better than with rhythmic methods and gadgets in the mouth.

My attention was first drawn to the masking technique in 1957 by Professor E.T. Jones, a physicist who played a major role as a scientific boffin during World War II. At his suggestion I visited a laboratory in northwestern England to test a prototype of a masking instrument consisting of a heavy tape recorder delivering loud continuous white sound (mixed frequencies) to a pair of large earphones. My speech at that time was very disfluent, but the continuous noise at a level of about 100 decibels enabled me to read aloud fluently in the clinic. Unfortunately, the benefit faded when I tried the instrument at home. I could still read aloud and recite, but couldn't combine my thoughts and speech to convey information, because the stuttering cues in the words still overrode the effects of the sound. The noise gave me a headache and, instead of getting used to it, I became irritated by it. Continuous white sound is now known to be less effective in increasing fluency than low frequency (500 Hz) sound delivered only when the stutterer speaks.

In 1976 the masking technique was refined by Ann Dewar and her colleagues at Edinburgh University, Scotland,[17] but I didn't consider testing it because I was responding well to other speech therapy, although I still had great difficulty using the telephone and speaking to audiences of more than a few people.

I instinctively distrust gadgets, particularly those used in

speech therapy, but when I heard that Ann Dewar's Edin-
burgh Masker was being manufactured by Findlay, Irvine
Ltd., at Penicuik, Scotland, and distributed in Canada by
Cantechs Ltd., of St John, New Brunswick, and in the
United States by the Foundation for Fluency, Inc., of
Chicago, Illinois, I decided to test the instrument for a
month.

The Edinburgh Masker consists of a neat little electronic
sound-producer or buzzer about the size of a packet of
cigarettes, a throat microphone, a small junction box, and
ear-pieces. The sound producer makes a low-pitched hum, of
about 500 Hz, which is modified by the pitch of the speaker's
voice and has a noise level of about ninety decibels. When a
person speaks, the throat microphone turns the buzzer on
and turns it off again when he stops, with a small lag to allow
for normal pauses in speech. The buzzer unit has a manual
switch that can override the throat microphone when necessary. Some ear-pieces are of the stethoscope type, but more
comfortable skeletal ear-moulds are available. The sound is
conveyed from the buzzer to the ear-pieces by small tubes
made of clear plastic, and the conventional throat microphone is attached to a point just below the Adam's apple by a
fabric tape. The microphone gets uncomfortable on hot days,
but it can be replaced by a smaller throat microphone attached by two-way sticky pads to the throat. If a person is
wearing a collar and tie or a turtle-neck sweater, the apparatus is no more obtrusive than a hearing-aid. (With an
open-neck shirt, however, it looks as though the wearer has
had a tracheotomy.)

The noise level is fairly high, and there was the possibility
that the masker would damage a user's hearing. Taking into
account the average number of hours the stutterers wore the
masker (3.3 hours per day) and the average period they spoke
(about 7.5 minutes per hour) Ann Dewar found that the
sound exposure was within the official limits for workers.
Careful monitoring of seventeen patients' hearing for up to
three years failed to detect any reduction in hearing acuity at
any sound frequency.[18]

The Edinburgh University team found that a lawyer and a
pharmacist spoke very little (2.8 to 3.2 minutes each hour)

during an ordinary working day, a university lecturer spoke much more (9.3 minutes each hour), while a retail salesman, a physiotherapist, and an interior decorator all spoke a great deal (11.6 to 13.4 minutes each hour). Nobody spoke much more than three hours each day, so the exposure to the noise was relatively short.[19]

Sixty-seven users of the masker were tested in Britain over a two-year period; 42 per cent received great benefit, 40 per cent considerable benefit, and 18 per cent slight benefit. Some objected to the appearance of the instrument, and others didn't like the noise. However, most thought that the benefits outweighed the disadvantages. About 70 per cent of the patients found that the instrument remained effective for a year at least; others found that the benefit declined. Five patients became fully fluent and discarded the instrument.[20]

The Edinburgh Masker's effects surprised me. I expected the blanking out of my speech by the sound to produce fluency for a while; but since I regarded it as a mere distraction and my stutter is an intractable type, I didn't expect much more. I had used distractive techniques before and their effects soon faded.

I tested the masker in stores and on the telephone, and there were a few failures, some the result of minor malfunctions of the instrument and others of my own attitude. I tried, without realizing it, to hear my own voice above the noise, in a desperate attempt to get feedback. When I succeeded, I stuttered. I tended to use the override too much, relying on the continuous noise rather than larynx-activated noise, but I stopped this when I learned to trust the throat microphone.

I had some early difficulties controlling the loudness of my speech and varying my voice's pitch. I tended to speak in a loud monotone like some deaf people, but I mastered these problems in two days. The noise was irritating at first, but I soon became used to it.

Since my family tells me that I talk too much even with my stuttering, I had to curb the urge to monopolize the conversation. I couldn't hear interruptions when I spoke, and it didn't give people a chance to chip in. I learned to watch people as I spoke and to let them have their say. The instrument worked best for me if I spoke in the slow, prolonged manner I had been taught by the excellent speech therapists at the Royal Ottawa Hospital. Without the masker I had to keep an iron control on my speech to use the techniques, but with the instrument it was much easier, and I could relax a little. There was less tension and less need to focus my attention on the approach to every sentence. Somebody who knew me said, 'What's happened to your speech?' and hadn't noticed the ear-moulds and throat microphone. I was fairly fluent apart from normal disfluency and fumbling for the right word.

It appears that the masker, quite apart from its distraction, removes the effect of most of my stuttering cues. I can read aloud, and words beginning with 'm,' 'p,' 'b,' and 't' no longer cause my stomach to tense as I prepare to cope. I don't anticipate a struggle. It helps my automatic speech and defuses most of my anxiety about stuttering.

Some cues still make me block even with a masker. If I visualize my name in writing, I have to make a great effort to keep control by using prolonged speech even though I cannot hear myself, but when I say my name automatically without seeing the words I am fluent.

My controllable rate of speaking has risen to 140 words a minute, which is easier on the listener. I was also startled to find that, after using the masker for several hours, I was much more fluent for a day or more afterwards, even when I did not use the device.

The machine isn't foolproof, and you don't just switch it on and speak. The user has to learn to stop trying to hear himself, and avoid visual images of his cues to block.

So far, so good. I intend to test the masker in more challenging situations – in committee meetings, on radio and television, and when speaking in public. The benefit may fade, but the masker makes me much more fluent on the telephone, which was always my worst cue to stutter, so I am cautiously optimistic. I shall also maintain the speech techniques I learned earlier.

Some therapists vehemently oppose the use of portable masking devices, and Sheehan[21] pointed out that they lend themselves to quackery. The masker does not help some people, and with others the benefit sometimes fades. The possibility that the masking sound may act merely as a distraction or avoidance raises the hackles of some therapists, and the haphazard, unguided use of the masker is not recommended. I just describe how it works for me.

Why the masker helps I don't know. It is not undoing previous therapy, or changing my attitudes. I have a verbal limp, and the masker helps me, like a walking-stick rather than a crutch, over the rough ground. If the masker continues to work I shall be delighted, and if the effect fades I shall be philosophical. To deny older stutterers who have been through the therapeutic mill a little help on the grounds of principle seems a little dogmatic.

Some younger stutterers find that a masking device helps them to lead normal lives, and good luck to them so long as they realize that they may need treatment for behavioural and attitudinal problems. If wearing a funny nose and plastic vampire teeth helps them to communicate and keeps them happy, I'd still say good luck.

The use of the masker, without previous professional assessment, by children, adolescents, and young adults is ill-advised. It's rather like giving a walking-stick to someone with an untreated paralysed leg. People with severe stutters often need rehabilitative therapy quite apart from modification of the speech.

The machine could be improved. There are still minor bugs such as kinked tubes, faulty cables, and erratic microphone contact, and ways of using it need tailoring to the individual. Nevertheless there are grounds for cautious optimism.

Some successful users report a complete change in their lives and attitudes, but I have not found this to be the case. It is easier to speak to people, interview editors, talk on the telephone, and order meals, but I used to do all these things before, stutter or no stutter. The masker just makes life easier and reduces anxieties about speaking.

Magic pills

At one time I kept a collection of pills that various physicians had prescribed for my stuttering over a period of ten years.

Many of the bottles remained unopened. All were kept in a locked cupboard because some were remarkably potent. There were enough tiny phenobarbitone tablets to put a small village to sleep. Beside them on the shelf were two brown bottles labelled 'Serenase' and 'Stematil.' Serapasil (or reserpine) kept company with the stimulant Benzedrine, and a small, dark, sinister bottle containing sodium amytal had a paper tag on which I had written 'Not Bloody Likely!' There were some little yellow pills that were supposed to improve a spastic's co-ordination (they made me sick after my one and only dose), vitamins B and C, and several unopened bottles of the tranquillizers chlorpromazine and Meprobamate. I never spent money on these pills because the physicians were a little casual about drugs and gave me pills off their sample shelves like candies. After a few unfortunate experiences I became cautious, and eventually the pills were flushed down the lavatorial bend.

The physicians who provided the drugs meant well, but they had no expertise in speech pathology. Many worked on the vague premise that relaxing a stutterer would cure his speech. Some doctors also had the idea that, since people who stutter severely sometimes look depressed (who wouldn't if they couldn't speak?) they just need a good belt of Benzedrine to tune up their systems.

About that time researchers were testing drugs on stutterers, and the physician who prescribed the Serpasil (reserpine), chlorpromazine, and Meprobamate had probably kept up with the scientific literature. These drugs reduce anxiety and tension in stutterers and have been beneficial as part of other therapy. Nevertheless, the results from the experiments were conflicting, and there is no unquestionable evidence that the drugs alleviate stuttering. [22]

While drugs such as tranquillizers can be useful in speech therapy and the treatment of other disorders, whether they are used depends upon the balance between the adverse side effects and the potential benefits. Some drugs have slight effects while others are potent, selective toxins.

Serpasil (or reserpine) has been widely used to treat high blood pressure and to sedate tense stutterers. This drug is now suspected of being associated with breast cancer and can have a wide range of side effects, including nausea, depression, sleeplessness, nightmares, drowsiness, and dizziness. Many other drugs react with reserpine in a harmful manner.

Meprobamate releases tensions, but can result in hives, clumsiness, drowsiness, blurred vision, diarrhoea, headaches, tiredness, and nausea and is not prescribed for pregnant women. It can slow the speech, suggesting some effect on the speech or language centres, and reacts with such drugs as antihistamines, narcotics, and barbiturates. Use of chlorpromazine, one of the phenothiazines, can cause muscle spasms, restlessness, tics, trembling, and sometimes fainting. The side effects vary from person to person, but many people adjust to these medicines after a short time. [23]

Other types of medication besides tranquillizers have been used to help stutterers. Heavy doses of vitamins B and C apparently benefit some people who stutter, but information on the duration of the improvement is hard to find. A physician prescribed for me large quantities of vitamin B-complex capsules, which resulted in a feeling of well-being but had no effect on my speech. The capsules are not, of course, as potent or effective as the massive vitamin injections given to some stutterers. It is difficult to see how vitamins can deal with the numerous factors that mediate a stutter.

So far nobody has invented the magic pill that will make stutterers completely fluent, and it isn't likely that anyone will do so, unless the predisposition to stutter is found to have an organic, neurological origin in some abnormality in the brain's speech centres. Neurological abnormality could possibly be treated by hormones or biochemicals that modify neurotransmitters. Even if this were possible it may not help adults with their Pandora's boxes of haunting anxieties about speech opened in childhood by the key of society's demands.

It is now clear that simple relaxation, by chemical or other means, will not resolve many stutterers' problems outside the clinic, and stimulants aren't likely to help, either; the stutter itself stimulates most people who stutter more than they wish. Perhaps, as the new schools of behavioural biology and physiology unravel the biochemical mysteries of our emotions and behaviour, they will shed light on the biochemical processes of anxiety-conditioned disabilities like stuttering and show us how to deal with them.

The power of suggestion

Surely somebody can persuade stutterers that there's no need to be anxious about the bats in their vocal belfries, and that they should stop all the fuss and bother of avoiding stuttering and get on with the business of automatic, fluent, controlled speaking. I trained a budgerigar under a black cloth to say 'Douglas (my brother), silly boy,' so it shouldn't be too hard to put me in a dark room and persuade me to mimic fluent speech.

A few people may have been made fluent by hypnosis. Unfortunately, the effect doesn't usually persist beyond the hypnotic trance, and the speech can relapse to a worse state than before. It is not as though the practitioners of hypnosis are trying to correct organic disorders like blindness or deafness, because a stutterer shows by his spells of fluency that he has all the necessary articulatory equipment. It should be possible to persuade him to use it. Sad to say, hypnosis doesn't usually work.

Suggestion plays a hidden role in most modern speech therapy. When the therapy includes psychotherapy and counselling, a skilled clinician will guide a stutterer to persuade himself to adopt certain attitudes and to speak in certain ways. One patient went to a qualified practitioner with a view to using hypnotic suggestion to reduce his hang-ups about speaking. After a few months of discussion, the patient asked when the hypnosis would start. The doctor replied that it had nearly finished, because the patient had used suggestion on himself and was greatly improved.

Every therapist uses non-hypnotic suggestion in speech classes, because it takes a great deal of gentle persuasion to get the stutterer to carry out projects like stopping strangers on the street to ask the way to the bus station or post office while repeating sounds deliberately. The nervous patient is likely to hide in a coffee shop. The therapist cannot bludgeon the stutterer into carrying out the painful tasks. She must make him feel that they are worthwhile and helpful. Some therapists I know could persuade people to take winter holidays on Baffin Island. In the right therapist's hands, suggestion and persuasion are potent tools.

Therapy by suggestion is not a closed book. As Charles

Van Riper points out, stutterers can sometimes generate enough will-power to refuse to stutter for a short time. Nobody knows why it happens. A stutter cannot be cured by powerful self-persuasion alone, but stutterers can, at the end of successful therapy, be taught to resist the urge to stutter if avoidance of speaking is no longer a problem.

The stutterer is asked to read in unison with the fluent therapist, which he does very easily. Then the therapist stutters deliberately and challenges the patient to keep fluent. The stutterer must resist the therapist's suggestion to revert to old stuttering behaviour, and gradually the patient is persuaded to build up resistance to stress. In a similar way, delayed auditory feedback can be used to challenge the stutterer who has responded to therapy to keep fluent by will-power, even though the delayed sound tends to disrupt his fluency.[24]

This is, of course, very different from hypnosis, but there is a strong element of auto-suggestion. It does not support the views of people who say 'You can stop stuttering if you really want to,' because self-persuasion is only effective as part of other therapy.

Injudicious use of hypnosis to cure a stutter in the music-hall situation can be very damaging. If hypnosis is used at all it should follow a careful assessment of the stutterer by a qualified professional in a clinical situation. There are first-class hypnotists, but there are enough quacks to stock a duck farm.

The mind-benders: psychotherapy

PSYCHOANALYSIS

With the plethora of doubts about whether stuttering is caused by organic disorders, and the overwhelming amount of evidence that stuttering develops under social pressure and is maintained by anxieties about speaking and responses to stuttering cues, you would think that the psychoanalysts would have come up with more answers than they have. Most stutterers who received intensive therapy in the 1940s and 1950s found themselves at one time or another sitting opposite a Freudian psychiatrist who probed for evidence of neurosis by asking them personal questions about their childhood and love life. Few found it helped their speech. Earlier this century Brill had some success psychoanalyzing stutterers. Most of his sixty-nine patients responded, but the number of subsequent relapses was disappointing.[25] Such analysis is not a sure-fire cure.

These days fewer psychologists and psychiatrists carry out in-depth analyses to find the alleged neurotic causes of stuttering. There are many causes, all of them interacting, and a neurosis may or may not be one of them. The more common approach is to treat the stutterer as he is today, reduce his tensions and fears about speaking, modify negative attitudes, and teach him better ways of speaking.

You could expect that the daily trauma experienced to a greater or lesser degree by all severe stutterers would result in a definite 'stuttering personality,' even a neurotic one. In spite of a great deal of research, there is no real evidence of such an entity. According to H.R. Beech and Fay Fransella, 'If the stutterer has a unique personality pattern this would have been abundantly apparent by this time.'[26] It is hard for a psychotherapist to develop general principles and know precisely what to treat.

All psychotherapy encounters the problem that in order to treat the patient it is necessary to establish a dialogue, and stutterers find it so hard to speak that this can be remarkably difficult to achieve. Sometimes a stutterer can give misleading answers when he avoids difficult words. The classic story of the stutterer who, when asked by a waiter which salad dressing he wanted, said, 'Roque____, Roque____, Roque____, Thousand Islands,' gives a good example of word substitution. It is easier for most people with stutters to say 'Yes' than 'No.' If the patient tends to favour the response 'yes,' regardless of the question, the clinician is led into a maze of contradictions.

Nevertheless, psychoanalysis can help a stutterer respond to other therapy. Dealing with 'frozen feelings' is one area in which psychoanalysis is useful. Some stutterers are so adept at freezing their feelings when approaching a traumatic speaking situation that it becomes a way of life, spilling over into all their daily relationships. All people discipline their feelings to deal with their fears or they couldn't perform, but these emotions may catch up with them later. The trouble with people who stutter badly is that fears beset them so often that they discipline their feelings all the time and all too well. They never let go.

In 1943 a German fighter aircraft carried out a low-level, surprise attack on southeastern London during the lunch break. It had a persistent Spitfire on its tail. The intruder carried a 250-pound bomb beneath its fuselage, and the pilot dumped the explosives at random to reduce the plane's weight and increase its manoeuvrability. Tragically, the bomb landed on a primary school dining-room and blew many small children to pieces.

During the cleaning-up operation the workers did their job in silence, with expressionless, mask-like faces. The horror was too great for them to bear consciously, so they froze their feelings to allow them to do their jobs. In the evening they congregated in a nearby pub, where some just sat and stared into space over their untouched beers, while others openly wept. Each reacted in his own way. Those who accepted the pain of their emotions and wept were lucky, but some of those who remained frozen would never accept the penalty of their outraged feelings and would stash them away in locked closets in their minds. Some would have nightmares for many years unless they faced the horror squarely.

People who stutter deal with a multitude of lesser horrors and nightmares every day. If they continually store away and deny decades of unfelt pain it can make them very tense indeed. Psychoanalysis and counselling can help them to face their memories' spectres. Some people plagued by stuttering had such terrible experiences in their first years at school that they blot this period out of their minds. In-depth analysis can help them to accept the pain of the memory, see themselves as a whole, deal with any lingering deep resentment of their childhood tormentors, and get on with the speech therapy. Many adult stutterers dealt with their feelings themselves during their childhood, but for some it was too much to bear.

Psychological counselling can help those who stutter to deal with emotions (not necessarily neuroses) that come to the surface during other therapy. Stutterers respond in different ways to their disability, and some have deep-seated anger toward their parents, siblings, peers, or any segment of society that torments them. Sometimes they have good reason to be angry; but anger and bitterness, with violent verbal or even physical explosions, can become a way of life.

Psychotherapy can help a stutterer, or any other person, to manage anger in a productive, positive way. There are two schools of thought about how to do this. During the last decade many psychiatrists interpreted Freud's ideas to mean that all repression is bad and that to repress anger is dangerous to a person's mental health. These practitioners have encouraged people to express their hostility openly by screaming and throwing tantrums to 'let it all out'. Such quickie solutions to mankind's frustrations have in my opinion helped to generate our permissive, spoiled-brat society.

Carol Tavris has debunked the idea that it is wrong to control anger in her refreshing book *Anger: The Misunderstood Emotion*.[27] She points out that openly expressing violent anger and 'having it out' with your antagonist does not defuse the anger or make the exploder feel any better. There are better ways than fury and abuse to deal with injustice or insult.

The problem that many stutterers face is that they are not sufficiently fluent to use sharp-edged syntax as a defence against rudeness. In spite of this, some handle it very well. A burly man with a severe stutter went up to the counter of a coffee shop and blocked badly when he ordered a cup of coffee. A man who belonged to one of those charitable organizations that wear funny hats and help paraplegics was sitting nearby. He mimicked the stutterer's speech and laughed. The large stutterer went over to him and disfluently but calmly said, 'Why did you do that? Do you find my stutter funny? I don't. You people provide wheelchairs for the physically disabled and help the blind, deaf, and mentally retarded. What's so different about people who stutter? You wouldn't ridicule or mimic a person in a wheelchair.'

The man was shattered. He apologized, asked about the problem and how it was treated, and volunteered his help. He was just an ordinary, decent person programmed by Western society's mores to ridicule stuttering. The highly explosive situation was defused when the stutterer managed his intense anger in a constructive way.

Van Riper has said that deep psychoanalytic procedures 'have not been shown to be particularly effective with the stutterer,'[28] but Bloodstein has concluded that 'psycho-analytic treatment of stutterers to date ... appears to have been too good to permit us to reject this method summarily, and too poor as yet to warrant any substantial amount of satisfaction.'[29]

Whatever the initial cause, the stutterer may well have outgrown the original stimulus to stutter and left it far behind. His main problems are usually his anxiety about speech, society's reaction to his disability, and his inner and outer response to that reaction.

There are many ways of carrying out psychoanalysis, and it is not appropriate to describe them here. The earlier Freudian approaches seem to be giving way to behavioural methods. Now that some behaviourists are under attack for too close adherence to Skinnerian 'Operant Conditioning,' new avenues are being explored. Undoubtedly some stutterers have neuroses that need resolution by psychoanalysis, just as some blind people need psychiatric help; but most stutterers respond well to less detailed, short-term counselling and reduction of their sensitivity to stuttering cues and frustra-tion. Gestalt therapy in various forms is used frequently as an adjunct to other therapy, so it is worth describing here.

GESTALT THERAPY

This approach is based on the principle that people are healthy when they are in touch with themselves and their sur-roundings. It emphasizes pattern, organization, and wholes, and involves the study of unanalysed personal experience rather than reflective introspection. The whole is looked on as quite different from the sum of the individual parts. The word 'gestalt' is hard to translate into English, but gestalten means a holistic pattern.

Gestalt therapy has been used to treat stutters by dealing with speech behaviour in relation to feelings and attitudes. The stutterer is made conscious of what he does when he stut-ters (stops breathing, purses the lips, lifts the tongue to the roof of the mouth), so that he can accept personal responsibility for the way he speaks and realize that, with guidance, he can modify his stuttering behaviour by continuing airflow and reducing lip and tongue tensions.

Many stutterers feel that there is a perverse little manikin inside them that makes them stutter, when in fact the stutterer himself is responsible for his stutter. He is shown that he can learn to choose whether he tenses lips and tongue or approaches speech in a gentle manner, stops breathing or continues his airflow. He can learn to choose between stuttering and fluency.

In order to be responsible for the way he speaks and to modify his speech patterns, he must stay in contact with his audience and not go off into the detached trance with which so many blocked stutterers remove themselves mentally from the intolerable situation. He is shown how to focus on the solution rather than the problem. A stutterer can't focus on anything if he has floated off into the protective never-never land of the severely disfluent. Gestalt therapy helps the stutterer to take more risks by testing unfamiliar ways of speaking in many different situations.

Gestalt therapy guides the stutterer to be aware of his conflict about wanting to speak yet not wanting to because of his stutter, and to stay in touch with his feelings, his audience, and his surroundings. The therapy deals with anxiety by persuading the stutterer to stop worrying about what is going to happen (don't anticipate the day's traumatic speaking situations) and to direct his attention and energies to present problems and their solutions. The over-all goal is to keep the stutterer in touch with his feelings and surroundings, and to modify attitudes that increase or reinforce his abnormal speech.[30]

Therapy similar to the Gestalt approach is used in most speech clinics, although not always under a Gestalt label. Treatment of avoidances, conflicts, awareness, and anxiety are the core of many modern therapies. Helping the stutterer to stay in contact, to understand what he does when he stutters, and to realize that he can choose to use the better speaking techniques offered by the therapists is important if the stutterer is to gain any freedom from the fear that is part of the problem. Supportive psychotherapy helps to clear the clutter from the stutterer's workbench so he can get on with the business of reconstructing his speech.

CONDITIONING AND FLUENCY SHAPING
Conditioning therapy is more favoured by clinicians than by the general public, who tend to associate it with brainwashing. Nevertheless new conditioning techniques are having great success.

A person with a stutter is conditioned to respond to numerous cues that trigger stuttering. One stutterer I knew in the Armed Forces savagely blocked whenever he saw a floral fabric because whenever he stuttered a sadistic schoolteacher had draped him over a chair covered with the fabric and beaten him for lazy speech, allegedly to help him. Most stuttering cues (particular sounds or words) are less dramatic, and it is fair to assume that what has been conditioned can be deconditioned by appropriate therapy. If an experimental rat can be taught to press a lever to obtain food or avoid pain, surely a person who stutters can be taught to speak in a normal way. Therapy that uses conditioning can reduce stutterers' sensitivities to cues, anxiety, and frustration. Even so, it is not as straightforward as many people think.

I am aware that many of my cues are indirect. Even pictures of objects or types of places or people associated with traumatic stuttering in the past can trigger a stuttering phase. Just the sight of a building can set me off. This became apparent when a clinician screened a series of slides and asked me to talk about them. Pictures of lecture halls, telephones, police cars, adolescents, customs officials, and people chatting socially, gave me great trouble until I was desensitized by repeated exposure. I didn't fear any of these images, but past associations made them trigger my stuttering. I was conditioned to respond to them and had to be desensitized systematically.

A classic example of indirect conditioning is the 'Albert's fear of furry objects' case. In the early 1920s a small American child called Albert was conditioned to be scared of furry objects by first frightening him with the noise made by striking a steel bar and then pairing a furry object with the noise. Although Albert was initially scared of the noise and responded to it, he later responded fearfully to furry objects without the noise. I can't help wondering what happened to Albert and speculating about how many furry objects scared him in later life.[31]

The conditioning techniques used to remove old bad habits and instil new and better ones mostly come under the broad heading of 'operant conditioning,' the principle of which is that when you behave in a certain way and there are consequences, these consequences influence your future behaviour.

When the consequences involve a reward (positive reinforcement), the behaviour is likely to be repeated. If the behaviour results in punishment (negative reinforcement), the behaviour is often avoided or weakened. A punishment following a form of behaviour can be made to reduce the behaviour, which is the principle underlying civil retribution for acts against society. Behaviour that removes the penalty or prevents it from occurring can be strengthened.[32]

The earlier work on operant conditioning tended to skim over innate factors like genes and the urge to seek novelty and assumed that any animal could be conditioned to do anything. Although this is now questioned, there is no doubt that experience affects fear and our responses to it. A subject's fear can be reduced if the feared situation is repeated without penalty (a technique used in speech therapy under the heading of 'desensitization') or if it is apparent that certain behaviour can end or prevent pain.

Whatever reduces a stutterers' fear of speaking has potential as a therapeutic tool, and operant conditioning, with its rewards and punishments for speech behaviour, has been used to improve stutterers' fluency. Rewards and punishments seem to have worked at least temporarily for some, but I am glad that it is one form of therapy I missed. There are more than enough penalties for stuttering already.

The effects of operant conditioning on stuttering were studied by Flanagan and his colleagues.[33] They subjected three patients to a punishing 105-decibel noise every time they blocked, and the subjects' disfluency was reduced considerably. It was also found that when the noise was continuous except when switched off briefly if a patient stuttered, stuttering increased. In other words the patients who stuttered became more fluent to avoid the noise penalty in the first case, and then stuttered to get subsequent peace and quiet in the second case. The speech responses were thought to be due to the consequences of stuttering – noise or silence.

Martin and Siegel found that when stuttering was penalized by electrical shocks from electrodes strapped to the patient's wrist, disfluency was markedly reduced. The improvement continued in the clinic without the shocks if the electrodes were simply attached, but the speech broke down when they were removed. One patient remained fluent when he wore a plain wrist-strap reminiscent of the punitive electrodes. In another situation a patient who stuttered became temporarily more fluent when he was simultaneously shocked and exposed to a blue light each time he stuttered. His fluency increased with the blue light alone, but the stuttering returned when both electrodes and the blue light were removed. Verbal punishment and rewards ('Not good' or 'Good') were also effective in reducing stuttering in the clinic, and a simple wrist strap to remind the stutterer to say each word as fluently as possible helped to maintain fluency.[34] These studies were research rather than therapy. They aimed at studying the effects of rewards and penalties.

In 1969, the Speech Foundation of America sponsored a conference at Montego Bay, Jamaica, to discuss the use of operant conditioning in stuttering therapy. The participants included such respected therapists as Joseph G. Sheehan and Charles Van Riper, who revolutionized stuttering therapy in North America, as well as professors of other university speech departments.

The experts were cautious about the desirability of using punishment to achieve fluency. As Van Riper reminded the participants, 'These stuttering clients of ours are not Skinnerian pigeons hatched from laboratory eggs. They are not Pavlovian dogs suspended from experimental frames. They are subject to other controls more powerful than those we can mobilize in the therapy room. Stutterers come to us with long histories of past conditioning ... Behaviour therapists have difficulty working with stutterers.' In similar vein,

Joseph Sheehan asked, 'Why should children stutter when the behaviour is apparently more punished than rewarded?' If punishment were an effective stuttering deterrent there would be few stutterers in Western society.[35]

Conditioning in benign forms is widely used today under the title of 'Fluency Shaping Therapy.' Operant conditioning and programming principles, with the reward-punishment aspects well hidden, are used in this therapy, which differs from therapies that attempt to treat the stutterer as a whole person. Fluency shaping therapy takes a direct approach. It assumes that the stutterer makes the sounds of speech incorrectly and that reasons for this are beside the point. Researchers of this school of thought have carefully examined what a stutterer does incorrectly and look upon stuttering as part of a speech spectrum ranging from severe disfluency to normal speech. The therapy is designed to push the speech toward the normal end of this spectrum by carefully graded exercises that emphasize the control of speech rate, gentle initial approaches (easy onset) to sounds, and prolongation of words to achieve fluency within the clinic. Later the techniques are transferred to everyday life.[36]

This technique was used by Ronald L. Webster, of Hollins College, Virginia, and his innovative approach evolved after a series of experimental programs. The earlier programs used delayed auditory feedback to achieve fluency, and the later schemes tried to overcome the fact that the stutterer tended to use the clinician as a crutch. The final treatment consisted of teaching the patient how to handle single sounds, followed by whole words, transition from word to word, prolongation, and an impersonal monitoring system.

This system minimizes the frequency with which the therapist must tell the stutterer what to do next. When the patient speaks correctly, a light flashes to indicate that he can move on to other exercises. If the light does not flash, the stutterer repeats the sound or word until it is correct. The frequency of disfluencies is recorded to assess improvement.

All tasks are carefully graded, and even the sounds are ranked according to difficulty. Vowels are the easiest; vowel-like consonants ('l,' 'r,' 'y,' and 'w') are a little harder; fricatives ('f' and 's') harder still; and stop-consonants (the plosives 'p,' 'b,' and 'd') hardest of all. The aim is to instruct the stutterer to start his sounds gently, handle 'silent' consonants correctly, and increase the duration of sounds.

Early in the therapy the duration of sounds is very exaggerated, but the prolongation is reduced until the rate of speaking is about 100 words or more per minute, which is slow but socially acceptable. The transfer of these techniques to everyday life was found to be unusually good, and positive results were obtained after only forty to sixty hours in the clinic. A set of twenty patients aged from eight to fifty-two years responded remarkably well. After treatment, nineteen reported better speech. Only one person felt that his stutter was the same. After therapy many of the stutterers talked more, as you would expect, were better able to take part in a wider range of social activities, and found their work easier to handle.[37]

The Webster or Hollins method[38] has aroused considerable interest and is now an important component of many programs. It may not help stutterers who hide their stuttering and refuse to stutter openly. The Webster method can greatly help the more open stutterers.

I recently revisited my old *alma mater*, the Royal Ottawa Hospital, and was greeted by the sound of slow, melodic chanting, as though somebody were intoning mantras. Closer inspection revealed the patients sitting in front of electronic boxes with flashing lights, holding all their syllables for one or two seconds. There was great emphasis on the gentle approach to words.

The sessions were remarkably relaxed. The highlight of the visit was when the group chanted 'Happy Birthday to You' holding each syllable for two or three seconds. Try it some time!

The well-known Monterey Program for stutterers employed by the Behavioural Sciences Institute in Monterey, California, also involves conditioning. It uses two approaches: GILCU (gradual increase in length and complexity of utterances) and delayed auditory feedback (DAF).

The patient progresses step by step from easy words to hard words. If he is fluent he is rewarded ('Good!'). If he stutters he is penalized ('Stop! Do it again.') He graduates from single words, to word pairs, to triplets, and then to whole sentences. Reading is followed by monologues and then conversation. He learns to transfer his fluency to the outside world. When patients find this approach to fluency difficult, DAF is used, and the goal is 0.5 stuttered word or less per minute for a period of five minutes. Results have been promising but maintenance of the improvement is still a problem.[39]

A clinician must decide which type of treatment is suitable for particular patients. It is usual to carry out an analysis of the patient's stuttering behaviour and engage in trial therapy before deciding whether or not fluency shaping therapy is the right approach. The speech is recorded on tapes, and the number of words or syllables stuttered per minute counted. Rate of speaking in words per minute may also be estimated. The severity of stuttering can be assessed in several ways, and therapists use various scales for rating the severity of stuttering. The clinician tries to assess the stutterer's attitudes about himself and his speech, and to what extent the disability is affecting his life, work, and happiness. She may use an informal, qualitative approach or a more precise, quantitative rating.[40]

The trial therapy assesses how well the patient responds to therapeutic procedures by speaking slowly and prolonging words. If the stutterer does not appear to be plagued by strong emotions about his speech, is accepted by family and peers, doesn't find that the stutter interferes a great deal with his life, doesn't disguise his stuttering, and is comfortable with using prolonged speech, he is probably a candidate for treatment by fluency shaping procedures. If the stutterer has been heavily penalized by society for his disability, is not readily accepted at home or school, hides his stutter, is uncomfortable with slow prolonged speech, and is obviously unhappy with or constrained by his impediment, he may respond better to therapy that treats the whole person, which may help him deal with his anxieties. Sometimes a combination of fluency shaping therapy and other methods is appropriate.[41]

In fluency shaping therapy there is little need for the stutterer to try to perform tasks that arouse great fear, because the approach is carefully structured. The therapists for this treatment are also relatively easy to train. One disadvantage is that the method requires the stutterer to speak in an abnormally slow, prolonged fashion until fluency is achieved in the clinic, and some stutterers find this both objectionable and remarkably difficult. The structured and more impersonal approach is less interesting for the therapist than techniques with more personal involvement.

Stuttering modifiers

Stuttering modification therapy is based on the idea that a person stutters because he struggles with or avoids disfluencies, feared words and sounds, and feared situations. The therapy is designed to reduce avoidances, anxieties about speaking, and negative attitudes about speech, and to help the stutterer *modify* his disfluency. The stutterer is taught to avoid fighting his blocks, to smooth out his stutter, to reduce tension, and to stutter more slowly in a relaxed and deliberate way. The therapy has a considerable psychotherapeutic content in addition to speech modification and, in contrast to fluency shaping therapy, attempts to treat the person as a whole instead of dealing exclusively with faulty speech habits.

A great deal of this therapy was developed at the University of Iowa Speech Clinic and at Western Michigan University. It is sometimes called the 'Iowa Method.'

Stuttering modification therapy in its many forms has revolutionized speech therapy in North America and its influence has been felt all over the world. During the 1920s it was all too clear that people with stutters were not responding well to psychoanalysis or to such conventional speech therapies as relaxation and distraction. Most of the patients relapsed. Carl Emil Seashore, a well known psychologist, who was Dean of the Graduate College at the University of Iowa, recognized the need for a better scientific understanding of speech and hearing disorders. In 1927, he selected Lee Edward Travis as Director of the Iowa Speech Clinic with a mandate to focus the skills of several university departments on hearing and speech problems, to establish a firm scientific basis, and to develop a program on a wider front than before.[42]

Following Travis's appointment there was a period of intense speculation about the origins of stuttering and experimentation with methods of treatment. Techniques evolved that tried both to reduce fears and avoidances and to change speaking patterns. Patients were taught to stutter openly with minimal abnormality and without fear.

Bryng Bryngelson, Wendell Johnson, Charles Van Riper, and Joseph Sheehan were the key figures who brought about this revolution in speech therapy. In the 1930s Bryngelson taught his patients to repeat sounds deliberately in a controlled way (voluntary controlled repetition, or VCR), and to stop avoiding stuttering and become objective about it. He stressed the group approach and encouraged the stutterers to take the techniques out of the clinic into real-life situations.

On a different tack, Wendell Johnson used voluntary controlled repetition to reduce the stutterer's caution about speaking, and to teach him to speak without tension until the disfluency resembled the pauses and hesitations of a normal speaker. Johnson felt strongly that the way a stutterer perceives his speech makes him stutter. He tried to make people with stutters responsible for their own speech instead of blaming their problem on something beyond their control. I have often said to myself that I block because my airflow ceases and my tongue rises in my mouth and becomes inflexible, but this is nonsense. My *tongue* doesn't rise; I *make* it rise, for some reason or other. I stutter because of what *I* do, not because of what my tongue decides to do. This may appear to be mere semantics, but the 'General Semantics Theory' of Polish philosopher, mathematician, and engineer Alfred Korzybski played a major role in Wendell Johnson's methods.

This theory is concerned with the relationships between the language people use and the way they think and act. Wendell Johnson drew upon Korzybski's ideas about why education, politics, and philosophy have progressed so slowly compared with science. Korzybski felt that science had progressed because precise information had been passed from one generation to another in such a manner that what was said matched the facts. In contrast, other human affairs have developed on the chaotic basis of inheritance of false but un-questioned assumptions, traditions, habits, attitudes, beliefs, and doctrines. As he said, 'It is not an exaggeration that it (language) enslaves us through the mechanism of semantic reaction,' and he suggested that the structure of our language affects the nervous system.

Johnson applied this theory to the stutterer's false assump-tions that any disfluency is socially unacceptable, that speak-ing is difficult, and that stuttering is caused by something (other than himself) that stops him speaking. His therapy tried to dispel these false assumptions by letting the patient observe what happened when he spoke fluently. He could see and hear both that he could be fluent and that normal speakers could be disfluent. Johnson's therapy involved a great deal of group discussion of the stutterer's perception of his abnormal speech, and the patient was encouraged to assume that there was no uncontrollable organic or emotional reason why he should be abnormally disfluent.[43]

These approaches helped many stutterers, but in spite of the emphasis on adopting new attitudes and using better speaking techniques in real-life situations, stutterers still tended to relapse. It is difficult to keep an eye on your at-titudes and mode of speaking all the time during a working day. Old fears about speaking and well-established stuttering cues all too frequently penetrate the chinks in the stutterer's newly acquired armour of objectivity.

Charles Van Riper established a speech clinic at Western Michigan University, carried out numerous experiments on stuttering, varied the therapy, and kept long-term records to discover how well patients maintained their speech improve-ment after therapy. His approach included elements of the Iowa method (like reducing anxiety about stuttering and modifying stuttering behaviour by a patient's analysis of his own speech) and emphasized the need for stutterers to stutter fluently rather than to try to speak completely fluently and normally. He tried to minimize the abnormality without com-pletely removing it.[44]

Van Riper's stuttering modification methods have been

remarkably successful. Five years after treatment, about 50 per cent of the stutterers he treated were very fluent, didn't exhibit fear of their stuttering, and didn't avoid hard words or difficult speaking situations. Many other patients greatly improved their speech and developed attitudes that enabled them to live more normal lives. The carry-over into everyday life of the speech improvement resulting from Van Riper's modification of the Iowa method was much better than with previous therapies.

Van Riper looked upon a stutter as a self-perpetuating, learned behaviour, regardless of the original causes. He felt that this behaviour arose from fearful anticipation and frustration resulting from past episodes of abnormal disfluency. He attempted to teach patients to stutter more normally. Although he used voluntary controlled repetition for speech exercises, he emphasized the use of smooth, prolonged speech that simplified the stuttering and made the speech more continuous. Prolongation of sound is widely used in modern therapy.

The technique was not easy to learn, and the stutterer's inclination to approach difficult words with pre-set lips and tongue and anxious anticipation still tended to disrupt the continuity. Van Riper realized that the short period of expectancy before saying a word was important and developed ways a stutterer could respond to this expectancy by preforming a better set of lip and tongue positions in place of the old, destructive sets. When a stutterer expected difficulty, he was to place his lips and tongue at rest and say the first sound so that it led into the next sound. Voice and airflow were started immediately. Van Riper worked to alter the stutterer's preparatory sets so that he could stutter more fluently.

Although this method gave good results, there were still problems. The stutterer had to watch his speech closely all the time and sometimes didn't change his approach to words as he should have done. To overcome this, Van Riper taught stutterers to pull out of their blocks with smooth prolongation. Again, this worked well, but stutterers still tended to get firmly entrapped in a block before they could organize their speech to pull out of it, so Van Riper developed methods of cancelling blocks. When the stutterer's speech stuck because he didn't use prolongation and pull-outs correctly, he was taught to pause, examine his feelings and speech behaviour, and try again.

The new techniques of preparatory sets, pulling out of blocks, and pausing when difficulties were encountered constitute the core of Van Riper's therapy, which also deals effectively with a stutterer's guilt, hostility, penalties, frustrations, fears of words and situations, morale, low self-esteem, and misconceptions.

His therapy does not involve psychoanalysis. Nevertheless, it is a psychotherapeutic approach that takes into account the many facets of the stuttering syndrome, reinforcing those that help a stutterer and removing those that make him lose control of his speech. Van Riper realized that penalties, frustration, anxiety, guilt, hostility, situation fears, word-phonetic fears, and the importance of what was being said could all make a stutter worse. In contrast, good morale, a strong ego, and past experience of fluency could improve a stutter. He designed individual therapies to reduce the factors that make a stutter worse and strengthen those that make it better, recognizing that the importance of individual factors varies considerably from one stutterer to another.[45]

A therapist treating young stuttering children with Van Riper's methods concentrates on a whole complex of things: reducing penalties; reducing a child's frustration; building up his tolerance to frustration; reducing anxiety, guilt, and hostility; releasing forbidden feelings; counselling parents individually and in groups; reducing the stresses and demands of communication; and increasing the amount of fluency a child experiences so that he can respond to it. In some children it is necessary to improve their self-regard and morale. When a child becomes aware of his stuttering, and the repetitions and abnormal prolongations impede his communication, treatment of frustration will become a necessary part of the therapy. He may not fear speech as much as older stutterers, and a child's stutter is far less complex than the full-blown, severe stutter of an adult, but his abnormal disfluency can make his life difficult.

There are a great many ways of treating children's stutters along these lines. If the child is treated when very young, his chances of achieving socially acceptable fluency are high. It is not possible to discuss all the techniques but some of those described by Van Riper in his excellent books, *Speech Correction: Principles and Methods*, 5th edition (1972), and *Treatment of Stuttering* (1973), are of particular interest.

A child finds it difficult to express his feelings about his speech and himself and, when he attempts to do so, he is all too often penalized or ignored by an impatient adult. Play therapy lets the child either say or act out his deep feelings and needs to a caring therapist. The therapist, in the role of a new parent, helps the child to recognize his fears and desires so that he can re-evaluate them.[46] The slightly different approach of 'Creative Dramatics' encourages children to improvise a play, invent the dialogue, and select parts to give them the opportunity to express their intense feelings.

Van Riper quotes a children's play about King Midas and his Golden Touch. One of the children, a boy, acted the part of King Midas by portraying him as a cruel man who shouted at the servants, hit the table, and ordered impossible things. The plot of the story was lost in the ranting and raving. When asked why he played the role in this way, the boy said he thought King Midas was a cruel man, as mean as his teacher.[47] Many people who stutter will recognize an echo of their own early experiences with impatient teachers at school.

The advantage of dramatics is that the child can express himself in front of a sympathetic group, and the method is used as a back-up to play therapy. It is not regarded as a suitable approach for children whose contact with reality is tenuous and who tend to fantasize and play roles , but Van Riper did find creative dramatics useful in resolving problems of sibling rivalry, teasing by playmates, and dealing with bullies.

Some children either do not respond well to the co-ordinated approaches of Van Riper and proponents of the Iowa method or have parents and teachers who cannot or will not modify their damaging responses to the children's abnormal speech. Desensitization therapy, which is used in different ways with both children and adult stutterers, teaches the stutterer to become less sensitive to the rejections, impatience, or worse by adapting to these adversities.

When parents are effectively counselled and ease the pressures on a stuttering child at home, the child may lower his level of tolerance. This can be disastrous in the classroom. The therapist helps the child to adopt and feel a basic fluency and then exposes him to increasing pressures of the type that precipitate his stuttering. As soon as the child shows signs of impending disfluency by increased rigidity and jerkiness, the therapist goes back to the basic fluency. This is repeated and gradually the child is able to tolerate more and more disruption. In these sessions, the child's fluency is carefully maintained under pressure and the effects seem to carry over into situations outside the clinic. Obviously, it requires a sensitive and skilful therapist and the trust of the child.

When treating a confirmed stutterer with many years of abnormal disfluency, Van Riper took into account anxieties about particularly difficult words and speaking situations. The adult stutterer's fears about words and situations tend to overshadow other factors – like penalties, frustrations, anxiety, guilt, and hostility – that increase stuttering. Many therapists focus on treating these word and situation fears and on strengthening the stutterer's morale and experiences of fluency.

Stuttering modification therapy and Van Riper's extension of it are widely used today in North America. The details vary, but in general the therapist makes a total attack on all the factors that increase stuttering. The adult stutterer is not penalized for stuttering, which is encouraged so long as it is done in a prolonged, fluent manner. Every attempt is made to reduce the penalties a stutterer has incurred because of his stuttering. The effects of frustration are reduced by permitting the patient to stutter, and efforts are made to build up his tolerance to frustration. Group discussions help the patient to share his experiences, good and bad, with others, to air his feelings, and to act out conflicts. Together with professional counselling and, if necessary, psychotherapy, this helps the adult stutterer to reduce his problems of anxiety and guilt.

The stuttering modification approach is complex and contains a large element of psychotherapy and counselling. It is rooted in many qualitative assumptions, and the therapy requires considerable skill on the part of the therapist – far more than that required to prescribe the pills and potions upon which modern medicine relies so heavily. A good stuttering modification therapist shares a stutterer's fears and frustrations and helps him to deal with them. She may also incorporate psychotherapy and fluency shaping to achieve the planned goals.

An eclectic form of therapy, including stuttering modification with its echoes of Bryngelson, Johnson, Van Riper, and Sheehan, together with some of the elements of fluency shaping is described in detail in *Clinical Manual for the Comprehensive Stuttering Program* (1984), by Einer Boberg and Deborah Kully of the Department of Speech Pathology and Audiology at the University of Alberta in Edmonton. Their supplementary *Client Manual* will help patients understand what is ahead of them.[48]

The Iowa developments led to an appreciation of the stutterer as a person. The approach is more humane than the regimentation and browbeating associated with so many of the earlier therapies. The stutterer is led to his solution rather than bludgeoned into temporary fluency by threats and criticism. The fact that some of the originators of these new, humane approaches – among them Charles Van Riper – were themselves stutterers increases the confidence of people who stutter in the techniques. Doubtless their success results from these clinicians' deep understanding of how a stutterer perceives his speech, himself, and the world around him. A person is likely to be better equipped to dispel the barrier of a stutterer's glass tower when he has been imprisoned within such a tower himself.

A problem facing all therapists is that of logistics. There are many millions of people in the world who stutter. By no means all of them come for therapy, even in North America and Europe; even so, in the more affluent Western societies there are more applications for treatment than the clinics can handle.

Stuttering modification therapy often takes one or more years and, because of the necessarily close relationship between the therapist and the patient, classes tend to be small and the turnover slow. It is not a therapy for mass application. Fluency shaping therapy takes only a month or so, apart from later maintenance. It has a much more rapid turnover and is more suitable for the treatment of large numbers of people.

The short-term success of some therapies, particularly conditioning therapies, has led to an almost evangelical attitude in some clinicians. Comments like, 'My therapy is the only one that works,' and 'All other therapies are bunk,' occasionally appear like graffiti on the clinical fabric. Even in the newsletters of stutterers' self-help organizations, professionals and near-professionals acridly denounce each other's views. Like most evangelists, their hearts are in the right place. They want to help people and feel strongly that their way to salvation is best. The ones to look out for are the speech-pathology equivalents of those articulate, hard-eyed, grey-suited evangelists on television who want to save your soul and reduce your bank balance at the same time.

In spite of all the difficulties, the incidence of successful therapy is increasing. Whether it will level off in the face of our ignorance about the causes of the malady remains to be seen. A better understanding of the neurology of stuttering should help to remove the remaining barriers. In the past decade a vast amount of research on stuttering has been carried out, and information is accumulating at an incredible rate. It just needs a genius to put it all together.

Will the benefits of speech therapy last forever?

This is the knottiest and most frustrating question of all. It all comes under the heading 'maintenance,' a word that causes therapists and stutterers alike many sleepless nights, heartaches, and even nightmares.

Some patients with relatively mild stutters go to a clinic, learn new speech techniques, and apply them in real life. No trouble at all. They never look back as they fluently chatter their way through life.

Then there are those like myself with stuttering so firmly riveted into their psychological bulkheads that it needs a therapeutic blow-torch to loosen it and let the words flow.

I had been in the audio-visual lab most of a hot summer's day. Even with television cameras trained on me, my therapist hadn't been able to shake my beautifully controlled speech. It was solid as the Rock of Gibraltar. A telephone assignment had been tough, but apart from a little tension it went remarkably well. Four years of therapy were yielding their fruit.

Thirsty after all the talking, I went to my usual watering hole where they keep a good line in draught beer. Full of confidence I sat at my usual glossy plastic table and signalled my favourite waitress, thinking of the frosted, frothy tankard ahead. When her pencil was poised over her pad I happily started to ask for my beer. I say 'started,' but that was as far as it went. Not a sound came out. Not a whisper. Just the faint gagging noise of a massive block which wafted my attention aloft into the never-never land of a stutterer's detachment, where he can think of anything except how to get out of the mess he's in.

I gradually fought my way out of the detachment and at last managed to cancel the block with a long sigh of released air. Smiling ruefully at the waitress I said with no effort at all, 'All I'm trying to do is order a darned draught beer!' We both laughed.

Back to the drawing board for another year or more.

Maintenance is so important that there's a whole 284-page book about it, *The Maintenance of Fluency* (1981), edited by Einer Boberg of the University of Alberta. It describes the views of the world's foremost speech pathologists about how to design therapies with longer lasting benefits. [49]

The sad fact is that many people who stutter go for treatment, revel in their new-found fluency in the clinic, and then face the heartbreak of a relapse. Relapse rates are much lower than they were a few years ago, but they are still uncomfortably high.

In order to maintain his better fluency a person with a severe stutter must practise the new way of speaking for about one hour every day, try it out in new situations, be philosophical about failures and encouraged by successes, and return to the clinic periodically for reinforcement of the methods and removal of any sloppiness. Many find it a great help to participate in self-help groups that will monitor speech.

It needs courage, discipline, and determination, and not all people have the inner resources.

At one time I practised speaking techniques for eight hours every day, soon cutting it to five, and eventually down to one. At this level of reinforcement I kept fairly fluent.

Since then my speech has been generally better, but I've become sloppy and lazy, finding it hard to think about my speech all the time for years on end. Consequently I still fall into verbal traps. However, the earlier therapy helps me to pull out of the chasms of major speech blocks. I no longer go into the free fall of tense silence that I used to experience many times every day.

Yes, the improvement achieved at the clinic can be maintained by many people, but for some it is not an easy road.

Which treatments are most successful?

Anybody embarking on the painful voyage of intensive therapy needs some idea of the chances of success. It is not possible to generalize, because so much depends on the type of stutter the patient has, his personality, the effort he is willing to make, and the skill of the therapist. Nevertheless there is evidence that some therapists are more successful than others.

Gavin Andrews and his colleagues at the University of New South Wales, Sydney, Australia, used a statistical method, meta-analysis, to compare the effectiveness of several techniques, including breath control (airflow), attitude therapy, biofeedback, desensitization, gently approaching sounds and words (gentle onset), prolonged speech, rhythm, and slow speaking.[50] They concluded that for adults prolonged speech and gentle onset to sounds and words were more effective than any other techniques in both the short and the long term. Rhythmic therapy had good initial results, but the benefit tended to fade considerably. Prolongation and gentle onset are combined with speaking slowly in many therapy programs, for example in Webster's fluency shaping and the Iowa school's stuttering modification.

This does not mean that the other techniques are useless. Biofeedback and desensitization are both in their infancy and may prove to be valuable therapeutic tools, and attitude therapy helps a great many stutterers.

Andrews and his colleagues feel that the clinical evidence does not support the widely held idea that stuttering is ill-understood and difficult to treat. A great deal is known about the possible causes of stuttering, the different methods of treatment, and the likely outcome. The facts are there; the only mystery is how to fit them together. The chances that therapy will improve a stutterer's speech are high, and getting better every year. We are no longer in the Dark Ages of stuttering therapy; the prognosis for people who stutter is encouraging.

If a stutterer can't get any therapy at all, therefore, it seems that the best thing he can do is speak very slowly, prolong his words, and approach the beginnings of words as gently as possible.

SIX

Where can a stutterer get the right kind of help?

'To help all created things, that is the measure of our responsibility; to be helped by all, that is the measure of our hope.'

Gerald Vaun

Stutterers who refuse to participate in formal therapy are likely to read this book. They usually read all books on stuttering, good and bad, that they can get their hands on, searching for a glimmer of light at the end of their handicap's tunnel. Doubtless they will read the menu of treatments and be tempted to try out rhythmic and other distractive methods. They will be delighted with the initial results and shattered when their speech falls apart.

This is *not* a self-help book and should not be used as such. Different types of stutterers need different types of treatment, and an effective, systematic approach is best designed by a competent professional after a full assessment of the problem. Some methods, even the good ones, can have a profound emotional impact, and it is useful to have psychological counsellors available to help smooth the therapy path and pick up the pieces when necessary. Going it alone with speech therapy without professional guidance is as wise as choosing your own pills in a pharmacy. By sheer luck you may get relief, but the side effects could be devastating.

Finding the best clinic

If an adult stutterer decides to seek help, what does he do? The obvious step is to go to the family doctor who will refer him to the nearest rehabilitation centre in a large hospital. Most rehabilitation departments provide treatment for a variety of communication disorders, including stutters. For some people this is the best approach, but there are several difficulties. A large rehabilitation centre is usually in a city. Since the early, intensive part of therapy involves regular visits, people living in outlying districts find it hard to attend and persist with the treatment. Some hospitals offer intensive courses of two or three weeks followed by less frequent visits. Even if the treatment is free, the sessions involve spending money on accommodation and meals. Over a period of four years I spent more than $5,000 (Canadian funds) on travel alone. A major problem is the amount of time the therapy takes. I used up a great deal of my leave going to and from the clinics.

Many of the speech therapists working on their own in small towns and rural areas are highly competent, but they are not likely to have the audio-visual equipment and electronic monitors that play such an important part in modern speech therapy. The smaller hospitals' budgets are limited, and these centres do not usually have on staff a psychologist who specializes in speech disorders to help when the going gets tough. Smaller facilities are excellent for subsequent speech maintenance, but may be less effective for initial therapy than hospitals with more resources.

The family physician may refer a patient who stutters to an unsuitable rehabilitation centre. There are good centres for treating stuttering and bad centres. Even an excellent family physician may not be well informed about stuttering or in a position to assess the quality of the treatment. A centre that deals with communication disorders in general may not have much experience of treating stuttering.

What does the stutterer do? He should do a little leg-work to find out about speech therapy in his own area before he sees his family physician. This is not usually as difficult as it sounds. Most countries have speech and hearing associations, which are good starting points. In the United States, the Speech Foundation of America (152 Lombardy Road, Memphis, Tennessee 38111), a non-profit charitable organization, provides guidance for stutterers and parents. This organization publishes and sells first-class, low-cost publications on stuttering and its early recognition and treatment written in non-technical language. The American Speech-Language-Hearing Association (ASHA) and its consumer branch can also be approached for information.[1] The Canadian equivalent is the Canadian Speech and Hearing Association (Royal York Hotel, Convention Mezzanine, 100 Front Street, Toronto, Ontario M5J 1E3), which is the parent body for its provincial satellites.[2] There are similar organizations in most countries. Most associations will answer enquiries about where therapy is available and which are the main centres, and some may indicate where progressive therapy can be found.

It is a great help to talk to other stutterers who have been treated at the different clinics. Sometimes you can find them in self-help groups. Other stutterers can often tell you whether a therapist is an inflexible authoritarian bully, or supportive, flexible, and progressive. Anyone who says they can *cure* the stutter should be looked upon with suspicion, because no responsible therapist will make that claim. An indication that a clinic relies completely on relaxation, medication, rhythmics, or distractions is also reason for caution. Evidence that a program involves a methodical rehabilitation of a stutterer's speech, using a flexible team approach with the stutterer helping others, and includes a follow-up program for speech maintenance is a good sign that the therapy is in touch with modern developments.

At this point a chat with the physician is needed. Some doctors may resent the fact that a patient has done research, but most will be glad to discuss the pros and cons of different types of therapy in the area. When the stutterer has been referred to a speech centre for assessment, he can meet the therapists and discuss the approach with them. They will know better than the stutterer what combination of treatments he needs, but at least he can assess whether or not they are using outmoded techniques that give short-term relief. Blind faith in any treatment is neither necessary nor desirable, but confidence in the therapist and the therapy is vital. There is no harm at all in going over the strategy of the therapy. The reluctance of some doctors to discuss with patients their prognosis and treatment is, or should be, obsolete.

If the stutterer likes what he hears, he needs the time, money, and motivation to embark upon the therapy, and the guts and discipline to persist with it over a period of months or even years. If he is seeking therapy he probably has good motives. He may be tired of society's rejection, discrimination, and cruelty, weary of not being able to participate in class discussions, or just interested in making more friends. One stutterer entered therapy after a horrendous session in court, during which the lawyer and judge had been unsympathetic about and critical of his disability. Many come for treatment only when they are desperate for help.

Self-treatment

The majority of stutterers do not have access to good speech therapy and cannot spare the time, money, and energy needed to attend clinics regularly. They have to rely on their own resources. This is not desirable, but it is a fact.

If a stutterer decides to treat his own disability with the help of his family and friends, he would be well advised to read Malcolm Fraser's booklet *To the Stutterer* and his excellent guide to self-treatment, sponsored and published by the Speech Foundation of America, *Self-Therapy for the Stutterer*.[3] The latter is endorsed by respected therapist Charles Van Riper, is based upon the treatments evolved by the Iowa and Michigan schools, and is easy to understand. The author assumes that stuttering is a form of behaviour that can be changed and describes how to analyse stuttering, control blocks, and face up to fears. Speaking slowly, using the easy-onset approach to words, stuttering openly and easily, ceasing to avoid situations or to substitute words, maintaining eye contact, using voluntary controlled repetition, cancellation, and easy pulling out from blocks are all advocated. All the elements of good modern therapy are there, but a speech therapist and a psychologist to encourage and guide the stutterer are absent. Other useful books are Ainsworth's *Counselling Stutterers*[4] and Irwin's *Stammering: Practical Help for All Ages*.[5]

Self-treatment is likely to be a long, hard road with many false starts and pitfalls and possibly periods of great distress and disappointment. The chances of success are lower than with systematic therapy designed and supervised by professionals.

Self-help groups

Although people who stutter come in all shapes and sizes, not many of them like working in groups. The effort of speaking is too great. Consequently stutterers' self-help groups are slow to get started, and many simply fade away.

Even the successful and progressive groups have remarkably few members considering the number of people afflicted by stuttering. The National Stuttering Project in the United States,[6] for example, is well established and active. It is efficiently run by full-time staff, but its membership of 1,500 is only about 0.06 per cent of the stuttering population. The situation in Canada is similar. Lack of funds is partly responsible for this, but the people who stutter are also responsible. They are reluctant to come out into the open and say, 'Here we are! We are ordinary people, but we can't speak very well. We'd just like a little help and understanding.'

I have tremendous admiration for a small self-help group of spastics in Victoria, British Columbia. The members have great difficulty speaking clearly and have problems with their muscle control, but they travel from church to church standing up and telling people about themselves. Without self-pity they try to show that behind the distressing physical and vocal facades there are warm, loving human beings with much to offer the world if society will let them. They don't ask a normal person to speak for them. They don't plead. They just describe the facts. It takes a great deal of courage.

If more stutterers would come out of their closets, join such groups, and learn to bear or even fight rejection, ridicule, and discrimination in good company, they would find the pain far less than the anguish of fear and self-inflicted loneliness.

The self-help organizations have numerous active chapters in the United States, Canada, Britain, Sweden, Germany, and Australia, but these groups can help only if the stutterers will contribute and participate. Some of the groups just provide a place where people who stutter can get together and talk without the ridicule and censure of society. It helps to know you are not alone. The relief of being able to talk openly about stuttering and the problems it causes can be tremendous.

Some groups take a somewhat militant stance. The P-club in Sweden for example, has taken action against inaccurate, damaging statements in the media about people who stutter. This group seems to be changing public opinion. Other groups are tied to a particular type of speech therapy or even to a particular hospital and provide ex-patients with a critical audience that helps them keep their speech techniques in line.

Anybody wanting help can contact these groups. A few addresses are listed in appendices. Talking with the members will give a good idea of where the best therapy can be found.

Speech therapists and patients: the informal contract

When a therapist accepts a stuttering patient for treatment there is an unspoken and unwritten contract. The therapist agrees to use her skills, and the stutterer agrees to work hard and persevere. Guiding a person with a severe stutter to better fluency is often painful and frustrating for both the therapist and the patient. The therapists invest a tremendous amount of themselves in their patients, particularly when they use stuttering modification therapy to treat the stutterer as a whole person. If the treatment fails, no matter how professional and objective the therapist is, there are likely to be feelings of guilt on both sides that need to be resolved. The therapist walks a razor's edge of emotional involvement. She must remain friendly with the patients without forming close friendships that would detract from the treatment. Speech therapy can be a very intimate and emotional business, and efforts need to be made by both therapists and patients to avoid the formation of bonds that are too close for comfort.

I was involved in an intensive course of speech therapy using innovative approaches that made great demands on the trust, courage, and emotions of the patients. We all felt shattered by the end of the second week, but most of us were much more fluent. A rising tide of emotional involvement was dealt with gently but firmly by the therapists, who were well aware of the tensions and ties that can develop between people sharing stress, fear, and pain.

Speech pathologists bring a degree of concerned professionalism to their work that has earned my unqualified respect.

What happens when speech therapy succeeds?

Adult stutterers like to daydream about what life would be like without a stutter. I could never understand what stopped anybody with normal speech from becoming Prime Minister, or at least a member of the Cabinet. Aiming a little lower, a person afflicted with a stutter may well think how pleasant it would be to be able to hold forth at committee meetings, ask questions at conferences, fluently court a pretty girl, and burn the ears of impudent telephone operators. He thinks of all the social situations he avoids because of the effort and embarrassment of having to talk and the signs of rejection on the faces of people he meets. He could get a date with the brunette he met on the ski slopes if only he could say all the right words without blocking. He could learn another language just for fun. He sees new vistas opening before him and may feel there would be nothing he couldn't do and nothing to fear if he were fluent.

The changes improved fluency make in a stutterer's life depend upon the person. If he is fundamentally a blockhead, he'll just become a blockhead without a stutter. If he's a genius, he'll still be a genius, but better able to tell people about it rather than hide his light under a bushel of uncontrolled repetitions and hesitations. A person with a slight stutter who achieves almost complete fluency will just be less nervous about the possibility that his speech will let him down. Someone who has had a severe, debilitating stutter for a long time may react profoundly to improved fluency. It depends upon how far the handicap has initially affected a person's life style and over-all social behaviour.

Most people who stutter severely delude themselves that their antipathy to the telephone, public speaking, large parties, committee meetings, and appearing on radio or television is wholly the result of their stuttering. They ignore the fact that many people with normal speech are terrified of the telephone, speaking in public, parties, and radio and television appearances. The improved fluency may or may not reduce a stutterer's hang-ups about situations he finds difficult. He may be so programmed to associate telephones with dislike that he cannot change.

All handicapped people who resolve their disability to the extent that it is no longer an appreciable handicap must deal with society's new perception of them and with their own changed perceptions of their surroundings. Recovery from a severe disorder can be a mixed blessing.

A freckled, red-haired boy, aged about seven, had been completely deaf and almost mute all his life until he had an operation that gave him normal hearing. I met him about a month after his surgery, when he was learning to speak. He was nervous and jumpy. When I spoke to him his eyes widened with fear, and it was clear that he didn't entirely understand what I said. This was to be expected in view of my partial disfluency and his previous deafness, but I was puzzled by his obvious fear until his mother explained.

The boy had never heard anybody speak, hammer in a nail, laugh, or sneeze, and the noise of the traffic, the wail of ambulance sirens, and the music on the radio were completely unfamiliar to him. He didn't yet associate speech with communication, music with pleasure, or sounds with activities and objects. I get jumpy at our cottage in the bush when I hear an unfamiliar noise in the middle of the night. Is it a raccoon, or a bear, or an intruder? The small boy had just encountered a host of unfamiliar sounds full of the menace of the unknown. He was sorting them out and learning to live in his new and noisy world. I was told he overcame this perceptual problem in a few months, his fears giving way to excitement.

A more extreme and tragic example of the difficulties a person with severely impaired perception experiences when adapting to newly restored faculties is the well-documented case of S.B., the fifty-two-year-old Englishman who lost his sight as a child and had it restored in 1958 by a brilliant eye operation. His response to being able to see was observed by the British psychiatrist Richard Gregory, who described the case in 'Recovery from early blindness: a case study.'[7] Richard Restak has also discussed S.B.'s case, in the context of perception of reality by man and other mammals, in his excellent and thought-provoking book *The Brain: The Last Frontier.*[8]

S.B. could see quite well, but had difficulty perceiving height and recognizing objects by their visible shapes. His drawings of objects left out important features, but he learned to associate things he knew from their feel when he was blind with what he saw with his eyes. Before he regained his sight he was a cheerful, confident, dominant man, who coped with heavy traffic and earned a good living repairing shoes. He was well adapted to his sightless life and enjoyed what he perceived by touch, smell, and hearing.

Soon after he regained his sight he began to deteriorate mentally and became a recluse, sitting in the dark for long periods. He found the visible world a drab place. His attempts to pull himself out of his downward slide failed. Everything disappointed him, and gradually he lost his peace of mind and self-respect.

When he was blind, every time he overcame his handicap it was an achievement, and the psychiatrist felt that, when S.B. could see, these triumphs seemed insignificant. S.B. became deeply depressed and died in 1960, less than two years after his eye operation. This is an extreme and sad case, but it illustrates the dangers of rehabilitating a person with a perceptual handicap if he is well adapted to his disability.

Recovery can be a mixed blessing, and it is unwise for a person who stutters to have false expectations about what life will be like when he becomes more fluent. He may be disappointed and find that some of the barriers between himself and society that he assumed were caused by his stuttering remain when he speaks more easily. A boy at my preparatory school, who threw up every time he became nervous, had a bad time with his peers and acquired the unenviable nickname of Spewky Sidney or S.S. He overcame his nausea, but still had a bad time because his large ears stuck out and he lisped. He kept his nickname. Blackbirds peck at birds of any other colour, not only white, and it doesn't always help to moult and grow more orthodox feathers.

I am not aware of any case history of the effects on the life of an adult with a severe, self-reinforcing stutter when he achieved a high degree of fluency. I know about mild stutterers who became very fluent and entered new and more challenging jobs. Some of these fluent stutterers enhanced their careers at the price of disrupting their families, but there could have been reasons other than the new fluency.

My own case is not clear-cut because I still stutter, but my speech control and social relationships have greatly improved in the last twenty years. My stutter was very severe and affected both my daily communication and my health. Now that I speak more easily and have arranged my life so that I speak less, my health has improved. This is, of course, welcome. The telephone is no longer a nightmare, and I use it frequently, which saves time. My temper has a longer fuse now that I can express my displeasure. I can interview and be interviewed more freely, and I don't avoid public exposure. People say that I am more outgoing, and I am conscious of being more relaxed about life. I no longer need to fight for survival every day.

All these can be listed on the credit side of the ledger. The debit side contains one item that I share with the unfortunate S.B. When I was very inarticulate, any successful communication was a major achievement, and overcoming almost insurmountable obstacles gave me daily kicks. Even such a small speech success as ordering breakfast in a restaurant was deeply satisfying. I miss the daily sense of achievement and have taken on new challenges – one of which is writing this book.

Some people who stutter develop acute senses and an exceptional ability to receive and send the unspoken part of communication. I was afraid that I would lose this if I became more fluent, but if anything these senses have sharpened now that speech is a larger part of my communicative amalgam. My case is very different from S.B.'s. He was completely adapted to his blindness and enjoyed his other senses. I coped with my stuttering and adapted in many ways, but no person who stutters severely fully adapts to the rejections of society.

As speech therapy improves and we learn more about the

cerebral processes involved in speech and emotion, people with severe stutters may become much more fluent with less effort. When this happens it may be necessary for therapists to extend their mandate so as to help recently fluent patients deal with their new perceptions, roles, and relationships with society.

SEVEN

The odyssey to fluent stuttering

'... a journey into the future, a hunting after happiness.'

William Stakhel

There is a wide gap between reading about stuttering theory and the reality of intensive treatment. If I had known what was ahead when I decided to have intensive speech therapy I doubt that I'd have had the courage to start the long journey to fluent stuttering. When I walked the high mountains in winter and fought fatigue, wind, and bitter cold, I often exclaimed, 'What the hell am I doing here?' During the more demanding parts of speech therapy, I said the same thing many times.

All my previous treatments had been fairly brief – about six months or less – and were carried out in the cosy, supportive confines of the clinics. I was not aware that my new treatment would persist for several years. Moreover, although I knew that situational and group therapies were involved, I had no real idea what they meant. Unwittingly, I was embarking on an odyssey in a leaky cockleshell of a boat of stuttering theory accompanied by a crew I didn't know. The skipper, to my dismay, would hand over the boat to the bewildered crew as soon as we were out of harbour so she could concentrate on therapeutic navigation.

The word 'situation' didn't bother me, but the thought of group therapy certainly did. It appalled me. Not being a groupie, I preferred to work and play with a few companions and was reluctant to involve myself with masses of humanity.

I felt that all medical treatment should be a private affair and was never especially keen on being a patient in those teaching hospitals where they bring students to view the ailing bodies while nurses flourish enema tubes in the background. Proposing that I should cold-bloodedly expose my speech – and my feelings about it – to a large group of strangers was like asking me to go to a nudist colony where the world would see all my moles, warts, and goose bumps. My first reaction was, 'Group therapy? Forget it!'

It turned out that the group work was the most enjoyable part of the therapy, and I made many lasting friends. It was the situational therapy that gave all of us the most trouble. It is all very well to expose your articulatory weaknesses to other people with stutters in the clinic, but taking these weaknesses out onto the street or displaying them on national television at prime time takes a great deal of *chutzpah*. This Yiddish word, which means shameless audacity, best describes what is demanded of patients in situational therapy. They need the audacity to approach strangers and stutter openly, deliberately, and fluently without feeling ashamed of their way of speaking. Without *chutzpah* the stutterer is lost.

During my preliminary assessment at the Royal Ottawa Hospital, the attractive speech therapist was coolly efficient, but when I unfolded my history of unsuccessful treatment a wary look came into her eye. Consider her position. Here was I, a talkative, stuttering scientist who had responded poorly to forty years or more of treatment and who clearly had reservations about speech therapy and even about speech therapists in general. It might be that I was an unusually resistant patient who couldn't or wouldn't co-operate; or it might be that I'd just had the wrong kind of treatment. What were the chances of even partial success? Obviously the prognosis was not good. No wonder she looked wary. Should she invest her time and the government's money in a lost cause? Much later she confessed that she was not at all keen to take me on.

She passed me to another attractive woman clinician, a psychometrist – the type of psychologist who measures the relative strength of your mind. My past experience of psychologists and other types of mind-benders had been mixed, and my feelings were ambivalent. I wasn't keen on another Freudian probe into the murkier corners of my libido, so I was cautious and parried some of the preliminary questions with a nimble riposte or two learned on past therapeutic battlefields. I relaxed when the conversation didn't stray below my chin, and it became apparent that this particular clinician was taking a refreshingly empirical, behavioural approach rather than asking me to wade ankle deep in the suppositions of a Freudian quagmire. Best of all, she had a puckish sense of humour and a fine nose for the ridiculous, so I knew we would get along as sparring partners. Unknown to me, she didn't share my enthusiasm, and she admitted later that she was shattered by the thought of having me as a patient. She went home and cried.

I nearly flunked my assessment. I thought I'd behaved myself remarkably well during the cross-examinations. I hadn't let on that I knew a little about the etiology and treatment of stuttering, because no clinician likes a smart aleck for a client. I politely shut up and let the therapists have their say and regarded myself as the perfect potential patient. The therapists' collective misgivings puzzled me.

Maybe it was the challenge or possibly just plain compassion, but they let me reach first base and try a few preliminary sessions. After they realized that I was co-operative, we all got along famously during the several years of treatment. All the therapists at the ROH's Speech Rehabilitation Unit (now Communication Disorders) were, and still are as far as I know, highly efficient and dedicated young women. The fact that they were also lively, intelligent, and attractive did not detract in the least from the therapy.

The early part of the treatment was on a one-to-one basis. At first the clinician tested my vocal capabilities and designed a plan of attack. My stuttering wasn't causing me too many problems in my daily life, although I found talking all the time in my job exceedingly tiring. Stress was building up, but in retrospect it was probably largely caused by the frustration of working for a bureaucracy. I had some difficulty reducing my rate of speaking, prolonging words, and using voluntary repetition in the early therapy sessions and was strongly conditioned to stutter in response to many word and situation cues – even in my sleep. I also had a deeply ingrained anxiety about stuttering and was tense before and during speaking. In retrospect, I was a prime candidate for integrated therapy consisting of both stuttering modification and fluency shaping.

It turned out that I received therapy to reduce anxiety, modify my attitudes, learn to prolong sounds and words, practise easy onset to beginnings of words, develop smooth verbal continuity using voluntary controlled repetition (VCR), reduce my rate of speaking, learn to relax before and during speech, respond better to stuttering cues, and increase my tolerance to speech frustration. Desensitization, group discussion, and exercises for transferring the new speech techniques to real situations with all their tensions were also included. These methods contain elements of the treatments designed by Bryng Bryngelson, Wendell Johnson, Joseph G. Sheehan, Charles Van Riper, and Webster, together with a spot of psychotherapeutic counselling. A novel element in the therapy was that as soon as a patient improved he was permitted to monitor other stutterers until, finally, when he had much better control, he graduated to Hospital Volunteer (with free parking privileges) and helped himself by helping others. This could be regarded as a form of operant conditioning, the Hospital Volunteer status being the reward, but there was little evidence of penalties. Whatever the basis, for many patients it was a highly effective treatment.

The therapy involved practice, practice, practice. There are many examples of patients who received therapy and later became speech therapists themselves so they could maintain their fluency by constant exposure to the speech techniques they taught. It is quite believable, because the best results come from constant practice.

The therapy was complex, but it was carried out in such a skilful, orderly way that there was no confusion. Each component of the treatment supplemented the others at the right stages and the emphasis of each phase could be shifted to suit the needs of individuals. It was a flexible, many-pronged approach on a wide front.

For a few weeks, the therapy was low key and consisted of designing graduated daily exercises, starting with short sentences and progressing to stages of increasing difficulty. I taped my disfluency and listened to my new speech, which soon became – at least in the clinic – a smooth flow like a meandering river instead of my usual verbal rapids, eddies, and whirlpools. I was gradually exposed to speaking situations in the hospital that involved talking to staff and patients. Success varied, but I developed a lot more nerve and learned a great deal about people.

The nerve developed because I was asked to go into the busy hospital dining room, select someone at random, introduce myself and say, 'May I sit here? I am receiving speech therapy and would like to practise my speaking techniques.' This took a great deal of guts – more than I thought I had. You never knew what kind of person you would get. Some were welcoming and co-operative, others said, 'Yes, I do mind! Get lost!' A panicky few fled to the washroom; some valiantly stuck it out but were clearly embarrassed; and one woman ignored me completely. Once I sat with a young psychiatric patient who was friendly and chatty but emphasized his philosophical points by stabbing the table violently with his fork until it bent, just inches from my chest.

There are some people who can walk up to strangers and start chatting. I am not one of them. I was so conditioned by my stoic British education, where it was 'just not done' and a 'poor show' to thrust yourself upon a stranger, that I had to make an enormous effort just to say 'Good morning' to a passer-by. It was not shyness, just custom. All these social inhibitions were cast to the winds during the first few weeks of therapy as I learned to chat to perfect strangers at the drop of a hat, stutter and all.

During this phase I visited the hidden side of society's moon, the world of the handicapped. Everybody knows the disabled are there, but most people prefer them out of sight and out of mind. At that time the Royal Ottawa Hospital Speech Rehabilitation Unit was housed in the same complex as other units for helping people severely handicapped by automobile accidents and strokes to cope with their disabilities. The situational speech exercises allowed me to meet young people who, with no hint of self-pity, cheerfully faced the consequences of terrible injuries, and older people, partly paralysed and nearly speechless from cerebral thromboses and aneurisms, who faced their limited futures with courage and dignity. It was a heart-rending yet heart-warming experience. It would be salutary for people who drink and drive to be compelled, as part of their sentences, to visit or even assist patients in the rehabilitation wards, where physiotherapists work so hard to help accident victims with spinal or cerebral injuries to lead more normal lives.

With a great deal of effort I was able to speak to many individuals in the hospital using the new methods. The speaking situations were carefully graded until I was able to talk to audiences of several people. The supportive atmosphere of the clinic improved my speech considerably within a few weeks, the only real remaining bugbear being the telephone.

Nobody can imagine the difficulties a person with a stutter has on the telephone unless they stutter themselves. Direct dialling has, of course, been a help. Before it was introduced it was exceedingly difficult for a stutterer to reel off long numbers to impatient operators. For many the telephone was not a viable means of communication. Even with direct dialling it is sometimes necessary to give a credit-card number for a long-distance call, and this is nearly impossible for a person with a severe stutter. At some stage you have to say who you are and what you want. There is no escaping the fact that the purpose of the telephone is to speak to somebody.

The first spoken words on the telephone at the clinic were voluntarily repeated in a slow, prolonged manner to signal the listener that the speaker had a speech impediment and no doubt about it. If a person with a stutter tries to hide his disability, the listener gets nervous and may think the speaker is drunk or making a silent, heavy-breathing, obscene phone call. Hundreds of times people on the telephone have said to me, 'There seems to be something wrong with the line,' when nonplussed by my silent blocks. My usual reply is, 'The line's okay. I have a stutter,' which I can usually say quite fluently.

Once a person knows you stutter, there's a fair chance of a reasonable response, but not always. The preliminaries were always the hard part, and it took tremendous concentration to speak and voluntarily repeat words and sounds fluently instead of blocking. Thereafter it was necessary to keep the rate of speaking down below sixty words a minute, to approach words gently and smoothly, and to keep up the flow during the dialogue.

The early telephone calls within the hospital were not too difficult, but when calls were made outside the clinic, most patients, including myself, had a great deal of trouble. As far as possible I made real-life outside calls to my bank, hotel, or office, but sometimes I faked it and tried calls to restaurants, hotels, car-hire firms, bus terminals, travel agents, and airline offices. The airlines were the best, because they usually replied with a recorded message saying they were busy and would the caller please call back – it enabled me honourably to cop out of an assignment that produced a cold sweat.

Hotels and restaurants varied in their difficulty. The telephone operators in the large, expensive hotels are trained to be polite and cope dispassionately with fires, earthquakes, cranks, and people struggling with a stutter. Calling was easy. I awarded the first prize for difficulty to telephone operators in small motels in Hull, across the river from Ottawa. They were usually so rude when you stuttered that they were a marvellous challenge. Fortunately they couldn't see my digital gestures (body language?) while I calmly and politely persisted with my questions, using voluntary repetition of sounds and prolonging the words. Busy bus companies were tough to deal with; they were impatient rather than rude, and I appreciated their reasons for being so. Salesmen wanting to sell you something, as at the car-hire firms, were pushovers. They'd have been polite if you'd asked the cost of hiring a Cadillac for a month in disfluent Kurdish.

These assignments provided insights into the ways different sectors of society respond to a stutter, even a controlled stutter, with its prolonged words and repeated sounds. In general, people who were under great stress or who belonged to ethnic groups that normally speak very quickly (e.g., Italian, French, and Spanish) responded badly to disfluency, which is understandable. I learned to arrange my unwitting telephone audiences into carefully graded degrees of difficulty.

Succeeding with the telephone can be quite a shock. A sixty-year-old executive had never been able to call his wife on the telephone because of his severe blocks. During a carefully controlled phone assignment he spoke fluently to her for about ten minutes, put down the telephone, and unashamedly wept.

Gradually the components of the therapy began to fall into place. It was like learning to drive a car. At first there were too many things to remember. It was vital that each step was carried out in the right sequence or the speech engine stalled. After a great deal of practice everything became more or less automatic, but you couldn't afford to relax your vigilance. If you did so you sooner or later collided with a difficult word and blocked your verbal traffic.

About this time I developed what I called the Stutterer's Credo as an *aide mémoire*.

The Stutterer's Credo

I believe that I can maintain fluent speech provided that:
I *prolong* my words and *speak slowly* at a rate I can manage;
I use *voluntary controlled repetition* to signal people that
    I stutter and to help me past potential blocks;
I approach the beginnings of words *gently* and slowly;
I *never push past blocks*;
I *pause (i.e., cancel) when I block*, and try again,
    approaching the word slowly and smoothly, using
    voluntary controlled repetition when necessary;
I *never* try to avoid a block by *substituting* an easy
    word for a hard word;
I *remain in contact* with the audience and myself, and keep
    sufficient eye contact not to cause embarrassment;
I *never avoid a speaking situation* just because I
    stutter (within the limits of common sense);
I *never hide my stutter* from myself or other people;
I *practise* good speech technique as often as possible
    in order to stutter in a fluent manner that will
    not interrupt communication.

I added another private component later: 'I shall *never* lose my temper with people who react rudely to my stuttering but, for the sake of other stutterers, I must *never* let them get away with it.'

The voluntary controlled repetition is the hardest part for me to maintain. Van Riper's cancellation of blocks is in the credo, and so is avoiding avoidance, which both work when I remember them. The gentle approach (easy onset) to words has echoes of fluency shaping therapy, and the attitude components reflect the psychotherapeutic aspects of speech modification therapy.

Over the years the therapy has continued to evolve and is still changing. In recent years therapists have placed much greater emphasis on the type of fluency shaping described by Webster,[1] but this varies from one clinic to another.

I used the Stutterer's Credo as my guiding light for several years. I still use it to refresh my memory about what I should be doing when I stray away from the path of vocal righteousness, which I do all too frequently.

If Moses could have included the credo in his famous tablets, maybe his stuttering would have improved. In any case he had an excellent therapist: 'And Moses said unto the Lord, "O my Lord I am not eloquent ... but I am slow of speech, and of a slow tongue." ... And the Lord said unto him ... "I will be with thy mouth ... and will teach you what ye shall do." '

Moses did something that makes most therapists shudder. He let his brother Aaron speak for him (Exodus 4:10–15; 27–30). He *avoided*.

Once I had grasped the basics, I soon became remarkably fluent within the hospital and was ready for greater challenges. When I was introduced to the main group it needed a major effort to overcome my antipathy to talking to large audiences. My speech became incredibly brittle and kept collapsing without warning, because the new and larger audience seemed to prevent me from using the speech techniques I had learned. The problem of audience interaction reared its head and became the heart of future difficulties.

I knew that when I used the new speech techniques I could stutter fluently in a manner that did not disrupt communication, but in difficult situations something prevented me from using the techniques. It was like being given a key to a locked chest full of my most precious possessions that only opened the lock when I was on my own and jammed when I wanted to open the chest to show the contents to other people. The precious possessions were the multitude of things I wanted to say. On my own I could say them, but could not always do so with other people present.

I chipped away for months at the solid wall that prevented me from using the wonderful new way of speaking. Eventually, the barrier disappeared, but even today it tends to return without warning and makes it difficult for me to use the techniques. In the most difficult situations I use the Edinburgh Masker. Although some therapists look upon it as a cop-out, or distraction, or a form of avoidance, I feel it is common sense to use it when the likelihood of speech failure is very high.

The speech therapist and psychometrist worked valiantly to remove this *something* – the wall that stopped me using the techniques. It would have helped if we had known what the something was! It was clear to me that this was the factor that had prevented me from responding to earlier therapy. Speculating, it seems likely that the wall was built during the many years of associating certain circumstances with stuttering and was constructed from a multitude of conditioned responses to difficult speaking situations. This subliminal conditioning is very hard to break, and the wall was a tangible, frustrating reality, an almost impermeable block to progress.

The power of the mental block is illustrated by what happened to me on one outside speech assignment in a shopping plaza. I went from store to store trying to use prolongation, repetition, and slow speech. Without warning my mind blanked out the well-learned methods for about fifteen minutes. I couldn't remember anything about the Stutterer's Credo or my therapist's guidelines. It took some time to get back in gear.

With months of practice and gradual desensitization, the wall began to crumble. My diary at that time says 'I tell myself to prolong and repeat, but sometimes nothing happens. I have been given a key that doesn't quite fit the lock. Chipping at this wall week after week has made some dents in its face, but the wall tends to return. Each time, however, the chips get larger and the wall gradually crumbles, leaving debris on the ground. At first I tripped over the pieces when I was careless or tired, but now I can chart my way around the remaining obstacles without too much trouble.'

This was one of the hardest tasks I have ever undertaken, and it made great demands upon my inner resources. Without the help of the therapists and the support of my companions in the group I don't think I could have persevered. By no means all stutterers have these barriers to using the prescribed speaking techniques, and some, particularly the younger people, seem able to use them quite freely.

A small group of about ten selected patients underwent concentrated therapy for ten hours or more every week-day for two weeks. Some sessions lasted until 11 PM, and by the end of the course both the therapists and the patients were visibly wilting. Every day started with simple word and sentence exercises to reinforce the prolongation and voluntary controlled repetition techniques and get the feel of different rates of speaking (40, 60, 80, or 100 words per minute) using stop-watches and tape recorders. Each day there were sessions on closed-circuit television, but in the afternoons we went in pairs to the shopping plazas, restaurants, and government offices to try out the techniques. Evenings were spent in group sessions discussing the philosophy of the therapy and refining the method. The grand finale was the challenge of a ten-minute presentation in front of an audience of thirty people. At the end of the two weeks we were all much more fluent in the clinic and had better carry-over in the outside world. We had taken a big step, but still had a long way to go.

It is worth giving more details about one or two points that came up during the course. My block about using the techniques was tackled intensively with desensitization sessions. I had many stuttering cues to contend with, but we managed to focus on a few of the main ones, which included taxis, hotels, lecture theatres, crowds, and, of course, the telephone. For hours on end, I was shown colour slide after colour slide illustrating these situations and I had to talk about each of them. At first my mental block inhibited the use of speech techniques, but gradually, when I was nearly exhausted and my eyes burned from looking at the slides, I found that I was using the speech techniques much more freely. This did carry over to the outside world.

My problem with the stuttering cues presented by telephones and lecture theatres still persists to a lesser degree, but ever since this therapy I have had little or no trouble with taxis, hotels, and other situations covered during these tiring sessions. My inhibiting blocks had dissolved in the solvent of pure boredom during the slide sessions. It was, of course, a form of conditioning, but it seemed to be the only quick way to dissipate the effects of inhibiting cues. It was very hard on the clinician.

The television sessions were terrifying at first, but they were invaluable once we became used to the gadgetry. The patient was videotaped while reading aloud or discussing his speech with the therapist; later he saw the playback. The first and last tapes were useful demonstrations of the change in our speech during the treatment. Most of all, however, the TV sessions forced the patient to accept the reality of his stutter, to scrutinize his speech in great detail, and to recognize bad habits. At first the replays in front of the group were embarrassing, but we soon learned to trust each other and to become more objective.

The videotapes brought us down to earth with a bump. I was horrified that my face looked like that of a stranger much less interesting than myself. I stuttered in minor ways (quite apart from the major blocks) much more than I had realized – I was so used to the lesser disfluencies and so adept at self-deception that they did not register. My nose, bashed about in past rugby encounters, looked like a crooked lump, and the resonant voice I thought I heard every day came over as a plummy English accent. I was disillusioned with my television image and, on the first replay, cried, 'Is that me? Oh, my God!'

When I stuttered on the screen, I didn't like it at all. It hardened my resolve to change my speech behaviour. When I went over the tapes I could compare what I did when I was fluent with what happened when I blocked. Gradually, I modified my speech behaviour. We all found it a challenge to meet our true selves, accept our stutters, and do something about it. At the end of the session I was interviewed by another stutterer for twenty minutes about photography during World War II. By using the speaking techniques, we managed to give a virtually flawless performance.

A few of us were selected to carry this television work over into the all-too-real world in a way that would terrify anybody. A national television network wanted some of us to show the public how the therapy was carried out and how the techniques were used outside the clinic. I was selected for the situation exercise.

I set up a session in a florist's shop and self-consciously walked into the store and asked a girl about how to look after plants while cameras, mikes, and lights hovered around. Although I was jittery, I used voluntary controlled repetition, cancellation, and prolongation without too much difficulty. The session ended, and I thankfully wiped the sweat from my brow and walked outside. To my horror I was interviewed again in front of a large crowd of curious onlookers attracted by all the paraphernalia of the media. I felt sick, but managed to maintain the speech techniques for a remarkably long ten minutes until it was all over. In retrospect, it went very well. The stress wasn't caused by stage fright, but by the effort of maintaining the speech techniques in such a challenging situation. I hoped they'd cut my clip from the television program, but I had no such luck. I appeared three times on the news at prime time and groaned every time I saw it.

The evening after this television trauma I went shopping in a large plaza on the other side of town. To my surprise, several strangers came up and congratulated me on the performance. Best of all, some of them said, 'I never understood what was involved in a stutter and how hard it is to treat. Where can we find out more about it?' It was worth every shattered nerve.

Most patients were nervous about testing the speech techniques in public, because failures were embarrassing. But when the techniques did succeed it was amazing how store clerks responded to controlled, prolonged, deliberately repetitive speech instead of an uncontrolled series of stumbles and blocks. As long as continuous communication was maintained, even with an unusual amount of repetition, the disfluency didn't matter. The audiences did not become tense and difficult, and the better feedback helped the stutterers' speech. The therapists had told us that people responded better to controlled disfluency than uncontrolled stuttering, but not all of us believed them. Nevertheless they were right.

The clinicians put us through these difficult therapeutic hoops, so it was only fitting that they should show us how to do it. I greatly admired their courage when, although they had normal speech, they went into stores and acted as though they had, first, uncontrolled stutters, and then controlled disfluency, so that we could see the differences in feedback. As the therapists struggled not to appear embarrassed they came in for a great deal of good-natured ribbing from the patients.

These public speech exercises were sometimes funny. One class was at the stage of deliberately repeating the first sounds of nearly every word all through the day. A group of them stood talking like slow machine-guns on a crowded escalator in a shopping plaza. A stout man just ahead heard this extraordinary chatter and turned around to stare as the steps bore him downwards. He was so fascinated that he forgot to step off the escalator and fell on his bottom at the end with all the other people piling on top of him in sheer pandemonium.

A tall burly farmer was asked by the therapist to go to busy Elgin Street in Ottawa and ask people the time, or directions to stores or restaurants, using his new techniques, just for practice. He accosted several people and was doing remarkably well until he saw across the street a scruffy-looking individual bumming quarters from passers-by. He was making angry gestures and clearly objected to the farmer trespassing on his territory. The large stutterer crossed the street and, looming over the vagrant, said in a low conspiratorial voice with perfectly controlled deliberate repetition, 'You bum this side, bud, and I'll bum the other.'

My most expensive situational-therapy experience occurred when I went into an art shop to try out my controlled repetition. It worked all too well. I walked out clutching a $250 painting of a winter scene.

After the intensive course of therapy, most of us had much better speech, but in the following weeks the benefit tended to fade under the pressures of the outside world. The real work of maintaining the speech began.

It was a long, slow slog and involved doing speech exercises for many hours a day at home, with regular visits to the clinic to reinforce the technique when it became sloppy. Some of the patients relapsed, others went on to much better speech, and most of us fought to hold onto our gains. The better speech increased confidence and reduced stress, and the truth of Van Riper's theory that *felt fluency* helps the stutterer became apparent. Before therapy, a stutterer's speech would plunge into an uncontrollable downward spiral to inarticulacy, the poor speech making the speech worse. After therapy, many of us could control the spiral and avoid the previous severe regressions that could last for several weeks.

After therapy, any adult who has stuttered severely for many years needs to be continually vigilant. When his speech regresses, he gets out his tape recorder, listens to what he is doing wrong, and practises the correct methods. Some stutters disappear almost completely, but not many adults have that much luck.

Some of us have been on refresher mini-courses to keep us on track. During these courses, it was obvious that speech therapy is evolving, with more emphasis on easy, gentle approaches to words, slower speech, and prolongation, and less concern with voluntary stuttering. The methods used by the different clinics vary. In the best of them, the approach is innovative, experimental, and empirical. The stuttering syndrome is so complex that we still have a long way to go before therapy can be placed on a firm scientific basis.

People who have been on these intensive courses develop a tremendous respect for the therapists. The clinicians operate within definite therapeutic guidelines, but need to be sensitive to a stutterer's needs and to use their intuition to forecast how the patient will respond to certain patterns of treatment. Some therapists seem to know what is going on inside a stutterer's head and to be able to predict his fears, but treatment sessions can be exhausting and frustrating. Genuine, qualified therapists (not the quacks) undergo rigorous training, require great skill, and work incredibly hard.

EIGHT

Living with an albatross around your neck: stutterers and society

'A man cannot be measured by the colour of his skin, or by his speech, or by his clothes or jewels, but only by his heart.'

Mika Waltari

A few years ago there was a story going around spastic circles in Canada about a severely disabled young man who was taken in his wheelchair to a shopping plaza. His disability was obvious: he had great difficulty controlling the movement of his limbs; his head tended to loll to one side; and when he tried to speak, his face contorted and the sounds that emerged were hard to understand. As his chair was wheeled past the stores, he was suddenly confronted by a burly, red-faced man who angrily shouted, 'Why do you filthy, ugly people come here? Stay away! Stay in the institution where nobody can see you.'

Many handicapped people encounter rejections that are not quite so traumatic, but if their handicap is obvious people tend to avoid them and occasionally react violently. A young man in Victoria, British Columbia, who is a spastic, was beaten up by louts as he walked home from therapy with a friend, simply because he walked and talked in a strange way. I learned as a young man to be wary when I spoke in certain bars because my stuttering attracted attention and sometimes triggered a fracas. It is the old story about society's reaction to someone who is different. The more obvious the difference, the greater the reaction.

A person with a mild stutter may have a few social problems, and at one time it was even fashionable to stutter – wealthy aristocrats in Britain cultivated a vague, stuttering, stumbling way of speaking as a mark of their status. Nevertheless, a person with a very severe stutter who grimaces, twitches, and contorts his face in his efforts to speak is likely to encounter social difficulties.

A young woman in a wheelchair who found it difficult to set up house with other handicapped people in an Ottawa suburb because of local residents' objections, said on television that 'Canadians just don't like the handicapped.' It is not only Canadians who react adversely to the disabled, and it is not just a case of liking or disliking. In this case, the residents were probably afraid that a colony of handicapped people would reduce real-estate values; but usually the reasons for such behaviour are more complex. It is easy to apply such words as 'insensitive,' 'selfish,' and 'cruel,' but unreasoning fear of the unfamiliar, the unknown, and the uncontrolled runs through people's behaviour toward the handicapped. There is some truth in the old English proverb that cruelty is a tyrant that is always attended by fear. Those who respond well to the handicapped are able to override their fears by intelligence, humanity, compassion, and a felt need to probe beneath the surface and understand.

Some sociologists say that society's response to the handicapped is a reflection of the inbuilt attribute of animal populations to reject or attack any individual who looks, acts, or smells different from the norm. However, man has a well-developed brain. He is more than just an animal responding unthinkingly to fear and uncertainty. We may have inherited a rag-bag of nasty behavioural traits, but our large convoluted, cerebral cortex enables us to monitor and modify these urges. If it didn't, no nubile female would be safe on the street. Man is not just the slave of inherited behaviour. Society may have inbuilt responses to the handicapped, but individuals possess brains that permit choices of behaviour.

A wealthy woman, one of the Beautiful People, once said to me, 'I try to be kind to handicapped people I meet, but *really* ... ! I just can't stand to see them. I simply tell them to go away. What else can I do?' She responded to her feelings of revulsion and fear without any visible signs of other cerebral activity. She had the choice of rejecting the handicapped or of making an effort to look beyond the surface and establish contact. She chose the easier course. I reminded her that I was a handicapped person with a severe speech defect. She looked startled and retorted, 'You're different. I've known you since you were a child,' and thereby put her finger on the problem of her relationship with the disabled. It was her fear of the unfamiliar and unpredictable that disturbed her, not just the disability.

Some people may argue that severe stuttering, with its on-and-off occurrence, cannot be regarded as a disability in the same way as the physical handicaps of paraplegics, the deaf, and the blind; but very severe stuttering can be as disabling as many major problems of limb control, hearing, and even sight. I was once asked, 'If you had the choice of having a severe, debilitating stutter or being blind, which would you take?' The question seemed an easy one to answer, but it took me several minutes to think about it. My reply was that I'd rather be blind, because society to some extent accepts blind people and allows for their disability. Sightless people, although they miss a great deal, can communicate effectively and participate in society in many ways. A person who stutters very severely is denied effective communication most of the time, and the attitudes of society limit his social activities unless he is very determined indeed. He can all too easily be forced to live in the dark, lonely cave of his own mind.

Adverse responses to stuttering often arise because most people do not appreciate the difficulties a person with a stutter encounters in the ordinary, daily communication that fluent speakers take for granted. Most people have no idea of the stutterer's hidden, everyday world.

The paradox

People in Western societies live in an age of enlightenment. Social services help the aged, the sick, the poor, and the disadvantaged. Research is funded by governments – sometimes grudgingly – to find ways of reducing the physical and mental woes of mankind. The brutality of nineteenth-century society toward many of its members seems mere history: mentally handicapped people are no longer chained in the squalor of Bedlam; eccentric women aren't burned as witches; and crippled people no longer need to beg – at least not in public.

Governments cannot provide for all the needs of the disadvantaged, and large numbers of organizations run by business people work hard to provide extra funds. Unfortunately, many of the same people who spend large sums assisting the disabled carefully avoid close contact with recipients of their largesse. Not all firms are willing to employ people who stutter severely, and the busy captains of industry more often than not respond coldly to handicaps of any kind.

Psychologists, sociologists, and anthropologists have theorized about this paradoxical rejection of handicapped people. Some feel that our society establishes largely material goals, and, in the fight for status, security, and approval, anybody who gets in the way is liable to be trampled underfoot in the impatient mêlée. The corporate urge to help the disabled has been described as an attempt to dissipate the feelings of guilt that arise from maltreating them in the workplace. Rather like running for a bus, pushing a man on crutches into the traffic, and paying someone else to take him to the hospital. Others feel that people who assist the handicapped do so from a feeling of, 'It could happen to me.' It may be that people are simply reluctant to look the harsher realities of life in the face. They push aside the visible evidence, yet want to help at the same time.

Rejections of stutterers by society can be remarkably subtle. Every person who is severely disfluent has experienced the unspoken brush-off by someone who greets him in a friendly, open manner and then, when he blocks, adopts a withdrawn, guarded expression. It may only be a slight change in expression, but it signals that the glass wall is being firmly bolted in place between the stutterer and his audience. When a stutterer becomes more fluent it is quite a shock when this shift in expression doesn't occur.

Surviving childhood and adolescence

The young teacher at the boarding school had little experience of dealing with children who stuttered. His patience was wearing thin as the twelve-year old boy tried to read his part as Brutus in Shakespeare's *Julius Caesar*. Blocking badly on every line, the boy held up the play, and the other children in the class became restless. The teacher suddenly exploded, 'Sit down, you stupid boy! If you haven't the brains to speak you shouldn't be here.'

This happened in several successive classes and the teacher made a point of ridiculing the boy and calling him 'stammer-mouth.' The other students naturally followed his cue. Understandably, the boy became sullen and withdrawn. The teacher eventually went too far, whereupon the youngster stood up, said loudly, firmly, and fluently, 'Unless you stop this and apologize I refuse to answer any more of your questions,' and sat down, dry-eyed but shaking with fury.

He kept his word. Although he spoke to other teachers and students, he ignored his tormentor. When asked a question he looked straight ahead and remained silent. He was taken to the principal, chastised, and repeatedly kept in after school, but he stuck it out until the principal finally told him that the teacher would never apologize. During the lunch break the boy walked out of the school, trudged the twenty miles home, and flatly refused to return. He'd tried the fight response and it had failed, so he took the other alternative, flight.

Was this the action of a disturbed child? Perhaps a better interpretation is that a very angry and determined boy took the only sensible course of action open to him. Incidentally, he did very well at his next school.

Many children who encounter such teachers – and in spite of our enlightenment such individuals still exist – may not have anywhere to escape to, or the will to do so, and their lives can be a misery at school. It is not likely that they will do well scholastically, and their stuttering will probably get worse.

Fortunately, there are some fine teachers with the perception and humanity to look beyond the stutter. I was remarkably lucky. From the age of fifteen to seventeen I came under the wing of David Hodgkinson, a young teacher with whom I shared a fondness for mountains and wild places. He subtly widened my perception and introduced me to literature, poetry, Greek philosophers, the lives of great men, and the intricacies of Bach. Besides providing me with a rich basis upon which to build my life, he managed to persuade other teachers to make allowances for my speech handicap. I was not asked to do the impossible. Unfortunately David died very young, which was a great loss to the young people he could have taught.

Most teachers fall between these two extremes as they struggle to cope with all the different youngsters in their care. Children are expected to conform to certain standards. With increasing dependence on the spoken rather than the written word, students with communication disorders fare badly. For some it is impossible to speak at length during oral examinations, or to give seminars, or to involve themselves in public speaking without the support of effective therapy. If teachers appreciated a stutterer's limitations and permitted him to communicate in other ways, it would relieve the stress. There must be thousands of stutterers who have seen on their school reports, 'Fails to participate actively in the class.' 'Participate' usually means standing up and asking questions, and most people who stutter severely find this very difficult indeed.

If the boy with a stutter is handy with his fists he won't have too much trouble from kids of his own age, although there are always a few bigger boys who will beat him up and continue to taunt. A better approach is to develop an exceptional skill in either the classroom or a sport, particularly the latter, which commands the respect of others. Although I've never enjoyed hunting animals for pleasure, I was a competition-grade marksman from the age of thirteen years. The medals, badges, cups, and other trophies I won reflected well on my peer group and stood me in good stead, relieving some of the pressures and reducing my need to respond aggressively to other kids' jeers about my speech.

People who stutter learn early in life that in order to survive in the classroom, in university, or in a job they must not only be as good as others, but considerably better. Their disability means that they are frequently labelled 'stupid,' and their basic differentness tends to push them outside the herd. They must prove themselves much more than other children.

I learned this at about nine years of age when we were given a written history examination of ten questions. It dealt with the Battle of Hastings in 1066. Nine out of ten of my answers were completely correct, but I blocked badly when we were asked to read our answers aloud and failed the test. Even today I remember my anger and explosive protest to the teacher, who just shrugged her shoulders. As a result I became an 'over-achiever,' and wrote in a letter to my brother, 'I'll show the old cow!'

Most of the severe stutterers I have met who managed to lead full lives had similar experiences. The 'I'll show 'em' belligerence can be exceedingly effective, but it is a two-edged blade that can wound the wielder. Cold-blooded determination to 'show 'em' means that a child does well for the wrong reasons and may derive little pleasure from school achievements beyond a wry, one-in-the-eye satisfaction. I soon realized that my gritted-teeth approach to learning at school was unproductive and relaxed to the point of idleness by thirteen when I realized that I could get good marks by more careful planning and less hard work.

Other severe stutterers in my schools seemed to reach a crossroads at the age of about ten. At that point the impediment either crushed them into inarticulate, lonely unhappiness or began to spin a tough web of determination and single-mindedness throughout their mental fabric. The determined children with stutters became the survivors, but paid the price of excessive stress. Teachers and parents naturally praise the successes of the over-achieving children with partial disabilities, but tend to ignore the tremendous pressure it puts on a child. Perhaps teachers can find ways to reduce the pressures by creating an environment where there is no need for the partially disabled child to 'show 'em.'

The route a child with a stutter follows, whether it be withdrawal or determined achievement, can greatly affect the number of optional courses he takes at school. The children in the regular class get used to a stutterer and cease to bait him after a while, accepting him as a member of their herd. They may even actively support him by helping to fight his battles. Taking optional courses means moving to other groups and meeting new students and teachers. The first few days in a new group can be hell for a stuttering child. It takes sheer guts to expose yourself to it and persist. Children crushed by their stuttering may flatly refuse to take other courses, while the determined stutterer grits his teeth and looks upon the courses and the new situations as challenges – battles to be won. The other people in the new class may find the stutterer edgy and abrasive at first, but this usually disappears as he proves himself, and they accept him. The problem is that a determined child who stutters has to prove himself repeatedly.

It is difficult for a concerned teacher or parent to know what a stuttering child can do and what he cannot do. They may try to avoid exposing the child to situations he cannot handle, but sometimes, with the best of intentions, they underestimate his ability to cope and close doors to his progress. There was a bright senior boy in a school who exhibited leadership qualities, but he was barred from becoming a prefect because the principal felt he would find it hard to maintain discipline. Later in life, still with a stutter, he became a leader and had no difficulty maintaining order. This problem arises in the job situation where the abilities of stutterers to communicate and perform are frequently underestimated by potential employers.

At a time when big is still beautiful in the eyes of some educators, many school classes are still too large for teachers to provide individual attention. If the large classes were broken down into units small enough to allow teachers to educate children and allow for their diversity, partially handicapped children could be given more teacher time. Some schools and teachers insist on oral rather than written communication for certain tests. More flexibility to permit disfluent pupils to communicate in writing would ease pressures. Siphoning off stutterers and other partially handicapped pupils into special classes or schools is not the answer, because young people with partial communicative disorders must learn to perform in the context of society. Isolating them denies them needed opportunities for integration and acceptance.

I never enjoyed the word games and amateur theatricals that other children seemed to find such fun, although at six I played a goblin in a Hallowe'en play and managed to say 'Tonight's the night, aha!' without stuttering. Even today I carefully avoid social occasions where quiz games are played, and I still dislike playing card games involving bidding. All of these involve speaking, and in some games you must speak more quickly than other people to win. I can cope these days, but the games are associated with too many unpleasant memories to evoke pleasure.

Word games, oral spelling, and reciting at junior school were daily nightmares because no allowances were made for my stuttering. This helped to consolidate a minor disfluency into a major, self-reinforcing stutter – although it could have been avoided by a little common sense on the part of the teachers. These days the classroom environment is more enlightened, but a child who stutters is bound to have difficulties where oral performance is rewarded.

Not many people who stutter severely are likely to do well in languages. How I passed my French oral examination is a mystery. My inflexible Latin teacher gave me zero for my reading of Julius Caesar's *Conquest of Gaul*. Gaul was apparently divided into three parts *('Gallia est omnis divisa in partes tres.')*. I managed the *'Gallia est omnis ... '* but ground to a halt on *'divisa,'* which, since it was in the first sentence, somewhat truncated the examination.

The child who stutters severely is an oddball in the classroom, and the way others react to this disability may push him even further outside school society. Children enjoy both mental and physical challenges, but a child who stutters may find the impediment such a challenge in itself that he gets fewer kicks out of other activities. I played such games as rugby, cricket, and field hockey well enough, but did not enjoy them or find them a challenge. If you were to climb Everest frequently, the everyday, commonplace hills would be a bore.

Some stuttering children find that they enjoy activities of little interest to the majority (I loved bugs and fossils) and this may alienate their peers. In later life, these unusual interests can be a strength or a weakness depending upon the circumstances. Deep down, most children want to be one of the herd, and this can be very hard for a child with a severe stutter.

Many embarrassing situations can be avoided if teachers give a little thought to planning games that involve speaking. If there is a child who stutters badly in a group, there are often ways of letting him participate without speaking. Teachers should put themselves in the kid's position and try to imagine what it would feel like to have a fifty-fifty chance of blocking on a key word and inviting ridicule. It is tricky, because the child doesn't want to be pushed out of the game, or exposed to disaster. Sometimes it helps just to ask the child what he wants to do.

A stuttering child frequently collects a circle of friends who look beyond the disability and appreciate the person within. I had many intensely loyal friends who took my side against bullies and unpleasant teachers. These good companions were the salt of the earth. Sadly, few of them survived World War II.

When a teacher meets a child it is almost impossible for her to assess what is going on behind the surface mask. I recently looked at pictures of myself as a nine-year-old. The face of the calm-eyed kid with a faint smile completely hid an inner turmoil of anxieties and a burning determination to succeed and survive.

If teachers with stuttering children in their classes would avoid pretending that there isn't a problem and seek qualified advice, it is likely that fewer small children with minor stutters would later develop severe stutters. Even adolescents would have a greater chance of recovering spontaneously or responding to therapy. The classroom may be a jungle, but there is no need for a teacher to be one of the predators.

Living with a stutterer in the family

The attitudes of family members can have as much influence on a stutter as the pressures at school. It seems obvious that a stutterer would feel more relaxed about his speech at home where he knows the people and moves in familiar surroundings, but this is not always the case. During therapy, many stutterers said they found transferring the new speech techniques to the home situation more difficult than using the techniques with strangers in stores. I have always found it exceedingly difficult to use voluntary controlled repetition, prolongation, and cancellation when talking with my three daughters.

The reasons for this anomaly are varied and complex. In my case I feel it is a question of role. We all have images of ourselves acting within a group. Using the speaking techniques creates an unfamiliar person that is just not me – at least, within the family. It needs a great effort to change my identity.

It is easy to be critical of parents who cannot cope with a stuttering child, but most of them do their best. Many stutterers I have known who had severe problems with their mothers and fathers came from well-to-do, upward-striving, middle-class families with materialistic goals. The parents had neither the time nor the patience to worry about their struggling offspring. Other stuttering friends who had bad times came from families where the father was more concerned about his macho image than about his child. The majority of stutterers with parental problems, however, have mothers and fathers who are just nonplussed by the handicap and have no idea what to do about it. If they seek help at all it is generally from the family doctor, who is not always in a position to give good advice about stuttering, however competent he may be in other areas. Some parents just ignore the problem and hope the child will 'grow out of it.' Sometimes the child does, but if I had a stuttering child I wouldn't bet on it.

Sibling rivalry within the family is unavoidable and, as in any other competitive situation, does not involve much compassion. Any weakness is likely to be used in the battles between brothers and sisters. My brother had a large head, size seven and three quarters, and when I was angry I frequently called him 'Big Head.' He replied in kind about my stutter. The no-holds-barred sibling battles were good training grounds for the competitive realities of adult life where the opposition uses any weakness against you.[1]

I was lucky with my family. My brother and sister were not unusually nasty, and I gave as good as I got. A supportive and well-intentioned mother did her best and exposed me to a variety of bad speech therapies – the best available – that helped to turn a mild stutter into a severe one. My father ignored the fact that I stuttered, but did not ignore me. He was a theatre buff, and we went to innumerable shows that entranced a young boy with spectacular performances of the *Student Prince, Chu Chin Chow, White Horse Inn*, and endless Gilbert and Sullivan operettas (compared to which I find modern musicals insipid). I loved to meet the actors in their fancy dress after the shows.

He did the wisest thing he could by exposing me to all types of people and situations. His business friends were a bit dull, but he had financial interests in theatres, circuses, and horses, so I met acrobats and knife-throwers, rode on elephants, played with painted clowns in baggy pants, and rode ponies bareback. It was a small boy's magic world that still brings me happy memories. He took me to the tropics, where he taught me to fish for sharks. He managed to instil in me a self-confidence that stood me in good stead later in life. He was no softie. As an Edwardian father he firmly believed in judicious retribution for all major sins, but he was a better therapist than most of the professionals I met at the time.

People with severe stutters encounter new problems when they acquire families of their own. Most married people I know who stutter severely have been fortunate in their marriage partners. This is not surprising, because any person taking on someone who can hardly speak as a marriage partner must have considerable courage, as well as the more than usual insight it takes to see beyond the tense, disfluent facade and love the person within. Stuttering tends to run in families for reasons that are not fully understood. The non-stuttering partner's parents may not take kindly to having a person with a stutter grafted onto their family tree.

A non-stuttering partner has not only to learn to share the pain that is the stutterer's daily lot, but also to accept the fact that stuttering may limit a person's ability to earn money and provide for the family. A non-stuttering partner had better be a survivor.

Some people who marry disfluent partners don't know what they are letting themselves in for. If they don't have the ability to adapt to the situation, the marriage is liable to disintegrate. I am lucky. My wife, Joan, shares all my problems and looks upon them as a challenge. Before we married, I carefully but nervously laid all the cards on the table and described to her the stresses of living with disfluency. Incredibly, she took me on. Fortunately her parents had met stutterers before, so there was no problem in that area.

The prospect of having children made me distinctly anxious. As an adult I had never hit it off all that well with kids, because their responses to my stutter were unpredictable and sometimes hard to handle. Small children of eight years or less looked wide-eyed and asked honest questions like 'Why do you talk funny?' I handled these by telling them that some people walked in funny ways, or looked funny, and I just talked funny. They usually accepted the explanation. Adolescents were, and still are, more difficult. Some can be very rude and abusive about disfluency and, although it is tempting, it isn't practicable to swat them like irritating blow-flies. I usually resort to my steely-eye-and-chilly-silence routine.

I was aware of the danger that stuttering might develop in our children so, not having access to reliable counsellors, I developed my own approach. There was no hiding the fact that I stuttered severely, but I was careful to show no hint of anxiety or stress about my disfluency. If I blocked I'd say, 'Oops! Better try again!' or laugh when my tongue tangled in a knot. I didn't want the children to associate speaking with stress and fear.

People who stutter severely sometimes feel isolated in the family because they can't read to their children, recite nursery rhymes, or invent stories, but I was determined to communicate using my limited verbal faculties. When the children were very young, my wife and I would read to them in unison, and, occasionally, I fluently told them 'secret' stories in a whisper, which most stutterers can handle. I was always able to sing to them, and car trips were continuous, noisy sing-songs. When my speech was in a good phase I managed to tell them short stories, particularly Kipling's *Just So Stories* ('How the Elephant Got His Trunk' was a great favourite), but I was walking on verbal eggs. As the children grew older and were learning to read, we read slowly together, which was not difficult. When they reached adolescence they preferred television to father's boring stories, so I was able to go off reading duty.

The approach must have worked, because my daughters, who are now adults, have few recollections that I had a speech problem. Even when they reached the age of twenty or more they found it hard to accept that I had difficulties. None of them developed stutters. All of them speak so rapidly and at such great length that I can barely squeeze in a word when we get together.

The wife of someone with severe, uncontrollable stuttering finds herself taking on tasks her husband cannot handle. It makes no sense to be dogmatic about his-and-her roles. If a job involves speaking at length, the guy will need help. The wife of a severe stutterer is likely to find herself doing most of the telephoning. Even today, when I can use the telephone fairly freely, I dislike it to such an extent because of past memories that I tend to leave it to my wife. She's a telephone addict – one of those people who dread the day Bell Canada begins charging for local calls – so she doesn't find it much of a hardship.

When we are outside the house and approach a speaking situation, we decide who will do the talking before we start. From past experience she talks to policemen and customs officers, since they tend to be suspicious of and unpleasant to people who stutter. Some business people are impatient with stutterers, and occasionally my wife deals with them to spare them the fleas they are likely to get in their ears if they were to be obnoxious. Sometimes she deals with government officials, who also tend to respond badly. Dealing with disfluency is not in the regulations.

Sometimes it is hard for a wife to know to what extent she should help. There is always the danger that she will be overprotective, but frank discussion can overcome this kind of difficulty.

Performers, like musicians, who have stutters and become public figures sometimes let their wives read their speeches at social gatherings. The stuttering husband may seem to lean on his fluent wife, but the wife may become dependent on her role as speaker and find it difficult to adapt to the new situation when the stuttering spouse responds to therapy and is able to handle his own affairs. There are many stories of women leaving their husbands when the men became fluent. The wives didn't feel their husbands needed them any more. Maybe the speech challenge was all they had in common.

Living with a stutterer in the family needs understanding and goodwill on both sides. Even without the fractured speech it is not always easy to maintain family harmony.

Friends and lovers

Considering how society treats people with speech disorders, it is amazing that most of the stutterers I meet are warm and friendly people. They may be cautious with strangers and can be a little edgy, but on the whole they are not as withdrawn as most people think.

Some young men with stutters take offence when none is meant. Quite a few people who try to be friendly but nervously giggle when confronted by a stuttering, grimacing youth are fed an undeserved knuckle sandwich. At the age of twenty-three, when my speech was almost completely useless, I was a little explosive myself, and apologized to more than one innocent person after taking great exception to what I thought was ridicule. Fortunately, most people who stutter grow up and become less sensitive. When I am not sure that I'm being ridiculed or patronized, I give the other person the benefit of the doubt. When I am certain that someone is being offensive, my better control of speech and temper enable me to use both carefully chosen syntax and body language, which are much more effective than tapping their claret.

People with stutters can accumulate a circle of valued friends if all concerned are prepared to make the social effort. These friends are exposed to a lesser degree to the same embarrassments, frustrations, and rejections as the stutterer when they are in his company. Only exceptional people can stay the course. At one time when I was in the Armed Forces my speech used to attract trouble like a magnet, and my good, muscular friends helped to save my skin many times.

When a stutterer first meets a stranger the question usually at the back of his mind is: 'How will this person react to my speech?' He may not admit it, but the question is there. Many times I have carried on a friendly, fluent conversation with someone and got along famously until I blocked. Even one block can do it. The person just doesn't want to know you and flees for cover. This used to bother me as a young man, but not any more. Some friends you win and some you lose.

The other side of the picture is that, after the first startled response, some people pull themselves together and persist with the conversation. Sometimes the persistence is sheer curiosity to find out what makes this oddball tick – which is fair enough. When they feel at ease, the merely curious start to ask the kind of questions described in the second chapter of this book. These questions can be genuine or offensive, and the stutterer treats them accordingly. I usually answer unsolicited questions about my speech with stock answers and platitudes until I am sure that the inquiry is genuine. At this point you can usually guess whether or not there will be a future rapport. A stutterer isn't likely to make a friend of a tactless noodlebrain who asks, 'Doesn't it embarrass you when you stutter and people think you are stupid?' My answer to this type of question is, 'Why do you ask that question?' Nevertheless, I welcome genuine inquiries and interest in speech problems.

During these preliminaries, a stutterer feels his way cautiously until both parties are comfortable and can relax, thereby providing a basis for potential friendship. A dialogue is not always sufficient, and acquaintances sometimes fall by the wayside when they share the problems generated by society. The friends who survive these traumatic experiences are pure gold.

The trickiest 'friends' for any handicapped person to recognize and deal with are the patronizers. There are a few people around who, because of their own hidden weaknesses, make friends with the disabled in order to feel better about themselves. Such a relationship can be damaging to a person with a severe stutter, whose self-confidence and self-esteem may not be all that strong, because the patronizer inflates his own ego by subtly putting down the handicapped person. This type of individual can be difficult to recognize. You can't go around questioning everybody's motives. If the 'friend' is upset when the handicapped person can do something better than he can, or makes light of his disfluent companion's successes, there is reason for suspicion. Some lonely stutterers, and other handicapped people whom society has treated cruelly, seek friendship at any price, and they all too easily get into bad company.

It is not advisable to generalize about the relationship between stutterers and members of the opposite sex. Some perfectly normal men with all their faculties in working order find it difficult to establish relationships with women, and vice versa. Stuttering is just another complication in an already complex picture.

It comes as a surprise to many male stutterers when girls reject them for reasons other than their speech. Soon after World War II, I was a member of a university class consisting largely of men who had been battered by war, demobilized early, and sent to college to keep them out of mischief. This influx of mature servicemen increased the competition for university girls to fever pitch, so I focused my attention on the town population.

I developed a passion for a girl who looked like Ava Gardner and worked behind the counter in a pharmacy. My speech was in a bad way, so I was a bit nervous about asking her for a date. I visited the pharmacy several times a week for a month or more and accumulated a vast supply of Ever-Ready razor blades, which were not all that easy to come by at that time. They were all I could afford, and I must have cornered the market. When I summoned enough courage to ask her out she accepted, suggesting that we first have dinner and then go to the local dance hall.

It was our first and last date. She turned out to be a ballroom dancer who had won all kinds of competitions. She said that I danced as though I had three feet. She didn't mind my stuttering in the least, but took the greatest exception to my slow fox-trot. Philosophically, I turned my attention to a girl who also looked like Ava Gardner and worked in a bookstore. She was a Shakespeare buff, and, in spite of my stutter, I managed, by judicious use of the bard's sonnets, to establish a relationship that was entirely satisfactory – until she turned to Chaucer, who was beyond my linguistic ability.

About this time I encountered an attitude that was entirely unexpected. I had a colleague, a cheerful, fair-haired, beefy lad who had been a flying-boat navigator until he was injured. He was not noted for his tact. My stuttering was causing me problems and one day, after I forcibly expressed my feelings about my fractured syntax, he said, 'Don't worry! One day you'll find a girl who can put up with your stuttering and go out with you. Who knows, you might even get married. Anything is possible!' It hadn't entered my head that my disfluency would impede my progress with girls, but he clearly thought that anyone with such a bizarre disability was at the end of the line as far as girl-friends and wives were concerned.

There is no doubt at all that stuttering scares off some young girls, particularly when they are at the age when appearances, normality, and belonging to the in-group are of paramount importance. When young people date they want to feel proud of the companions they introduce to their families and friends. Sometimes a girl with a stuttering boy-friend is forced to make a choice between him and her family, and not many have the strength to withstand that kind of pressure. A pleasant young man in Ontario with a severe, grimacing stutter became firm friends with an attractive girl and accompanied her to many social functions. The girl introduced him to her parents who were perfectly normal farm people. They were polite to the stutterer, but distant. The next time he asked the girl for a date she regretfully turned him down, because her parents had ordered her to get rid of her stuttering friend.

This situation is not uncommon. I went sailing with a girl, but met her father first. He was a practical, down-to-earth business man ('Where there's muck there's money, lad.'), and plainly thought his daughter had brought home a dangerous kook. While we sailed, he had a pair of binoculars trained on us in case I ravished his daughter in the bilges, causing a great deal of on-board hilarity. I solved the problem by looking back with my own binoculars. After a minute or so of staring at each other eyeball to eyeball, he disappeared. I was not asked to stay for dinner.

Some stutterers whose feelings have been trampled and abused by society find it difficult to establish deep relationships with people, particularly those of the opposite sex. They may have many friends and acquaintances, but the relationships move in shallow water, the stutterer being unwilling to go out of his depth and explore the unknown. It is largely a matter of trust. Any deep emotional attachment involves showing another your inner self and assuming the person won't abuse that trust. Some stutterers have inner conflicts that they are not prepared to reveal to others. The disfluent can build their own glass walls for self-protection and never come out into the real world. Sometimes it is up to a friend or lover to break down the walls and establish the trust. You don't have to stutter to have problems about trusting people. Our frenzied society, grasping for monetary will-o'-the-wisps, can be cruel to people with no functional disabilities at all.

The withdrawn stutterer needs to learn to gamble a little, to make mistakes, and to burn his social fingers, accepting that rejection and unkindness are just a part of life. How you deal with them is all that matters. I was saved from withdrawal by an insatiable curiosity about life and people that made me willing to pay the price, however painful, to find out what makes the world tick. Part of me is sociable, and part is solitary. At times I must spend periods alone to recharge my mental batteries. Like other people, stutterers may withdraw for productive purposes, and this has nothing to do with their speech impediments.

People who stutter sometimes avoid social gatherings, and a casual observer may interpret this as shyness or pathological withdrawal. This is not necessarily the case. After talking at work and trying to cope with my stutter, I was usually tired by the end of the day. The last thing I wanted to do was go on talking, however congenial the company. Coping with disfluency can be very tiring indeed, and many stutterers who speak a great deal at the office prefer some non-vocal recreation like swimming, skiing, riding, walking, going to a movie, or engaging in a hobby.

Some stutterers find conversation in large groups difficult, particularly where there is rapid repartee. A disfluent person just cannot get in his word before he is cut off. He finds it impossible to contribute to the conversation, and this can make a chatty social evening very boring. On a few such occasions I have accidentally fallen asleep. Sometimes, to my embarrassment, I have snored loudly.

The academic rat race

There always seemed to be a great many students with stutters when I was at university after World War II – at least one in any group. They all seemed to do well in their examinations. It was easy to conclude that people with stutters are more intelligent than others. While this is incorrect as far as the general population is concerned, there is an element of truth in the case of university students.

University students in the United States and Britain were repeatedly surveyed in the 1930s because most of the speech research was carried out at universities, and the students were convenient to study. Not only were stutterers much more common at American universities (1.8 to 2.8 per cent) compared with the population in general (about 1 per cent), but stuttering university students had consistently higher scores on intelligence tests than fluent students. This apparently superior intelligence possibly reflected the segment of the population at university in those days (upward-striving, middle-class), or the fact that to succeed in school and get into university a stutterer had to be better than others and determined to succeed. Because of difficulties with oral examinations and presentations, the grades of stuttering children tend to be lower than average.[2] The child who gets as far as university must have the wits and the will to beat the odds.

When a person enters university, the highly competitive academic systems make few allowances for a stutter. The student copes or gets out. A severely disfluent student will have a hard time coping with a law course, where oral, Socratic methods of question and answer are used. A disfluent medical student may find it impossible to stand up and describe case histories to a highly critical audience. High grades mean good jobs, and the stutterer had better be a survivor in the more competitive faculties.

I went to universities in Britain at a time when oral seminars and presentations were of minor significance compared with written reports. There are chilling stories of stutterers who went to universities in Europe where all the examinations consisted of standing alone and answering orally the questions posed by committees of cold-eyed professors. Stutterers cannot survive in such oral systems. Even today, most universities in North America require students to give seminars, whether they stutter or not, even when the subject is something like forestry, horticulture, or soil science where verbal disabilities are not likely to be too much of a problem. I waded my way through a few seminars, oral examinations, and defences of theses, but it was no joy either to the examiners or to myself.

The fact that a student who stutters badly cannot cope with the oral demands of degree courses in subjects like law and medicine may indicate that the profession is just not for him. In some cases, however, the methods used in university faculties prevent a disfluent student from pursuing a career he could easily manage. Articulacy does not necessarily indicate academic ability.

I was permitted to write when possible, and when I had to speak I used a variety of visual aids – graphs, charts, and tables – to minimize the amount of speaking. My colleagues said they found my talks brief (of necessity), to the point (I cut out the garbage), and preferable to many presentations by more wordy peers. This latitude is not available at some present-day universities, and the oral demands place an unnecessary strain on the disfluent student. The rigidity of academic, bureaucratic, and governmental institutions is one of the numerous ills of our time and prevents the varied needs of individuals being met.

Earning a living: the hidden discrimination

Going for a job interview was as enjoyable for me as visiting my school principal's study after being found guilty of such a major transgression as walking with my hands in my pockets. In both instances I knew that the next few minutes were sure to be painful.

As a young man I applied for a job breeding raspberries at

a horticultural station in England. I bristled with degrees, know-how, intelligence, and energy, and was shaken when I was defeated by a quiet young woman in thick tweeds and brogue leather shoes. The interviewers were civilized and polite in a reserved British way, and you could see they were trying to remember that the King, God bless him, shared my problem. Nevertheless, it was clear that they had reluctantly concluded that anyone who stuttered as badly as I did couldn't possible have all his marbles. When the kindly, elderly man said I would hear from them, and the tweedy girl was taken to lunch, I knew I'd blown it.

I went through interview after interview, but it was clear that nobody wanted a well-qualified ex-serviceman with a stutter, although they seldom said the stuttering was the problem. Even the fact that I had been to the right kind of school, spoke with the right kind of accent, and knew that you passed a port decanter to the left didn't cut any ice with the establishment. I was astonished therefore when, after a perfunctory interview, I was offered a job growing palm trees by a company making soap and margarine. The salary was four times what I expected, with a house, several servants, an automobile, and six month's leave every two years. My knowledge of palm oil was so limited that I thought copra was something you mined, so I was a little suspicious. Delving into a gazetteer revealed that I was destined for some death hole in the swamps of West Africa where they could put up with my stuttering for the year or so of my life expectancy. I resumed the job hunt.

In retrospect, these depressing interviews were the best thing that could have happened to me. In order to eat I wangled a grant to do research for a post-graduate degree and spent six years on my own talking to deer and pine trees in the Highlands of Scotland, a stutterer's idea of paradise.

Later, with another degree to put on my shingle, I had a further spell of interviews and tried unsuccessfully to get work growing trees in Wales, extracting perfume from lavender in the south of France, and studying water in a waterless part of Australia. Gradually, I learned the art of interviewing and landed a disagreeable job at Oxford University for a few years before embarking on a career of ecological research in Britain's beautiful Lake District where my disability was not much of a handicap.

In spite of all the talk about equal opportunity and civil rights, employers faced with choosing between two people with equal qualifications, one of whom stutters and one of whom doesn't, are likely to select the fluent applicant. In a way this is discrimination, but employers should be able to hire the people they want.

The probationary period is a useful instrument. If employers would give stutterers and other handicapped people a chance to show whether they can handle a job, this would help. If they can't do the job, replacing them is sensible rather than discriminatory. Far too many employers write off an applicant at his first block, forgetting that his speech is likely to be at its worst at a job interview, particularly the hot-seat type of screening where you sit on a hard chair in the middle of a horseshoe of impatient interrogators.

After many painful interviews I learned to act a variety of roles. When the board consisted of bureaucrats, I became a bureaucrat and trotted out the jargon they love, peppering my speech with words and phrases like 'objectives,' 'collective bargaining,' 'decentralization,' 'cost effectiveness,' 'mandatory,' 'critical paths,' 'lines of command,' and 'conceptualization.' With scientists I put on the brilliant-but-eccentric act; and with business people I became a thrusting executive, obsessed with cash flow, rates of return, cost effectiveness, and linear programming. My performances were so effective that people forgot the stuttering and began to offer me jobs.

I was playing roles. Therapists may frown at role-playing to achieve better fluency, but I'd have danced the part of the Sugar Plum Fairy to get a good job.

I was lucky. I had the education and the skills, and my family could house and feed me while I hunted for work. Not all stutterers are so fortunate.

There is no doubt that in the job market there is a great deal of hidden discrimination against people with severe stutters, quite apart from their actual fitness for the work. Stutterers make some people feel uncomfortable. They may not fit in a work group, either because of their stuttering or their tendency to over-achieve and compete aggressively. Employers wanting a contented work force tend to get rid of the odd man out, and it is their prerogative, since they pay the bills. Nevertheless, it would help if employers appreciated what a disfluent person can do rather than what he cannot do. People with stutters and other handicaps can do first-class work. They are often great planners and strategists – they have to be to survive – and this can be an asset.

Stuttering makes you resourceful. You instinctively think about things that could go wrong and devise ways of dealing with them before they happen. A simple problem like having the car break down in a remote area and trying to get help can be traumatic. You walk up to a farm and knock on the door. Someone opens it and at your first block is liable to slam it in your face. If you get as far as the telephone you're likely to block, and the person on the other end may hang up on you. The disfluent and stranded traveller has to sit down and think of a solution. I always carried a pad, a pencil, and a small tape recorder.

People can cope with most things if they curb their urge to take flight. I had just driven to Quebec City when I received a message telling me to represent Canada at an international meeting in the southern United States concerning a subject about which I knew very little. There were no briefings, no guidelines, no time to do any homework, and no allowance for my disability. I just had to be there. An hour before the meeting I alternated between feeling sick and numb, but when I entered the room and adopted the role of government scientist, all the tension disappeared. I blocked and stuttered, but my eccentric-scientist act saved the day. The meeting went remarkably well, and the bottle of Jack Daniel's sour mash in my room soon quieted my jangled nerves. At the time it never entered my head that even a fluent person would have been nervous when faced by such a challenge.

There is no easy solution to the problems stutterers encounter in looking for and keeping jobs. It is necessary to be realistic, but a greater attempt to be open about the problem and deal with it honestly instead of pretending it isn't there would benefit all concerned.

Foreign travel

A few years ago an intelligent, slightly built young man with fair hair set out from Canada on a private adventure, hitch-hiking across Europe and Asia Minor to Afghanistan. He managed to reach his destination and to return home all in one piece. This still amazes me, because he had a very severe stutter and distorted his face as he struggled to speak.

My stutter has landed me in trouble many times on my travels. Customs officers are the worst. I suppose they look for signs of anxiety and tension in guilty passengers carrying contraband. When my stutter was in a bad phase I probably gave the impression of being agitated when all I was doing was trying to say 'I've nothing to declare.' Once, on returning to Britain from a visit to a research laboratory in the Netherlands and being asked by the customs officer if I had anything to declare, I blocked on the word 'No.' He passed my bags; however, when I was leaving the building an official in plain clothes hustled me into a nearby office where, in more ways than one, they left no stone unturned as they looked for diamonds. I was interrogated at gun point at the border between France and Italy because I blocked. In New York's Kennedy Airport a cold-eyed lout in uniform opened and up-ended my suitcase, scattering belongings everywhere, looking in the linings, and saying, 'What are you so nervous about?' and ignoring my explanation that I was not nervous, I just stuttered. Spanish customs officers in Madrid were suspicious, snarky, and belligerent about my disfluency, but they were like that with everybody.

Even entering Canada from the United States was a problem. If I blocked when I answered the customs officer's questions, my car was sure to be pulled over and searched. There were exceptions, and some customs officers were helpful and courteous. In one of the banana republics, where customs officials are over-officious, blocking severely could mean mouldering in a rat-infested dungeon for years.

Trying to cope with a foreign language is bad enough without a stutter. When I was in Italy I fluently asked a young woman in a store for Virginia cigarettes to avoid smoking their acrid Nationales. I had looked up the words in my little Italian dictionary and couldn't understand the shouting and fist-shaking that followed my request – until someone told me I'd muddled the grammar and asked the girl if she were a virgin.

A stutterer will experience abroad all the problems he meets at home, but on a bigger scale because of the language barrier. Asking for food in restaurants and merchandise in stores in a foreign language can be traumatic even for fluent people, as many Americans find when they visit Quebec City thinking it's the same as New Orleans. Taxi drivers can be a pain. Some try to charge you double fare if they think you can't or won't argue (I can and do!).

I like seeing new places, meeting new people, and participating in new cultures, but for me travelling has never been as enjoyable as other people seem to find it. For many years I travelled all over the world on business, and now that I don't have to do so it is something of a relief. I was offered an interesting short-term job in Paris a year or so ago, but turned it down because I couldn't bear the thought of battling in French with hotels, taxi drivers, and officials for three months. Some severe stutterers love travelling and don't seem to mind the hassle.

Stores and restaurants

The majority of people take speaking, like their heartbeats, for granted. If they want something, they ask for it. If they want to ask a question, they ask it. If they want to protest, they protest. A stutterer never takes speech for granted even in his fluent phases. He may have had good therapy, but he must always watch his way of speaking and plan for possible failures. Stutterers can ask for things, question, and protest, but, like porcupines making love, only with the greatest care.

Stores and restaurants present a severe stutterer with a multitude of problems. Store clerks vary in their responses, but many are hostile and some are downright rude. In some restaurants if you stutter at the headwaiter when you arrive he is liable to try to fob you off with a table between the wash-rooms and the kitchen door if you let him – which I don't. As a young man I just pointed at the menu for dishes I wanted to order and even acted mute to avoid unpleasantness from the waitress. Many times I ordered dishes I didn't want because they were easy to say. I still can't ask for pressed duck.

When my speech was very bad indeed I was completely lost without my pencil and scribbling pad, because I couldn't order anything in a store without writing it down. Occasionally, I encountered someone who was blind or couldn't read, which really put gravel on my gears. After countless bad experiences in these situations, I found trying to use speech techniques in stores and restaurants incredibly difficult, but these situations cause me few difficulties today.

Public transport

Public transport is not usually a major problem for severely disfluent people unless they have to ask for directions or tell the driver where to go in front of other passengers. Airport buses can be a trial because the drivers stand up at the front and ask for destinations. If the name of the hotel is difficult to say I am in trouble, particularly if it's in French. Taxis used to be difficult. Even if I wrote the address on a piece of paper, the driver would ignore it and ask where I wanted to go. If I had trouble speaking, the drivers were less than polite, and I was not all that tolerant of their bad manners.

Railway trains were fine. You got your ticket, sat in your seat, and shut up. Nobody bothered you. Air travel can be tricky; it depends on whom you get beside you. Some passengers are a delight to talk to, like the very old lady in her eighties who, when I was in my mid-forties and doing calculations on a pad, leaned over and said, 'You'll be one of them young students!' and told me about her adventures as a nurse in the Arctic fifty years ago.

Passenger aircraft are full of young executives who read too many books on psychology and tend to suffer from verbal incontinence and impertinent curiosity. They ask questions like, 'Is it true that all people with communication disorders have castration complexes?' unaware that my wishful thinking about them includes more than a complex in their futures. I avoid sitting next to young men with expensive brief-cases, manicured finger-nails, Holt Renfrew pin-stripes, glossy shoes, and dollar signs glittering in their eyes.

Hotels

Hotels that are large and expensive frequently have well-trained staffs that are used to dealing with eccentric and even objectionable people. If you spend money and don't muck up the room, set the place on fire, pinch the towels, or offend the other guests, you are welcomed with open arms. They won't mind if you're a stuttering Martian with seven legs provided you have the right credit card. If you stutter and offer to pay with real money, then you're in deep, deep trouble ...

The arrival part is not too bad. Even if I blocked badly on my name at the reception desk I could always shove my credit card under their noses so they could identify me. The difficulties arose when I reached my room and wanted to take advantage of the hotel's services. You ask for most services by telephone. That darned telephone!

I stayed at hotels for twenty years before I used room service. I was so disfluent and conditioned to block on telephone calls that if I wanted a maintenance man to repair a leaky faucet, I just put up with the drip. It was no use going down to the desk and asking for a plumber. They just referred me to room service. So the tap dripped. Ordering meals or drinks in my room was impossible, so I invariably ate elsewhere. Asking for an early call on the phone by giving the room number and the time was out of the question, so I learned to carry an alarm clock. Making a long-distance call through the hotel operator was a major battle. First you had to give your name and room number, and then the digits. I usually ground to a halt on my name until the operator cut me off. The family learned not to expect calls from me when I was away, but some business calls were unavoidable. My speech was usually not bad once I connected with my target, but the process of getting there was exhausting.

I learned to use verbal aids. I could, if I spoke with great care, tape messages on my own, so I bought a small tape-recorder and recorded what I wanted to say to the operator, with two repeats in case she didn't hear the first time. I lifted the receiver, dialled the operator, played the tape to get over the vital message of name, room, and number, and ad libbed from then onwards. It took a bit of practice, and I once played the operator a recording of the Glasgow Orpheus Choir by mistake, making matters worse by going off into peals of laughter. But usually it worked remarkably well.

The staff of many small hotels run as family businesses are most courteous and helpful, and these hotels can be gems. The best we ever stayed at nestled in the middle of a peach orchard in Pennsylvania, near to the village with the unusual name of Intercourse. The Amish people who ran the place were not in the least put out by my stuttering, and we spent a tranquil night in spite of the bangs of the bird-scarers. In contrast, many of the cantankerous receptionists at dingy dumps in the boondocks are incredibly unpleasant to fluent customers and intolerable if you block. After a preliminary effort to be polite, it is sometimes necessary to be outspoken. The angrier I used to get, the more fluent I became. With my vast vocabulary of synonyms that I used to substitute for difficult words, I managed to make my feelings known, stutter or no stutter. If you have trouble speaking, this kind of hotel usually makes you pay in advance and may not accept your credit card. Nevertheless, I prefer to stay at small places rather than those twenty-storey monsters in which you fry to a crisp if some fool smokes in bed and sets the place alight.

I used to get angry with rude receptionists, but now I just feel sorry for them. They are just tired, bored, afraid of the unfamiliar, and behave in the only way they know.

It would help even in the best hotels if a person who has difficulty speaking could go to the information desk and ask for room service or an early call. The major hotels are proud of their facilities for the handicapped, including ramps for wheelchairs, specially designed washrooms, and chains and pulleys to help a person get into and out of bed and the bath. This is fine, but there are handicapped who have no trouble using their limbs. No allowance is made for the stutterers, the aphasics, the deaf, and the mute who, once in their rooms, tend to be trapped by the glass walls of their handicaps. Hotels can be lonely places.

In the near future we are likely to see telephones in homes and hotels linked to computer terminals, video displays, and printers. I envy the stutterers of the future who will be able to key-punch their messages to room service or the information desks without struggling to speak. A room or two in a hotel with a computer link would make the stay much more enjoyable for those with speech and hearing disabilities.

The telephone nightmare

To a greater or lesser extent, the telephone haunts all people who stutter. The mere sight of the instrument can recall a multitude of humiliations. The ring of a telephone that needs answering can arouse sheer panic. I discovered to my surprise that a great many people with normal speech are scared by the telephone, and that most callers become exceedingly nervous when an answering machine asks them to leave a message. Stuttering just amplifies the fears.

The telephone is such an impersonal way of communicating. You can't see the speaker and read the body language that plays such a large role in a stutterer's communication. The telephone message is conveyed by mere words. There may be information in the tone of voice, but the spoken words are the main thing.

When I stuttered very badly I'd pick up the phone, dial the operator, and try to say the number. I inevitably blocked, and more often than not she'd say, 'Please put your telephone down and dial again. We have a bad connection.' cutting me off before I could explain that it was me, not the phone, that had a bad connection. This was repeated three or four times until I bellowed, 'Hold it a minute, god damn it! Keep the plug in and listen!' This I could say fluently if I was mad enough. When I had all her attention, I tried to say the number careful digit by careful digit, but there were long silences between syllables. She never got the number right the first time, so I battled through the digits over and over again. Some valiant souls stayed the course, but many operators hung up in despair. For me the telephone was not a practical form of communication. I coped at the office, but didn't willingly make a social call for twenty-five years.

In Britain most of the operators were polite; at the worst they were impatient. My most memorable call was to a rural exchange near the resort of Os in Norway. The male operator's English was non-existent and my Norwegian was tourist gibberish, but I managed to read the carefully rehearsed digits from my dictionary. Of course I blocked; it still amazes me how any Scandinavians get their tongues around their vowels. The man became abusive, so I put down the telephone and looked up in my dictionary a few of the words he had used. Most of them referred to the nether parts of farmyard animals so I carried out more careful research. I dug from the dictionary a few choice Norwegian nouns and adjectives about unlikely ancestry, picked up the phone, dialled, and fluently returned his serve. Match and game. I never did make the call.

In France, Italy, and Spain telephoning was impossible. I could say the words with a passable accent, but when I hesitated the blast of grapeshot that came over the wire would put anybody off.

North American responses are patchy. In New York State and Massachusetts the operators are so impatient that they don't seem to be able to cope with people who stutter, or anybody else for that matter. Soft-spoken operators in Georgia are wonderful. They just wait patiently until the number emerges and even have a chat afterwards, hoping that I enjoy their fair state.

Canada is a country of contrasts, and this applies to telephone operators. In British Columbia, Alberta, and Saskatchewan, they generally treat my disfluency with the greatest courtesy and patience; even in Ontario a stutterer using the phone will have few problems west of North Bay. The nearer you get to Ottawa, the harder it is for a stutterer to use Ma Bell's facilities. Maybe it's the feisty, Gallic temperament, but as soon as I hear an operator with a French accent I think, 'Here we go again!' I had no problems at all when I stuttered in both English and French while I worked in Quebec, except on the telephone.

One young man stuttered when he contacted an Ottawa

operator. Following the guidelines of his therapy he paused and said to the operator, 'I have a stutter. I shall probably repeat words, and pause. Please hold on!' To his amazement the male operator began to jeer at him and imitate his speech, so the stutterer lost his temper and slammed down the phone. He should have asked for the supervisor and reported the incident, but even if he had done so it's doubtful that it would have done much good. I've reported abusive operators several times. Only once did I get a reply, and the letter just made polite, placatory noises.

It is a mystery to me why some operators respond this way. As a rule a person's reaction to stuttering seems to be rooted in fear, so maybe the operators are scared of not being able to cope with a stutterer; or perhaps they mistake him for a drunk. Bell has expressed concern for the handicapped and has devised electronic equipment to help disabled people to use the telephone more easily. I just wish they'd take a closer look at the human factor and teach more of their operators good manners and how to deal with callers who cannot speak very well. It's not too hard. Just wait. The words will come eventually.

Even telephoning can be funny. I was taking therapy in Ottawa and was at the stage when you deliberately repeat every first sound three times (voluntary controlled repetition). I wanted a long-distance number, and there was no direct dialling, so I contacted the operator and fluently said, 'Six, six, six, one, one, one, three, three, three, five, five, five,' until I heard choking sounds on the line and realized what I was doing. I burst out laughing, explained the problem, and we both enjoyed the joke.

Despite lighter moments and even with improved fluency, I dislike the phone. The rude, impatient responses of some of the operators to even minor pauses and disfluencies still raise my hackles. Until the entire system is automated, and a person with a stutter can dial all numbers, the only answer is better education for the operators.

I often wonder what the snarky ones look like. When they put video screens on the phones I may be surprised to find that some of them don't sit pulling the wings off wriggling, helpless flies.

The faceless bureaucracy

Bureaucrats tend to manage their affairs by the rule books, and there don't seem to be any guidelines about how to deal with the vocally disabled. Managing employees who differ from average is a human problem, and the last concern of all the government regulations I have read seems to be the problems of humanity. Give the public service an administrative riddle to solve and it will succeed – expensively, perhaps, but nevertheless succeed. Give the service a human problem and it will flunk the test.

The Income Tax Office in Ottawa has facilities for the handicapped, but when you enter the advisory room, you take a number. When you are called, you stand in a kind of cattle stall facing a flinty-eyed tax officer behind a plastic counter. You can't sit, but stand like a penitent so that all the waiting victims can hear your financial confessions. Imagine that you have a stutter and block on every fourth word. You try to explain your tax problem in the bureaucratic bafflegab that is the only language the clerks understand. It's hard enough for a fluent person to cross this hurdle, but for a stutterer it can be a nightmare. All the supplicants behind you hear your blocks and repetitions and get an earful about your problems of cash flow. You lose your privacy and dignity as well as your money. Why can't they provide the privacy of cubicles with four walls?

At the Passport Office the person behind the counter tends to get difficult if you block, and the rigmarole of swearing in for citizenship is about as hard for a stutterer as taking marriage vows. In any government office you meet, besides the usual bureaucratic shell-game, blank-eyed unhelpfulness when you block. Some people with stutters find the bureaucracy easier to deal with than others, but most people who stutter very badly tell a sad tale of rudeness and obstruction. Fluent people get the same run-around, but a stutter makes the problem worse.

The move to bilingualism in Canada has placed many civil servants who stutter in a difficult position. They may have done a good job for years, but the regulations demand that public servants in management positions or who deal with the public be proficient in French. Whether you see a franco-phone once every two years is beside the point. Many older people find it hard to learn French – which is why the lists of executives in the federal government telephone books read like the Paris directory – and many stutterers find the oral methods used in language schools impossible to handle. The language regulations virtually bar employees with severe stut-ters from promotion to more senior positions they could han-dle efficiently.

By fancy administrative footwork I managed to avoid the French courses and still get promoted, but many disfluent employees are less fortunate and are limited by blind applica-tion of discriminatory regulations. More flexibility in the language program to allow for the fact that some employees have linguistic problems would at least indicate a little con-cern for the people involved. There's not much hope that the situation will change in the near future because, as L.J. Peter wrote, 'a bureaucracy defends the status quo long past the time when the quo lost its status.'[3]

The arm of the law

It was difficult to drive in the rush hour on the ice-covered, granite cobblestones of Aberdeen, Scotland, without sliding into other vehicles, and I cursed the police car when it abruptly cut in front and signalled me to stop. A red face framed by a chequered police cap peered suspiciously in at the window sniffing for evidence of alcohol and asked if I knew that one of my rear lights had blown and that travelling without all my lights was breaking the law. I promised the policeman I would go to a mechanic on the way home. Un-fortunately, 'm' is difficult for me to say and I blocked badly on 'mechanic.' I was promptly arrested and carted off to the cop shop where I had the devil of a time convincing the law that I was sober.

Police tend to associate disfluency with drunkenness, and before the breathalyser tests it was hard for a stutterer to prove that he was sober. Earlier in this century, the test for drunkenness was to walk a straight line and reel off tongue-twisters like, 'The Leith police dismisseth us.' A person who stuttered was sure to fail the test. A great many people were detained merely because they tangled their words.

About the time of my arrest a well-known scientist found himself in a British court. He was brilliant, one of those academicians who seemed to be good at everything. His lucid pen described physics, mathematics, and mechanics in a manner everybody could understand and enjoy. Like many exceptional people he was eccentric, and when he spoke he bumbled. He was so inarticulate that he was hard to understand. The police arrested him in his car in London. Although he was stone cold sober, a charge of drunken driving stuck as far as the courts, where it was dismissed when witnesses testified that he always spoke that way.

As a young man I was detained twice for stuttering. In addition, because of my impediment, I have had difficulties with the police so many times that I've lost count. Police deal with the seamy side of life and tend to be suspicious of anybody who acts in a way that is outside their usual experience. I now realize that many police in North America are frightened by unfamiliar situations and unusual people. A lone New York State police trooper stopped to find out why our car, which had conked out, was parked beside the turnpike in the pouring rain. He was plainly terrified when I blocked badly, and he became belligerent, virtually accusing me of stealing my own car.

There are many fine police officers (and I knew one policeman who stuttered and had quite a time in court), but on the whole I avoid contact with the law. The odds are too high that there will be unpleasantness. The police have the guns and the law on their side, and a stutterer is likely to come off second best in any altercation.

The only way to solve this problem is for the police to be taught that about 1 per cent of the population stutters and that there are many others – stroke victims with aphasia, clutterers, people with cleft palates, and the totally deaf – who speak in strange ways that are sometimes hard to understand. Altogether there must be five million people in North America who, for one reason or another, have difficulty speaking, and the majority of these are respectable, law-abiding citizens. There is no need for the police to give them a hard time.

I knew two pretty girls who were totally mute, but who both had boy-friends and managed to lead fairly normal lives. I asked them if they had encountered any problems with the police, and they both replied, in writing, that although they had met officers there had been no trouble at all. On my next encounter with the police, I pretended to be mute and wrote my answers to their questions on a pad. It worked, and the tough-looking officers were courteous and helpful. It seems to be all right if you shut up but far from all right if you talk in a strange way. I was tempted to remain mute in future encounters, but you can't go around acting false roles all the time.

In the days when I stuttered very badly I avoided the courts at all costs and was reluctant to appear as a witness. This attitude arose from my experience of court proceedings in Britain when I was in the Armed Forces. We were granted week-end passes to the nearest town, and during a night out with the boys my money ran out as the beer poured in – our pay was only two pounds a week at the time. Rather than sit in draughty Church Army canteens or read uplifting books sitting on hard chairs in Salvation Army hostels, I used to watch the court proceedings. It was the cheapest show in town.

At two of the sessions stutterers were involved. One stutterer was accused of child abuse, and the prosecution's lawyer used the defendant's inarticulacy as evidence that he had mental problems, was an unreliable member of society, and could have committed the crime. The objections by the defence were disallowed by the judge. The trial went on for several days, so I never heard the outcome, but it was a gross misinterpretation of the implications of stuttering.

At another session, the main witness for the defence, was a quiet, shy, wispy-haired little man who stuttered badly. The prosecution's lawyer fired questions at him rapidly, and the poor guy's speech gradually fell apart. The lawyer implied that the stutterer was not mentally equipped to be a competent witness ('M'lud, the witness seems unwilling or unable to reply to questions pertinent to the case'), and the witness was dismissed.

The figure of justice has a sword in one of her hands, and the legal profession is not noted for its humanity. In most courts the opposing barristers are adversaries, and in this competitive situation no holds are barred provided they are legal and comply with the regulations that govern court proceedings. Any weaknesses of the defendant, plaintiffs, and witnesses are exploited by the battling lawyers. A stutterer can come off very badly indeed.

Judges and barristers should realize that people who stutter are, apart from their speech, average citizens. It should be possible for a person with a communication problem to reply in writing or other ways suited to his handicap. There are indications that courts dealing with the rights of spastics and other impaired citizens permit unusual forms of communication, and this is a step in the right direction.

I never liked the idea of justice being blindfolded, because it implies that justice relies only on what it hears. What you hear from disfluent people can give the wrong impression, and it is necessary to open your eyes and look more deeply to get at the facts. Aristotle once said that the law is reason free from passion. Unfortunately it is also free from compassion in too many cases.

The two masks of the media

When I went to the theatre as a small boy I was fascinated by the plaster reproductions of early Greek theatrical masks that decorated the frieze above the stage. In most theatres there were two masks, one a laughing face representing comedy, and the other a face with the mouth and eyes distorted by grief representing tragedy. I learned later that theatrical comedy can be tragic and that the two masks cannot always be separated.

Writers, artists, and actors who entertain the masses mould public opinion for good or evil. Today television and the cinema wield enormous power. For thousands of years authors and actors have cashed in on the idea that audiences find disabilities funny, further reinforcing this point of view by their performances.

When the Roman Empire was at the peak of its power, a man called Balbus Blaesius was locked in a cage beside the Appian Way, the main thoroughfare to Rome. He had a very severe stutter and was only one of many disabled unfortunates on exhibition for the entertainment of passers-by. For a small coin Balbus would talk to wayfarers and delight them with his tangled tongue. Inhuman? Certainly, but the exhibition was part of a long tradition of poking fun at handicapped and misshapen people.

We are supposed to be more enlightened today, but a few years ago I watched a television show about a fair where one of the main attractions was a young man with cluttering, stuttering speech who earned his living by shrilly mangling his words for the paying public in the tradition of Balbus Blaesius in his cage. At these fairs people still pay to see dwarfs and bearded ladies, just as I used to pay my sixpence to see two-headed snakes and five-legged calves when I was a small boy fascinated by the incongruities of the world.

It is difficult to understand how adults can derive entertainment from looking at or listening to people with disabilities. It is too easy to say that people are basically sadistic. It is more likely that they think, 'Thank goodness it's not me.' Maybe that is why people go to see the deformed and disfluent – relieved thankfulness.

Open ridicule of handicapped people in movies and on television is not common today, but there are frequent implications that people who stutter are foolish, mentally retarded, or psychopathic. In many movies, a weak but sinister character is given a stutter to illustrate his psychopathic tendencies, and an actor playing a sadistic killer may well stutter to imply an unhappy childhood that caused his mental disturbance. Most of the characters on the media who stutter are portrayed as weak, stupid, and unreliable – as cowards, wimps, or dangerous criminals – and people begin to get the idea that this is the way things are.

Comedians can't help cracking jokes about a person who stutters, or who is deaf, or who has a wooden leg, but there are ways of doing it. Stutterers, deaf people, and those with wooden legs can get into some funny situations. Few of these people would object if people laugh *with* them. But none likes being laughed *at*. Jokes about people who are different can be fairly harmless. It depends upon the context. Canadians joke about 'Newfies,' Americans about 'Polacks,' the

English about the 'Micks,' and the Australians about 'Poms,' and the inferences are that the butts of the jokes are simple or stupid. I don't much like these jokes, but mostly they lose their sting because people know that the targets are anything but stupid. With a stutterer or deaf person they are not so sure, because the difficulty in communicating may suggest stupidity.

Jokes that imply that handicapped people are stupid are in poor taste, and also somewhat cowardly, since the target is seldom in a position to retaliate. Nevertheless, people should retaliate more. Whenever I see, hear, or read in the media suggestions that disfluent people are stupid, unreliable, or psychopathic I write letters pointing out the errors and the implications. I must have written hundreds of such letters, but have never had a reply. If more people expressed their distaste, the media might eventually get the message.

Disabilities are not funny. There are so many other ways of entertaining people that it shouldn't be too hard to cease the implied ridicule. In recent years, a few TV shows have handled stuttering unusually well. I remember one about a young boy with a stutter who fell in love with his school counsellor. The difficult topic was handled sensitively, with gentle humour. In another program a talk-show producer with a stutter addressed his staff using excellent word prolongation, cancellation, and easy onset. The script writer and producer knew their jobs.

More often, however, the implication is that anybody who stutters is an idiot. Many comedians seem to go along with Will Rogers's averral that everything is funny as long as it happens to somebody else, but Aesop put it better when he wrote, 'Clumsy jesting is no joke.'

Acceptance: the two-way transaction

There is no doubt that some stutterers deliberately withdraw from society, either because of the great effort it requires to speak or because of society's treatment of them. Unfortunately, as Shakespeare wrote in *Cymbeline*, 'Society is no comfort to one not sociable.' Unless the stutterer is willing to make the effort, however painful, he cannot expect people to accept him and co-operate with him. Neither can people expect the disfluent to become useful citizens unless individuals make the effort to calm the irrational fears that arise when confronted by a grimacing person trying to force his way through a speech block. These fears are the foundation of the glass wall that separates stutterers from other people. Acceptance is a two-way transaction. Society won't accept handicapped people unless these people are willing to be accepted.

Some people who stutter have been so battered by society that asking them to come out of their den to meet their tormentors and establish productive links is, in the stutterer's eyes, like asking a deer to hold a meeting with a pack of wolves. It may take time for the stutterer to develop trust and be assured of the new and unfamiliar goodwill. Some people with severe stutters live in a fairly hostile world because their mode of speech makes people nervous. Others find the world more benign; it depends upon the circumstances and the social circles in which they move.

There are no set rules about how to break down the walls between the disabled and society, but good starting points are patience, good manners, goodwill, and a desire to look beyond superficial appearances. Unfortunately, patience is rare in a busy world, many people look upon good manners as redundant, and the media have persuaded people to value superficial appearances rather than intrinsic qualities.

The stutterer himself must accept that employers have their likes and dislikes and are, to some extent, free to indulge them. Not all those who reject members of minority groups are bigots. An employer may have hired several people from the Outer Hebrides before, and if they gave him a bad time he's not likely to be enthusiastic about employing another of them. He forms his opinion and preferences on experience – incomplete perhaps, but experience none the less – and this is not necessarily prejudice. A person with a stutter, a paraplegic, a black person, or a woman, any of whom may have been rejected by an employer, should be sure of the facts before crying, 'Prejudice!'

Government institutions, in particular, need to take off their bureaucratic blinders, look beyond the regulations, and accept that blindness, deafness, and limb malfunction are not the only disabilities. In Canada, the income-tax department insists that people are only disabled for the purpose of income-tax deductions if they are blind or spend most of the day in a wheelchair or in bed. People who manage to get around painfully on prosthetic devices or crutches are not usually permitted to deduct the expenses they incur in overcoming their disability so that they can earn a living. An academic whose hands were so crippled with cerebral palsy that he could not write was not allowed to deduct from his taxable income the cost of hiring a secretary to type for him. People dragging their legs around on crutches were not permitted to use the handicapped tax deductions. The irony is that this bureaucratic brutality takes place within a federal organization that also contains a Department of Health and Welfare dedicated to helping the sick and disabled.

Trying to change the legislative and bureaucratic status quo is reminiscent of the Greek legend about poor old Sisyphus, who was forever condemned to roll a huge stone up a hill, with the stone always rolling back just before he reached the top. Getting past the bureaucratic fortifications can be frustrating. You get to the right person in one branch and he passes the buck to another branch. The Sisyphean toil is repeated on many hills and you seldom get anywhere unless you find a politician with the key that fits all the bureaucratic doors, or better, a hammer to bash them down.

Stutter power

A tall young man walked along the beach of an Ontario resort wearing a dark blue T-shirt with 'Stutter Power' written in yellow across the front. Clearly he had no hang-ups about revealing his disability to the whole world, but unfortunately the words were wishful thinking. Stutterers have little power to change the attitude of society or to end discrimination in the job market.

The harsh fact is that most stutterers find it hard to stand up in public and protest. If they tried they wouldn't be taken seriously because society has been conditioned to ridicule stuttering. If circus clowns were being discriminated against and appeared on television to state their case with painted, sad faces and bulbous noses, they wouldn't get much support. People would just laugh.

There are many organizations that help the physically and mentally disabled, the blind, the deaf, and the mute to get jobs and deal with discrimination. Unfortunately, nobody seems to help the *partially* disabled. Crippled people who get around without a wheelchair and try to earn a living, kids with very limited vision who press their thick glasses close to their school books, those with hearing that is so poor that hearing-aids only help a little, and the people with speech distorted by cleft palates, stutters, and stroke-induced aphasia get little consideration or help.

A young man at a reputable Canadian high school had a severe problem with his vision. He was not totally blind, but he was a slow reader and lived in a misty world that was always out of focus. At school he was poor at games and did not get high grades, so he was continually teased and punched by other kids and scolded by teachers for his slowness. His life at school was a misery. A few years ago his parents convened a meeting with an eye specialist, the school principal, and the boy's teachers. Few of the teachers bothered to turn up, and shortly afterwards the boy dropped out of the school system. Only his parents were willing to stand up and give him support. He wasn't totally blind, so nobody cared.

Even when partially disabled people go to see an ombudsman or other authority concerned with civil rights they are not likely to get much help, because the official may well hold the general view that partial disabilities do not cause people much distress. The idea of a militant stutterer may seem ludicrous to many, but it is high time the disfluent learned to speak out or get someone to speak for them.

Stutterers have formed self-help groups, particularly those which help people with stutters to maintain their better speech. Most of these groups are offshoots from the speech clinics. There have been attempts to form lay stuttering associations in Canada to express stutterers' viewpoints and promote their rights, but most fade away from lack of support. There are several successful, active groups in the United States, but few of the groups are militant.

Stutterers are a silent minority, generally avoiding public

exposure and finding it difficult to work on committees or function in large groups. Perhaps the huge numbers of people who stuttered at some time in their lives but later became fluent could co-operate with the disfluent to present their case more forcibly. They could put over the idea that there are more handicaps than being in a wheelchair or being deaf or blind, and that stuttering and other partial disabilities can cause people real hardship.

If there were legal and financial support, class actions could be brought against media people who condone or foster the idea that people who stutter are psychopathic or mentally incompetent. These slanders and libels reduce stutterers' opportunities in the job market. An organization that is not fearful of retaliation from the income-tax department could present a strong case for permitting stutterers and others with partial disabilities to deduct the costs incurred in hiring the help and purchasing the apparatus (tape recorders, maskers, assistants, transport, etc.) that help them earn a living.

During the seventeenth century Pascal wrote, 'The property of power is to protect.' If people with stutters feel they need more protection, they should persuade more articulate people to support them and use the power of group representations.

The elderly stutterer

There was an old farmer who enjoyed sitting on the front porch smoking his pipe and looking out at his fields and barns where he used to work so hard. He had stuttered badly all his life. A friend he hadn't seen for many years called in for a chat, and they walked over the farm talking about old times. The friend was astonished at the man's fluency. 'What happened to your stutter?' he exclaimed. 'Oh that,' the farmer smiled. 'These days I'm too old and tired to bother with stuttering. It's no trouble at all.'

There are several versions of this story, and they may all be apocryphal, but the tale illustrates an important point. Stuttering, the fighting to speak, is hard work. It takes youth and energy to wrestle the words into submission. Fighting to speak is so tiring that you only willingly talk at length when you are trying to make your way in the world, meet challenges, fight for acceptance, and scale life's pinnacles in spite of the verbal odds stacked against you. All this struggling inflates the tensions and anxieties that make the stutter worse in the distressing spiral of untreated disfluency.

In old age there is no longer the drive to succeed at your job and climb the corporate ladders. It's hard enough dealing with life's level ground without tackling the challenges of the heights. You let go a little and look back, maybe with a chuckle or two, at the enormous amount of effort you spent tilting at the windmills of your imagination, fighting adversaries that were really yourself, and seeking Holy Grails that turned out to be made of tin.

You are your own man and can choose to speak when and where you please. The telephone need no longer thrust a lance of ice into your guts. You no longer have to take part in meetings, justify yourself and your work, or go to large parties. Nobody is going to ask you to do the impossible. If you don't wish to talk you don't. You can sit on your porch, smoke a pipe, and look at your fields.

As the pressures ease, so the speech gets better. You still stutter, but it is no longer a fight to speak. You can choose your own verbal battle-grounds.

Although I am hardly in the first bloom of youth, the young person I used to be still lives within me and looks out at the world through my eyes. I don't consider myself old. Nevertheless, when I took early retirement to be my own master the relief was tremendous. The tensions of anticipating the talking involved in getting through an ordinary working day were greater than I realized at the time. After I left, my speech improved rapidly.

Since then I foolishly became involved in high-pressure talking from time to time, and the tensions built up again. After a week or so the speech began to fracture. I have learned to take the pressures off my speech and enjoy my fluency.

The way a stutter affects you in old age depends, of course, on what kind of person you are. If your stuttering has defeated you throughout your life and driven you into unhappy solitude, you will look back sadly with many regrets and still feel the pain of old emotional wounds that never heal. One of the saddest pictures I ever saw was an illustration of what the caption called 'An Old Stutterer' in one of the textbooks. He was well dressed, but the despair in his eyes and the tired, sagging features went straight to the heart. He had been utterly crushed by his stutter and society's cruelty.

I have met very few older stutterers who have been so totally defeated. Most of them are more like old soldiers, taking it easy after battle, with the pain of their honourable scars well under control. There may be some who look back with bitterness and wish that their lives could have been different unhindered by the ball and chain of disfluency, but the general feeling seems to be that life has been good and full of challenges and richness. Without the stutter they wouldn't have become the people they are. It has moulded them from infancy.

NINE

The road ahead

'Yesterday is not ours to recover,
but tomorrow is ours to win or lose.'

Anonymous

A stuttering friend who was a born pessimist was also some-thing of a blues singer. During World War II, he was sure that he was going to get the chop, and used to sit in the cold, damp Nissen hut strumming a tinny old banjo and singing a mournful little song:

'Ah went up on this mountain,
Saw as far as ah could see,
Ah went up on this mountain
'N the blues had me.'

He always sang the same verse from the same song. It was our only music apart from a rickety spring-driven turntable and a scarred old record of the Anvil Chorus, so we put up with it. He was wrong. He survived. As far as I know he's still wailing his pessimistic little dirge.

The great thing about people who stutter is that, unlike my woeful friend, so many of them are optimists. When one type of therapy fails, they try another, and then another. Hoping, always hoping. They may fall flat on their faces and make fools of themselves, but they pick themselves up and try a new tack against the headwinds of life. Give them a chance and they'll grab it and run with it.

What have people who stutter to look forward to in a world that has produced so many technical marvels but remains in such a state of political, economic and moral chaos? Will scientists soon find out what causes a child to start stuttering? Will somebody find a real cure? Will the new technology make life easier for the severely disfluent? Will society learn to accept people with speech and other disabilities more readily? Will the partially disabled have a louder voice in dealing with legal and bureaucratic injustices and prejudices? The answers to these questions will determine the future happiness and social effectiveness of millions of stutterers and other disabled people.

Technology is one of the things man does best, so it is fair to assume that there will be considerable advances in speech technology in the next twenty-five years, provided that governments allocate sufficient research support. The science of psychology and neurology are gradually unravelling the mysteries of the brain's processes and how they affect our behaviour, and the old qualitative type of psychology is giving way to a new science based on firmer neurological and biochemical foundations.

People who contend that stuttering is just learned behaviour may ask, 'Why bother about all this research? Why not treat the symptom?' Several intractable complaints – including depression, schizophrenia, malaria, poliomyelitis, tuberculosis, and smallpox – yielded to treatment once their causes were understood. Fifty years from now we shall probably look back on today's speech therapy as groping in the dark, which is how we have come to regard the older methods of relaxation and rhythmics.

Conditioning methods like fluency shaping therapy and combinations of speech rehabilitation and psychotherapy get better every year and will continue to do so unless therapists polarize into fluency shapers and stuttering modifiers. The more fanatical proponents of fluency shaping tend to look down their noses at the complex, personal approach of stuttering modifiers, and some of the latter have a hunch that the human brain has its own ideas about how far it can be conditioned. It is hoped that the clinicians will bring the best in both approaches to bear on the problem. When we understand the functions of the brain better, particularly the role of neurotransmitters at the nerves' synapses, and find out to what extent the ear is involved in the mechanics of speech, treatment will develop on a firmer basis.

There is no real barrier to finding out whether or not stuttering or the inclination to stutter is encoded in our genes. The information could be obtained from studies of twins and siblings living with natural and adoptive parents, by calculating the frequencies of stuttering in all these groups. This type of study has yielded important insights into schizophrenia. All it needs is the will, the time, and the money.

If stuttering proves to be genetically mediated this does not mean that nothing can be done about the disability. Each gene produces compounds that trigger psysiological processes. When the processes are understood, their abnormalities may respond to treatment. (Again, schizophrenia and other disorders mediated by neurotransmitters and enzyme systems come to mind.) Knowledge about the genetic basis of stuttering could provide an early warning system and enable children to be treated earlier.

A stutterer reading the literature about his problem comes across a few points that strike sparks of relevance in his mind. Some of the sparks fade as he reads further, but others continue to glow and illuminate the whole stuttering scene. A few of the points are old ones that have tarnished with time; they deserve polishing again in view of new knowledge. Good examples are laterality and its relationship to stuttering and the old organic idea of bugs in the brain's computer. Other points are more innovative – for example, the question of whether excessive anxiety about speech is encoded in our genes or associated with malfunctions in the areas of the brain concerned with our emotions. A reconsideration of the role of the middle-ear muscles in speech also raises glimmers of understanding and even of hope. Novel approaches to operant conditioning using biofeedback have great promise in treating anxiety-mediated disabilities like stuttering.

Laterality revisited

The cerebral dominance theory suggested that the left side of the brain's cerebral cortex, where the speech centres are usually located, must dominate the right side in order to time correctly the nerve impulses from the brain's motor centre to the muscles of the lips, tongue, and jaw and enable a person to speak normally. It was suggested that stuttering could be caused by a lack of dominance of the side of the brain dealing with speech. Many speech therapists clung to this neurological straw for decades, but the idea fell into disrepute. The results of recent research indicate that the theory is worthy of re-examination.

The ability to speak is relatively new in the evolutionary time scale, and speech is possible because man has two unique speech centres in the brain that enable him to put ideas into words. These centres are Broca's and Wernicke's areas.

Broca's area is on the left side of the brain a little above and to the front of the tip of the ear in most normal right-handed people. It is responsible for programming the mechanics of speech. Broca's area controls the motor cortex, a strip of specialized tissue arching over the brain from ear to ear like a headphone, which activates the muscles involved in speech and other movements. When Broca's area is damaged the speech is understandable but ungrammatical, slow, and hesitant. Verbs, pronouns, and connecting words like prepositions are left out. A typical sentence would be 'Church Sunday eleven o'clock sermon.' Damage to this area affects writing in a similar way.

Wernicke's area is concerned with language and plays a major role in speaking, comprehension of written and spoken words, and sentence construction. When this area is damaged the words may be spoken clearly and fluently with perfect grammar but make no sense at all.

Investigations of these brain areas have indicated that what someone is going to say is organized in Wernicke's area. If the word is read optically it travels from the eye to the visual area at the back of the brain and then to Wernicke's area along a nerve bundle – the 'angular gyrus.' If the word is heard, the signal travels from the brain's auditory area a little to the front of Wernicke's area and then onwards to the latter.

Wernicke's area is both a junction box and a signal processor. After it processes the signals, they pass on to Broca's area, which produces a detailed, co-ordinated program for speech and flashes messages to the nearby motor cortex, which in turn activates the articulatory muscles. All the nerve tissues, together with their linkages, need to be in working order for a person to say, 'Good morning. I would like three litres please,' to the milkman.

This simple model of speech tends to get a little scrambled when left- and right-handedness enter the picture, since it is now known that differences in handedness are associated with different positions of the speech centres in the brain. About 99 per cent, or more, of normal, right-handed people have their speech and language centres (Broca's and Wernicke's areas) on the left side of the brain. Their brain's right side is more concerned with matters of space, time, seeing things as a whole, and intuition. Some people's brains have a limited capability for language on the right side, but in right-handed people most of the language business is carried out on the left side. If the right-handed person writes with his right hand so that the nib points toward him, he may have his language centres on the opposite side of the brain – the right side. The reversed-pen stance is uncommon in right-handers, accounting for only about 1 per cent. By contrast to most right-handers, some left-handed people have their speech centres on the right side of the brain and the space-time-intuition function on the left. However, if the left-handed person writes with his left hand in such a way that the pen's nib points toward him, his speech centres tend to be on the left side, as with most right-handers. Eye movements and writing position reveal a great deal about the workings of the brain, and Dr Jerre Levy of the University of Chicago used this fact in her elegant experiments on brain laterality and asymmetry.[1]

An experiment to test whether stuttering is more common in people with the speech centres on the right side of the cerebral cortex than in those with speech centres on the left side would produce useful insights into whether stuttering is associated with reversed, abnormal brain circuitry. The implied complication of a reversal of speech centres in relation to the brain's visual and auditory centres and the motor cortex makes the mind reel.

My own case is complicated because I am partly ambidextrous. I throw with my right hand and do precision work with my left. I get on a bicycle on the right side and, in my riding days, I would have preferred to have mounted my horses from the right side, but they violently objected. I use my left hand for many tasks, but kick a football in the wrong direction with the right foot. The real tangle in the wool is that I write from left to right with my right hand, and scribble from right to left with my left hand, always with the pen's nib away from me. I can even, with a little practice, write with both hands at once, one script a mirror image of the other. I am in good company, because Leonardo da Vinci could do the same; he wrote all his notes with his left hand in mirror script. If my speech centres are associated with my handedness, I am not at all sure where they are located and just hope that I have Broca's and Wernicke's speech and language areas in the ordinary place, on the left side.

It is interesting that two of my daughters write with their left hands, and their pens' nibs point away from them, making it remotely possible that their speech centres are on the right side of the brain instead of the usual left. Neither of them stutters.

If stuttering proves to be associated with displacement of the speech centres or abnormal cerebral dominance and this appears to be one of the tributaries feeding the stutter's main stream, at least therapists will know what they are dealing with and can decide where to focus their attention.

The brain's neural network

Whenever I am accused by my wife of having a lot of nerve, I exasperate her by nodding in agreement, reminding her that I have about 10^{11} (or about 100,000 million) neurons or nerve cells with about 10^{15} (1,000 million million) nerve contacts – the synapses – in addition to billions of interlaced, short, thread-like fibres (dendrites) between the neurons.[2] The long fibres (axons) of the neuron cells are the main wires of the circuit, and each one has its own protective insulation – the fatty myelin sheath. A typical neuron may have 1,000 to 10,000 synaptic connections and receive information from 1,000 or more other neurons. The sheer number of units and connections in the circuitry is staggering, and the brain makes our most advanced computers look primitive by comparison.

This complex machine works by biochemical processes and electrical impulses. The neuron's chemistry sends an electrical impulse along the axon to a club-like junction (the synapse), which is connected to a receiving neuron. The two are not strictly connected, because there is a minute space between the receiver neuron and the receptive synaptic swelling. The swollen synapse stores a chemical transmitter (neurotransmitter), which is released into the small gap by the nerve's electrical impulse and changes the electrical state of the receptor neuron, which may fire and send its message, or not, depending on its function. If the chemical transmitter of the synapse does not work properly, the circuit misfires and the next neuron cannot pass on its electrical message. When the neuron's electrical discharges are out of synchronization, or the axons are damaged, the electrical circuits break down and we have problems.[3]

Fortunately, the brain can repair itself to some extent, so that people can function quite well after certain kinds of brain damage, although in some instances even minor injury can have devastating effects. It depends on where the problem lies and on the age of the individual.

When a person has a stroke, and the nerves that control the movements of muscles involved in speech (Broca's area) are damaged, the victim speaks poorly, although he can still sing with ease. This parallels the plight of people who stutter severely but can also sing. Damage to Wernicke's area results in fluent, grammatical nonsensical speech.

Damage to the speech areas does not necessarily mean that the speech will be out of action for ever. While it is true that Broca's and Wernicke's areas play a major role in speech and language, other areas of the brain can take over their functions to some extent. For example, a person with his main speech centres on the left side of the brain may have a limited speech capability on his right side that can help to some extent in a crisis. The damaged brain tissue cannot recover, but neurons near the damaged site may take over.[4]

If the zone damaged in Broca's area is small, the chances of partial recovery are quite good.[5] Children, in particular, recover remarkably well; and, curiously, left-handed people recover better than right-handers – laterality rears its puzzling head again. Moreover, a stroke victim with damage on the left side of his brain is often depressed about his disability, while patients with damage on the right side are often unconcerned about their predicament.[6] Speech disruption caused by lesions in the speech areas on the left side of the brain are likely to be associated with anxiety.

These are facts, but at this point it is necessary to wade into a swamp of speculation. Consider the case of a child who is slightly more disfluent than usual. In the absence of bad therapy, stress, penalties, and ridicule there is a good chance that the disfluency will disappear in later childhood, although this depends upon the severity of the stuttering. If the child is penalized, stressed, rejected, and ridiculed, he will be anxious about his speech, and it is likely that his stuttering will get worse and tend to reinforce itself. However, even when his speech is bad, he will be able to sing fluently most of the time.

The key points are that the child is disfluent but can sing, often recovers, and may be anxious. The question is whether this picture fits the template of a person with a left-side (speech-zone) abnormality of the brain in, for example, Broca's area. The answer is not exactly, but there are a few points of contact. If a left-side speech zone of a stutterer's brain were damaged or abnormal, neighbouring neurons or some other brain zone could in time take over some of the speech function, and the quality of the speech would depend upon the degree of damage. If this were the case, many children would recover – and, in fact, many stuttering children spontaneously lose their stutters. Many patients with damage in Broca's area can sing. Anxiety about the disability would be expected with left-side brain damage, and stutterers' anxiety about their speech is well known.

The behaviour of left-side stroke victims with damage in Broca's area will strike echoes in many stutterers' minds, and there is a little evidence of brain abnormality in the language areas of dyslexics' brains. There is a need to reconsider the question of whether organic abnormalities in the brain affect the onset of stuttering and to examine the possibility of left-side abnormalities in the speech areas in the light of evidence from stroke victims and dyslexics. Recent research is moving along these lines.

My wife and I knew a very old lady in England who liked to sit in her sunny room, look at the flowers, and cheerfully chat to visitors. When she was younger she was very articulate and talkative, and her friends described her as loving but fierce. Her speech centres or their connections had deteriorated in her old age, and she found it difficult to speak. Her speech was not the laboured articulation and telegraphic syntax of a person with damage in Broca's area, nor was it the fluent, grammatical, but nonsensical speech of a person damaged in Wernicke's area. She certainly wasn't a clutterer. When she spoke she made sense, but she repeated sounds and went into severe blocks of five seconds or more, just like a stutterer.

As we sat and talked to this fascinating woman we were both struck by the similarity of her speech to that of an adult stutterer, the only difference being her freedom from anxiety.

Experts will probably say that her so-called stutter was not a real stutter, but something like it. Nevertheless, except for her lack of fear, her speech fitted the stuttering pattern exactly. As I listened I heard a carbon copy of my own speech. The old lady was almost completely deaf, and the complications of anxiety and hearing were absent, so it seems that speech patterns very similar to stuttering can develop from deterioration of the tissues in the brain's speech areas. It is unwise to conclude from this that stuttering is simply due to brain abnormality, but it suggests that the possible association between brain structure and stuttering is worthy of close examination.

Understanding anxiety

It is not known whether a child's stuttering stems from anxiety or whether the anxiety is caused by the stuttering, but there is little doubt that anxiety contributes a great deal to the growth and consolidation of stuttering behaviour. It is fair to ask, therefore, whether better methods will be developed to understand and deal with this anxiety.

The obvious way to reduce a stutterer's anxiety is to

remove, reduce, or control his stutter, and this underlies the fact that increased fluency increases fluency. The stuttering modification therapy of the Iowa school focuses on these fears and tries to dispel them by teaching the stutterer to adopt realistic, objective attitudes and to *feel* his fluency. Many patients with severe stutters like mine can still be overwhelmed by unexpected fears about particular words even after years of therapy, to the extent that at times it seems like a phobia about speaking. If this so-called phobia has been learned, it can be unlearned – unless it is caused by an inheritance of excessive fearfulness about communicating. It must be remembered that a stutterer's fear of stuttering may be an appropriate response to disfluency, since society takes such exception to it. Nevertheless, the degree of anxiety may be abnormal.

There is evidence that excessive fearfulness can be inherited. The basenjis mentioned earlier inherited a fearful response to man, and laboratory rats were found to have distinctive genetic strains quite different in their fearfulness (reactivity), one strain being ten times more fearful than the other. Furthermore, hybridizing fearful and less fearful rats produces rats with intermediate behaviour, so genes seem to be involved. Animals inherit specific fears (e.g., of objects looming over them), as well as fears of many things that threaten their survival.[7]

Anxiety can be learned in infancy. At a very early age a child will respond fearfully when what he sees or hears does not match his previous experience. Although the relationship of fear to cognitive mismatch is complex,[8] it raises the question of whether a small child used to a fluent mother most of the day could be alarmed by hearing a disfluent, stuttering father communicating in a way that does not match the child's experience and expectation. There is some evidence that a child with a stuttering mother is more likely to develop a stutter than otherwise.

The possibility that abnormalities in the brain's nerve network cause excessive anxiety must be considered, but the chemical relationships between the different parts of the brain are so complex that it is hard to get a clear picture. In *The Tangled Wing*, Melvin Konner makes clear that abnormalities in the balance between the components of our centres mediating emotion (in the limbic system) and damage to the insulating myelin sheaths of the message-carrying axons could produce inappropriate or excessively fearful responses.[9] Nevertheless, much more information is needed before the biochemical and biological nature of fear is understood and before anxiety can be treated with confidence.

Several drugs can be used to treat anxiety. Valium (Diazepam) is a good example. This drug influences the release of a chemical neurotransmitter (gamma-aminobutyric acid) at synaptic junctions of message-carrying axon fibres in the brain. Unfortunately, although Valium reduces anxiety it also decreases alertness.[10] Alcohol affects the chemical signals of the nerves and reduces anxiety in a similar way to Valium, which is doubtless the reason why alcohol is so popular in our fearful world. Anxiety can be modified by drugs, but at the price of side effects many patients are reluctant to pay. Doubtless better drugs will evolve. Cimetidine, for example, is sometimes used instead of Valium, but all drugs are likely to have side effects.

Attempts have been made to treat some phobias by brain surgery, but it is to be hoped that this is not attempted with stutterers until more is known about the neurology of speech, and of fear, and about whether the anxiety of stutterers is a cause or an effect or both. The memory of tongue-butchering Dr Dieffenbach is still too fresh in many stutterers' memories.

For the time being, therefore, it seems appropriate for scientists to try to probe the role of anxiety in stuttering and for speech therapists to try to control the fears by conventional therapy (possibly assisted by better psychotherapy and carefully administered drugs), while realizing that excessive anxiety is only part of the complex stuttering syndrome.

I never cease to feel a sense of awe that I carry around with me an incredibly complex and efficient organic computer protected by my thick skull. The brain is *me*, and from it I look out upon the world and flash signals along my axons, relay the signals across the synaptic gaps, and activate my sight centres at the back of the brain that allow me to see. If I want to talk about what I see, signals are flashed to my language centre, which alerts Broca's area, which in turn signals the neurons that control my lip, tongue, and jaw muscles and make my larynx vibrate. All in a flash. As I see something else, new signals are generated and new words are spoken.

Every thought we have, every movement we make, and every emotion we feel are the result of billions of flashing electrochemical signals, sorted, co-ordinated, and monitored in the soft tissues of our brain. When I was a foetus my neural network miraculously grew from a few cells, the neurons' axons weaving their way in my brain tissues, nudged and coaxed by biochemical compounds to make the right connections with other brain cells. When the wrong connections were made they often aborted so that better connections could be made. Even after I was born, the slender, branched dendrites growing out from the nerve cells continued to grow, each new experience adding new branches.

It is amazing that most people get their brain circuits wired up more or less in the right way. The probability that something will go wrong as the network develops under the guidance of the biochemical stew generated by both our genes and our environment seems very high. Nature must be forgiven if she occasionally makes a mistake.

Sound and speech

In 1974 Ronald L. Webster of Hollins College, Virginia, said that investigation of the role of the middle-ear muscles was 'the most meaningful potential direction for the conduct of future research on the problem of stuttering.'[11] There is a wealth of evidence that delayed feedback of the sound of a person's speech can cause disfluency and that masking the feedback completely can make a stutterer fluent, so it is likely that the ear is involved in the act of speaking.

The middle-ear (tympanum) involves two small muscles (the tensor tympani and the stapedius) attached to three small movable bones – the hammer (malleus), the anvil (incus), and the stirrup (stapes). These bones form a lever that picks up the sound vibrations from the ear-drum, amplifies them, and relays them to an inner membrane, which vibrates and enables us to hear. The tensor tympani muscle, attached to the malleus, dampens loud noises and protects the fragile eardrum. It is activated by a nerve with a delay of about 150 milliseconds. The stapedius muscle, which shields the inner ear from an excessive amount of relayed sound, is attached to the stapes and responds in about 60 milliseconds. These two muscles also hold the three bones of the chain in position, and contract not only in response to sound but also about 65 to 100 milliseconds before a person speaks. The muscle contraction appears to be part of an involuntary preparation for the act of speaking. The middle-ear muscles seem to be involved in speech both in stutterers and in fluent speakers.

A study of the movements of the muscles of the middle ear of five stutterers indicated that the contractions occurred at the time of stuttering. However, when the stutterers spoke fluently, the muscles contracted in the normal way, just before speaking.[12] The timing of the ear's muscle contractions associated with stuttering may be abnormal. Caution is necessary in interpreting this fact, since a stutterer's tension can produce many abnormal physiological and muscle responses. Nevertheless, one stutterer who had the middle-ear muscles removed during an operation for some other disorder found that his stutter decreased from about 8–12 per cent disfluency to 1–3 per cent, and the improvement persisted even though he still had intact the middle-ear muscles in the other ear. His hearing was slightly reduced, but this was dealt with by a hearing aid.[13]

It seems possible, therefore, that the contractions of the ear muscles of stutterers may be erratic or out of phase and may disrupt auditory feedback to such an extent that they interfere with speaking. Whether the pre-speech ear-muscle contraction is vital to speech initiation remains to be seen. If this proves to be the case, it may lead to new treatment opportunities. However, some scientists feel that this middle-ear theory is a backwater rather than in the mainstream of current research.

It seems clear that sound and hearing are much more involved in speech than was previously thought, and that speech may be guided (or misguided) by specific auditory cues. Unfortunately, we still don't know how speech and hearing interact, and the operation on the stutterer's ear was a one-shot affair, so we are not likely to see people with stutters lining up to get the tiny muscles chopped out of their middle ears.

Biofeedback

These days it is very fashionable to sit with small circular electrodes attached to the muscles of your forehead listening to a biofeedback beeper signal that you have managed to persuade yourself to relax. When I worked in a city I used to survey people's foreheads for the hickies left by the tacky kisses of the biofeedback electrodes. There were more than you'd think.

The principles of biofeedback are not new. Any mental and physical activity causes changes in the body's electrochemistry. Tensed muscles send out different electrical signals than relaxed muscles; some forms of mental activity send out different electrical brain waves than others; and many processes modify our body temperature. If these signals can be measured and amplified into indicators a person can see, hear, or feel, then theoretically he can control the bodily activities that generate the signals by thinking in a passive way or by deliberately creating particular inner feelings.

Although this sounds like witchcraft, most people have at one time or another controlled their bodies with their minds to reduce anxiety, discomfort, or severe pain. On many of the occasions when I've shivered with cold I've thought warm thoughts and felt much better. People in great agony can sometimes consciously ride with the pain and convince themselves it is receding. When parents tell their children that they can do almost anything if they put their minds to it, they are not far wrong as far as the body's functions are concerned.

The most commonly measured signals of the body are temperature, muscle tension (EMG biofeedback), and alpha waves from the brain (EEG biofeedback). The last two are most relevant to stuttering.

Electromyographic (EMG) feedback has been used with some success to treat a wide range of disorders. Barbara B. Brown, in *Stress and the Art of Biofeedback*,[14] lists twelve emotional problems (including anxiety, phobias, tension headaches, insomnia, and depression), five psychosomatic problems (including asthma, hypertension, and intestinal disorders), and ten physical problems (including painful muscle spasms, spasticity, cerebral palsy, and migraines) that have responded to EMG biofeedback. Anxiety is particularly responsive to the technique, which consequently has promise as a treatment for stuttering.

For several days I sat plugged into a biofeedback machine having great fun making the monitor bleep to my changes in muscle tension. I became so good at it that I could play games and perplexed the therapist by bouncing around the readings just by thinking and feeling in different ways. I was a natural feedback patient and could relax myself into a near-trance while I spoke fluently. The trouble was that my control over my state of relaxation disappeared as soon as I walked out of the clinic.

I still feel that the biofeedback method can play a useful role in speech therapy. The assertion that felt fluency helps to keep you fluent is true, but some stutterers have never felt what it is like to speak fluently in a relaxed manner in public. It feels wonderful. You try and remember what the feeling felt like, but it's very difficult to measure, monitor, and use on demand.

EMG was tested by Guitar in his laboratory, using electrodes on the larynx, chin, upper lip, and the forehead's frontalis muscle. The electrical activity was amplified into a humming tone. Three patients tried to keep the tone as low as possible, and when the lowest level was achieved they read sentences that included difficult words. Similar trials were run without the feedback. In all cases the EMG biofeedback reduced stuttering, and the improvement persisted for several months, even with telephone calls.[15] Whether the muscle relaxation helped the speech, or the humming tone provided some form of distraction are points in question. Oliver Bloodstein commented that EMG feedback seems well suited to eliminate the excessive tension of stutterers and that it holds considerable promise.[16] Other scientists have studied the use of EMG biofeedback to treat stuttering, but the technique is still in its infancy.

Alpha-wave feedback is concerned with the variations of the alpha rhythms (9 to 12 Hz) from a person's brain. There are several types of brain waves, but high alpha activity is associated with a state of relaxed wakefulness and receptivity. This technique, also in its infancy, consists of attaching the EEG electrodes to the scalp so that the patient can learn to control his alpha waves by observing them on the screen and passively modifying them. Although there is often a great deal of interference with the waves, the method has helped many people with tension problems. In Texas, hyperactive children with stuttering and insomnia are said to have responded well to alpha-wave training.[17] If biofeedback can help stutterers to control their anxiety about speaking it may prove to be one of the more useful modern tools.

New information will provide fresh insights into the causes and treatment of stuttering, but more funds are needed to support research. People who stutter should make their collective, hesitant voices heard in high places and clamour for more attention to their problems. Ingenious man should be able to come up with a few answers after two thousand years of research on tangled tongues.

The information age

The world is changing rapidly, and stutterers, like other people, will need to adapt if they are to survive. The rapidly increasing world population, the spread of mechanization, and the scarcity of natural resources are likely to increase competition for food, homes, and jobs. These stresses will place more pressure on a stutterer's speech and may increase people's impatience with the disfluent and other handicapped. Technology is advancing more rapidly than our social values. If we make mistakes we can make them faster and more often. People who stutter will need all their resourcefulness to survive.

If we can believe the futurists, we are entering the Information Age, where communication will be paramount. A person with a stutter will find that some of the new technology will help him; but some situations may prove hard to handle.

Computers are here to be used and misused whether we like it or not. They have invaded our homes and schools, and communication by video screen and computer print-out will soon become commonplace. A stutterer could find that he needs to speak less. You don't have to be fluent to punch keys, look at screens, and read messages on pieces of paper.

People using computers tend to lean heavily on pure logic both at home and in the workplace. They tend to use the areas of the brain devoted to logic more than those from which derive the 'human' attributes of holistic thinking, intuition, compassion, and love. Logic can be so powerful and convincing that people tend to discount their better selves when convinced by cold figures. The brutalities of the slave trade were justified by the cold logic of economics and the quest for power. Humanity is left out of too many equations.

If the use of computers results in a coldly 'rational' society, handicapped people are in for a bad time. Fortunately computers can, when used as extensions to the mind rather than as minds themselves, process data very rapidly. They provide access to huge amounts of information, and this could be of enormous benefit in studies of stuttering. Complex, interactive computer models of businesses, forest ecosystems, and physiological processes have been constructed and work well in their own fields. All of these systems, like a stutter, involve many interacting factors. Perhaps one day a computer model of a stutter can be created and manipulated to discover better methods of treatment.

When I heard about electronic conferencing, mail, and noticeboards my heart sang at the thought of the imminent demise of my arch enemy, the oral telephone. I ran to the nearest computer store where some bright fellow plugged a modem into our computer and unplugged a great many dollars from our bank account. We were all set to Communicate.

The modem is called a Smart Modem because it is clever enough to operate in two gears, 300 bauds and 1,200 bauds, slow and fast. The problem was that I was not as smart as the modem, and the massive instruction manual defeated me. A colleague who kindly offered to advise left a gaggle of commands flying around my empty head, each of which escaped through one ear or the other in a very short time. I tried. I even achieved buzzing and clicking noises, but no messages. I was, however, entirely successful in promoting the cash flow of the telephone company. In two days of practice I ran up a $70 telephone bill.

So my modem with all its baudy potential sits on my desk, and the thick manual stands unsullied on the bookshelf beside my other tattered computer manuals. Back we went to the bosoms of old Ma Bell's merry band of telephone operators.

In spite of my dim-witted disappointment, electronic conferencing could help people who stutter if they and their colleagues have the wherewithal to buy the hardware, the type of minds that can understand computerese, and the cash flow to keep paying the telephone bills.

If a stutterer takes the trouble to become computer literate, many new job avenues will be available to him where his disfluency will not be a major handicap. The Information Age could benefit the disfluent and other disabled considerably if they have the courage to plunge into this new world.

The silent minority: not so minor

In times of economic crisis the political economists look hungrily at the funds allocated to hospitals, schools, universities, pensions, and programs for the handicapped. Soon after any election, the headlines appear in the press: 'Plans to Cut Social Services.' This is perplexing, since most people are under the impression that politicians are elected to serve society.

Fortunately, the electorate can do something about it. The handicapped have a more powerful lobby than they realize. Quite apart from obvious, severe disabilities, there are many that are partial or periodic but nevertheless disabling. About 1 per cent of people stutter; about 1 per cent are dyslexic; 1 per cent have schizophrenia; and many more have agoraphobia, severe sight or hearing disabilities, and damage to the brain's speech centres by ruptured aneurysms or cerebral embolisms. If someone took the trouble to calculate the numbers of people disabled to the extent that it interferes with their ability to work unaided and to participate effectively in society, the so-called disabled minority would turn out to be not so minor after all.

Without taking into account the elderly, at least 6 per cent of the population have functional disabilities of one kind or another. In North America alone there must be fifteen million disabled people who can vote or will vote in the future. This would be doubled if the disabled old people were taken into account, and doubled again if the parents, siblings, husbands, wives, and friends of the disabled were included. A total of about sixty million people could have a loud voice in the policies of the nations of North America if they made the effort.

There is increasing evidence of militancy among the old and the disabled. The elderly have appeared on the streets waving banners protesting reductions in pensions, facilities, and rights. Unfortunately, their voices have not been loud enough. They can't go on strike and they haven't the money to take cases to court. Their efforts are dissipated. The only way disabled people can be heard is to act in a large group to get political clout. This shouldn't be necessary, but we don't live in Shangri-La.

Charters of human rights of one kind or another exist in many countries. The people who seem to benefit most from these rights are criminals and other public nuisances who howl 'Discrimination!' when they feel the hand of retribution on their shoulders. Nevertheless, the mechanisms for the disabled to assert their rights are there to be used. We should learn how to use them. There is no need to put up with blatant maltreatment and discrimination. Every few years the voters can elect men of conscience into positions of power – if they can find them.

Shifting attitudes: the quiet revolution

In spite of the materialism of the world's developed countries, there has been a quiet revolution in people's attitudes since 1950. Old values have been reconsidered and rejected, accepted, or modified. Gross exploitation of natural resources regardless of its effect on the environment is no longer accepted as unavoidable; progress is no longer measured just by economic growth; some economists include values other than dollars in their calculations of costs and benefits; women are less frequently regarded as second-class citizens; and efforts are being made to secure the rights of all people, regardless of race, sex, age, creed, or colour. Many citizens have opted out of the race for power, possessions, and money to live simpler, more satisfying lives and are attempting to raise their children to share their values. The 'Back to Basics' movement at times became a little too basic, but the idea of re-evaluation is both welcome and refreshing.

The growth of new religious sects and the popularity of evangelists, both good and bad, suggest that people are looking for new sets of values (or new ways of looking at old values) and are prepared to spend time, money, and energy on consolidating and spreading their new beliefs. Certainly, the barbarians are still with us. Predators still prey on the weak and defenceless, but the growth of grass-roots movements to think and do things in better ways is encouraging. People of goodwill and conscience have votes. The old walls of established and outmoded attitudes can be cracked.

Society's attitudes toward the disabled are immeasurably better than they were fifty years ago. I have clear, childhood memories of destitute amputees in the 1930s pushing themselves around on low wooden trolleys and begging for pennies; and of processions of jeering children following severely disabled spastics down the street. Hunchbacks were fair game for gangs of youths out for an evening's mischief, and albinos and individuals with harelips or cleft palates were openly ridiculed. Today these brutalities are much less open and less frequent. Most of today's discrimination is indirect, hidden, or unintentional.

During the 1940s, my wife, Joan, went to a girls' school in England where good manners were high on the list of priorities. On one occasion a teacher said to Joan, 'What would you do if you met a person in a wheelchair or someone who was severely deformed? You wouldn't turn away would you?' The implication was that, whatever your fears, you treated the disabled like anyone else, with courtesy and consideration. Other ways of behaving were just not imaginable. She was not ordered to behave in a particular way, but was shown that there was no other acceptable course of action. She and the teacher took it for granted.

Society has basic standards of behaviour that include honesty, truthfulness, and finding non-violent solutions for problems. Laws exist to see that these standards are enforced. In general only major infringements of law reach the courts, and it is impossible to legislate to outlaw minor dishonesties, lies, and acts of aggression. You could fill the bookshelves with legislation to deal with injustices and discrimination, but no amount of legislation will compel people to cease their rudeness, rejection, and insensitivity when they meet the disabled unless they want to. It is necessary, therefore, to 'raise society's consciousness' about such matters.

Most people are willing to listen, learn, and change their attitudes when they know the facts. If stutterers are to live without the glass wall between themselves and society, they must make sure that the facts reach the public. School is the obvious place to start, but the radio, press, and television offer tremendous opportunities for informing and influencing the public. It will take time, but society's attitudes toward people with tangled tongues can be changed for the better without punitive, unenforceable legislation. Stutterers and their families and friends, as well as the various speech associations, could have a tremendous impact on the public through the media if they were to make the effort.

The outlook for changing society's behaviour toward the disfluent is promising, but it won't just happen on its own.

Conclusion

This book has been a long journey. During its writing I resurrected old memories, some painful, some warm, some funny. Like any other journey, it was an education, and assembling the information gave me new insights into my speech. At times I walked on dangerous ground. Some of the chapters caused my speech to deteriorate temporarily, and at times it was hard to write objectively, but I was sustained by the memory of the warmth and courage of all the hundreds of stuttering children, adolescents, and adults I have met, and of the dedicated therapists with whom I worked. And how we worked!

People who stutter deserve better from society, and maybe this book will help in a small way to achieve this. I still find it an effort to speak, but can look back over fifty-five years of hesitant, unpredictable speech and more than fifty years of therapy not with regret, but with a sense of quiet jubilation that I have met so many wonderful people, lived such a rich life, and encountered so many challenges. I have seen the darkest and the brightest sides of humanity, and the bright side reigns supreme.

Notes

The abbreviation *JSHD* used in these notes refers to the *Journal of Speech and Hearing Disorders*.

PREFACE

1 Many therapists are sceptical about the use of the Edinburgh Masker and deplore excessive claims in the media about its usefulness. Other therapists recognize the value of the masker for some stutterers, particularly those who have impediments that have not responded well to treatment. The incident described in this Preface explains how it worked for me on a particular occasion. This does not imply that it is the answer to all stuttering. The masker is discussed later in the book in more detail.

2 Although 'stammering' is the present Old World term for the New World's 'stuttering,' the term 'stut' has a long and honourable pedigree. In 1627, Sir Francis Bacon, the scientist, philosopher, and man of letters, wrote in *Sylva Sylvarum*: 'Divers, we see, doe Stut. The Cause may be ... the Refrigeration of the Tongue; Whereby it is lesse apt to move ...; And we see that those that Stut, if they drinke Wine moderately, they Stut less, because it heateth ... it may be (though rarely) the Driness of the Tongue which maketh it lesse apt to move, as well as Cold; For it is an Affect that it cometh to some Wise and Great Men; as it did unto Moses, who was *Linguae Praepiditae*.'

  Bacon's suggestion that stuttering was caused by the coldness or dryness of the tongue perpetuated a myth originating in the teachings of Aristotle and Hippocrates. The term 'stammering' was used by Benjamin Alexander, MD, as early as 1769 in his translation of Morgagni's *Treatise on Stuttering*.

3 A great many terms, many of them poorly defined, were used for 'stuttering' in the early literature. Hippocrates' *'trauloi'* seems to refer to speech defects in general, but Aristotle's *'ischnophonoi'* was used specifically for stuttering. Stuttering and cluttering were

grouped under the title of *'psellismus'* in the seventeenth century. *'Balbus,' 'balbuties,'* and *'batarismus'* were used for stuttering, but the usage tended to be erratic. Stuttering in early times is described in some detail by R.W. Rieber and J. Wollock in 'The historical roots of the theory and therapy of stuttering,' in R.W. Rieber, ed., *The Problem of Stuttering* (New York: Elsevier 1977).

4 'Cluttering' is best described as a disability consisting of rapid, jerky, slurred, jumbled speech, with words repeated or left out. The words come in rapid spurts. Most clutterers can speak fluently when they speak slowly and carefully, which is not necessarily true of people who stutter severely.

CHAPTER 1

1 United States Department of Health and Human Services, *Stuttering: Hope through Research* (Washington, DC: National Institute of Health, Publication 81-2250, 1981)

CHAPTER 2

1 A. Mehrabian, 'Nonverbal communication,' *Nebraska Symposium on Communication* (Lincoln, Neb.: Nebraska University Press 1972); and R.P. Harrison, 'Nonverbal behavior: an approach to human communication,' in R.W. Budd and B.D. Ruben, eds., *Approaches to Human Communication* (Rochelle Park, NJ: Spartan Books 1972), 253–68

2 J. Fast, *Body Language* (New York: Pocket Books 1975); D. Morris, *Man Watching: A Field Guide to Human Behavior* (New York: Abrams 1977); Harrison, 'Nonverbal behavior'

3 O. Bloodstein, *A Handbook on Stuttering*, 3rd ed. (Chicago, Ill.: National Easter Seals Society 1981), 87, 99

4 Ibid., 80; and W. Johnson and associates, *The Onset of Stuttering* (Minneapolis, Minn.: University of Minnesota Press 1959)

5 Bloodstein, *Handbook on Stuttering*, 3rd ed., 160–1

6 J.O. Graf, 'Incidence of stuttering among twins,' in W. Johnson and R.R. Leutenegger, eds., *Stuttering in Children and Adults* (Minneapolis, Minn.: University of Minnesota Press 1955)

7 S.E. Nelson, N. Hunter, and M. Walter, 'Stuttering in twin types,' *Journal of Speech Disorders* 10 (1945): 335–43

8 Bloodstein, *Handbook on Stuttering*, 3rd ed., 99

9 L.F. Buscaglia, 'An experimental study of the Sarbin-Hardyck test as indexes of role perception for adolescent stutterers,' *Speech Monographs* 30 (1963): 243

10 C. Cherry and B.McA. Sayers, 'Experiments upon the total inhibition of stammering by external control and some clinical results,' *Journal of Psychosomatic Research* 1 (1956): 233–46

11 C. Van Riper, *Speech Correction: Principles and Methods*, 5th ed. (Englewood Cliffs, NJ: Prentice-Hall 1972), 284

12 J.G. Sheehan and M.M. Martyn, 'Spontaneous recovery from stuttering,' *Journal of Speech and Hearing Research* 9 (1966): 121–35
13 P.J. Glasner and D. Rosenthal, 'Parental diagnosis of stuttering in young children,' *JSHD* 22 (1957): 288–95
14 Sheehan and Martyn, 'Spontaneous recovery from stuttering'; and O. Bloodstein, *A Handbook on Stuttering*, 1st ed. (Chicago, Ill.: National Easter Seals Society 1969), 78–80
15 P.B. Ballard, 'Sinistrality and speech,' *Journal of Experimental Pediatry* 1 (1912): 298–310
16 J.E.W. Wallin, 'A consensus of speech defectives among 89,057 public school pupils – a preliminary report,' *Sch. Soc.* 3 (1916): 213–16
17 Bloodstein, *Handbook on Stuttering*, 3rd ed., 143
18 Ibid., 11
19 Ibid., 18
20 The Hector Speech Aid is manufactured and distributed by Peter Graham Partnership, 10 Eastway, Epsom, Surrey, England KT19 8SG. The author has never used this speech-rate meter and cannot comment on its value.

CHAPTER 3

1 Some speech pathologists and teachers may feel that the classroom trauma described in this chapter is exaggerated. It is true that schools have changed for the better in their treatment of the handicapped. It has also been said that British children are, on the whole, less kind to each other than their North American counterparts. Nevertheless, I still hear about young people with stutters in North America who find their schooling a time of fear, frustration, and humiliation, even in the community colleges where the students are old enough to know better.
2 A.K. Bullen, 'A cross-cultural approach to the problem of stuttering,' *Child Development* 16 (1945): 1–18; and Bloodstein, *Handbook on Stuttering*, 3rd ed., 102
3 J.C. Snidecor, 'Why the Indian does not stutter,' *Quarterly Journal of Speech* 33 (1947): 493–5
4 Ibid.
5 E.M. Lemert, 'Some Indians who stutter,' *JSHD* 18 (1953): 168–74
6 J.L. Stewart, 'The problem of stuttering in certain North American Indian societies,' *JSHD*, Supplement 6 (1960)
7 W. Johnson, *Speech Handicapped School Children* (Minneapolis, Minn.: University of Minnesota Press 1967); and Bloodstein, *Handbook on Stuttering*, 3rd ed., 106–8
8 M.L. Aron, 'The nature and incidence of stuttering among a Bantu group of school-going children,' *JSHD* 27 (1962): 116–28
9 Toyoda, cited in C. Van Riper, *The Nature and Treatment of Stuttering* (Englewood Cliffs, NJ: Prentice-Hall 1971), 39
10 Personal communication, Tokyo Speech Clinic, 1984
11 Bloodstein, *Handbook on Stuttering*, 3rd ed., 80

CHAPTER 4

1 Van Riper, *Speech Correction*, 277
2 H.E. Beech and F. Fransella, *Research and Experiment in Stuttering* (London: Pergamon Press 1968), 55
3 Bloodstein, *Handbook on Stuttering*, 3rd ed., 41–2
4 Ibid., 94
5 Johnson and associates, *The Onset of Stuttering*
6 J. Shields, L.L. Heston, and I.I. Gottesman, 'Schizophrenia and the schizoid: the problem of genetic analysis,' in R.R. Fieve, D. Rosenthal, and H. Brill, eds., *Genetic Research in Psychology* (Baltimore, Md.: Johns Hopkins University Press 1975)
7 S.S. Kety, D. Rosenthal, P.H. Wender, and F. Schulsinger, 'The types and prevalence of mental illness in the biological and adoptive families of adopted schizophrenics,' in D. Rosenthal and S.S. Kety, eds., *The Transmission of Schizophrenia* (Oxford: Pergamon Press 1968), 345–62
8 Bloodstein, *Handbook on Stuttering*, 3rd ed., 98–9
9 Ibid., 101–2
10 L. Chan and B.M. O'Malley, 'Mechanism of action of the sex steroid hormones,' *New England Journal of Medicine* 294 (1976): 1322–8, 1372–81, 1430–7
11 J.P. Scott and J.L. Fuller, *Genetics and the Social Behavior of the Dog* (Chicago, Ill.: University of Chicago Press 1965) Some scientists feel that no form of behaviour is heritable, in spite of mounting evidence to the contrary. Some accept that a nervous disposition may be inherited, but question that specific anxieties (e.g., about speaking) are encoded in our genes. Nevertheless, it is known that young rodents inherit an instinctive fear of a moving shadow overhead (it could be a predatory bird). Even human beings seem to have inherited, from their tree-dwelling ancestors, a fear of falling. This complex subject is discussed in some detail by Melvin Konner, *The Tangled Wing: Biological Constraints on the Human Spirit* (New York: Holt, Rinehart and Winston 1982), 208–35.
12 D.B. Lindsley, 'Bilateral differences in brain potentials from two cerebral hemispheres in relation to laterality and stuttering,' *Journal of Experimental Psychology* 26 (1940): 211–25; and L.C. Douglass, 'The study of laterally recorded EEG's of adult stutterers,' *Journal of Experimental Psychology* 32 (1943): 247–65
13 E. Boberg, L.T. Yeudell, D. Schopflocher, and P. Bo-Lassen, 'The effect of intensive behavioural program on the distribution of EEG alpha power in stutterers during the processing of verbal and visuospatial information,' *Journal of Fluency Disorders* 8 (1983): 245–63
14 P.T. Quinn, 'Stuttering, cerebral dominance and the dichotic word test,' *Medical Journal of Australia* 2 (1972): 639–43
15 W.H. Moore and W.O. Haynes, 'Alpha hemispheric asymmetry and stuttering: some support for segmentation dysfunction hypothesis,' *Journal of Speech and Hearing Research* 23 (1980): 229–47

16 Boberg et al., 'Effect of intensive behavioural program on EEG'
17 Bloodstein, *Handbook on Stuttering*, 3rd ed., 10–17
18 R. West, 'An agnostic's speculations about stuttering,' in J. Eisenson, ed., *Stuttering: A Symposium* (New York: Harper and Row 1958)
19 Eisenson, *Stuttering: A Symposium*; and Bloodstein, *Handbook on Stuttering*, 1st ed., 39
20 Konner, *The Tangled Wing*
21 J. Langone, 'Deciphering Dyslexia,' *Discover* (August 1983): 34–42
22 Cherry and Sayers, 'Experiments upon the total inhibition of stammering'; and S. Sutton and R.A. Chase, 'White noise and stuttering,' *Journal of Speech and Hearing Research* 4 (1961): 72
23 C.P. Stromsta, 'A methodology related to the determination of phase angle of bone conducted speech sound energy of stutterers and non-stutterers' (PH D diss., Ohio State University 1956); abstracted in *Speech Monographs* 24 (1957): 147–8
24 Bloodstein, *Handbook on Stuttering*, 3rd ed., 68
25 Ibid., 283–4
26 Ibid., 279
27 G. Fairbanks, 'Systematic research in experimental phonetics I. A theory of the speech mechanism as a servosystem,' *JSHD* 19 (1954): 133–9; and Bloodstein, *Handbook on Stuttering*, 3rd ed., 66–8
28 Bloodstein, *Handbook on Stuttering*, 1st ed., 66–8
29 L.E. Travis and L.B. Fagan, 'Studies in stuttering III. A study of certain reflexes during stuttering,' *Archives of Neurology and Psychiatry* 19 (1928): 1006–13
30 M. Palmer and A.M. Gillett, 'Sex differences in the cardiac rhythms of stutterers,' *Journal of Speech Disorders* 3 (1938): 3–12
31 C.H. Ritzman, 'A comparative cardiovascular and metabolic study of stutterers and non-stutterers,' *Journal of Speech Disorders* 7 (1943): 367–73
32 C.W. Starkweather, 'Stuttering and laryngial behavior – a review,' *ASHA Monographs* (Rockville, Md.: American Speech-Language-Hearing Association, Publication 21, 1982)
33 Beech and Fransella, *Research and Experiment in Stuttering*, 105; and Bloodstein, *Handbook on Stuttering*, 1st ed., 105–6
34 Bloodstein, *Handbook on Stuttering*, 3rd ed., 116–7
35 Beech and Fransella, *Research and Experiment in Stuttering*, 88
36 Ibid.
37 R. Cabanas, 'Some findings in speech and voice therapy among mentally deficient children,' *Folia Phoniat.* 6 (1954): 34–9
38 J.R. Knott, W. Johnson, and M.J. Webster, 'Studies on the psychology of stuttering II. A quantitative evaluation of the expectation of stuttering in relation to the incidence of stuttering,' *Journal of Speech Disorders* 2 (1937): 20–2; and W. Johnson and J.R. Knott, 'The moment of stuttering,' *Journal of Genetic Psychology* 48 (1936): 475–9
39 Bloodstein, *Handbook on Stuttering*, 3rd ed., 44

40 Johnson, *Speech Handicapped School Children*; W. Johnson, 'The role of evaluation in stuttering behavior,' *Journal of Speech Disorders* 3 (1938): 85–9; and Bloodstein, *Handbook on Stuttering*, 3rd ed., 54–6

41 J.G. Sheehan, *Stuttering: Research and Therapy* (New York: Harper and Row 1970)

42 C. Van Riper, *Speech Correction: Principles and Methods*, 3rd ed. (Englewood Cliffs, NJ: Prentice-Hall 1972), 329–30

43 Bloodstein, *Handbook on Stuttering*, 1st ed., 40–5

44 C. Van Riper, 'Study of the thoracic breathing of stutterers during expectancy and occurrence of stuttering spasm,' *Journal of Speech Disorders* 1 (1936): 61–72; Knott, Johnson, and Webster, 'Studies on the psychology of stuttering II'; and R. Milisen, 'Frequency of stuttering with anticipation of stuttering controlled,' *JSHD* 3 (1938): 207–14

45 Bloodstein, *Handbook on Stuttering*, 3rd ed., 224–5

46 E.J. Brutten and B.B. Gray, 'Effect of word cue removal on adaptation and adjacency: a clinical paradigm," *JSHD* 26 (1961): 385–9.

47 W. Johnson, R.P. Larson, and J.R. Knott, 'Studies in the psychology of stuttering III. Certain objective cues related to the precipitation of the moment of stuttering,' *JSHD* 2 (1937): 23–5; and A.E. Goss, 'Stuttering behavior and anxiety as a function of experimental training,' *JSHD* 21 (1956): 342–51

48 S.F. Brown, 'The loci of stuttering in the speech sequence,' *Journal of Speech Disorders* 10 (1945): 181–92

49 Bloodstein, *Handbook on Stuttering*, 1st ed., 186

50 S.F. Brown and A. Moren, 'The frequency of stuttering in reading,' *Journal of Speech Disorders* 7 (1942): 153–9

51 Bloodstein, *Handbook on Stuttering*, 1st ed., 193–210

52 N.H. Berwick, 'Stuttering in response to photographs of selected listeners,' in Johnson and Leutenegger, eds., *Stuttering in Children and Adults*

53 J.G. Sheehan, R. Hadley, and E. Gould, 'Impact of authority on stuttering,' *Journal of Abnormal Psychology* 72 (1967): 290–3

54 Bloodstein, *Handbook on Stuttering*, 1st ed., 158

55 H.J. Heltman, *First Aids for Stutterers* (New York: Expression Company 1943)

56 A.E. Goss, 'Stuttering behavior and anxiety as a function of the duration of the stimulus words,' *Journal of Abnormal Social Psychology* 47 (1952): 38–50

57 R.L. Webster, 'A behavioral analysis of stuttering: treatment and theory,' in K. Calhoun, ed., *Innovative Treatment Methods in Psychopathology* (New York: John Wiley and Sons 1974)

CHAPTER 5

1 R.W. Rieber, ed., *The Problem of Stuttering: Theory and Therapy* (New York: Elsevier 1977), 135–6

2 Ibid., 128
3 H. Mercurialis, 'Treatises on the diseases of children,' J. Wollock, trans., in Rieber, ed., *The Problem of Stuttering*, 127–40
4 Ibid.
5 R. Luchsinger and G.E. Arnold, 'Voice speech and language,' in *Clinical Communicology: Its Physiology and Pathology*, 1st ed., G.E. Arnold and E.R. Finkbeiner, trans. (Belmont, Ca.: Wadsworth Publishing 1965), 739–69
6 Ibid.
7 M. Katz, 'Survey of patented anti-stuttering devices,' in Rieber, ed., *The Problem of Stuttering*, 181–206
8 Ibid.
9 Van Riper, *Speech Correction*, 5th ed., 278
10 Ibid., 280
11 H. Geniesse, 'Stuttering,' *Science* 82 (1935): 518
12 Bloodstein, *Handbook on Stuttering*, 3rd ed., 250
13 Beech and Fransella, *Research and Experiment in Stuttering*, 171
14 V. Meyer and J.M. Mair, 'A new technique to control stammering: a preliminary report,' *Behaviour Research and Therapy* 1 (1963): 251–4
15 Ibid.; and Beech and Fransella, *Research and Experiment in Stuttering*, 176
16 I. Goldiamond, 'Stuttering and fluency as manipulatable operant response classes,' in L. Krasner and L.P. Ulman, eds., *Research in Behavior Modification* (New York: Holt, Rinehart and Winston 1965); and G.A. Soderburg, 'Delayed auditory feedback and stuttering,' *JSHD* 33 (1968): 260–7
17 A. Dewar, A.D. Dewar, and H.E. Barnes, 'Automatic triggering of auditory feedback masking in stammering and cluttering,' *British Journal of Disorders of Communication* 11 (1976): 19–26
18 A. Dewar, A.D. Dewar, W.T.S. Austin, and H.M. Brash, 'The long-term use of an automatically triggered auditory feedback device in the treatment of stammering,' *British Journal of Disorders of Communication* 14: 3 (1978): 219–29
19 Ibid.
20 Ibid.
21 J.G. Sheehan, 'Reflections on the behavioral modification of stuttering,' in M. Fraser, ed., *Conditioning in Stuttering Therapy – Applications and Limitations* (Memphis, Tenn.: Speech Foundation of America, Publication 7, 1981), 123–36
22 Beech and Fransella, *Research and Experiment in Stuttering*, 91–6
23 United States Pharmacopeial Convention, Inc., *About Your Medicines* (Kingsport Press: distributed in Canada by Canadian Pharmaceutical Association 1981), 336–9, 235–8, 297–301; and J. Graedon, *The People's Pharmacy* (New York: St Martin's Press 1976), 47, 269
24 Van Riper, *Speech Correction*, 5th ed., 333–5
25 A.A. Brill, 'Speech disturbances in nervous and mental disease,' *Quarterly Journal of Speech Education* 9 (1923): 129–35

26 Beech and Fransella, *Research and Experiment in Stuttering*, 105–24
27 C. Tavris, *Anger: The Misunderstood Emotion* (New York: Simon and Schuster 1982), 121–50
28 Van Riper, *Speech Correction*, 5th ed., 275
29 Bloodstein, *Handbook on Stuttering*, 1st ed., 241–2
30 J. Hoffman, 'The application of Gestalt therapy principles to therapy with an adult stutterer' (Mimeo abstract, Ontario Speech and Hearing Convention 1976)
31 J.B. Watson, *Behaviorism* (New York: W.W. Norton 1924, cited in Konner, *The Tangled Wing*, 219
32 Konner, *The Tangled Wing*, 383–4
33 B. Flanagan, I. Goldiamond, and N. Azrin, 'Operant stuttering: the control of stuttering behavior through response-contingent consequences,' *Journal of Experimental Analysis of Behavior* 1 (1958): 173–7
34 R.R. Martin and G.M. Siegel, 'The effects of response contingent shock on stuttering,' *Journal of Speech and Hearing Research* 9 (1966): 340–52; and 'The effects of simultaneously punishing stuttering and rewarding fluency, *Journal of Speech and Hearing Research* 9 (1966): 466–75; and B. Biggs and J. Sheehan, 'Punishment or distraction? Operant stuttering revisited,' *Journal of Abnormal Psychology* (1970), cited in Bloodstein, *Handbook on Stuttering*, 3rd ed., 50
35 Fraser, ed., *Conditioning in Stuttering Therapy*, 12, 132
36 B. Guitar and T. Peters, *Stuttering: An Integration of Contemporary Therapies* (Memphis, Tenn.: Speech Foundation of America, Publication 16, 1980), 13
37 Webster, 'A behavioral analysis of stuttering'; also R.L. Webster, 'Empirical considerations regarding stuttering therapy,' in H.H. Gregory, ed., *Controversies about Stuttering Therapy* (Baltimore, Md.: University Park Press 1979)
38 Bloodstein, *Handbook on Stuttering*, 3rd ed., 365–6
39 B.P. Ryan, *Programmed Therapy for Stuttering in Young Children* (Springfield, Ill.: Charles C. Thomas 1974); 'Stuttering therapy in a framework of operant conditioning and programmed learning,' in Gregory, ed., *Controversies about Stuttering Therapy*, 129–73; Webster, 'A behavioral analysis of stuttering'; and Webster, 'Empirical considerations regarding stuttering therapy'
40 F.L. Darley and D.C. Spriestersbach, *Diagnostic Methods in Speech Pathology* (New York: Harper and Row 1978)
41 Guitar and Peters, *Stuttering*, 33–6
42 Bloodstein, *Handbook on Stuttering*, 3rd ed., 343–53
43 W. Johnson, *People in Quandaries* (New York: Harper and Row 1946); Johnson, 'The time, the place and the problem,' in Johnson and Leutenegger, eds., *Stuttering in Children and Adults*; and Bloodstein, *Handbook on Stuttering*, 3rd ed., 347–9
44 C. Van Riper, 'Experiments in stuttering therapy,' in Eisenson, ed., *Stuttering: A Symposium*

45 Van Riper, *Speech Correction*, 5th ed., 248–340
46 Ibid., 291–2
47 Ibid., 292
48 E. Boberg and D. Kully, *Clinical Manual for Comprehensive Stutter-ing Program* (Edmonton, Alberta: University of Alberta 1984); and E. Boberg, 'Intensive adult therapy program,' *Seminars in Speech, Language and Hearing* 1: 4 (1980): 365–73
49 E. Boberg, ed., *The Maintenance of Fluency*. Proceedings of the Banff Conference, Banff, Alberta, June 1979 (New York: Elsevier 1981); and Boberg, *Clinical Manual*
50 G. Andrews, B. Guitar, and P. Howie, 'Meta-analysis of the effects of stuttering treatment,' *JSHD* 45 (1980): 287–307

CHAPTER 6

1 ASHA is essentially a professional association, but has a consumer branch called the National Association for Hearing and Speech Action (NAHSA) at 10801 Rockville Pike, Rockville, Maryland 20852, U.S.A. Telephone: (301) 638-6868 and (301) 897-8682. Helpline: (800) 638-8255 (or 6868). This is an active organization with a full-time staff.
2 The Canadian Speech and Hearing Association (CSHA) is a profes-sional organization, but the local branches will point stutterers toward suitable clinics. There is a need for a consumer-oriented branch in Canada.
3 M. Fraser, ed., *To the Stutterer* (Memphis, Tenn.: Speech Founda-tion of America, Publication 9, 1972); and *Self-Therapy for the Stut-terer*, 3rd ed. (Memphis, Tenn.: Speech Foundation of America, Publication 12, 1981); Malcolm Fraser has written and edited many excellent publications for the Speech Foundation of America in Memphis, Tennessee. Many of these are designed for use by non-professionals.
4 S. Ainsworth, *Counselling Stutterers* (Memphis, Tenn.: Speech Foun-dation of America n.d.)
5 A. Irwin, *Stammering: Practical Help for All Ages* (Markham, Ont.: Penguin Books 1980)
6 National Stuttering Project, 1269 7th Avenue, San Francisco, California 94122. Telephone: (415) 566-5324 or (415) 647-4700. Issues a newsletter.
7 R.L. Gregory, 'Recovery from early blindness: a case study,' in R.L. Gregory, ed., *Concepts and Mechanisms of Perception* (London: Duckworth 1974), 65–129
8 R.M. Restak, *The Brain: The Last Frontier* (New York: Warner Books 1979), 96–102, 407–9. Excerpts by permission of Doubleday & Co., Inc. Copyright 1979, Richard M. Restak.

CHAPTER 7

1 Webster, 'A behavioral analysis of stuttering'

CHAPTER 8

1 The inevitability of sibling rivalry in the family was questioned by one reviewer. She pointed out that my childhood was spent in Britain and that British children tend to be more unkind to each other than North American children. This may be true, but from what I know of human nature and with experience of how small brothers and sisters compete and call each other names, I feel that the rivalries are usually there. It is just a matter of degree.
2 Bloodstein, *Handbook on Stuttering*, 3rd ed., 108–9
3 L.J. Peter, *Peter's Quotations: Ideas for Our Time* (Toronto, London, New York: Bantam Books 1979), 57

CHAPTER 9

1 J. Levy, 'Perception of bilateral chimeric figures following hemispheric disconnection,' *Brain* 95 (1972): 61–78; 'The origins of lateral symmetry,' in *Lateralization in the Nervous System* (New York: Academic Press 1977); and Interview with J. Levy described in J. Restak, *The Brain*
2 F.H.C. Crick, 'Thinking about the brain,' *Scientific American* 241: 3 (1979): 219–32
3 C.F. Stevens, 'The neuron,' *Scientific American* 241: 3 (1979): 54–65
4 N. Geschwind, 'Specializations of the human brain,' *Scientific American* 241: 3 (1979): 180–99
5 J.P. Mohr, cited in Geschwind, 'Specializations of the human brain'
6 Geschwind, 'Specializations of the human brain'
7 J.A. Gray, *The Psychology of Fear and Stress* (New York: McGraw-Hill 1971); and Konner, *The Tangled Wing*, 220–1
8 Konner, *The Tangled Wing*, 220–5
9 Ibid., 223–7
10 J.F. Tallman, S.M. Paul, P. Skolnick, and D.W. Gallagher, 'Receptors for the age of anxiety: pharmacology of the Benzodiapines,' *Science* 207 (1980): 274–81
11 Webster, 'A behavioral analysis of stuttering'
12 W.M. Shearer, 'Speech: behavior of middle-ear muscle during stuttering,' *Science* 152 (1966): 1280; and Webster, 'A behavioral analysis of stuttering'
13 Webster, 'A behavioral analysis of stuttering'
14 B.B. Brown, *Stress and the Art of Biofeedback* (Toronto: Bantam Books 1981), 65–6
15 B. Guitar, 'Reduction of stuttering frequency using analog electromyographic feedback,' *Journal of Speech and Hearing Research* 18 (1975): 672–85
16 Bloodstein, *Handbook on Stuttering*, 3rd. ed., 366–7
17 M. Karlins and L.M. Andrews, *Biofeedback: Turning on the Power of Your Mind* (New York: Warner Books 1976), 57

Glossary

Anyone who attempts to define the terms used in psychology, neurology, pharmacology, and speech therapy is sure to get into hot water, but it is essential that a reader knows precisely what the author means when he uses unfamiliar words. Many glossaries, dictionaries, and textbooks were consulted to try to tie down precise meanings of words, but few experts seemed to say the same thing.

The words in this glossary are defined in the sense that they are used in this book and some are explained in more detail in the text. There are other meanings, and shades of meaning, and some definitions are over-simplified or over-generalized. The word 'stuttering,' for example, has three pages of definitions in Malcolm Fraser's glossary (see the following paragraph), and the psychologists seem to have difficulty saying exactly what the words 'psychologist,' 'psychiatrist,' and 'psychotherapy' mean.

Readers interested in a wider vocabulary about stuttering are referred to Malcolm Fraser's excellent booklet, *Stuttering Words – A Glossary of the Meanings of Words and Terms Used or Associated with Stuttering and Speech Pathology* (Memphis, Tenn.: Speech Foundation of America, Publication 2, 1980).

albumins A group of proteins soluble in water and coagulated by heat.

ambidextrous, ambidextrality The ability to use either hand with equal efficiency.

anticipatory struggle The abnormal feelings and behaviour of a stutterer as he prepares to speak and tries to avoid expected speech difficulties.

aphasia Partial or complete loss of the ability to speak in a comprehensive way, to understand spoken words, and to formulate, understand or express meanings as a result of injury, disease, or other abnormalities of the brain.

auditory feedback The sensations produced by the stimulation of the ear by the sound of one's own speech transmitted by air or bone.

axon The nerve fibre that transmits messages from one nerve cell (neuron) to another. The axon transmits; the dendrites receive (see 'dendrites' and 'neuron').

Broca's area (or **Broca's convolution**) The area in the brain responsible for programming the speech signals to the brain's motor tissues that control the movements of lips, tongue, jaw, larynx, etc. Sometimes called the speech area.

cerebral dominance The dominance of one side of the brain's cerebral cortex for a particular function (e.g., speech). See also 'laterality.'

chlorpromazine A phenothiazine drug used to treat nervous, mental, and emotional disorders.

cluttering Rapid, jerky, disjointed speech, with slurred or jumbled articulation. Thought to be due to a neurological disorder.

cognitive mismatch A mismatch between what a child sees or hears on one occasion and what he has experienced before.

conditioning Procedures used to elicit specific responses to situations, objects, etc., in order to modify behaviour. In general it means 'learning.'

creatinine A chemical compound (methylglycocyamidine) in muscle and urine.

creative dramatics Use of drama in psychotherapy and speech therapy to identify areas of conflict and provide release by playing roles.

decibel (Db) A unit of sound-wave intensity.

delayed auditory feedback The hearing of one's speech after a brief time interval.

dendrites Fine branches of the nerve cell (neuron) that receive signals from other nerves.

desensitization See 'systematic desensitization.'

disfluency Speech that is not smooth and fluent to a degree that can be normal (all people hesitate when they speak) or excessive (as in a stutter).

distraction Diverting the attention from the speech and thereby reducing the speaker's fear of stuttering.

dyslexia A perceptual disorder making it difficult for a person to read, write, spell, and, in some cases, speak.

easy onset Starting a sound, syllable, or word slowly and gradually without tension. Synonymous with 'easy initiation.'

echo speech See 'shadowing.'

Edinburgh Masker A portable electronic instrument that prevents a stutterer from hearing himself as he speaks.

endocrine glands Glands that secrete and release hormones (e.g., adrenalin and insulin) that affect the organs of the body.

epilepsy A disorder of the nervous system involving periodic fits, paroxysms, and loss of consciousness.

etiology The predisposition, development, and maintenance of a complaint (e.g., a stutter).

extrovert A person with an attitude that directs the consciousness towards the external objective world (antonym = 'introvert'). Jung recognized a distinct, extroverted type.

eye contact Looking the listener in the eye while speaking to him, and receiving visual feedback.

fluency shaping therapy Speech therapy that applies benign conditioning techniques to modify the speech behaviour of stutterers (easy onset to words, prolongation of sounds) by graded tasks, without treating the origins of the stutter or the anxiety about speaking.

fricative Sound made by forcing air through an orifice narrowed by tongue and lip movement (e.g., 'th,' 'f,' 'v,' and the sibilants 's,' 'z,' 'sh').

general semantics The relationships between the language people use and the way they act. Used in speech therapy to define and treat a stutterer's false assumptions about his speech.

Gestalt psychology A system of psychology concerned with patterns and the whole person.

globulins A group of proteins that dissolve in salt solutions but not in water (globulin, fibrinogens, fibrin, etc).

hertz (Hz) A unit of frequency of one cycle per second.

incus (anvil) A bone shaped like a tooth with two roots. Located in the middle ear.

introvert A person with an attitude that directs the consciousness toward the inner, subjective world. (Antonym = 'extrovert'). Jung recognized a distinct introverted type.

laterality The relationship between brain-sidedness and left- and right-handedness and speech. The 'laterality theory' is that a shift in handedness or confusion in sidedness is involved in the onset and maintenance of stuttering. See 'cerebral dominance.'

learned behaviour A persistent change in the responses of nerves, muscles, emotions, speech, and behaviour in response to external stimuli in the environment and clinic.

malleus (hammer) A small bone with an oval head and spur located in the middle ear.

masker An instrument emitting a sound used in masking to prevent the speaker hearing his own speech (e.g., 'Edinburgh Masker').

masking Interference with the perception of sound by the ears so that the speaker cannot hear his own speech. Sometimes used in the sense of changing the patterns and quality of sound the speaker hears.

masseter An elevator muscle of the lower jaw.

meprobamate A systemic drug used to treat nervousness and tension.

middle ear (tympanum) The part of the ear just inside the ear-drum that contains the three-boned lever (ossicular chain), and the muscles that control and support it, involved in the amplification and transmission of sound to the inner-ear membrane.

motor cortex The parts of the brain concerned with movement of lips, tongue, head, limbs, etc.

mute A person who cannot speak.

myelin A white fatty substance that forms the protective sheath of nerve fibres (axons).

neuroleptic drug A drug that affects the central nervous system's chemicals ('neurotransmitters') that transmit messages across the junction of one nerve with another.

neuron A nerve cell. Neurons are the building blocks of the brain. Each one consists of a roughly spherical or pyramidal cell body with numerous fine branches (dendrites) radiating from it and receiving signals from other nerve cells. A nerve fibre (the axon) extends from the cell body and transmits signals to other nerves.

neurosis A personality disorder causing a person to have irrational fears, obsessions, and compulsions, and preventing him from dealing effectively with reality.

neurotransmitters The chemical compounds that carry the nerve signals across the synaptic gap where one nerve cell connects with another (e.g., dopamine).

nonfluency See 'disfluency.'

non-verbal communication Messages conveyed not by spoken or written words but by involuntary movements of the face and limbs and by posture.

operant conditioning The form of conditioning in which a person's response allows reinforcement of behaviour (i.e., rewarded behaviour is likely to be positively reinforced and punished behaviour negatively reinforced).

ossicular chain The chain of small bones (the malleus, incus, and stapes) involved in sound transmission and amplification in the middle ear.

perseveration The abnormal persistence of a mental or motor (movement) process after the situation that caused it has ceased to exist.

phenobarbitone (or **phenobarbital**) A drug that depresses the activity of the central nervous system.

phobia An excessive, irrational anxiety about an object or situation.

phonetics The science of speech sounds.

play therapy The use of play activities in the psychotherapy and speech therapy of children.

plosive A sound created by interrupting air flow, building up air pressure, and releasing it, as in 'd,' 'b,' 'p,' 't,' etc.

preparatory set The hidden and often involuntary preparation or rehearsal for speech by pre-setting the positions of lips, tongue, etc.

prolongation The lengthening of speech sounds or lip, tongue, etc., postures.

propositional speech Speech containing meaning and implication.

psychiatrist An expert who applies specialized knowledge to treat mental and nervous disorders; covers both psychotherapy and psychology. *Note*: In this book the word refers to practitioners with a medical degree (MD).

psychobiology The study of psychology in terms of biological brain processes.

psychologist An expert who applies psychology for therapeutic purposes. *Note*: In this book the word refers to practitioners without a medical qualification (MD).

psychotherapy Treatment of mental illness, personality maladjustments, and harmful attitudes by psychological means.

pull-out Voluntary, controlled release from a stuttering block.

rhythmic therapy Treatment of stuttering using rhythm (a metronome, marching, etc.) as part of the speaking pattern. Regarded by many as a form of distraction.

schizophrenia A mental disorder involving conflicts between or separation of different aspects of personality and affecting the emotions and behaviour.

semantics The scientific study of the meaning of words.

shadowing Speaking at the same time as another person, or with a slight delay. Synonymous with 'echo speech.'

sociobiology The biology of social behaviour.

stammering See 'stuttering.'

stapedius A small muscle in the middle ear.

stapes (the stirrup) A stirrup-shaped small bone in the middle ear.

stematil One of the phenothiazine drugs used to control nervous, emotional, and mental conditions.

stuttering A speech disorder consisting of excessive and conspicuous involuntary hesitations, repetitions, prolongations, and blocks that interrupt the speech flow, together with struggling to speak, anxiety about speaking, and avoidance of words and speaking situations. *Note*: There are many other definitions.

stuttering modification therapy Speech therapy designed to reduce avoidance of speaking and hard words, lessen anxieties about speech, modify attitudes about speech, and help the stutterer change his pattern of disfluency.

synapse The connection of one nerve cell to another. At the junction there is a gap across which chemical compounds (neurotransmitters) carry the nerve signal.

syndrome A group of symptoms typical of a complaint (e.g., a stutter).

systematic desensitization Weakening of an undesirable response by repeated, gradual exposure to the situations that cause it.

tensor tympani A small muscle in the middle ear.

tympanum See 'middle ear.'

voluntary controlled repetition (VCR) The deliberate, voluntary, repetition of a sound, syllable, or word in a smooth, prolonged effortless manner to replace uncontrolled, involuntary repetition (stuttering) and reduce fear and avoidance of speaking.

voluntary stuttering See 'voluntary controlled repetition (VCR).'

Wernicke's area The tissue in the brain responsible for language formulation and comprehension.

Suggested reading

The Speech Foundation of America Publications described below can be purchased for about $1.50 to $2.00 (U.S.) from the Director, Speech Foundation of America, 152 Lombardy Rd., Memphis, Tennessee 38111.

General Reviews

Bloodstein, Oliver. *A Handbook on Stuttering*. 3rd edition. Chicago, Ill.: National Easter Seals Society for Crippled Children and Adults 1981
  This is a first-class review. The approach is technical, but the book is written in simple English and is easy to understand.
Van Riper, Charles. *The Nature of Stuttering*. Englewood Cliffs, NJ: Prentice-Hall, Inc. 1971
  A very readable general treatment of stuttering.
- *Speech Correction: Principles and Methods*. 5th edition. Englewood Cliffs, NJ: Prentice-Hall, Inc. 1972.
  Describes many speech defects and their treatment. Aimed at clinicians, but the simple style will appeal to the layman.

Guidance for Parents with Stuttering Children

Ainsworth, Stanley. *Stuttering: What It Is and What to Do about It*. Lincoln, Neb.: Cliff's Notes n.d.
  A low-cost booklet giving more details than the following publication.
Ainsworth, Stanley and J. Fraser-Gruss. *If Your Child Stutters – A Guide for Parents*. Revised edition. Memphis, Tenn.: Speech Foundation of America, Publication 11, 1977

An excellent low-cost summary written for the layman. Available from the Speech Foundation of America, Memphis, Tenn.

Self-help

Barbara, Dominick A. *A Practical Self-Help Guide for Stutterers*. Springfield, Ill.: Charles C. Thomas 1983.
Useful counsel about attitudes.
Fraser, Malcolm. *Self-therapy for the Stutterer*. Revised edition. Memphis, Tenn.: Speech Foundation of America, Publication 12, 1981.
Probably the best book on self-help. Its cost is low, it is simply written, and up to date. See also several articles in: Fraser, Malcolm, ed. *To the Stutterer*. Memphis, Tenn.: Speech Foundation of America, Publication 9, 1972.

Guidance for Teachers and School Clinicians

Fraser, Malcolm, *Stuttering – Treatment of the Young in School*. Memphis, Tenn.: Speech Foundation of America, Publication 4, 1982.
Mainly written for public-school speech therapists, it provides the non-specialist with guidance about what to do and what not to do when dealing with stuttering children.
Leith, William R. *Handbook of Stuttering – Therapy for the School Clinician*. San Diego, Ca.: College Hill Press 1980

Guidance for Stutterers

Fraser, Malcolm, ed. *To the Stutterer*. Memphis, Tenn.: Speech Foundation of America, Publication 9, 1972
A remarkable, encouraging book written by twenty-five experts. Covers attitudes, therapy, self-help, and dealing with fear.

Modern Views and Therapies

Curlee, Richard F. and William H. Perkins, eds. *Nature and Treatment of Stuttering. New Directions*. San Diego, Ca.: College Hill Press 1984

An up-to-date review of the treatment of stuttering. Describes promising methods for the future. Valuable for the clinician and informed layman.

Ingham, Roger J. *Stuttering and Behaviour Therapy – Current Status and Experimental Foundations.* San Diego, Ca.: College Hill Press 1983

A first-class review of treatment for stuttering written mainly for the clinician but also useful for the informed layman.

Self-help and consumer organizations

Self-help organizations tend to come and go, but there are a few hard-core national organizations that have many local chapters. These organizations create opportunities for timid stutterers to come out into the open and meet people who will not mock their strange way of speaking. They provide a forum for airing feelings, views, and complaints, and opportunities to test newly learned ways of speaking. These groups help to dispel the loneliness of many stutterers trapped in their glass towers.

A stutterer who is fearful about approaching a doctor about his problem but who wants to be helped will find that these organizations, some of which have clinicians as members, are a good starting-point. He is likely to be greeted with sympathy and understanding, and will be given gentle but hard-nosed advice.

The addresses given are those provided in 1984. They tend to change.

SELF-HELP ORGANIZATIONS

Australia

Australian Speak Easy
  Association
PO Box 113
Maclean
New South Wales 2463

Speak Easy Association
Victoria Branch
GPO 1173 K
Melbourne, Victoria 3001

Speak Easy Association
New South Wales and
ACT Branch
PO Box 1004
Parramatta
New South Wales 2150
(Speak Easy has branches in
other parts of Australia.)

Canada

Speak Easy, Inc.
95 Evergreen Avenue
Saint John, New Brunswick
E2N 1H4
Telephone: (506) 696-6799
Newsletter: *Speaking Out*
(There are several local
branches)

L'Association des bégues du
Canada (l'ABC)
3600 Fullum 26
Montreal, Québec H2K 3P6
Newsletter: *Speaking Out*

Denmark

P-Klub, Föreningen for
Stammere i Denmark,
(P-Club, Association for
Stutterers in Denmark)
c/o Taleinstitutte
Tjornevej 6
DK-8240, Risskov

Finland

Finska Stammares Förening rf.
(National Association of
Finnish Stutterers)
Box 60
SF-00131, Helsinki

Japan

Japanese Association of
Stutterers for Help and
Friendship
Shinjo Fukano
A-44-306 Khoro 5
Otokoyama, Yahata-shi
Kyoto 614

Norway

Norsk Interesseorganisasjon
for Stamme (NIFS)
(Norwegian Fellow-
Organization for Stutterers)
Postbox 878
Sentrum, N-Oslo 1

Sweden

SSR (Sveriges Stamnings-
föreningars Riksförbund)
(Stutterers' Clubs Organization
of Sweden)
Box 755
S-101 30 Stockholm 1
(There are eleven local chapters
of the Swedish P-Club:
Blekinge, Dalarna, Göteborg,
Norrboten, Jönköping,

Upplands, Kronoberg, Skåne,
Stockholm, Västmanlands,
and Östergötland.)

Switzerland

Vereinigung für Stotternde
und Angehörige (Versta)
Postfach 437
CH 8042, Zurich

United Kingdom

Association for Stammerers
21a Pound Lane
Epsom, Surrey
(Several local chapters.)

Association for Stammerers
86 Blackfriars Road
London SE1 8HA
Newsletter: *Speaking Out*

United States

National Stuttering Project
1269 7th Avenue
San Francisco, California
94122
Telephone: (415) 566-5324 and
647-4700
Newsletter: *Letting Go*
(There are many branches of
this organization in the
United States.)

National Council of Adult
Stutterers
Speech and Hearing Clinic

Catholic University of America
Washington, DC 20064
Telephone: (202) 635-5556

Council for Adult Stutterers
11435 Monterrey Drive
Silver Spring, Maryland 20902

National Association of
Councils of Stutterers
1724 North Troy Street
Nr. 772
Arlington, Virginia 22201

Speakeasy International
233 Concord Drive
Paramus, New Jersey 07652

West Germany

Der Kieselstein (The Pebble)
Mitteilungsblatt Deutsch-
sprachiger Stotterergruppen
Bundesvereinigung Stotterer-
Selbsthilfe
Baustrasse 2
5650 Solingen 11
Newsletter: *Der Kieselstein*
(Chapters in forty-two German
cities.)

Bundesvereinigung Stotterer-
Selbsthilfe
Postfach 110222
5650 Solingen 11
Telephone: 02122-73075

CONSUMER ORGANIZATIONS

There are two consumer-related organizations in the United States that provide information and advice for stutterers. They both have full-time staff and provide excellent service.

National Association for Hearing and Speech Action (NAHSA)
10801 Rockville Pike
Rockville, Maryland 20852
Telephone: (301) 638-6868 and 897-8682
Helpline: 800-638-8255 (or 6868)

The seventy-year-old NAHSA is the consumer affiliate of the professional American Speech-Language-Hearing Association (ASHA). NAHSA deals with communication disorders in general, including deafness, aphasia, and stuttering. The Helpline telephone link provides toll-free communication with the experts.

A small annual fee is charged for members. The group enables people with communication disorders to influence government policy, keep informed about the most modern types of treatment and new devices, tap NAHSA's extensive information system about speech disorders, and become part of a network of people working to help people who cannot communicate effectively. A newsletter, *NAHSA News*, is published quarterly.

The Speech Foundation of America
152 Lombardy Road
Memphis, Tennessee 38111
Telephone: (901) 452-0995

The Speech Foundation of America provides advice and publishes low-cost booklets about speech disorders, particularly stuttering. Some of the booklets are for clinicians, but many are designed to advise and help parents and teachers of stuttering children and the stutterers themselves. The booklets are well written in simple language and contain sound advice.

Parents bewildered by their children's speech behaviour but reluctant to approach a clinician will find some of the booklets invaluable.

Both of these organizations provide people who have speech and hearing defects with a first-class lifeline. It is hoped that similar organizations will develop in other countries.

Organizations concerned with stuttering therapy and research

The organizations in different countries concerned with stuttering and other speech disorders are listed below to provide points of contact for those interested in treatment and the more technical aspects of speech pathology. Some organizations are professional associations for speech pathologists; and others are involved in research, or treatment, or both.

It would be impossible to list all the centres. There are about 24,000 clinicians treating speech disorders in the United States alone. The centres listed are to some extent chosen arbitrarily and reflect the replies to a one-year survey carried out with the help of the different embassies. No information is provided about the quality of the therapy provided. The larger hospitals treat stuttering in most countries, but the degree of specialization and type of therapy vary considerably.

There are many private clinics and free-lance therapists, but it should be remembered that the objective of most of these private enterprises is to make money. Some of these commercial establishments are genuine and helpful, but a person with a stutter seeking help should get professional advice before spending his money on treatment that may at best provide only a short-term benefit, and may at worst do lasting damage. *Caveat emptor*!

International

General Secretary
International Association of
  Logopedics and Phoniatrics
  (IALP)

European Chairman:
Dr E.F. Stournaras
Erasmus University
Overschiese Kleiweg 498
3045 PS Rotterdam
Netherlands

North American Chairman:
  Dr E. Conture
400 Scott Avenue
Syracuse, New York 13210
U.S.A.

Australia

Australian Association of
  Speech and Hearing
253 Hampton Street
Hampton, Victoria 3188
Telephone: 598-0097

Prince Henry Hospital
Anzac Parade
Little Bay
New South Wales 2036
Telephone: 661-0111

Cumberland College Health
  Sciences
PO Box 170
Lidcombe
New South Wales 2141
Telephone: 646-6444

Office of the Principal
South Australia College of
  Advanced Education
46 Kintore Avenue
Adelaide
South Australia 5000
Telephone: 08-228-1611

Most states in Australia have
several clinics that specialize in
stuttering therapy. The speech
pathology departments of most
major hospitals will direct
people to centres for advice,
information, and treatment.

Austria

Arbeitsgemeinschaft
  Österreichischer Phoniater
p.A. OA Dr med H. Hoffer
II HND-Univers. Klinik
Garnissongasse 13
A 1090 Wien

Österreichische Gesellschaft für
  Logopadie, Phoniatrie, und
  Pädaudiologie
I HND-Univers. Klinik
Dept. Phoniatrie
Lazarettg. 14, A 1090 Wien
Telephone: 4800-3316,
  3317 DW

These are the addresses of the
professional organizations of
speech specialists in Austria.
Stutterers are treated at the
ear, nose, and throat clinics of
the major hospitals, and there
are no special centres for
speech therapy.

245 Organizations for therapy and research

Belgium

French-speaking Area
Centre du Langage
Service d'oto-rhino-
   laryngologie
Cliniques Universitaire St
   Pierre
1000 Bruxelles

Service de Rééducation de la
   Parole et du Langage
Service d'oto-rhino-
   laryngologie
l'Hôpital de Bavière
Université de Liège
Bld de la Constitution
4000 Liège

Centre Universitaire d'Audio-
   Phonologie Paul Guns
Clos Chapelle aux Champs 30
BTE 30, 40
1200 Bruxelles
Telephone: 762-34-00
   Ext. 32.40

Flemish-speaking Area
Katholieke Universiteit (Speech
   Pathology)
Leuven

Vrije Universiteit
   (Neurolinguistics)
Brussel

Katholieke Vlaamse Hoge-
   school
J. De Bomstraat 11
2000 Antwerpen

HIPB (Speech Pathology)
St-Lievenspoortstraat 143
9000 Gent

HRIPB (Speech Pathology)
De Pintelaan 135
9000 Gent

HTI (Speech Pathology)
Spoorwegstraat 12
8200 Brugge

Vlaamse Verenining voor
   Logopedisten
Antwerpsesteenweg 154
2350 Vosselaar

Federatie voor Revalidatie-
   centra
Kasteelstraat
2700 Sint-Niklaas

Rehabilitation Centre for
   Speech and Hearing
   Disorders
UZ St-Rafael

Canada

Alberta
Alberta Speech and Hearing
   Association
308 Corbett Hall
University of Alberta
Edmonton T6G 0T2

Department of Speech
   Pathology
411 Garneau Professional
   Building
University of Alberta
Edmonton T6G 0T2

Department of Speech
  Pathology and Audiology
University of Alberta
400-11044 82 Avenue
Edmonton T6G 0T2
Telephone: (403) 432-5990

Department of Neuro-
  psychology
PO Box 307, Alberta Hospital
Edmonton T5J 2J7

Stuttering Clinic
Department of Speech
  Pathology and Audiology
University of Alberta Hospitals
83rd Avenue and 112th Street
Edmonton T6G 2B7

Alberta Society for Stuttering
  Research
c/o Department of Speech
  Pathology
400 Garneau Professional
  Centre
University of Alberta
Edmonton T6G 0T2

Alberta Children's Hospital
1820 Richmond Road SW
Calgary T2T 5C7

British Columbia
British Columbia Speech and
  Hearing Association
2125 West 7th Avenue
Vancouver V6K 1X9

Speech Pathology Department
Lions Gate Hospital
230 East 13th Street
North Vancouver V7L 2L7

South Okanagan Health Unit
PO Box 340, Kelly Avenue
Summerland V0H 1Z0

Manitoba
Manitoba Speech and Hearing
  Association
PO Box 474
Winnipeg R3C 2J3
Telephone: (204) 489-7143

Speech Therapy Department
Seven Oaks General Hospital
2300 McPhillips Street
Winnipeg R2V 3M3

New Brunswick
New Brunswick Speech and
  Hearing Association
180 Woodbridge Street
Fredericton E3B 4R3

Speech Therapy Department
St John Regional Hospital
PO Box 2100
St John E2L 4L2

Newfoundland
Newfoundland Speech and
  Hearing Association
PO Box 8201, Postal Station
  'A'
St John's A1B 3N4

Speech Pathology Department
L.A. Miller Centre
Forest Road
St John's A1A 1E5

Speech Pathology Department
Sir Thomas Roddick Hospital
Stephenville A2N 2V6

Nova Scotia
Speech and Hearing
   Association of Nova Scotia
PO Box 775, Postal Station
   'M'
Halifax B3J 2V2

Speech and Hearing
   Association of Nova Scotia
PO Box 975
Truro B2N 5G8
Telephone: (902) 895-1511

Nova Scotia Hearing and
   Speech Clinic
Fenwick Place
5599 Fenwick Street
Halifax B3H 1R2

Speech Clinic
Yarmouth Regional Hospital
Yarmouth B5A 2P5

Ontario
Canadian Speech and Hearing
   Association
Royal York Hotel
Convention Mezzanine
100 Front Street
Toronto M5J 1E3
Telephone: (416) 368-8132

Disfluency Program
Speech and Language
   Pathology
Children's Hospital of Eastern
   Ontario
401 Smyth Road
PO Box 8010
Ottawa K1H 8L1
Telephone: (613) 737-7600

Communication Disorders
Royal Ottawa Regional
   Rehabilitation Centre
505 Smyth Road
Ottawa K1H 8M2
Telephone: (613) 737-7350

Precision Fluency Shaping
   Program
Clarke Institute
Speech Pathology Department
250 College Street
Toronto M5T 1R8
Telephone: (416) 979-2221

Speech Pathology
Department of Rehabilitation
Toronto General Hospital
101 College Street
Toronto M5G 1L7

Speech Pathology Department
Hospital for Sick Children
555 University Avenue
Toronto M5G 1X8
Telephone: (416) 597-1500

Department of Language
   Pathology
University of Western Ontario
339 Windermere Road
PO Box 5339, Postal Station
   'A'
London N6A 5A5

Speech Pathology
Scarborough General Hospital
3050 Lawrence Avenue East
Scarborough M1P 2V5
Telephone: (416) 438-2911

Many of the school boards and major hospitals in Ontario are concerned with speech disorders.

Prince Edward Island
Prince Edward Island Speech and Hearing Association
c/o Department of Health and Social Services
Social Services Branch
PO Box 2000
Charlottetown C1A 7N8

Co-ordinator, Speech and Hearing Program
Department of Social Services
PO Box 2000
Charlottetown C1A 7N8

Quebec
Le Corporation professionelle des orthophonistes et audiologistes du Québec
4770 rue de Salaberry
Montreal H4J 1H6
Telephone: (514) 332-9090

School of Human Communication Disorders
McGill University
1266 Pine Avenue West
Montreal H3A 1A1

Department of Speech Pathology and Audiology
Montreal General Hospital
1650 Cedar Avenue
Montreal H3G 1A4

Ecole d'orthophonie et d'audiologie
Université de Montréal
2375 Côte Ste-Catherine
Montreal H3T 1A8

Sir Mortimer B. Davis Jewish General Hospital
Department of Audiology and Speech Pathology
3755 Chemin de la Côte Ste-Catherine
Montreal H3T 1E2

There are about a hundred centres (school boards, universities, hospitals, etc.) concerned with speech disorders in the Province of Quebec. Not all of them focus on stuttering.

Saskatchewan
Saskatchewan Speech and Hearing Association
79 Rawlinson Crescent
Regina S4S 6B7

Czechoslovakia

Dr F. Sram
Nad Privozern 11
1, Prague 414700

Denmark

Inspectorate of Special Education
(Inspectionen for Special-undervisningen)

Speech Handicapped Division
Vester Voldgade 117
1552 Copenhagen V.
Telephone: (01) 12-89-93

France

Hôpital neurologique de Lyon
Laboratoire de neuro-
  psychologie et de réeducation
  du langage
24 quai St Vincent
69001 Lyon

Fédération Française des
  orthophonistes
39 rue Pascal
75013 Paris

Institut des bégues
185 Boulevard President
  Wilson
33000 Bordeaux

Greece

Ministry of Health and
  Welfare
Health Protection and
  Promotion Division
17 Aristotelous Street
Athens

There are no special centres
for research and treatment of
stuttering in Greece. Treatment
is undertaken by local mental
health units. There are no
Greek stutterers' self-help
groups.

Israel

School of Communication
  Disturbances
Chim Shiba Medical Centre
Tel-Hashomer

Italy

Societa Italiana di Audiologia
  e Fonatria – SAF
Via Ticino 7
00198 Roma

Japan

The following list gives the
location of speech pathologists
in Japan who have been
certified by the American
Speech and Hearing
Association. Information
about the organizations
concerned was not available in
all cases, so in some cases
individual contacts are named.

Ministry of Health and
  Welfare
2 Kasumgaseki 1 Chome
Chiyoda-Ku
Tokyo

Sachiyuki Hamamoto
Tokyo Speech Clinic
1-17 Jingumae Shibuya
Tokyo

Dr Vchisugawa
4-12-15 Honkugenvma
Fujisawa-shi
Kanagawa-ken

Tsukuba University
1-1-1 Tennodai
Sakuramura
Niihari-gun
Ibarragi-ken

M.Q. Denny
18-13 Minami-Senju
Arakawa-Ku
Tokyo 116

C.C. Elliott
3-11-53 Minami Azabu
Minato-Ku
Tokyo 106

S.S. Ladd
c/o Deloitte, Haskins, and
  Sells
CPO Box 1193
Tokyo 100-91

C.A. Shimizu
4-12-14 Yushima
Bunkyo-Ku
Kokyo

R.J. Dunham
Nagamino Dai 2 Chome
Nada-Ku Kobe

M.L. Mason
PSC Box 2104
Yokota Ab
APO 96328SF
Yokota

Netherlands

Nederlandse Vereniging voor
  Logopedie en Foniatire
(Netherlands Association for
  Logopedics and Phoniatrics)
Oosthaven 52
2801 PE, Gouda

Stichting Institut voor
  Slechthorenden en
  Spraakgebrekkigen
(Foundation of People with
  Hearing and Speech Defects)
Jaltadaheerd 63
9737 HK Groningen

New Zealand

New Zealand Speech
  Therapists Association
1 Pere Street
Auckland 5

New Zealand Speech
  Therapists Association
Speech Therapy Clinic
George Street Normal School
Dunedin

Poland

Akademia Medyczna W.
  Pozania
60-355
Poznan

Republic of South Africa

Department of Speech
  Pathology and Audiology
University of Pretoria
Pretoria 0002

Department of Speech
  Pathology and Audiology
University of the
  Witwatersrand
Milner Park
Johannesburg 2001

Department of Speech and
  Hearing Therapy
University of Durban-Westville
Private Bag X54001
Durban 4001

Department of Logopedics
University of Cape Town
7 Dalston Road
Observatory 7925

The South African Speech and
  Hearing Association
PO Box 31782
Braamfontein 2017

Sweden

Swedish Association of
  Logopedics and Phonetics
Danderyds Sjukhus
182-88 Danderyd

Svenska Logopedforbundet
Foenatriska Avdelningen
Regionjukhuset
581-85 Linkoping

Institutionen for Logopedi och
  foenatri
vid Sahlgrenska Sjuhuset
Foenatriska Avdelningen
Goteborgs Universitet
413-45 Goteborg
Telephone: 031-60-10-00

Switzerland

International Society of
  Logopedics
Avenue de la Gare
CH-1003, Lausanne

Dr J. Sopko
34 Killmattenstrasse
CH-4105 Basel

Abteilung für Sprach- und
  Stimmstörungen der ORL-
  Klinik
Universitätsspital Zurich
Bergstrasse 94
CH-8032 Zurich

Phoniatrische Abteilung des
  Kantonsspitals Basel
Petergraben 4
CH-4000 Basel

Hör-, Stimm- und Sprach-
  abteilung der ORL-Klinik
Inselspital
CH-3010 Bern

Phoniatrie der ORL-Klinik
Kantonsspital
CH-6004 Luzern

Abteilung für Gehör-, Sprach-
  und Stimmheilkunde der
  ORL-Klinik
Kantonsspital
CH-9000 St Gallen

United Kingdom

College of Speech Therapists
6 Lechmere Road
London NW2 5BU

Stammering Research
Department of Physiology
University Medical School
Edinburgh University
Teviot Place
Edinburgh, Scotland EH8 9AG
Telephone: 031-332-3607

Centre for Personal Construct
Psychology
132 Warwick Way
London SW1V 4JD

Department of Linguistic
Science
University of Reading
Reading, Berkshire

Warneford Hospital
Oxford, Oxfordshire

Speech Therapy Unit
The City Literacy Institute
Keeley House
London WC2

Bloomsbury, Hampstead, and
Islington Speech Therapy
Services
Finsbury Health Centre
Pine Street
London EC1
Telephone: 01-278-2323
ext. 325

People needing advice or
treatment outside London can
apply to local health centres
for appraisal and therapy
under the National Health
Service.

United States

Alabama
The Chairman
Department of Communicative
Disorders
University of Alabama
University, Tuscaloosa 35486

Speech and Hearing Clinic
1199 Haley Center
Auburn University
Auburn 36849

Arizona
Department of Speech and
Hearing Sciences
University of Arizona
Tucson 85721

California
Communicative Disorders
University of Southern
California
Los Angeles 90008

Department of Speech
Pathology (Communicative
Disorders)
California State University
Long Beach 90840

Department of Speech and
Hearing
University of California
Santa Barbara 93106

Florida
Speech Pathology
University of Tampa
Tampa 33606

Communicative Disorders
University of Florida
Gainesville 904

Georgia
Speech Pathology
University of Georgia
Athens 30601

Illinois
Department of Communicative
   Disorders
2299 Sheridan Road
Northwestern University
Evanston 60201

The Director
Stuttering Programs
Department of Language and
   Speech Pathology
Northwestern University
Evanston 60201

Foundation for Fluency Inc.
4801 West Peterson Avenue
Suite 218
Chicago 60646

Iowa
The Director
Department of Speech
   Pathology
University of Iowa
Iowa City 52242

Kansas
Department of Communicative
   Disorders and Sciences
PO Box 75
Wichita State University
Wichita 67208

Maryland
American Speech-Language-
   Hearing Association (ASHA)
10801 Rockville Pike
Rockville 20852
Telephone: (301) 897-5700

Massachusetts
Department of Communication
   Disorders
Boston University
48 Cummington Street
Boston 02215

Special Education Department
Boston University
Boston 02215

Michigan
National Council of the
   Stutterer
PO Box 8171
Grand Rapids 49508

The Director
Language, Speech, and
   Hearing Clinic
Department of Speech
   Pathology and Audiology
Western Michigan University
Kalamazoo 49008

Speech Pathology
Eastern Michigan University
Ypsilanti 48197

Minnesota
Department of Communication
   Disorders
115 Shevlin Hall
University of Minnesota
Minneapolis 55455

Missouri
Department of Sociology and
   Anthropology
University of Missouri
St Louis 63121

Montana
Speech and Pathology
University of Montana
Missoula 59801
Telephone: (406) 243-0211

New Hampshire
Speech and Pathology
University of New Hampshire
Durham 03824
Telephone: (603) 868-5511

New York
The John Jay College
City University of New York
444 West 56th Street
New York 10019

Behavioral Sciences
Cornell University Medical
    College
925 East 68th Street
New York 10021

Department of Speech
Brooklyn College
City University of New York
Brooklyn 11210

Hofstra University Speech and
    Hearing Center
Hempstead 11551

Speech Department
Karen Horney Clinic
New York 10001

North Dakota
Speech, Language, and
    Hearing Clinic
PO Box 8040 University Station
Grand Forks 58202
Telephone: (701) 777-3232

Ohio
Speech Pathology
Bowling Green State University
Bowling Green 43402
Telephone: (419) 353-8411

Pennsylvania
Department of Speech
    Pathology
University of Pittsburgh
Pittsburgh 15260

Speech Pathology
Temple University
Philadelphia 19104

Tennessee
Stadium and Yale Hearing and
    Speech Center
Knoxville 37916

Texas
School of Communication
    Disorders
Central Campus
University of Houston
Houston 77004

Stuttering Center
Baylor College
Houston 77004

Utah
Department of Speech
  Pathology and Audiology
University of Utah
1201 Behavioral Science
  Building
Salt Lake City 84112

Virginia
Division for Children with
  Communication Disorders
The Council for Exceptional
  Children
1920 Association Drive
Reston 22091
Telephone: (703) 620-3660

Department of Psychology
Hollins Communications
  Research Institute
Hollins College
Roanoke 24020

Washington
Department of Speech and
  Hearing Sciences
Eagleton Hall
University of Washington
Seattle 98195

Department of Speech
Washington State University
Pullman 99163

Washington DC
The Speech Foundation of
  America
5139 Klingle Street
20307

Army Audiology and Speech
  Center
Walter Reed Army Medical
  Center
20307

Wisconsin
Speech Pathology
Marquette University
Milwaukee 53233
Telephone: (414) 344-1000

USSR

Professor S. Taptapova
Vspolniiperd 16 K 2 KV 86
Moscou K1

West Germany

Bundeszentrale für gesund-
  heitliche Aufklärung
Ostmerheimerstrasse 200
D-5000 Köln 91
Postfach 91 01 52

Klinik für Kommunikations-
  störungen
Langenbeckstrasse
Mainz

Deutsche Gesellschaft für
  Sprachheilkunde e.v.
Rostocker Strasse 62
2000 Hamburg 1

Zentralverband für Logopadie
Goethestr. 9
5000 Köln 41
Telephone: 02234179651

Index